Examination Guidelines

HEALTH ASSESSMENT

A NURSING APPROACH

SECOND EDITION

HEALTH ASSESSMENT

A NURSING APPROACH

SECOND EDITION

Jill Fuller, RN, PhD

Vice President
Professional and Diagnostic Services
St. Joseph's Hospital
Minot, North Dakota

Jennifer Schaller-Ayers, RN,C, MNSc, PhD (Candidate)

Assistant Professor of Nursing
University of Texas at El Paso
El Paso, Texas

J.B. Lippincott Company
Philadelphia

Sponsoring Editor: Donna L. Hilton, RN, BSN
Coordinating Editorial Assistant: Susan M. Keneally
Project Editor: Tom Gibbons
Indexer: Ellen Murray
Design Coordinator: Doug Smock
Interior Designer: Susan Hess Blaker
Cover Designer: Ilene Griff
Production Manager: Helen Ewan
Production Coordinator: Kathryn Rule
Compositor: Pine Tree Composition, Inc.
Printer/Binder: Courier Book Company/Westford
Color Insert Printer: Walsworth Publishing Company
Cover Printer: Lehigh Press Lithographers

6 5 4 3 2 1

Library of Congress Cataloging in Publications Data

Library of Congress Cataloging-in-Publication Data

Fuller, Jill.
    Health assessment : a nursing approach / Jill Fuller, Jennifer
Schaller-Ayers. — 2nd ed.
        p.   cm.
    Includes bibliographical references and index.
    ISBN 0-397-55003-0
    1. Nursing assessment. 2. Physical diagnosis. I. Schaller-
Ayers, Jennifer. II. Title.
    [DNLM: 1. Nursing Assessment.   WY 100 F966h 1994]
RT48.F85   1994
616.07′5—dc20
DNLM/DLC
for Library of Congress   93–30471
                                                     CIP

Preface

Health Assessment: A Nursing Approach is a modern day textbook designed to teach the nurse the "habit of observation," the skills of inquiry and investigation, and the aptitudes required for clinical judgment. It provides a strong foundation for assessment and diagnosis, integrating the nursing process, interviewing techniques, health history taking, diagnostic study interpretation, physical examination skills, environmental evaluation, and growth and development concepts. But this text is more than a book of assessment skills and techniques. It is a foundation for clinical practice that illustrates the scope and responsibility of today's professional nurse with emphasis on nursing's distinctive domain in health care.

CONCEPTUAL FRAMEWORK

Health Assessment: A Nursing Approach is a unique text that provides a *nursing model* for health assessment. This text will clarify the relationship of assessment to nursing diagnosis and nursing process to medical treatment. It uses the frameworks of *functional health* and *nursing diagnoses* while incorporating traditional physical examination techniques and clinical problem identification. The intent is to prepare a practitioner who can effectively evaluate persons with varying health concerns both in multidisciplinary and autonomous practice settings. Health assessment is presented in a way that is congruent with the nursing goals of gathering and analyzing data about a person's state of *wellness, functional ability, physical status, strengths,* and *responses to actual or potential health problems.*

The conceptual framework of functional health and nursing diagnoses is appropriate regardless of the nurse's philosophy or practice setting because it represents a way of organizing the nursing data base, not a theoretical model for practice. This conceptual framework also ensures a *holistic* approach to assessment with consideration of all aspects of human function. This text provides the traditional emphasis on assessing *physical health status* as well as other dimensions of health, including *health perception and health management, sleep and rest, self-concept, roles and relationships, sexuality, stress and stress responses,* and *values and beliefs.*

As nursing evolves as a discipline with a unique body of knowledge, nurses are increasingly questioning traditional assessment methods based primarily on a medical model and the relevance of such methods for nursing. *Health Assessment: A Nursing Approach* is committed to refining and evolving a distinctive nursing approach to health assessment.

ORGANIZATION

The text is organized in three main sections: Unit I, *Overview of Health Assessment and Clinical Competencies;* Unit II, *Health Assessment of Human Function;* and Unit III, *Health Assessment Across the Life Span.*

Unit I presents the foundational professional and clinical concepts required for health assessment, including a discussion of the nature and scope of a nursing health assessment; the principles of interviewing and history taking; basic physical examination techniques and instrumentation; the sequence and documentation of a comprehensive physical examination; diagnostic reasoning and documentation guidelines; and vital sign assessment techniques.

Chapter 4, "The Physical Examination," presents an overview of a complete physical examination, including a *full-color photo presentation of a head-to-toe physical examination.* This sets the stage for subsequent chapters in which procedural aspects of the physical examination are discussed in detail. The student is shown the "big picture" and how the various elements of the physical examination fit together before learning detailed examination procedures and the relationship of the data to clinical diagnosis. Chapter 4 also illustrates how functional health as an assessment data collection framework can be easily and comfortably interchanged with the traditional methods of body systems and head-to-toe examination sequences.

Chapter 5, "Diagnostic Reasoning and Documentation," emphasizes *critical thinking* as the basis for health assessment. Diagnostic reasoning is presented as an intellectual process for formulating judgments about health status based on assessment data. Subsequent chapters apply the critical thinking concepts presented in Chapter 5 through discussions of nursing diagnosis and clinical problem identification as well as through discussion questions in the critical thinking exercises at the end of each chapter.

Unit II presents guidelines for assessing functional abilities and physiologic status. The chapters are organized according to 11 functional health areas rather than by body systems or as a sequential head-to-toe method of physical examination. This approach was chosen because nurses today collect assessment data to focus on nursing diagnoses, level of wellness, personal strengths, and physiologic alterations as manifestations of the patterns of human function. Guidelines are presented for evaluating human function using interview data, nursing observations, results of diagnostic studies, and physical examination data.

The organization of all Unit II chapters is similar. Each chapter begins with an *introductory overview* that describes the *assessment focus* for the functional area being discussed and lists the *nursing diagnoses* that might be identified after thorough evaluation of that particular function. The assessment focus describes what the nurse assesses to evaluate a particular functional area thoroughly. The first table in each chapter further illustrates this assessment focus by specifying assessment goals for the functional pattern and related data collection methods. This table illustrates how various types of interview, diagnostic, and physical examination data are used to make judgments about the functional area being assessed. If all of the areas presented in the chapter are assessed, the nurse has screened for the signs and symptoms associated with the nursing diagnoses listed in the chapter.

The next section of each chapter is called the *knowledge base for assessment.* This section provides the theoretical basis for assessing a particular functional pattern. The knowledge base section presents definitions of terms and concepts and reviews pertinent physiologic processes or theoretical underpinnings. For example, in Chapter 13, "Assessing Self-Concept," this discussion highlights the definition of self-concept proposed by nursing and other disciplines. In addition, variables that may affect the development of self-concept are identified. The knowledge base in Chapter 8, "Assessing Nutrition and Metabolism," focuses primarily on reviewing the physiologic processes involved in nutrition and metabolism. In all chapters, knowledge base concepts lend greater significance to the assessment data obtained through the methods highlighted in each chapter.

Assessment methodology in each Unit II chapter begins with a discussion of the *health history* that is required to gain a thorough understanding of the functional health area being discussed. Interview guidelines are provided in each chapter to assist the nurse in obtaining data corresponding to indicators for each nursing diagnosis listed at the beginning of the chapter. Situations in which it would be appropriate to use screening questions in place of a comprehensive interview are identified. The significance of the types of data obtained by interviewing is discussed in detail in the text.

A discussion of the *diagnostic studies* that may contribute to an overall understanding of a particular functional area follows the health history discussion. Pertinent diagnostic studies may focus on the significance of laboratory values, special imaging, or psychometric measurement. For example, in Chapter 8 the laboratory studies used to make judgments about nitrogen balance, an indicator of protein metabolism, are discussed. In Chapter 12, "Assessing Sleep and Rest," particulars of a sleep laboratory evaluation are highlighted. In Chapter 16, "Assessing Stress and the Stress Response," the diagnostic study section focuses on surveys or questionnaires the nurse might use to evaluate stressors and the stress response.

Each chapter then discusses the pertinence of observational or physical examination data to the functional area. This section is indicated by the headings *physical examination* in Chapters 8 through 11 and 15, and *nursing observations* in Chapters 7, 12 through 14, 16, and 17. In addition to the types of general appearance observations that are helpful in determining a person's level of functioning in a particular area, detailed *examination guidelines* are presented for this section of Unit II. The examination guidelines may focus on physical examination techniques or specific types of observations that are informative for a particular functional area.

Following each examination guideline is a discussion that focuses on *documenting examination findings.* Examples are provided to assist the nurse with the documentation of both normal and abnormal findings. Finally, the *nursing diagnoses* and *clinical problems* associated with data that may be obtained from each examination process are discussed. This section focuses on how data are used to identify and support a particular clinical diagnosis.

Each chapter concludes with an *assessment profile* and a *critical thinking exercise.* This clinically oriented assessment profile presents a situation related to the functional area examined in the chapter. A brief clinical scenario introduces a person with functional alterations. The critical thinking required to arrive at conclusions about the person's profile is then discussed. This serves to illustrate concepts presented in Chapter 5, "Diagnostic Reasoning and Documentation." The critical thinking exercise provides additional material related to the chapter content and uses discussion questions to further stimulate higher-level cognitive processes relevant to assessment.

Finally, a *research highlight* illustrates nursing research pertaining to a subject discussed in the chapter. The highlight emphasizes the relevance and usefulness of nursing research in relation to health assessment.

Unit III presents specialized aspects of health assessment, including approaches that should be used for different age groups—infants, children, adolescents, and the elderly—and those that apply to different practice settings and contexts. Chapter 19, "Health Assessment of Infants, Children, and Adolescents," and Chapter 20, "Health Assessment of Elderly Persons," focus on normal age-related physical findings, examination skill modifications for different age groups, and growth and development concepts in relation to functional areas. Chapter 21, "Assessing in Special Situations," provides specific guidelines for assessment in the acute care setting, trauma assessment, assessment in the chemical dependency treatment setting, and assessment in bladder retraining programs. The intent is to illustrate the types of modifications and special skills that might be required in a variety of different practice settings. For example, in the acute care setting, nurses conduct bedside head-to-toe examinations to screen for illness complications and to monitor treatment responses. Additionally, the nurse requires special skill for evaluating the technology that is often associated with medical treatment in this setting. Chapter 21 provides practical guidelines for modifying assessment techniques learned in Unit II to fit with the real, and often hectic, world of nursing practice.

KEY FEATURES

Health Assessment: A Nursing Approach presents the essential concepts, processes, and skills that help students build a solid foundation for a nursing-oriented health assessment pertinent to a variety of health care settings. To achieve this goal, the text emphasizes the following key features:

- *A strong nursing process and nursing diagnosis framework.* Assessment is viewed as the initial step in the nursing process that concludes with the diagnosis of a person's health or illness status. The relevance of assessment data to nursing diagnoses is highlighted throughout the text.

- *A holistic and transcultural approach to health assessment across the life cycle.* By using the framework of 11 functional health areas, students learn the focus of a holistic assessment that emphasizes physical status as well as psychosocial and cultural aspects of the person. Developmental concepts are presented to illustrate assessment strategies applicable across the lifespan.

- *Health and wellness.* A specific chapter emphasizing the assessment of health perception and health management practices helps the student relate health and wellness concepts to assessment. The nature of normal findings is emphasized throughout the text to further illustrate these concepts.

- *Varied data collection methods, including interviewing, diagnostic testing, observation, and physical examination.* The approach to health assessment advocates the use of multiple and varied data sources and methods. The relevance of diagnostic test findings to the interpretation of health status is added to the traditional armamentarium of interviewing and physical examination.

- *Clinical relevance.* Special assessment methods are provided to guide the nurse in the evaluation of common or special clinical concerns, including edema, wound healing, suicide potential, crisis, pain, physical changes of pregnancy, and equipment functioning.

PEDAGOGIC FEATURES

To reinforce and enhance learning and involve the student in the learning process, numerous pedagogic aids summarize or highlight text information.

- *Assessment Terms* listed at the beginning of each chapter alert students as to what to expect in the chapter and help them focus on chapter content.

- *Assessment Focus tables* emphasize specific assessment goals for a particular functional area and related data collection methods.

- *Interview Guides* for each functional area indicate the types of questions the nurse should ask when eliciting a health history.

- *Anatomy and Physiology Overviews* precede each physical examination section to enhance understanding of physical examination techniques and findings.

- *Examination Guidelines* are arranged in an easy-to-read two-column format: the left column outlines the step-by-step procedure for conducting the examination, and the right column highlights the clinical significance of various aspects of the physical examination, including normal findings and deviations from normal.

- *Displays of Abnormal Findings* expand on the material in the examination guidelines section to help the student recognize, sort, and describe abnormal findings. An extensive collection of original art illustrates these displays.

- *Documentation Samples* of normal and abnormal findings illustrate the language that may be used to ensure complete yet brief descriptions of findings. A variety of formats are illustrated, including narrative, SOAP, and charting by exception.
- *Nursing Diagnosis and Clinical Problem sections* provide additional discussion of factors to consider when making a diagnosis.
- *Assessment Profiles* present clinical scenarios and take the student through the critical thinking processes required for formulating accurate and valid nursing diagnoses.
- *Critical Thinking Exercises* provide discussion topics that require the application of higher-level cognitive processes such as application, analysis, synthesis, and evaluation.

- *Research Highlights* illustrate the relevance and usefulness of nursing research in relation to health assessment.
- *Abundant illustrations and photographs* clarify the text and enhance understanding.

TEACHING LEARNING PACKAGE

The *Instructor's Manual* includes an abbreviated overview of chapter content, learning objectives, classroom teaching-learning strategies, and a complete test bank of questions. Transparency masters are provided to enhance the use of the text and provide a template for an instructor-designed syllabus.

Jill Fuller, RN, PhD
Jennifer Schaller-Ayers, RN,C, MNSc, PhD (Candidate)

Acknowledgments

We are grateful to the many people who lent their support, help, and inspiration to this project. We acknowledge the following persons with special appreciation:

The nursing students to whom we have taught health assessment courses and our nursing colleagues at St. Joseph's Hospital, Minot, and the University of Texas at El Paso (especially Patricia Castiglia, Janet Mayorga, and Teresa Smiley). Their support convinced us to promote a nursing model for health assessment.

Friends at St. Joseph's Hospital (especially Dean Mattern, Alice Schiele, and Stephanie Witwer) who helped more than they realize in seeing this project to completion.

The reviewers of the first edition and second edition manuscripts, whose insights helped us to improve our product.

Brad Nelson from Medical Illustration at the University of Utah Medical Center, Salt Lake City, for his excellent photography and Larry Ward for his artistic talent with the line illustrations. A special thank you to Julia Klein and Susan Baggaley for assisting with the photo shoot for the second edition. We also wish to thank the people who appeared in the photographs.

Donna Hilton and Diana Intenzo for their editorial support and insights. Their interest, expert guidance, and encouragement were essential for the completion of this project.

The many experts behind the scenes at J.B. Lippincott, especially Susan Blaker, Tom Gibbons, and Susan Keneally.

Contents

A color insert, "Ophthalmoscopic and Otoscopic Examination," appears between pages 334 and 335.

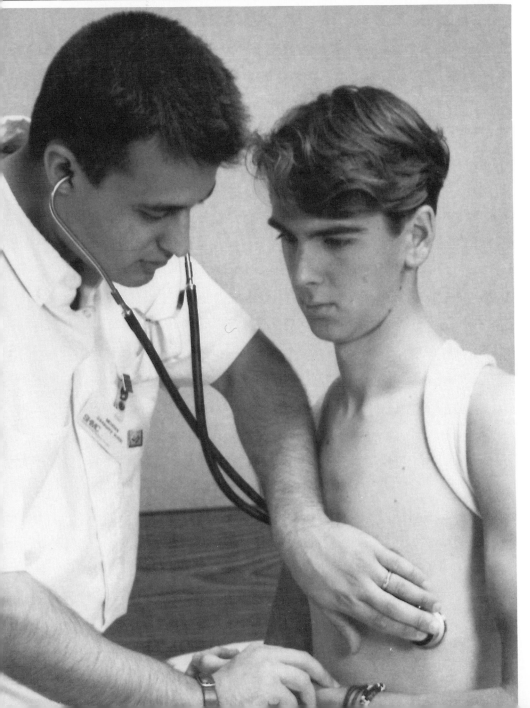

Unit I

Overview of Health Assessment and Clinical Competencies

Introduction to Health Assessment

Assessment Terms

Data Collection

Subjective Data

Objective Data

Assessment

Nursing Diagnosis

Functional Health Patterns

Comprehensive Health Assessment

Admission Data Base

Focused Health Assessment

Screening

Reassessment

INTRODUCTORY OVERVIEW

Health assessment is a process by which you, the nurse, analyze and synthesize collected information in order to make judgments about health status or to determine a person's need for nursing care. Assessment allows the nurse to accomplish the following:

- Determine strengths that promote health behaviors and wellness
- Identify needs, clinical problems, or nursing diagnoses that form the basis of nursing care

Data collection refers to the process of obtaining uninterpreted data or information on a client, such as the body temperature, blood pressure, height, medications used, self-care abilities, feelings about illness, lung sounds, or skin color. Data collection could be thought of as the process of obtaining measurements related to an individual's health status. Various tools and techniques can be used to measure and collect this information, including interviewing, observing, listening, physical examination, reviewing records, and reviewing results of diagnostic tests.

The client should be considered the primary data source, and other sources, such as family members, medical records, and other health care professionals, should be considered secondary sources. You should attempt to elicit data from the client and then validate information as needed through secondary sources.

Data are usually classified as subjective or objective. *Subjective data* represent the client's perspective and are communicated to the nurse by the client. You cannot measure or directly observe subjective aspects of the client's condition. You can make inferences about the

Jill Fuller and Jennifer Schaller-Ayers:
HEALTH ASSESSMENT: A NURSING APPROACH, Second Edition.
© 1990, 1994 by J. B. Lippincott Company.

client's condition, however, based on his or her statements. Examples of subjective data include the client's descriptions of pain, nausea, dizziness, and fear.

Objective data include information obtained by observation, measurement, or physical examination. Such data can be verified by another observer. The nurse can collect objective data by observing, listening, feeling, smelling, or measuring. Examples of objective data include a grimace during a dressing change, a potassium level measurement of 4 mEq, crackles heard during lung auscultation, and a decubitus ulcer measuring 4 cm in diameter.

Assessment follows the data collection and requires the practitioner to draw upon a specialized knowledge base in order to make valid judgments about the health of the person being evaluated. For example, "lung crackles" might be an example of data obtained during the physical examination, whereas "impending respiratory failure" might be the nursing assessment of that person. The assessment or judgment of "impending respiratory failure" requires that the practitioner is not only able to detect the lung crackles on physical examination but is able to analyze and synthesize that information along with other signs and symptoms and information, validate perceptions regarding the person's health, and use diagnostic judgment.

Although skill and competence are required in collecting data, it is clear that using these data in conjunction with other patient information to make a diagnostic judgment requires special education and training; thus, additional professional qualifications may be required for those making assessment. Recently, the Joint Commission for Accreditation of Healthcare Organizations (JCAHO) has established standards regarding who is qualified to assess patient needs for nursing care (JCAHO, 1994). One of those standards states that "Each patient's need for nursing care related to his/her admission is assessed by a registered nurse." The purpose of this standard is to assure that a patient's initial assessment is the responsibility of a qualified registered nurse. Although other qualified individuals may collect patient data, including licensed practical nurses, aides, and technicians, this standard identifies the registered nurse as having the necessary education and training to make the initial assessment of the patient's needs for nursing care.

The following review of nursing history demonstrates how both data collection and health assessment have been emphasized.

EVOLUTION OF HEALTH ASSESSMENT IN NURSING

Florence Nightingale

Florence Nightingale considered assessment an essential nursing function, and referred to this process as "observation of the sick" (Seymer, 1954). Nightingale believed nurses needed to develop technical data collection skills such as measuring and recording vital signs and observing vital functions. Nightingale also emphasized the importance

of interviewing patients to obtain pertinent information about health and illness states. Moreover, she believed in assessing the environment and living conditions of the patient. Nightingale stressed that assessment required judgment rather than mere data accumulation.

Nursing historians state that Florence Nightingale was well ahead of her time, for although her nursing peers had begun to discuss the importance of nurses' observational skills, patient assessment and related judgments were considered more within the domain of medicine than nursing.

Expanded Nursing Roles

Nursing roles continued to expand in the late 19th century as more hospitals were built in response to urban and industrial growth. As the need for nurses in hospitals increased, so did the number of nurse training programs. Public health nursing, which developed in the early 1900s, focused on health assessment and preventive health care. Public health nurses practiced in homes and in the community, especially in rural areas, to promote health and identify problems requiring intervention. Consequently, they needed additional skills to screen people for health problems. Postgraduate courses were developed to emphasize health assessment of environments, families, groups, and individuals.

During the 20th century, nursing roles continued to develop. Some nurses began to specialize in primary care, acute care, long-term care, and intensive care, each requiring greater skill in data collection and assessment. In the 1970s, the development of nurse-staffed intensive care units expanded nursing roles to include surveillance of patients with acute pathologic conditions. Nurses were expected to make on-the-spot diagnostic judgments about a patient's physiologic status.

The nurse practitioner role emerged during the same period, as a result of two programs: a nurse-run ambulatory clinic program at the University of Kansas Medical Center (Lewis & Resnik, 1967) and the first pediatric nurse practitioner program, established at the University of Colorado (Ford & Silver, 1967). The nurse practitioner's responsibilities evolved to include providing primary health care to certain underserved groups, especially children and women, rural communities, and the elderly. In providing primary health care, nurse practitioners began performing comprehensive physical examinations, a service that traditionally had been considered a medical function. Increasingly, nurses used physical examination skills to obtain data pertinent to patient care.

Whether nurses should use physical examination skills and whether the resulting data contributed to nursing's goals were debated during this time by both nurses and physicians. Many nurses believed they should use physical examination skills while maintaining a nursing focus (Kramer, 1971):

> The real question is not whether the nurse should check a child's ears with an otoscope (that is, a means), but what is her purpose (her end) in doing so?

Education for Health Assessment

In response to expanding nursing roles, data collection competencies, including the ability to conduct a complete physical examination, were incorporated into undergraduate nursing education programs in the 1970s. Influenced by nurse practitioner programs, most undergraduate nursing programs used a medical model to teach health assessment. This model included a specific interview format (chief complaint, history of the present illness, general health history, family health history, review of systems) and physical examination according to body systems. Although a medical model of assessment enabled nurses to formulate diagnoses relevant to medicine, it did not provide a means of systematically assessing a person's need for nursing care. Nevertheless, the medical assessment model dominated nursing education and nursing literature during the 1970s and into the present.

Assessment and the Nursing Process

Lydia Hall first conceptualized nursing as a process in the 1950s. Thereafter, many nurse scholars began to describe nursing activities in the context of a nursing process. Yura and Walsh defined the nursing process in phases: assessing, planning, implementing, and evaluating (Yura & Walsh, 1967). Since then, each nursing process component has been extensively discussed and developed, and assessment has been divided into assessment and diagnosis.

During a 1967 conference on the nursing process, two scholars presented papers dealing extensively with assessment (Yura and Walsh, 1967). Black (1967) stated that a nursing assessment was focused on assessing "patient needs." Nursing needed greater guidance, however, if such assessments were to be useful and accurate. Merely saying that patients had physical, psychological, social, and spiritual needs " . . . fails to point to particulars that are specific enough to guide us in a detailed assessment of needs" (Black, 1967, p. 1). Instead, Black advocated referring to Maslow's hierarchy of needs (1968) as a framework for nursing assessment, and specified assessment parameters for each of Maslow's categories. When assessing physiologic needs, for example, the nurse should collect data about food and fluid intake, oxygenation, rest, physical activity, waste elimination, and sexual satisfaction.

At the same conference, Harpine (1967) emphasized that nursing assessment should actively involve the person whenever possible. Only after making observations about the person, and then exploring those observations with the person as a means of validating the nurse's perceptions, should the nurse enter the judgment phase of assessment.

Consequently, certain aspects of a nursing health assessment have been established:

- Assessment initiates the nursing process.
- Assessment is a systematic, deliberate, and interactive process.
- A nursing health assessment focuses on specific individual characteristics, especially functional abilities and the ability to perform activities of daily living.
- Data are collected from several sources by various methods.
- A nursing health assessment includes data collection, validation of perceptions, and diagnostic judgment.

NURSING DIAGNOSIS

Nursing diagnosis is a more recent addition to the nursing process. Before the early 1970s, when nurses began to classify nursing diagnoses, diagnosis was implicitly understood to be part of assessment. The judgment phase of assessment does imply diagnosis because data analysis enables the nurse to identify the person's problem or need for nursing care. Since the 1970s, human requirements for nursing intervention have been termed *nursing diagnoses.*

Because nurses are responsible for analyzing health problems addressed by nursing diagnoses, it is essential to know what data must be collected and how they should be analyzed in order to make nursing diagnoses.

NURSING PROCESS MODELS

A contemporary model of the nursing process outlined by Gordon (1987) illustrates principles of data collection and assessment (Fig. 1-1). Assessment begins by deciding what aspects of the person should be the focus for data collection. Gordon suggests that having some type of conceptual model (*e.g.,* a nursing perspective or view of the person) will suggest broad areas for data collection. Gordon chooses Human Functional Health Patterns as a framework for data collection but other models might be just as helpful.

Gordon is not alone in proposing that nurses have a framework to guide data collection. For example, JCAHO standards suggest that assessment by nurses include consideration of the following factors: biophysical, psychosocial, environmental, self-care, educational, discharge planning, and significant others. On closer examination, it appears that similar types of data would be collected by using either the framework of functional health patterns or the more generic framework provided by JCAHO. The point is to have some idea of what type of data should be collected in order to make judgments about requirements for nursing care.

Before the practitioner arrives at a diagnosis based on the data, several other cognitive processes are required; for example, the nurse must decide whether or not the data represent a normal or abnormal pattern (see Fig. 1-1). If the nurse recognizes something abnormal, the nurse must give additional thought to determining the specific nature of the problem and then decide whether the problem represents a need for nursing care (nursing diagnosis) or requires intervention by another discipline.

Assessment is an ongoing and circular process. The nurse should monitor the client's progress in attaining desired outcomes. If the predicted outcome is not attained, the nurse must reevaluate the diagnoses and prescribed interventions and formulate new ones. Hence, the process is continuous (see Fig. 1-1). Gordon's nursing process model illustrates that assessment is indeed an analytic process requiring skill and knowledge.

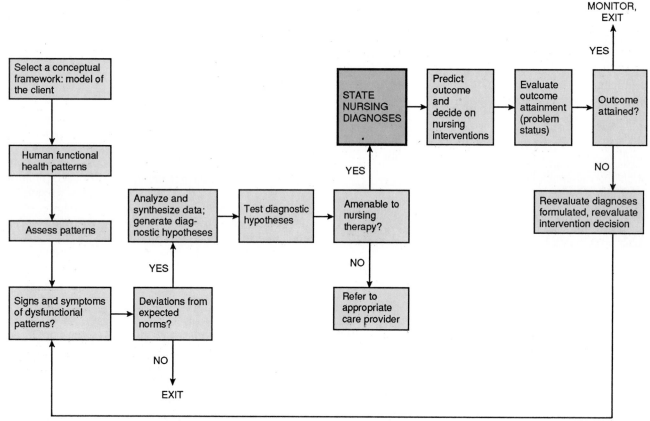

Figure 1-1. The nursing process. A nursing process model advocating the use of a nursing conceptual framework (functional health patterns) to direct data collection and assessment. (Gordon, M [1987] *Nursing diagnosis: Process and application* (2nd ed.). New York: McGraw-Hill)

FUNCTIONAL HEALTH PATTERNS

Gordon proposed functional health patterns as a guide for establishing a comprehensive nursing data base. These 11 categories make possible a systematic and standardized approach to data collection, and enable the nurse to determine the following aspects of health and human function:

Health Perception and Health Management. Data collection is focused on the person's perceived level of health and well-being, and on practices for maintaining health. Habits that may be detrimental to health are also evaluated, including smoking and alcohol or drug use. Actual or potential problems related to safety and health management may be identified as well as needs for modifications in the home or needs for continued care in the home.

Nutrition and Metabolism. Assessment is focused on the pattern of food and fluid consumption relative to metabolic need. The adequacy of local nutrient supplies is evaluated. Actual or potential problems related to fluid balance, tissue integrity, and host defenses may be identified as well as problems with the gastrointestinal system.

Elimination. Data collection is focused on excretory patterns (bowel, bladder, skin). Excretory problems such as incontinence, constipation, diarrhea, and urinary retention may be identified.

Activity and Exercise. Assessment is focused on the activities of daily living requiring energy expenditure, including self-care activities, exercise, and leisure activities. The status of major body systems involved with activity and exercise is evaluated, including the respiratory, cardiovascular, and musculoskeletal systems.

Cognition and Perception. Assessment is focused on the ability to comprehend and use information and on the sensory functions. Data pertaining to neurologic functions are collected to aid this process. Sensory experiences such as pain and altered sensory input may be identified and further evaluated.

Sleep and Rest. Assessment is focused on the person's sleep, rest, and relaxation practices. Dysfunctional sleep patterns, fatigue, and responses to sleep deprivation may be identified.

Self-Perception and Self-Concept. Assessment is focused on the person's attitudes toward self, including identity, body image, and sense of self-worth. The person's level of self-esteem and response to threats to his or her self-concept may be identified.

Roles and Relationships. Assessment is focused on the person's roles in the world and relationships with others. Satisfaction with roles, role strain, or dysfunctional relationships may be further evaluated.

Sexuality and Reproduction. Assessment is focused on the person's satisfaction or dissatisfaction with sexuality patterns and reproductive functions. Concerns with sexuality may be identified.

Coping and Stress Tolerance. Assessment is focused on the person's perception of stress and on his or her coping strategies. Support systems are evaluated, and symptoms of stress are noted. The effectiveness of a person's coping strategies in terms of stress tolerance may be further evaluated.

Values and Belief. Assessment is focused on the person's values and beliefs (including spiritual beliefs), or on the goals that guide his or her choices or decisions.

OUTCOMES OF THE HEALTH ASSESSMENT PROCESS

Analyzing data from a nursing perspective leads to one or more of the following outcomes:

- The person's state of wellness is affirmed. No problem exists.
- The person's strengths are identified.
- Nursing diagnoses are formulated.
- Problems that can be treated collaboratively by the nurse and other health professionals are identified.

SCOPE OF A NURSING HEALTH ASSESSMENT

The American Nurses' Association (ANA) Standards of Nursing Practice (1985) direct nurses to establish a comprehensive data base for persons requiring nursing care. (Display 1-1). The nurse must obtain pertinent information about all parameters specified by a particular standardized assessment tool or structure. A comprehensive data base using functional health patterns, for example, requires the nurse systematically to collect data on all 11 health patterns.

Display 1–1
Assessment Standard for General Professional Nursing Practice

Standard 1

The collection of data about the health status of the client/patient is systematic and continuous. The data are accessible, communicated, and recorded.

Rationale

Comprehensive care requires complete and ongoing collection of data about the client/patient to determine the nursing care needs of the client/patient. All health status data about the client/patient must be available for all members of the health care team.

Assessment Factors

1. Health status data include
   - Growth and development
   - Biophysical status
   - Emotional status
   - Cultural, religious, socioeconomic background
   - Performance of activities of daily living
   - Patterns of coping
   - Interaction patterns
   - Client's/patient's perception of and satisfaction with his health status
   - Client/patient health goals
   - Environment (physical, social, emotional, ecological)
   - Available and accessible human and material resources
2. Data are collected from
   - Client/patient, family, significant others
   - Health care personnel
   - Individuals within the immediate environment and/or the community

3. Data are obtained by
   - Interview
   - Examination
   - Observation
   - Reading records, reports, etc.
4. There is a format for the collection of data that
   - Provides for a systematic collection of data
   - Facilitates the completeness of data collection
5. Continuous collection of data is evident by
   - Frequent updating
   - Recording of changes in health status
6. The data are
   - Accessible on the client/patient records
   - Retrievable from record-keeping systems
   - Confidential when appropriate

(American Nurses Association. [1991]. *Standards of clinical nursing practice*. Washington, DC: ANA.)

Realistically, however, you cannot always generate a comprehensive nursing data base. You may not have time for such comprehensive data collection, or you may need to focus attention on the client's most threatening problem. The scope of health assessment, including the frequency of reassessment, is influenced by your goals and by the person's health status. Data collection and assessment may be comprehensive or focused.

Comprehensive Health Assessment

A *comprehensive health assessment* is usually conducted to identify a person's requirements for nursing care. This may be part of the admission process in a hospital or the focus of the first visit between nurse and client in a home setting. Often, this type of assessment is a prerequisite to establishing a nursing care plan.

Data required for a comprehensive assessment are often recorded on standard forms. These forms may be referred to as the *admission data base.*

You should consider the person's condition before initiating a comprehensive assessment. If he or she is in pain, in need of sleep or rest, or physiologically or psychologically threatened, postpone the comprehensive assessment or use an alternative approach. For example, for a patient recently admitted to a coronary care unit with the medical diagnosis of acute myocardial infarction, pain relief, drug administration, and EKG monitoring may take precedence over comprehensive health assessment. Furthermore, the patient may find a lengthy interview intrusive and irrelevant in such a life-threatening context.

Even so, you have the responsibility for, and the patient has the right to, comprehensive nursing assessment. Rather than omit the comprehensive assessment, modify the format. For example, if you use a standardized form to establish the nursing data base, you may fill in selected parts of the form with data collected during ongoing nurse–client interaction. You may collect data while providing care. While giving the patient a dinner tray, for example, you may ask several questions about usual diet or special problems with eating or digestion. While assisting the patient with a bedpan or commode, you may ask questions about usual patterns of bowel or bladder elimination. Considerable skill is required for this approach. You must remember what data to collect when standardized questionnaires and forms, which might be intrusive during routine nursing care, are not at hand, and remember the information in order to record it on the data base later.

Focused Health Assessment

The assessment process may also be less comprehensive than that required to establish a nursing plan of care. A more focused assessment is indicated when the primary goal is to screen, reassess, or identify specific problems.

Screening involves evaluation of data to identify specific risk factors associated with various health problems. For example, blood pressure is measured to identify hypertension, and stool specimens are evaluated to screen for colorectal cancer (see also Chap. 7).

Reassessment is necessary for persons receiving ongoing nursing care to determine if baseline parameters are changing and to evaluate responses to nursing interventions. The frequency of reassessment depends on the urgency of the patient's condition. For example, a patient in shock would be reassessed more often than a healthy person awaiting outpatient surgery. Reassessments are more focused than a comprehensive assessment because attention is placed on the abnormal conditions discovered during the initial comprehensive assessment or on the detection of common complications.

A focused assessment is also indicated when the goal is to identify and evaluate a specific problem. For example, when a patient presents to an emergency room with trauma, the initial assessment, called the primary survey, is focused on the status of the airway, breathing, circulation, and cervical spine. The secondary survey takes into account the status of other major body systems. The intent is to determine whether or not there are life-threatening injuries. A comprehensive assessment to establish a nursing plan of care is postponed until the patient is stable.

Another example of a focused assessment to identify a specific problem is when the nurse may want to assess a patient to determine whether or not pain medication has been effective. This type of assessment usually requires minimal data collection and may be recorded differently in the medical record than information required for the admission data base. Other special situations in which focused assessments are indicated include acute care settings or rehabilitation settings, or during discharge planning for home care (see Chap. 21 for additional discussion).

Chapter 1 SUMMARY

A nursing health assessment involves obtaining and analyzing data describing a person's state of wellness, strengths relative to health promotion, and needs for nursing intervention. Assessment, the first phase of the nursing process, involves analysis of data to make judgments about health status.

Several factors have influenced nurses as they developed skill and competency in relation to data collection and health assessment:

- *Nightingale's insistence that nurses develop skill in observing the sick (1859)*
- *The expansion of nursing roles, especially in hospital*

nursing and public health nursing (1900 to the present)
- The development of the nurse practitioner role, which required nurses to develop specialized data collection skills to serve as primary care providers (1960s)
- The incorporation of physical examination skills into undergraduate nursing curriculums (1970s to the present)
- The conceptual development of the nursing process; specifically, the designation of assessment as a distinct phase of the process (1960s)
- The development of a classification system for nursing diagnoses (1970s to the present)

Currently, a nursing health assessment is characterized by increasing clarity of purpose, and consensus exists regarding the following ideals:
- Conceptual nursing models should provide focus and direction for health assessment.
- Assessment should enable the nurse to recognize health problems that concern nursing.
- Assessment scope should vary according to the nurse's purpose.
- Multiple data sources and collection methods should be used to gain knowledge about the client's condition.
- A nursing data base should be the basis of a plan of nursing care.

✳ CRITICAL THINKING

Assessment is a key process of professional nursing practice. Nursing, as a discipline, has developed the assessment process to determine people's needs for nursing care, to monitor responses to illness and intervention, and to evaluate overall health and well-being.

Learning Exercises

1. Explain how the role of the nurse in health assessment has changed since Nightingale's time.

2. Identify and describe the type of knowledge required for health assessment.

3. Identify and describe the types of skills required for health assessment.

4. Defend the use of a conceptual model to guide the health assessment process.

5. If you had to design an original organizing framework to guide nurses in the process of health assessment, describe what it would look like.

6. Identify and discuss the advantages of using the functional health patterns conceptual model to guide health assessment. Identify and discuss disadvantages of choosing this model to guide health assessment.

BIBLIOGRAPHY

American Nurses Association. (1991). *Standards of clinical nursing practice.* Washington, DC: American Nurses Association.

Black, K.M. (1967) Assessing patients' needs. In H. Yura & M.B. Walsh (Eds.). *The nursing process: Assessing, planning, implementing, evaluating.* Washington, DC: The Catholic University of America Press.

Ford, L., & Silver, H. (1967). The expanded role of the nurse in child care. *Nursing Outlook, 15,* 43–45.

Gordon, M. (1987). *Nursing diagnosis: Process and application* (2nd ed.). New York: McGraw-Hill.

Harpine, F.H. (1967). Assessing the needs of the patient. In H. Yura & M.B. Walsh (Eds.). *The nursing process: Assessing, planning, implementing, evaluating.* Washington, DC: The Catholic University of America Press.

Joint Commission on Accreditation of Healthcare Organizations. (1994). *Accreditation manual for hospitals.* Oakbrook Terrace, IL: JCAHO.

Kramer, M. (1971). Team nursing—a means or an end? *Nursing Outlook, 19* (10), 648–652.

Lewis, C., & Resnik, B. (1967). Nurse clinics and progressive ambulatory patient care. *New England Journal of Medicine, 277,* 1236–1241.

Lynaugh, J.E., & Bates, B. (1974). Physical diagnosis: A skill for all nurses? *American Journal of Nursing, 74* (1), 58–59.

Maslow, A.H. (1968). *Toward a psychology of being* (2nd ed.). New York: Van Nostrand and Reinhold.

Nightingale, F. (1859). *Notes on nursing: What it is and what it is not.* London: Harrison.

Price, B. (1987). First impressions: Paradigms for patient assessment. *Journal of Advanced Nursing, 12* (6), 699–705.

Yura, H., & Walsh, M.B. (Eds.) (1967). *The nursing process: Assessing, planning, implementing, and evaluating.* Washington, DC: The Catholic University of America Press.

Yura, H., & Walsh, M.B. (1988). *The nursing process* (5th ed.). Norwalk, CT: Appleton-Lange.

Ziegler, S.M., Vaughan-Wrobel, B.C., & Erlen, J.A. (1986). *Nursing process, nursing diagnosis, nursing knowledge: Avenues to autonomy.* Norwalk, CT: Appleton-Century-Crofts.

Chapter 2

The Assessment Interview and Health History

A clinical data base consists of two main components: the health history and the record of the physical examination. The history reflects information obtained by inquiry—the person may be interviewed, a questionnaire may be filled out, records may be reviewed, or other practitioners may be consulted. The richest source of data for the health history is often the interview, because opportunities are provided for building a relationship between the nurse and the client that encourages disclosure and sharing of information. Of all the techniques for obtaining a health history, interviewing requires the greatest amount of skill because of the interpersonal interaction and communication expertise required. This chapter discusses interviewing and the use of questionnaires as a means of establishing the health history.

THE PURPOSE OF THE ASSESSMENT INTERVIEW

The primary purpose of an assessment interview is to collect data that may be used to make judgments about a person's health status. The assessment interview also provides the opportunity to establish a helping relationship between the nurse and client. A helping relationship is characterized by rapport, trust, and a feeling of care and concern. This type of relationship is the basis for mobilizing hope, finding an acceptable understanding of illness, pain, or anxiety, and providing emotional or spiritual support.

Indicators for nursing diagnoses or other clinical problems may be obtained through the interview process. The assessment interview provides the opportunity to identify the person's special concerns and perceptions about health, illness, health-promoting behaviors, and health care. Demographic information, as well as data pertaining to social background and support systems, are obtained. This information is the foundation for clinical judgment and diagnostic reasoning. Data collected during the interview are interpreted with consideration of other types of data, such as those obtained through observation and examination.

The assessment interview requires a systematic and comprehensive approach. Without thoroughness and attention to detail, the likelihood of making accurate diagnoses diminishes. Being systematic means using an organized approach with logical sequencing of questions. The nurse should know ahead of time what topics will be the focus of the interview, relevant questions to ask in relation to each topic, and ways to proceed smoothly from one topic to another.

The most comprehensive type of assessment interview is the admission assessment interview that occurs when the client first comes under the care of the nurse. During a comprehensive admission interview, the nurse should obtain data pertaining to all 11 functional areas. Detailed approaches for obtaining data pertaining to each of the 11 functional health areas are discussed individually in Chapters 7 through 17. An interview of this scope helps to establish the nursing data base. A well-developed data base serves as a baseline from which to evaluate the effectiveness of nursing care and note changes in the client's status. A comprehensive data base also facilitates care planning.

Occasionally, the person may question the relevance of some of the information requested during the interview. For example, a patient in the coronary intensive care unit may ask the nurse, "Why do you ask so many questions about my family? I don't have any family problems. I'm here because I had a heart attack. What do you do with all that information anyway?"

Remember that most people are socialized to think that health care focuses only on medical diagnosis and treatment. You may need to inform them of the role you play in helping them with health management. Because of nursing's focus on health management, questions about family relationships and other functional areas are germane. For example, if a person who has experienced a heart attack has strong family relationships, this may be a factor in promoting recovery. The family may provide some of the support and motivation that are necessary to ensure the person's compliance with a rehabilitation program. On the other hand, the lack of a family support system places the person at greater risk for noncompliance with therapeutic recommendations, so additional planning and intervention may be indicated. Explain that the questions you ask about the person's family help identify strengths and possible problems and assist in determining appropriate interventions, with the goal of improving the person's overall health.

The health assessment interview also provides information about how the person perceives his or her health. Although you may not agree with the person's perceptions, it is important to understand these perceptions when planning nursing care. For example, a person who believes that herbal remedies are an important part of recovery from surgery may need health care providers to acknowledge this belief and make appropriate accommodations. As another example, consider the person who believes that his or her

hospital stay will be at least 1 week following a surgical procedure; however, a typical length of stay for a person with the same diagnosis is usually 3 days. Knowing that a discrepancy exists between the person's beliefs and what is most likely to happen alerts the nurse to address this issue.

The health assessment interview is an intentional process and proceeds in a goal-directed manner. To assure that the desired information is obtained, most practitioners use forms with standardized questions to guide the interview. Even with these aids, an understanding of the interview process and skillful application of therapeutic communication principles are required to elicit information of a personal nature and to assure that the client's responses truly represent his or her real concerns. These therapeutic communication principles are discussed later in this chapter. An interview in which the practitioner applies therapeutic communication principles almost always yields more useful information than an interview that consists of simply reading questions from a form and recording the response.

THE INTERVIEW PROCESS

The assessment interview may be formal and structured to collect a wide range of information, or informal and focused on a specific area of concern. An admission assessment interview is usually formal and structured to establish a comprehensive nursing data base. During an informal interview, you may discuss specific concerns with the person while providing nursing care. Data collection through interviewing and questioning should be a continuous, ongoing process lasting as long as you and the person interact.

The health care setting may influence the scope of the assessment interview. In well-child clinics, for example, the interview usually focuses on routine health practices, nutrition, and normal growth and development, whereas in the intensive care unit, data collection focuses on physical symptoms and responses to threatening conditions.

Three interrelated phases constitute an effective interview: the introductory phase, the working phase, and the termination phase.

The Introductory Phase

The introductory phase sets the tone and direction of the interview and establishes a mutual understanding of the purpose of the exchange. The purposes of the introductory phase are as follows:

- To establish rapport
- To ensure a comfortable setting
- To state the purpose of the interview

Establishing Rapport. Rapport between nurse and client is an essential component of the helping relationship. Establishing rapport begins with demonstrating respect for the client as a person with problems, rather than regarding the person as a problem to be solved.

You should demonstrate respect at the beginning of the interview by extending a cordial greeting, addressing the client by name, and then introducing yourself by name and title. You should not address an adult client with his or her first name unless invited. Offering to shake hands is one way of demonstrating warmth and acceptance.

Nonverbal behaviors, especially on your part, may also help build rapport. Mutual respect can be expressed best when you and the client face each other and maintain eye contact. If possible, you should avoid standing over the person, because this may be intimidating. Of course, such a position may be appropriate if you are informally interviewing the person while providing care. If the interview is conducted at the bedside, you should sit beside the bed with the siderail down, leaning slightly toward the person. Nonverbal behaviors such as expressions of disgust, boredom, or impatience may interfere with establishing rapport or may imply lack of interest.

The interview should be conducted in a manner that implies you have adequate time to spend with the person. For example, do not say to the person, "I have to ask you all these questions before I finish my shift."

Beginning the interview with a brief, casual conversation that focuses on the person may help dispel tension or awkwardness. If your comments are predominantly self-centered, the person may feel neglected or unimportant.

Ensuring Comfort. If possible, you should conduct the interview in a private setting, free from interruptions or distractions. When privacy is difficult to maintain, such as in acute care settings, you can at least close the door or wait until other people have left the room before initiating the interview. Pulling the curtains or moving to the corner of the room also helps to promote a sense of privacy, even though these gestures may not necessarily prevent others from hearing what is said.

You should take every effort to assure the confidentiality of the information provided by the person. This includes limiting discussion of the information to appropriate persons and limiting access to the record.

Stating Purpose. State your purpose at the beginning of the interview. Tell the person you want to discuss his or her health in order to determine how, as a nurse, you can help. Encourage the person to participate in the interview. The person who answers questions, responds honestly, and shares relevant personal information is most likely to benefit from the health assessment interview.

The Working Phase

During the working phase of the interview, which is the most time-consuming phase, you should collect data that are pertinent to the person's overall health status. Such information will be invaluable in forming an appropriate care plan. Record both verbal responses and nonverbal behavior. The purposes of the working phase are as follows:

- To collect biographic data
- To collect data pertinent to the client's health status
- To identify and respond to the client's needs

The Structured Interview. A structured interview may be used to facilitate data collection during the working phase. Familiarity with the forms before the interview will enable you to concentrate on the person's responses. Formats for structured interviews vary. Traditionally, nurses have followed a medical model in conducting health assessment interviews. However, nursing models are now being used in many settings.

The structured interview usually begins with biographic information, including name, age and birthdate, sex, address, birthplace, marital status, and occupation. Although asking about previously recorded biographic information is unnecessary, you should always review such data, because it is relevant to the person's social identity and self-concept.

The next portion of the structured interview concentrates on determining the person's functional status. (Subsequent chapters discuss specific interview guidelines for each functional area.) You can proceed smoothly from one topic to the next by using transitional phrases such as "Now I'd like to discuss how you feel about your sleep habits," or "Now I'd like to ask some questions about your bowel and bladder functions."

The structured interview should proceed from general to specific. Gather general biographic information and data pertaining to health perceptions before discussing sexuality, personal values, and relationships. You must establish trust and rapport before discussing intimate topics.

If the person is reluctant to discuss specific topics, you should provide an opportunity to talk about what he or she feels is most important. Use broad opening statements such as, "Why don't you begin by telling me what brings you here," or "What's troubling you today?" Once the person has expressed immediate concerns, he or she is more likely to discuss other subjects.

View the structured interview as a guide rather than a rigid series of questions that must be asked in a set order. Excessive questioning may undermine rapport, inhibit responses, and encourage the person to assume a passive role of merely answering questions. Applying principles of therapeutic communication rather than direct questioning may result in a more productive interview, as is discussed in more detail in the next section. Such techniques encourage free expression about the topics raised.

Communication is also enhanced when both you and the client speak the same "language." The terminology used should be simple and appropriate and not based on medical jargon. When necessary, define terms and structure questions to allow time for the person to respond thoughtfully and meaningfully.

Completing the health assessment interview in one session may not always be possible. If the person shows signs of fatigue or a limited attention span, bring the interview to a close. Trying to continue under these circumstances would be nonproductive.

The Termination Phase

The termination phase serves to end the interview. Saying how long the interview will last at the beginning will prevent the person from experiencing a sense of premature closure at the end of the interview.

Presummary, summary, and follow-up techniques may be incorporated into the termination phase. Presummary involves providing cues to indicate that the interview is

Display 2–1
The Interview Process: Clinical Profile

Ann Jones, age 26 years, comes to the health clinic as a potential participant in the nurse-operated weight reduction program. Mrs. Jones is worried she will not be accepted for the program because she does not meet weight and height criteria for being overweight. Although she is reluctant to discuss it, Mrs. Jones explains that her weight stays as low as it does because she induces vomiting after eating.

The Introductory Phase

Nurse: Good afternoon, Mrs. Jones. I'm May Klein, one of the registered nurses associated with the weight program. (Smiles and extends hand.)
Client: Hello. Please call me Ann. (Accepts handshake but avoids eye contact.)
Nurse: I'd like to discuss the program you are interested in. Then, I'd like to ask you some general health and nutrition questions so you and I can decide if our program meets your needs. We have about 30 minutes. (States purpose, implies a mutual decision-making process, and states time limitations.)
Client: You probably won't take me into the program.
Nurse: You seem worried about not getting the kind of help you need.

At this point, the nurse focuses on the client's feelings, which should be clarified before questioning and data collection continue.

The Working Phase

The nurse is concerned with obtaining additional information about the client's nutritional practices and weight perceptions. Asking numerous questions may intimidate the client, especially Mrs. Jones, who is initially reluctant to share information. Note the techniques the nurse uses.

Nurse: So, you are interested in the weight reduction program.
Client: Yeah. I've heard from a couple of friends how successful it is. And the people are caring no matter how much or how little you need to lose.
Nurse: Yes. We try to help people achieve realistic goals and feel good about themselves in the process. To do this, I need to find out a little more about your goals and how you feel about your present weight. These are personal questions, but your answers will help me plan an individualized program.
Client: Well, I guess I only need to lose about 10 to 20 pounds. I'm not sure. My husband is upset with the way I look in a bathing suit—especially compared to his friends' wives or girlfriends.
Nurse: So your husband's reactions are one reason for coming here.
Client: Yeah, but I have been dieting and keeping my weight controlled. I just don't feel very healthy anymore.
Nurse: Most people I talk with use several methods for weight control. Some are successful and others aren't, and as you mention, feeling healthy is an important factor. Tell me more about some of your experiences.

The nurse is gathering data by techniques other than direct questioniing. She is also careful to avoid judgmental questions or statements such as, "Why would you want to lose weight?" or "Your husband is wrong." Such statements will probably inhibit honest disclosure.

The Termination Phase

The nurse is able to discuss the client's weight perceptions and to obtain data about her eating disorder during the working phase. The client is accepted into the weight reduction program with the understanding that weight maintenance, healthy eating habits, and self-esteem will be emphasized. After 25 minutes, the nurse initiates the termination phase.

Nurse: I see we have only 5 minutes left today. Before we finish, I'd like to review your situation and make plans for you to start the program.
Client: Okay.
Nurse: You are concerned that you weigh too much, although we haven't yet explored why in great detail. You usually watch your diet but sometimes engage in binge-type eating. When you binge, you purge. You see your behavior as unhealthful and desire to change. We discussed the goals of your plan and agreed to discuss how to proceed at the beginning of the program, 1 week from now.
Client: I feel ready to start this program. It's not going to be easy, though.
Nurse: Um-hmm. (Silence.) Let me give you an on-call number. If talking to someone on our staff will help before next week, please call. Or call if you have questions.

The nurse terminates with summary statements, and follow-up plans are made. Finally, the nurse shakes hands with the client and thanks her for her participation.

coming to an end. For example, you could say, "I see that we only have 10 minutes left. Is there anything else you would like to discuss before our time is up?" or "There are three more questions I'd like to ask." Planning additional interview sessions may be necessary if all relevant topics have not been adequately discussed.

Next, a brief summary of the points covered will allow both you and the client a chance to validate perceptions. Specific plans for follow-up or additional interviewing are discussed at this time.

THERAPEUTIC COMMUNICATION

During the interview, you should attempt to elicit as much relevant information as possible within a limited time frame. Therapeutic communication techniques, nonverbal as well as verbal, will promote a free flow of information. The effectiveness of the techniques used will vary from person to person and will depend on your skill as an interviewer. Overuse or forced use may actually stifle communication. Practice is the key to using therapeutic communication effectively.

You should be attentive to your general demeanor and presentation style as you interview the person. Being too formal may give the person the impression that you do not have time or genuine concern, and he or she may be hesitant to communicate freely. On the other hand, an overly casual approach may fail to instill confidence. Choose your words carefully, and remember that the person may easily misinterpret your comments.

Communication Techniques

Personalize the Interview. As you interview, remember that you are not only eliciting information but you are establishing a helping relationship. In order to do this, you must personalize the interview by portraying sincerity and focus on what the person is saying rather than on a form that needs to be completed. The best approach would be one in which the nurse glances at the questions on the form, establishes eye contact with the person while asking questions, looks at the person while the person is answering, and offers clarification of responses and additional probing when needed (Figure 2-1). The worst approach would be one in which the nurse does not look at the client but looks down at the form to be filled out and reads the questions verbatim from the form, without providing any clarification of answers or without probing for further clarification from the client. Note the approaches used in the following examples:

Example 1: Poor Technique

Nurse:	Do you have any problems with your usual activities, such as walking, housework, housework, or shopping?
Client:	No, not really.
Nurse:	Do you have enough energy to do your daily activities?
Client:	Yes.
Nurse:	Are you independent in all your daily activities?
Client:	Yes.

Example 2: Good Technique

Nurse:	You mentioned before that you were concerned about your recovery from your knee surgery you had 3 months ago. How are things going for you?
Client:	I initially seemed to be improving a little each day but now I think I've reached a plateau.
Nurse:	That must be frustrating for you. Tell me what you mean by reaching a plateau?
Client:	I seem to have made progress since my surgery but now I think I'm not making any more improvements; and I have more problems getting around than I did before surgery. It's especially hard to go down stairs and get up from a chair.
Nurse:	What happens when you do these things?
Client:	I need to use my arms to help me get up from a chair. I have to either pull myself up or push up off the chair with my arms. I go down stairs only one stair at a time and have to walk sort of sideways.
Nurse:	That sounds awkward and uncomfortable. What concerns do you have about your safety as you move around?

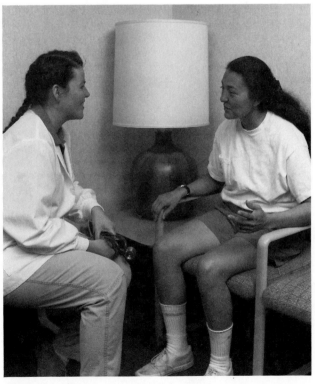

Figure 2–1. Establishing eye contact during an interview is an important communication technique.

Clearly, the nurse in example 2 is using better communication techniques to interview the client about activity and exercise patterns. Attempts are made to personalize the interview. The nurse begins by linking the questions to something the client has already talked about. Making these transition statements as you proceed through a lengthy interview helps keep the person focused.

Use Open-Ended Questions. Verbal therapeutic communication techniques are most effective if the questions asked are open-ended rather than closed-ended. Open-ended questions usually prompt full answers and provide more information, whereas closed-ended questions can be answered in one word, either "yes," "no," or "okay." The following are examples of open-ended questions:

"Tell me about your family."
"What are some of your concerns about caring for your new baby?"
"What do you do to stay healthy?"

You can see that these questions could not be answered by a simple "yes" or "no" but require that the person tell the interviewer more specific information. In example 1 (poor technique), you can see that every question was a closed-ended question. Although using closed-ended questions is often necessary, using all closed-ended questions makes the interview very impersonal and only gives a very limited picture of the individual's health. Closed-ended questions do not allow the interviewer and client to develop any personal rapport. In example 2 (good technique), the interviewer asks open-ended questions, which elicit much more helpful specific information and also allow more interaction between the interviewer and client, which is conducive to more open communication. Open-ended questions that ask "why" should be avoided because the person might feel threatened or intimidated and, thus, give a defensive response. For example, if parents who have brought a young child with an elevated temperature to the emergency department are asked, "Why didn't you bring your child to the hospital sooner?", the parents might feel that the health care provider is blaming them for the problem or accusing them of not acting in a responsible manner.

In certain circumstances, such as when requesting biographic information such as name, occupation, address, and marital status, closed-ended questions are appropriate. Closed-ended questions are also appropriate in emergency situations, when quick responses are required. For example, if a person arrives in the emergency room wheezing and out of breath, you would ask, "Do you have asthma? Are you allergic to anything?" rather than "Tell me about your shortness of breath."

Make Broad Opening Statements. Broad opening statements may be especially helpful in the earliest stages of the interview, but may be used at any time. This technique allows the client to play an active role in the interview and to establish the priorities for discussion. Examples of this kind of statement are as follows:

"Tell me about your accident."
"What brings you to the clinic today?"
"What would you like to discuss today?"

Use Reflection. Reflection is the technique of repeating or paraphrasing a person's words or questions in order to promote further explanation and discussion. For example,

Client:	My skin is driving me crazy.
Nurse:	Driving you crazy?
Client:	Yes. For the last week it's been itching and burning.
Nurse:	Itching and burning for 1 week?
Client:	Well, not constantly. And it seems to itch more than burn. I think it burns only after I've been scratching it.

Verbalize Implied Ideas. This technique involves restating what the client has said, and adding some interpretation. As with reflection, the purpose is to encourage further discussion in order to amplify the problem being explored. This technique also gives the client an opportunity to verify the meaning of what he or she has said. For example:

Client:	I don't know what's wrong with me. I used to sleep 6 or 7 hours a night without awakening.
Nurse:	You're concerned because you've noticed a change in your sleeping habits?
Client:	Yes, I've always been a good sleeper. Now I'm up and down all night.
Nurse:	This seems unusual to you?
Client:	Yes, even though I don't feel tired or take naps during the day.
Nurse:	You're getting enough sleep but you're still bothered by nighttime awakenings?
Client:	Yes. The nights are so long—just lying there, awake in bed, when I should be sleeping.

Provide General Leads. Another method for keeping the conversation going in a specific direction is to inject certain leading phrases or responses, such as, "Go on," "Um-hmm," "Oh?", "And then what happened?" or "How did you feel about that?"

Seek Clarification. Occasionally, the person being interviewed will make a vague or confusing statement. In such instances, it is important to clarify what has been said before continuing with the interview. A suitable response might be, "I'm not sure I understand what you're trying to say," or "What do you mean by unbearable?"

Use Silence. At times during the interview, the most appropriate response is silence. Silence allows you a moment to organize your thoughts and also indicates that talking is not necessarily a criterion for nurse–client interaction. Some interviewers, however, feel uncomfortable when nothing is being said. Self-confidence is needed to use this technique effectively. Periods of silence offer an opportunity to observe nonverbal cues such as posture, facial expressions, and body movements.

Use Open Body Language. You should also use nonverbal cues as a method of communication. Maintaining eye contact or sitting in a relaxed, nonthreatening posture conveys a sense of interest in what the client is saying. Sit with your arms unfolded and your body slightly relaxed, and lean toward the client. Keep your facial expression interested but neutral, avoiding expressions of disgust, anger, or boredom.

Listen Actively. Listening is a communication skill that enhances assessment because it concentrates attention on what the client is saying and enables you to consider subtle messages that the client may be conveying. Effective listening involves blocking out environmental distractions as well as your own prejudices. Attentive behavior and occasional verbal responses assure the client that you are listening.

Share Perceptions. It often helps to share your observation with the client in order to prompt further discussion. Statements such as, "You appear to have some physical discomfort today," or "I notice that you bring up your boyfriend frequently," or "It seems to me that you . . . " may open the conversation to a greater expression of feelings.

Confront Contradictions. When inconsistencies arise between the client's statements and behavior, you should explore the contradiction directly, as, for example, in the following statements: "You tell me that you're not upset about it, but you look like you're about to cry," or "You tell me that you are not tired but it looks like it's becoming more of an effort to keep talking."

Review the Discussion. Therapeutic interactions, especially health assessment interviews, should always close with some type of summary. The main points should be discussed and reviewed in relation to the goals of the interview. For example, you could briefly review the person's health strengths, perceptions, and any identified health problems.

Barriers to Therapeutic Communication

Offering Advice. Giving the client advice or voicing opinions is generally not helpful and may discourage decision making. Often when the client asks, "What would you do?", he or she is seeking assurance that you would do the same thing in the same situation. If your advice differs from what the client wants to hear, it may stir feelings of ambivalence. A request for advice can be turned into a therapeutic exchange, with a response such as, "What would you like to do?" or "It sounds like you need more information to make this decision. Let's talk about it some more."

Abruptly Changing Subjects. It is generally not a good idea to change subjects too quickly. Doing so can be disconcerting and can disrupt rapport. Pausing frequently during the interview and using transitional phrases when moving from one subject to another provide opportunities to think through responses and reactions.

Acting Defensively. If the person being interviewed lashes out at other members of the staff or even family members or friends, it is best not to defend the people being criticized. To do so would imply judgment and inhibit further expression of feelings.

Minimizing Feelings. Disagreeing with a person's feelings about a situation succeeds only in denying the person the right to his or her feelings. It is equally nonproductive to insist that there is nothing to worry about when, in fact, the person is expressing concern. Such a response demonstrates a lack of understanding or empathy.

Offering False Assurance. Offering false hope or promising quick solutions to complicated problems is unfair and unrealistic. Saying, "Everything will be okay," denies the reality of the situation and frequently forces the person to hide fear and anxiety, which are human responses that require nursing intervention.

Jumping to Conclusions. You should never make an assumption and act on that assumption without first checking out the facts. For example, you should not assume that a person who is overweight wants to lose weight. Neither is it wise to assume that a person who has breast cancer will automatically agree to the traditional treatment. Such conclusions represent your personal values and judgments, and may serve to antagonize the client.

CULTURAL CONSIDERATIONS

Culture has a profound effect on the way people communicate. Therefore, sensitivity to culture should influence how an interview is conducted. Cultural differences that have the greatest impact on communication are language, verbal communication patterns, and non-verbal communication patterns. People from the same culture will recognize and conform to the various norms of both verbal and nonverbal communication that exist in that culture. People from two different cultures, however, may have different "rules" for interaction, and therefore may misunderstand each other.

You should keep in mind that cultural differences may influence how verbal and nonverbal messages are interpreted. For example, a Southeast Asian woman may avoid eye contact when talking to a man. An American woman, on the other hand, may have no such compunction and may look directly at anyone with whom she is talking.

Culture also influences health beliefs and behaviors. Members of some cultures believe that disease can be cured by magic or rituals, or by eating certain foods. Therefore, it is important to determine the person's ethnic or cultural orientation and to ask about health beliefs.

Language and Meaning

Language barriers will obviously affect the length of the interview and may necessitate the presence of a translator. Allowing enough time for the interview, arranging for a translator, and maintaining a relaxed and unhurried attitude will facilitate communication. Family or friends may serve as ready translators but may not always be objective in what they communicate. Furthermore, when family is involved, confidentiality may be a problem.

Even when there is no language barrier, misunderstandings may arise, depending on how certain words are interpreted. For example, for today's teenagers, the word *bad* often means something that is respected or valued.

One way to determine if concepts or words must be clarified during the interview is to watch for nonverbal and verbal cues, such as a frown or a blank stare, that indicate misunderstanding. In such a case, you may say, "I'm not sure you understand what I mean when I ask if you have been dieting. Let me explain." To prevent misunderstanding, avoid slang expressions, especially when cultural differences exist.

Verbal Communication Patterns

Cultural traditions and norms also influence verbal communication patterns. Some cultures consider direct questioning to be the best way to gain information, whereas others view direct questioning as intrusive, rude, or embarrassing. Some cultural groups will respond to interview questions in a vague manner to avoid embarrassment and confrontation.

Verbal response to pain also varies among cultures. For example, many Anglo-Americans and Native Americans are taught not to cry in the face of pain because crying is considered to be childish or self-indulgent. On the other hand, Latin Americans are permitted by their culture to respond to pain in a physical and vocal manner.

You may have to adapt the interview style to account for such cultural variations. At the same time, you should make a special effort to maintain a nonjudgmental attitude toward different communication styles.

Nonverbal Communication Patterns

Gestures, body movements, and personal space are all influenced by culture and upbringing. In many Western cultures, direct eye contact may indicate interest and attention. In other cultures, eye contact may be viewed as an intrusion. Touching may be an accepted part of everyday interactions in some cultures; others consider touching among casual acquaintances to have a sexual connotation. Similarly, how close people stand or sit to one another is determined by the way their culture defines personal space. In many Middle Eastern cultures, people stand close when talking to one another, whereas Anglo-Americans prefer to maintain a greater distance when engaged in conversation.

DEVELOPMENTAL CONSIDERATIONS

The age of the person being interviewed can affect the way you should conduct the interview, especially if the person is very young or very old. For a child under 6, it is usually necessary to interview a parent or guardian, although the child's behavior should be observed for relevant verbal and nonverbal cues. Interviewing a parent or guardian involves employing communication techniques similar to those used when interviewing any adult. The feelings and concerns of the parents must be taken into consideration. Parents frequently feel guilty if their child becomes sick or injured, and may actually blame themselves for the child's illness. In such instances, you should use nonjudgmental questions to elicit pertinent data. Questions such as, "When did you first notice signs of fever?" are much more appropriate than "Why didn't you bring him to the clinic sooner?" Providing support and reassurance by empathizing with the parent's concern ("You seem very worried") may encourage a more open response and result in additional information.

A child over 6 years old can be interviewed directly; play and picture-drawing are alternative means to elicit data. Asking the child to draw a picture illustrating his or her experience in the hospital, a picture of a family member, or a self-portrait can serve as a basis for discussion. Children over 6 years should not be "talked down to" or treated as if they were babies. As when interviewing adults, you should maintain eye contact and assume a position that does not intimidate the child.

Parents may or may not be present when you interview a child. If a parent is present, you are afforded an opportunity to observe family interaction. If the parent is dominating the conversation, or coaching or coercing the child to make certain responses, you should address the child directly with comments such as, "Now I'd like to hear how you feel about the situation."

Similar considerations are necessary when interviewing an elderly person. Sensory problems need to be recognized. However, avoid raising your voice even if the person has a hearing problem. Loud voices can be distressing and even offensive. In the elderly person with a hearing loss, it is usually the high-pitched sounds that are not perceived, and raising your voice usually raises the pitch. Instead, to minimize sensory problems, make sure before the interview begins that the person is wearing his or her eyeglasses or hearing aids. Facing the person and speaking slowly and clearly can help improve communication by making it easier for the hard-of-hearing person to lip-read. Making sure the area is well lit, so that the speaker's face can be seen, and eliminating extraneous sounds, such as from televisions and radios, will facilitate better interaction.

Allow more time when interviewing an older person; more than one interview session may be necessary to collect all the appropriate data. An elderly person usually has more information to share than a younger person. On the other hand, older people tend to underreport or refrain from revealing pertinent symptoms, because they may consider the symptoms to be part of aging and therefore unimportant. Older people may also hesitate to share information if they consider you to be too young or the information to be too personal. Establishing rapport and credibility is one way to overcome this reluctance. One effective way to establish rapport is to encourage older clients to reminisce and to take pride in their past accomplishments.

QUESTIONNAIRES AS HEALTH HISTORY TOOLS

A questionnaire is a written form that contains questions to which a person is asked to respond, usually in writing. Questionnaires are usually self-administered and are therefore less interactive than verbal interviews. Questionnaires may be designed to elicit responses in various ways, such as with closed- or open-ended questions, checklists, or Likert-type scales in which clients are asked to agree or disagree with certain statements.

In health assessment, questionnaires are used in two ways. First, they are a quick way to elicit factual information such as name, address, age, other biographic data, medications taken, past and present illnesses or injuries, and family health histories. Such questionnaires are often designed for a specific setting or type of client. The type of information desired determines the questions or checklists presented. The questionnaire is usually followed by a personal interview during which the responses are reviewed, especially those perceived as indicating a problem.

Second, the questionnaire may be used to elicit data about personal characteristics such as attitudes, beliefs, opinions, learning needs, or behavior patterns. This type of questionnaire is usually presented in a standard form, and in many instances has been carefully developed by researchers to ensure its validity (in other words, to ensure that it fulfills its intended purpose).

Although research questionnaires have relevance for health assessment, they have certain disadvantages and must be used with caution. At best, they may accurately measure human responses, such as coping styles, anxieties, or self-esteem, although such data are usually obtained through the follow-up interview and by inference. The information obtained from the interview, however, may be incomplete or inaccurately interpreted. A well-worded questionnaire can be more reliable in such instances.

Questionnaires have other disadvantages. The impersonal format of the questionnaire may inhibit nurse–client interactions regarding complex health problems. Some questionnaires are lengthy and may require too much concentration and effort from an ill or fatigued person. Responding meaningfully to questionnaires also requires a certain level of literacy. If uncertain who will read a completed questionnaire a client may be reluctant to respond honestly and may put down answers he or she thinks are expected. Questionnaires are also subject to misinterpretation.

Chapter 2 SUMMARY

Interviewing is a data collection method that focuses on the following:
- Health states and health-promoting behaviors
- Cues indicative of health problems
- Perceptions about health or health problems

The interview process has three phases: introductory, working, and termination. Each phase is characterized by certain tasks and objectives.

Throughout the interview, you must consider the client's cultural and developmental background, and use appropriate verbal and nonverbal therapeutic communication techniques to facilitate data collection, such as the following:
- Personalizing the interview
- Using open-end questions
- Broad opening statements

- Reflection
- Verbalizing implied ideas
- General leads
- Clarification
- Silence
- Open body language
- Active listening
- Sharing perceptions
- Confrontation
- Summarizing

Questionnaires may be used as interviewing tools, especially to elicit factual data about the client or opinions, attitudes, or attributes. However, the shortcomings of questionnaires as a means of collecting data should be carefully considered.

✳ CRITICAL THINKING

You are admitting a 45-year-old female with metastatic breast cancer to the medicine service of a general acute care hospital. She has developed pneumonia. She is oriented but depressed and experiencing a great deal of pain.

Learning Exercises

1. Demonstrate how you would begin an interview with this person. Create a script of the first few sentences you might say.

2. Identify and describe an approach that could block therapeutic communication in this situation. Explain what's wrong with the approach you described.

3. If you could ask this person only three questions, decide what they would be and specify how you would ask them. Create a script for each question.

4. The patient states that she doesn't want to talk to anyone. Specify how you would respond.

5. The patient starts to cry when you ask her how she's been managing at home. Specify how you would respond.

BIBLIOGRAPHY

Braverman, B.G. (1990). Eliciting assessment data from the patient who is difficult to interview. *Nursing Clinics of North America, 25* (4), 733–750.

Cassell, E.J. (1989). Making good interview skills better. *Patient Care, 23* (6), 145–160.

Cormier, L.S., Cormier, W.N., & Weisser, R.J. (1984). *Intervention and helping skills for health professionals.* Monterey, CA: Wadsworth Health Sciences Division.

Helms, J. (1985). Active listening. In G.M. Bulechek & J.C. McCloskey (Eds.). *Nursing interventions: Treatments for nursing diagnoses.* Philadelphia. W.B. Saunders.

Kasch, C. (1986). Toward a theory of nursing action: Skills and competency in nurse–patient interactions. *Nursing Research, 35* (4), 226–230.

Leininger, M. (Ed.) (1988). *Transcultural nursing: Concepts, theories, and practice* (2nd ed.). New York: John Wiley & Sons.

Santora, A. (1986). Communicating better with the elderly: How to break down barriers. *Nursing Life, 6* (4), 24–27.

Travelbee, J. (1971). *Interpersonal aspects of nursing.* Philadelphia: F.A. Davis.

Whall, A. (1988). Therapeutic use of self. *Journal of Gerontological Nursing, 14* (2), 38–39, 46–47.

Chapter 3

Physical Examination Techniques

Assessment Terms

Inspection

General Survey

Asthenics (Ectomorphs)

Sthenics (Mesomorphs)

Palpation

Light Palpation

Deep Palpation

Bimanual Palpation

Percussion

Mediate (Indirect) Percussion

Immediate Percussion

Fist Percussion

Auscultation

OBSERVATION

The basic techniques of physical examination are inspection, palpation, percussion, and auscultation, together referred to as *observation*. These skills enable you to collect data systematically using the senses of sight, touch, hearing, and smell. Physical appearance, behavior, communication patterns, and activity abilities can all be observed, as can a person's environment and events that affect him or her. Observing facial expression for signs of discomfort, detecting odors that indicate infection, listening to chest sounds to determine airway patency, and touching the skin to determine body temperature are all examples of observation.

Inspection

Inspection is systematic and deliberate visual observation to determine health status. Begin the physical examination with a general survey or inspection of the person, including an assessment of age, posture, stature, body weight, grooming, and mobility patterns. Next, carry out a more thorough observation in a head-to-toe fashion. Note the shape and size of the head, hair distribution, general skin condition, and facial expressions. Inspect the face for symmetry of eyes and balance of facial expression. While inspecting the neck, note visible pulsations, bulges, or venous distention. Inspect the chest and abdomen, noting symmetry, masses, pulsations, skin condition, and visible signs of dis-

Jill Fuller and Jennifer Schaller-Ayers:
HEALTH ASSESSMENT: A NURSING APPROACH, Second Edition.
© 1990, 1994 by J. B. Lippincott Company.

comfort, such as holding the abdomen. Inspect the lower extremities, noting espeically ankle swelling and skin integrity.

Following the general survey, more detailed observations are made as the physical examination progresses to specific body parts or systems. Inspection always precedes palpation, percussion, or auscultation of a particular area. More specific guidelines on examination skills are provided in subsequent chapters.

Effective inspection is facilitated by good lighting and exposure. Occasionally, instruments such as the ophthalmoscope and the otoscope may be used as well.

GENERAL SURVEY

The general survey provides an indication of the person's overall health and outstanding physical features. The general survey is initiated on meeting the client and is usually the first step of a comprehensive physical examination. A number of judgments can be made about the person based on the general survey and are summarized below.

General State of Health. The person's general state of health may be indicated by statements such as "appears well," "appears chronically ill," or "appears acutely ill." Additional observations are necessary to validate these judgments. For example, poor nutritional status, especially muscle wasting (cachexia), sunken eyes, temporal wasting, and loose skin are features associated with chronic illness. The so-called chronic facial mask of pain is associated with a flat or fixed facial expression, lackluster eyes, and the appearance of fatigue. Acute illness may be associated with pallor, diaphoresis, an increased ventilatory rate or effort, and guarding of painful areas.

Signs of Distress. The general survey may reveal that the person is experiencing significant distress related to some condition that may require attention before proceeding with a general interview or examination. The following signs of distress should receive immediate attention:

- *Abnormal ventilatory patterns.* Severe dyspnea, labored breathing with use of accessory muscles, stridor (crowing sounds on inspiration or expiration), wheezing, and rapid breathing (tachypnea) may all signal problems with the cardiovascular or respiratory system.
- *Cyanosis.* Central cyanosis or bluish discoloration of the mucous membranes and the skin indicates inadequate oxygen saturation of arterial hemoglobin. Acute dysfunction of the cardiovascular or respiratory systems should be considered.
- *Acute anxiety.* Fidgety movements, restlessness, cold, moist palms, and tense facial expressions may indicate anxiety. Anxiety is associated with numerous conditions that may be either physiologic or psychological in nature.
- *Pain.* Pain is indicated by guarding or protecting the painful area, wincing, crying, moaning, and/or diaphoresis.
- *Visible trauma.* Bleeding, inflammation, or other signs of physical injury should be evaluated further before proceeding with an interview or physical examination.

Mental Status. The person's orientation to time, place, and person may be established during routine questioning that begins during the general survey and may continue through the physical examination.

Nutritional Status. General observations of the person's body weight can provide a great deal of insight into nutritional status and clues to associated health problems. Persons with cachexia have a wasted, walking-skeleton appearance and are usually suffering from chronic illnesses such as cancer or advanced pulmonary disorders. Obesity may indicate generally poor nutritional practices or be indicative of endocrine or metabolic problems. For example, people with Cushing's syndrome appear obese largely because of abnormal deposits of fat in the trunk, face (moon facies), and posterior neck area (buffalo hump).

Hygiene and Grooming. The person's hygiene and grooming are evaluated with consideration of cultural norms, age, and socioeconomic status. For example, many cultures do not include use of deodorant, a clean-shaven look for men, or women shaving their legs; women's makeup may vary depending on culture; children who make their own choices regarding what to wear may choose clothes that do not match; and people of lower socioeconomic status may wear outdated clothing.

It is also important to compare the appearance of one side of the body with the other. Inattention to grooming on one side of the body indicates one-sided neglect, which is associated with contralateral lesions of the cerebral cortex.

A decline in personal hygiene or grooming may be a sign of depression, dementia, or schizophrenia.

Odors. Note any general odors such as body odor and the odor of urine or feces. The examiner is especially attentive to breath odors such as alcohol, acetone, urine, and ammonia. Alcohol on the breath may indicate acute alcohol intoxication; acetone is associated with diabetic emergencies; urinous breath (uremic fetor) is a manifestation of chronic renal failure; an ammonia odor may indicate liver disease.

Gait and Posture. Abnormal gaits may be described as ataxic, hemiplegic, parkinsonian, scissors, spastic, steppage, or waddling. Detailed descriptions of these gaits and their clinical significance are found in Chapter 10 (see "Examination Guidelines: Musculoskeletal System"). Posture is evaluated by watching the person walk, sit, and change positions. Abnormal postures may be associated with disorders of the muscles, bones, or neurologic system. Certain conditions are characterized by typical postures, including chronic obstructive pulmonary disease, sciatica, and arthritis of the spine (see Chap. 10).

Body Habitus. People may be characterized according to a number of normal body types. The significance of body types is that certain diseases tend to be associated with certain body types. There are three primary body types: asthenics, sthenics, and hypersthenics. *Asthenics (ectomorphs)* appear thin and have poorly developed musculature. These individuals also appear tall with long necks, chests, and abdomens. *Sthenics (mesomorphs)* have an athletic appearance with average height, large bone structure, and good muscle development. *Hypersthenics (endo-*

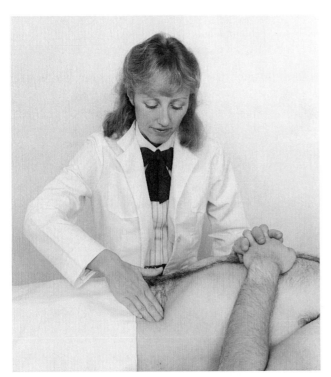

Figure 3–1. Light palpation. The fingertips are moved in a circular motion, depressing the body surface 0.5 to 0.75 inch (1 to 2 cm).

morphs) have a short, round appearance and good muscle development. These individuals tend to be obese.

Speech Patterns. Speech is noted with attention to pace, pitch, clarity, and spontaneity. Slurred speech may indicate neurologic disorders. Inappropriate use of words needs to be evaluated further during mental status testing. Slow, hoarse speech may be associated with hypothyroidism.

PALPATION

With palpation you rely on the sense of touch to make judgments about (1) the size, shape, texture, and mobility of structures and masses; (2) the quality of pulses; (3) the condition of bones and joints; (4) the extent of tenderness in injured areas or structures; (5) skin temperature and moisture; (6) fluid accumulations and edema; and (7) chest wall vibrations.

Different parts of the hand are used to palpate different types of structures. Breasts, lymph nodes, and pulses should be palpated with the fingertips, where nerve endings are most concentrated. The thumb and index fingertips are used to evaluate tissue firmness. Temperature can be quickly assessed with the back of the hand, where temperature sensory nerves are most concentrated and the skin is thin. Vibrations can be felt most strongly with the palm of the hand, especially along the metacarpal joints.

Palpation should be carried out in such a way as to avoid discomfort. Your hands should be warm and the client relaxed to avoid muscle tensing. Palpate painful areas last. The amount of pressure you apply is governed by the type

of structure you are examining and the degree to which palpation may cause discomfort. Any expression of distress or pain should prompt you to palpate lightly.

Palpation may be light, deep, or bimanual. *Light palpation,* the safest and least uncomfortable, involves exerting gentle pressure with the fingertips of your dominant hand, moving them in a circular motion (Fig. 3-1). Place your hand parallel to the part of the body surface you are examining, and extend your fingers to depress the skin surface approximately 0.5 to 0.75 inches (1–2 cm). Exert and release fingertip pressure several times over an area. Exerting continuous pressure would tend to dull the tactile discrimination senses.

Deep palpation, which is done after light palpation, is used to detect abdominal masses. The technique is similar to light palpation except that the fingers are held at a greater angle to the body surface and the skin is depressed about 1.5 to 2 inches (4 to 5 cm). A variation of this technique involves placing the fingertips of one hand over the fingertips of the palpating hand (Fig. 3-2). The top hand should press and guide the bottom hand to detect underlying masses.

Bimanual palpation involves using both hands to trap a structure between them. This technique can be used to evaluate the spleen, kidneys, breasts, uterus, and ovaries.

PERCUSSION

Percussion involves tapping the body lightly but sharply to determine the position, size, and density of underlying structures, as well as to detect fluid or air in a cavity. Tap-

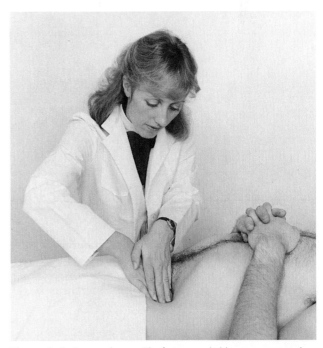

Figure 3–2. Deep palpation. The fingers are held at a greater angle to the body surface than in light palpation, and the skin is depressed 1.5 to 2 inches (4 to 5 cm). Deep palpation may also be done with only one hand.

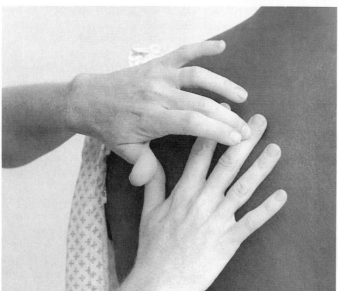

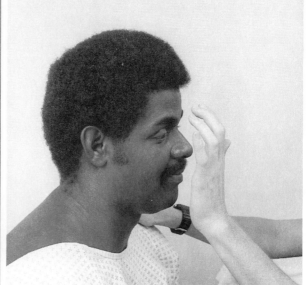

A

B

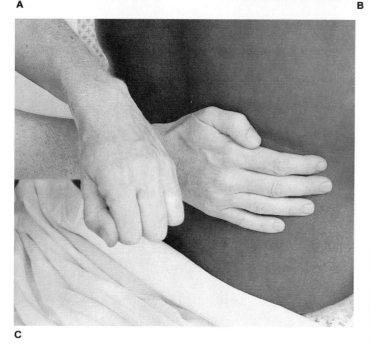

C

Figure 3-3. Three percussion methods. (**A**) Mediate percussion is performed with two hands, using the finger of one hand as the plexor and the finger of the other hand as a pleximeter. (**B**) Immediate percussion is performed by using the fingers of one hand to strike the surface. (**C**) Fist percussion involves placing one hand flat against the body surface and striking the back of the hand with the other hand.

ping the body creates a sound wave that travels 2 to 3 inches (5–7 cm) toward underlying areas. Sound reverberations assume different characteristics depending on the features of the underlying structures. Percussing the right upper abdominal quadrant, for example, will usually elicit dull sounds, indicating the presence of the liver; tapping over the lungs should reveal resonant sounds associated with air-filled spaces. Percussion should usually be performed after an area has been palpated.

Three percussion methods can be used: mediate or indirect, immediate, and fist percussion (Fig. 3-3). The method chosen depends on the area to be percussed. *Mediate or indirect percussion* should be used to percuss the abdomen and thorax, and can be performed by using the finger of one hand as a plexor (striking finger) and the middle finger

of the other hand as a pleximeter (the finger being struck). *Immediate percussion,* used mainly to evaluate the sinuses or an infant's thorax, involves striking the surface directly with the fingers of one hand only. *Fist percussion,* used to evaluate the back and kidneys for tenderness, involves placing one hand flat against the body surface and striking the back of the hand with a clenched fist of the other hand.

Procedure. Mediate or indirect percussion is the basic technique of percussion and is performed in the following manner:

1. Place the index or middle finger of your nondominant hand firmly against the surface being percussed. The other fingers, as well as the heel of this hand, should be raised to avoid contact with the body surface. Hold

the finger firmly against the body surface throughout percussion, even when it is not being tapped by the other hand.

2. Use the middle finger of your dominant hand as the plexor. Hold the forearm horizontal to the surface being percussed. Keep the forearm stationary and use wrist motion to make striking movements.

3. Quickly strike the distal phalanx of the finger that is positioned on the body surface with the tip of the finger of the other hand. Use only the wrist to generate motion, and quickly remove the striking hand after percussing to avoid muffling the percussion sound. You may percuss a single area two or three times before moving to the next area. Light tapping is more effective than heavy tapping.

4. Identify the percussion sound. Skillful percussion reveals one of five percussion sounds, depending on the density of underlying structures: flatness, dullness, resonance, hyperresonance, and tympany (Table 3-1). A *flat sound* is elicited by percussing over solid masses such as bone or muscle. A *dull sound,* which has a lower pitch than a flat sound, is elicited when the high-density structures, such as the liver, are percussed. *Resonance* is a hollow sound heard, for example, by percussing the lung. *Hyperresonance* is an abnormal sound with a pitch between resonance and tympany, and may indicate an emphysematous lung or pneumothorax. *Tympany* is a drum-like sound heard over air-filled body parts such as the bowel or stomach.

5. Proceed to the next percussion area. Move from more resonant to less resonant areas, because detecting a change from resonance to dullness is easier than detecting a change from dullness to resonance.

Common Errors in Percussing. The most common errors in performing mediate percussion are as follows:

- *Moving the forearm of the dominant hand.* Remember, all motion should be generated from the wrist.
- *Pressing the striking finger into the positioned finger.* Remove the striking finger immediately after tapping.
- *Causing injury to oneself or the client* by inadvertently striking the client or your own hand with a long fingernail. The fingernail of the plexor finger should be kept short.

- *Failing to hear the percussion note.* Eliminate environmental noise, including noise caused by bracelets or loose-fitting watches. If the note is still difficult to hear, check your technique.

Auscultation

Auscultation is the skill of listening to body sounds created in the lungs, heart, blood vessels, and abdominal viscera. Auscultation is usually the last technique used during the examination. The sequence usually progresses from inspection to palpation, percussion, and auscultation, except during the abdominal examination, when auscultation is the second step (following inspection).

Immediate auscultation involves placing one's ear directly on the skin, such as over the lung. This method is rarely used because environmental noise frequently interferes with hearing. The usual method is *mediate auscultation,* or using a stethoscope to detect sounds. The best results are gained using a good-quality stethoscope. You should eliminate extraneous noise such as televisions, voices, and equipment sounds before performing auscultation. Do not create noise by moving the stethoscope over body hair or clothing or by touching the stethoscope tubing.

Auscultated sounds are described in terms of pitch, intensity, duration, and quality. *Pitch* is determined by the frequency of sound vibrations and should be classified as high or low. *Intensity* refers to the loudness of the sound. *Duration* refers to how long the sound lasts or how long it takes to occur in relation to a physiologic event such as systole. *Quality* of sound must be described using subjective terms such as tinkling, harsh, or blowing. Specific auscultatory guidelines are discussed throughout the text.

SYMPTOM ANALYSIS

Symptoms are detected during the physical examination or identified during the interview. Symptoms that indicate a possible change in physical status include pain, nausea, dizziness, dysphagia, and dyspnea. Such symptoms are systematically evaluated to aid in diagnosing physiologic alter-

Table 3–1. Percussion Sounds

Sound	Pitch	Intensity	Quality	Location
Flatness	High	Soft	Extreme dullness	*Normal:* sternum, thigh *Abnormal:* atelectatic lung
Dullness	Medium	Medium	Thud-like	*Normal:* liver, diaphragm *Abnormal:* pleural effusion
Resonance	Low	Loud	Hollow	*Normal:* lung
Hyperresonance	Lower than resonance	Very loud	Booming	*Abnormal:* emphysematous lung; pneumothorax
Tympany	High	Loud	Musical, drum-like	*Normal:* gastric air bubble; puffed-out cheek *Abnormal:* air-distended abdomen

ations. Evaluate each reported physical symptom according to the following criteria (elicited by questioning the client):

- *Onset:* When did you first notice the symptom (time and date)? Was the onset sudden or gradual? Has this symptom occurred at other times in the past? What circumstances precipitated the symptom?
- *Location* (may be relevant only for certain symptoms): Where did the pain occur? (Ask the client to point to the exact location.) Does the pain radiate?
- *Quality:* How did you feel when it occurred? How would you describe it?
- *Quantity:* How intense was the symptom (mild or severe, or rated on a scale of 1 to 10)? Did the symptom interfere with your usual activities, such as walking, sleeping, or talking?
- *Frequency and duration:* How frequently did the symptom occur and how long did it last?
- *Aggravating or alleviating factors:* What makes the symptom worse or better?
- *Associated factors:* Did you notice any other changes when you noticed this symptom? (Ask about factors normally associated with the symptom, such as nausea with chest pain.)
- *Course:* How has the symptom changed or progressed over time?

PHYSICAL EXAMINATION INSTRUMENTS

The physical examination is conducted with the aid of several instruments. Some are simple, such as safety pins and cotton wisps used to evaluate sensory function. Others are complex, such as stethoscopes, which are used to evaluate heart tones. Some of the more complex, commonly used physical examination instruments are discussed in this chapter as well as in other chapters. During a complete physical examination, the instruments and equipment listed in Display 3-1 may be used.

Stethoscope

A stethoscope is used to evaluate sounds that are difficult to hear with the human ear, such as heart, bowel, vascular, and lung sounds. The stethoscope transmits sound to the ears while blocking out environmental noise (Fig. 3-4).

The chestpiece of the stethoscope is designed to detect high- or low-frequency sounds and consists of two main parts: the diaphragm and the bell. The flat, closed diaphragm filters out low-pitched sounds and is used to detect high-pitched sounds such as lung sounds. Best results are obtained by placing the diaphragm evenly and firmly over the person's exposed skin. Because the diaphragm has a relatively large surface, it transmits acute sounds over a wide area. The diaphragm should be at least 1.5 inches in diameter. Smaller diaphragm pieces are available for examining children.

The open bell portion of the chestpiece is used to detect low-frequency sounds such as diastolic heart murmurs. The bell should be at least 1 inch in diameter. The bell is placed gently on the person's skin. If too much pressure is applied, the bell will function as a diaphragm. Faint sounds may be difficult to detect with the bell because of its relatively small size.

The stethoscope tubing is made of flexible rubber or plastic that is thick enough to block environmental sounds.

Display 3–1
Instruments and Equipment Used for a Complete Physical Examination

Basic

Stethoscope	2 test tubes
Sphygmomanometer	Reflex hammer
Thermometer	Tuning fork
Ophthalmoscope	Vaginal speculum
Otoscope	Water-soluble lubricant
Nasal speculum	Gloves
Tongue blades	Flexible tape measure
Flashlight	and ruler
Snellen chart	Watch with second hand
Dental mirror	Safety pins
Gauze squares (4″ × 4″)	Beam balance scale
Cotton wisps	Paper, pencil, pen,
Cotton tip applicators	Recording forms

Optional

Schiotz tonometer	Guaiac filter paper and developer
Doppler flow detectors	Urine dipsticks
Jaeger charts	Hydrometer (urinometer)
Skin fold calipers	Glass slides and fixative (for Pap
Sterile/clean-specimen	smears)
containers	
Culture media	

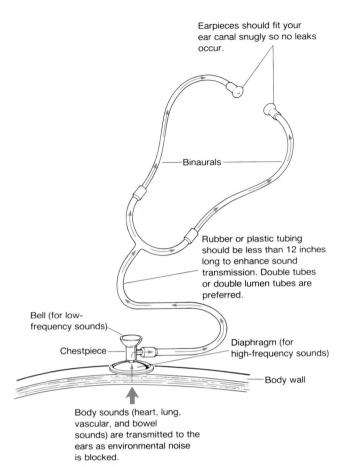

Earpieces should fit your ear canal snugly so no leaks occur.

—Binaurals—

Rubber or plastic tubing should be less than 12 inches long to enhance sound transmission. Double tubes or double lumen tubes are preferred.

Bell (for low-frequency sounds)

Chestpiece—

Diaphragm (for high-frequency sounds)

—Body wall

Body sounds (heart, lung, vascular, and bowel sounds) are transmitted to the ears as environmental noise is blocked.

Figure 3–4. The stethoscope.

Double tubes that are less than 12 inches long further enhance sound transmission.

The binaurals are placed in the ears and are positioned to project sound toward the tympanic membrane. The tips of the earpieces approximate the angle of the ear canal, and should fit snugly and comfortably. Manufacturers usually supply several earpieces so that a comfortable pair can be selected.

Doppler Probe

The Doppler probe is used to evaluate blood flow, especially when traditional methods such as pulse palpation or auscultation are inappropriate or ineffective. Common clinical applications include evaluating fetal heart sounds and peripheral pulses such as brachial, radial, femoral, popliteal, dorsalis pedis, and posterior tibial pulses (see Chap. 10). The Doppler probe, or transducer, is placed on the skin in order to send a low-energy, high-frequency sound beam (ultrasound beam) toward underlying red blood cells. Ultrasound waves are reflected off moving objects, in this case, the red blood cells, and return to the Doppler transducer, which also functions as a receiver. The Doppler probe detects the change in sound frequency as sound is

returned and converts the sound into an audible signal (Fig. 3-5). When blood is flowing through the vessel that is being evaluated, a pulsatile sound can be heard.

Doppler probes are available as pencil-shaped probes, flat discs, or stethoscope-like units. Each device usually has an on/off switch and a volume control dial. A small amount of gel can be applied between the end of the Doppler transducer and the client's skin to eliminate air interference. The probe is then placed gently on the skin over the vessel at approximately a 60-degree angle to the flow within the vessel. Excessive pressure applied to the skin may occlude the vessel.

Ophthalmoscope

An ophthalmoscope is used to inspect internal eye structures (see Chap. 11). The head of the ophthalmoscope is placed on a battery base, and may be exchanged for an otoscope head. To understand the effective use of this instrument, it is important to become familiar with the structures of the ophthalmoscope head (Fig. 3-6A).

Internal eye structures can be viewed by directing a light source toward the person's pupil and looking through the viewing aperture. Light is directed away from the headpiece by a front mirror window. The viewing aperture may be adjusted by turning the aperture selection dial. To see the different apertures available on the ophthalmoscope model (Fig. 3-6B), shine the light toward a piece of paper and adjust the aperture selection dial. Usually, the large aperture is selected if pupils are dilated, and the small aperture is chosen if pupils are constricted. The slit aperture may be used to examine the anterior portion of the eye and evaluate fundal lesion levels. The grid aperture may be used to characterize, locate, and measure fundal lesions. The red-free filter or green beam may be used to evaluate the retina and disc, especially for any hemorrhaging, which

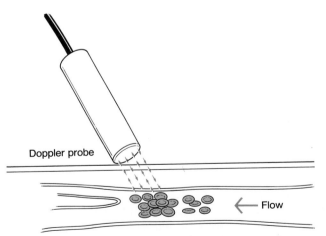

Doppler probe

← Flow

Figure 3–5. Doppler sound generation. The transmitting crystal emits an ultrasound beam through the skin to a vessel and moving red blood cells. The red cells reflect the ultrasound beam to the receiving crystal.

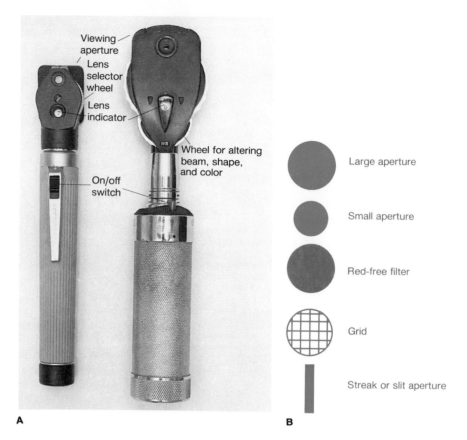

Figure 3–6. (A) Front views of two different ophthalmoscopes. **(B)** Five apertures contained within the viewing aperture.

appears black with this filter, whereas melanin pigments usually appear gray.

The ophthalmoscope lens can be adjusted to bring the internal eye structures into sharp focus, compensating for nearsightedness or farsightedness of the client or examiner. If necessary, you may wear contact lenses or glasses during the examination if the lens adjustment does not provide sufficient compensation. The lens can be adjusted by rotating the lens selection dial with the index finger while looking through the viewing aperture. At the zero diopter setting on the lens indicator, the lens neither converges or diverges light. The black numbers, obtained by moving the lens selection dial clockwise, have positive values (+1 to +40) and improve visualization if the client is farsighted. The red numbers, obtained by counterclockwise rotation, have negative values (−1 to −20) and improve visualization if the client is nearsighted.

Otoscope

An otoscope is used to inspect the structures of the internal ear (see Chap. 11). The head of the otoscope should be placed on a battery base and may be exchanged for an ophthalmoscope head. The structures on the head of the otoscope are depicted in Figure 3-7.

Internal ear structures should be viewed by looking through the illuminated magnifying lens and speculum.

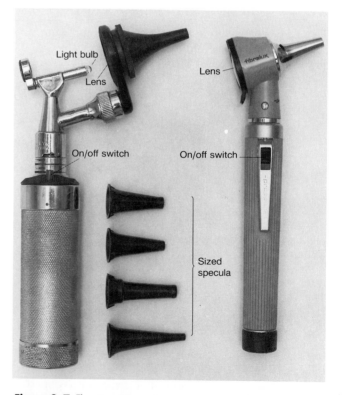

Figure 3–7. The otoscope.

The lens may be displaced to the side so that instruments can be inserted or foreign bodies removed. The size of the speculum should allow maximal visualization with minimal discomfort to the client.

Some otoscopes are equipped with pneumonic devices to introduce a small amount of air against the tympanic membrane, and may be used to evaluate the flexibility of the tympanic membrane.

Chapter 3 SUMMARY

Physical examination skills include
  Inspection, including the general survey
  Palpation
  Percussion
  Auscultation

Together, these techniques are referred to as observation. *In addition, a systematic approach to symptom analysis is used to evaluate a person's physical status.*

Common instruments used to augment observations during the physical examination include
  Stethoscope
  Doppler probe
  Ophthalmoscope
  Otoscope

The comprehensive physical examination is conducted in a systematic manner, usually in a head-to-toe fashion or according to major areas of the body.

✳ CRITICAL THINKING

A 23-year-old female presents to the hospital emergency room with severe abdominal pain. In addition to obtaining a brief history, a physical examination is required to adequately assess her and make the appropriate diagnosis.

Learning Exercises

1. Select and describe the key observations you would want to make during the general survey of this patient.

2. Explain how the general survey would help you prioritize and organize the physical examination.

3. As you percuss the patient's abdomen, she asks you what you're doing. Demonstrate how would you explain your actions.

4. Identify and defend the advantages of using a systematic approach as you examine each body area (*e.g.,* for each body area, you proceed by inspection, followed by palpation, auscultation, and finally, percussion).

5. Explain why an analysis of the patient's pain from her perspective is important.

BIBLIOGRAPHY

Baker, J.D. (1991). Assessment of peripheral arterial occlusive disease. *Critical Care Nursing Clinics of North America, 3* (3), 493–498.

Byers, V.B. (1973). *Nursing observation* (2nd ed.). St. Louis: C.V. Mosby.

Durbin, N. (1983). The application of doppler techniques in critical care. *Focus on Critical Care, 10* (3), 44–46.

Fitzgerald, M.A. (1991). The physical exam. *RN, 54* (11), 34–39.

Littman, D. (1972). Stethoscopes and auscultation. *American Journal of Nursing, 72* (7), 1238–1241.

Smith, C.E. (1984). With good assessment skills you can construct a solid framework for patient care. *Nursing '84, 14* (12), 26–31.

Chapter 4

The Physical Examination

Head-to-Toe Examination

Head-to-Toe Examination   Body Systems Examination

This chapter focuses on three aspects of physical examination: the sequence used for performing a comprehensive physical examination, documentation of the examination, and the relevance of physical examination data to the overall assessment process.

PREPARATION FOR THE PHYSICAL EXAMINATION

The physical examination usually takes place after the examiner has interviewed the client. The client should start the examination with an empty bladder. The examiner should assemble the necessary equipment and position it where it can be readily accessible, such as on the bedside table or Mayo stand.

The client is informed of the purpose of the examination and suitable explanations are given throughout the examination to optimize cooperation and decrease anxiety. For example, the examiner may say, "I'm going to examine you in order to evaluate your general health and follow up on some of the symptoms you reported during our previous discussion," or "I am going to listen to your heart and lungs to see how you are responding to your treatments."

Privacy and Exposure

The examination should be conducted in a private setting, preferably an exam room where the door may be closed. In hospital rooms, privacy curtains should be drawn during the examination.

The client should be completely undressed and covered by an exam gown. As each body area is examined, the area should be completely exposed. For example, during the examination of the anterior chest,

Jill Fuller and Jennifer Schaller-Ayers:
HEALTH ASSESSMENT: A NURSING APPROACH, Second Edition.
© 1990, 1994 by J. B. Lippincott Company.

the gown is removed to the waist. The examiner should only expose the body area being examined and cover the client as soon as possible after exposure. Sheets or drawsheets may be used to cover the body. For example, when the examiner raises the gown to examine the abdomen, a sheet may be used to cover the lower body.

Protection from Potentially Infectious Agents

During the physical examination, precautions should be taken to protect against transmission of blood-borne diseases and to prevent cross-contamination. "Infectious" body fluids for blood-borne disease include blood; semen; vaginal fluids; cerebrospinal fluid; synovial, pleural, peritoneal, pericardial, and amniotic fluid; and saliva.

Precautionary guidelines established by the Centers for Disease Control (1991) should be followed to prevent transmission of infectious agents during the physical examination. The following practices are recommended:

- Wash hands thoroughly before initiating the examination.
- Wash hands again after contact with contaminated surfaces or body fluids.
- If the examiner has an open cut or abrasion on his or her hands, wear gloves to protect the patient.
- Routinely wear gloves when contact with body fluids is likely. For example, wear gloves during the oral examination, the rectal examination, and the vaginal examination. Also, wear gloves when contact with soiled linens is likely.
- Wear gloves when examining open skin lesions or if the patient has a weeping dermatitis.
- Wear gloves to handle and clean soiled equipment such as vaginal speculums.
- Clean contaminated equipment using proper procedures and disinfectant agents.
- Wear gloves when collecting specimens (stool, urine, sputum, wound drainage).
- If safety pins are used during sensory testing, use a new pin for each patient and discard each pin carefully to prevent injury.
- Clearly label any body fluid specimens to indicate "Body Fluid Precautions."

Positioning

By convention, physical examination techniques are taught with the examiner on the right side of the client, who is positioned in bed or on an examining table. Probably the most important reason for encouraging the examiner to stand on the right side is to minimize the examiner's movements from one side of the patient to the other during the examination, which would be awkward. Moreover, most examination maneuvers are performed with the right hand,

even in left-handed examiners, making this position more convenient.

The patient's position will be changed several times during a comprehensive examination. The exam should be organized to minimize the number of times position changes are required, as this can be tiring. Whenever position is changed, the examiner should be attentive to any support needed as well as body alignment. For example, prolonged sitting should not occur without proper back support. Certain clients may require assistance in moving from one position to another.

THE EXAMINATION SEQUENCE: HEAD-TO-TOE VERSUS BODY SYSTEMS

Perhaps the most widely used method of approaching physical examination is the head-to-toe sequence, in which the practitioner systematically examines every part of the body, beginning at the head and progressing down the body to the toes. A detailed head-to-toe examination for an adult, ambulatory person is outlined in the Examination Guidelines on page 33. This sequence can and should be modified according to the examiner's preferences or because of the health status of the client, the setting, or the client's age. Some examiners prefer to examine the neurologic system completely before proceeding with other body areas, whereas others prefer to examine the neurologic functions while each body part is examined. An acutely ill person may be examined with greater emphasis on the organs and systems related to their illness, and hospital patients may be screened for signs typical of physical complications. A person being seen in a specialty clinic, such as an eating disorder clinic, might only receive a physical examination pertaining to nutritional status.

When examining infants and children (Display 4-1), the head-to-toe approach is commonly modified such that the least distressing aspects of the exam are conducted first, (e.g., listening to heart and lungs sounds), whereas the most invasive procedures are postponed to the end of the exam (e.g., examining the ears with the otoscope).

Some practitioners prefer to use a body systems approach to physical examination, which focuses on examining each of the body systems one at a time, including the neurologic, cardiovascular, respiratory, gastrointestinal, genitourinary, musculoskeletal, and integumentary systems. This approach is used most frequently when the purpose of the examination is to determine the function of a particular system. For example, for a person who has had an acute myocardial infarction, the nurse may choose to examine the cardiovascular system in order to make judgments about cardiovascular function. Physical examination components for four major body systems are shown in Table 4-1.

(See page 47 for Display 4-1 and Table 4-1.)

Physical Examination   *Head-to-Toe*

General Principles

The physical examination is performed in a systematic manner, such as in a head-to-toe fashion. The guidelines presented here apply to the comprehensive examination of an ambulatory adult. The examination sequence may be modified depending on your preference and the client's condition. Variations are usually recommended when examining people who are seriously ill or injured, or when examining infants, children, and frail elderly patients (see Chaps. 19 and 20).

Examination Methods

Physical examination methods are discussed in detail throughout this book, and chapter cross references are provided. The methods of general inspection are discussed in greater detail in the general inspection sections of Chapters 7 through 12. In addition, for guidelines to observe
- Musculoskeletal features and range of motion, see Chapter 10.
- Pulses, see Chapter 10.
- Skin integrity, see Chapter 8.
- Deep tendon reflexes, see Chapter 11.

Preliminary Evaluation

At the beginning of the examination, while the person is ambulatory and before he or she changes into an examining gown, you may evaluate the following:
- Height and weight
- Posture and gait
- Snellen visual acuity
- Cerebellar function

Sensory Testing

Sensory testing may be performed throughout the examination. See Chapter 11 for additional guidelines.

Examination Guidelines   *Head-to-Toe Examination*

Procedure

1. INITIATE THE GENERAL SURVEY.

   a. The general survey begins when you first meet the client, in the waiting room or examination room, or while delivering bedside care.

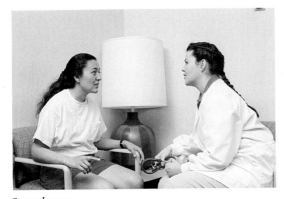

General survey

What To Observe and Record

- General state of health
- Signs of distress such as breathing difficulty, pain
- Awareness, behavior, facial expression, mood (Chap. 11)

GUIDELINES *continued*   ***Head-to-Toe Examination***

Procedure   **What To Observe and Record**

    b. Survey mobility and gait as the person walks into the room.   • Height, weight, nutritional status (Chap. 8)

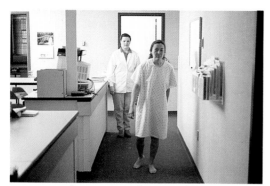

Surveying mobility and gait

    c. Continue the general survey as you examine each body region.

- Hygiene, grooming, clothes
- Skin condition (Chap. 8)
- Odors
- Posture, motor activity, physical deformities (Chap. 10)
- Speech pattern (Chap. 11)
- Apparent age vs. actual age

With the client seated on the examination table, bed, or chair,

2. MEASURE VITAL SIGNS (Chap. 6).

- Blood pressure
- Pulse
- Respiratory rate
- Body temperature

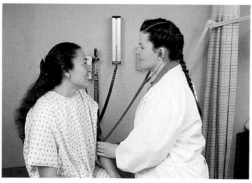

Measuring vital signs

3. EXAMINE THE HEAD.

    a. Inspect and palpate the cranium.

- Hair (Chap. 8)
- Size, shape, and symmetry
- Tenderness
- Scalp smoothness

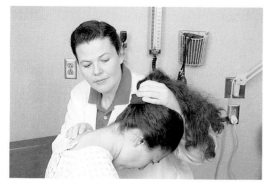

Inspecting the hair and scalp

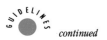 *continued*

Head-to-Toe Examination

Procedure

b. Palpate and auscultate the temporal arteries.

c. Inspect and palpate the face.

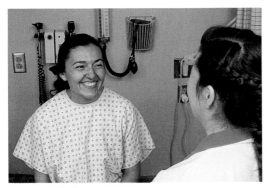

Inspecting the face

d. Test cranial nerves V and VII (Chap. 11).

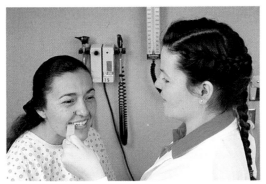

Testing motor function of cranial nerve V (trigeminal)

e. Inspect the nose and test cranial nerve I.

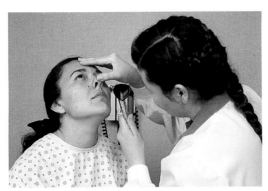

Inspecting the nose

What To Observe and Record

- Thickening
- Tenderness
- Bruits
- Symmetry
- Movements
- Tenderness
- Nodules
- Sinus tenderness (Chap. 8)

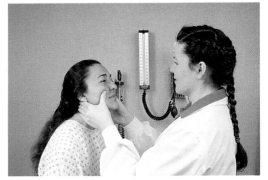

Palpating the face

- Motor and sensory responses

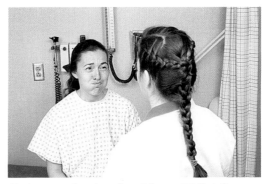

Testing motor function of cranial nerve VII (facial)

- Patency
- Septum
- Mucosa
- Sense of smell

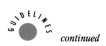

continued   ***Head-to-Toe Examination***

Procedure

4. EXAMINE THE EYES AND TEST VISION (Chap. 11).

   a. Inspect and palpate to evaluate external eye structures.

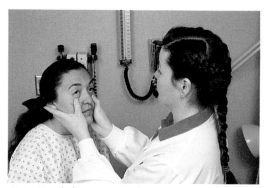

Inspecting the lower conjunctiva

   b. Evaluate visual acuity. Perform Jaeger chart testing of near vision now, or Snellen chart testing of far vision at the beginning of the examination.

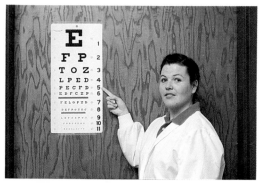

Testing visual acuity

   c. Test extraocular muscle function (cranial nerves III, IV, and VI).

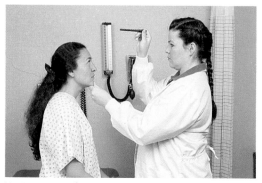

Testing extraocular eye movements

What To Observe and Record

- Shape and symmetry
- Eyelids and eyelashes
- Lacrimal glands, puncta, and lacrimal functions
- Upper and lower conjunctiva
- Lens, cornea, iris, and pupil

- Eye chart readings
- Peripheral vision

- Extraocular eye movements
- Eye movement during cover-uncover test
- Eye alignment and symmetry

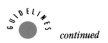

Head-to-Toe Examination

Procedure

d. Test pupillary reflexes.

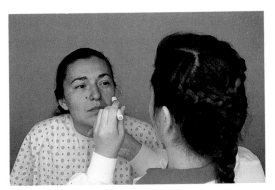

Testing pupillary light reflex

e. Inspect internal eye structures with the ophthalmoscope; darken the room if possible.

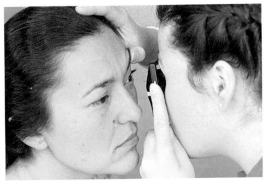

Inspecting the internal eye with the ophthalmoscope

5. EXAMINE THE EARS AND TEST HEARING (Chap. 11).
   a. Inspect and palpate the external ear.

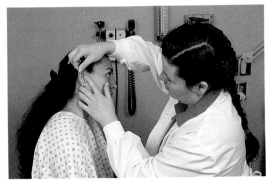

Palpating the external ear

What To Observe and Record

- Reaction to light
- Accommodation

- Retina
- Retinal vessels
- Optic disc
- Macula

- Skin integrity
- Structure, alignment, and symmetry
- Tenderness

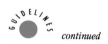

Head-to-Toe Examination

Procedure

   b. Evaluate hearing.

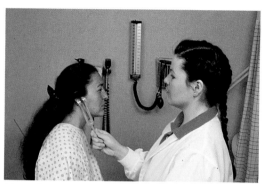

Testing hearing acuity

   c. Inspect the ear canal and tympanic membrane with the otoscope.

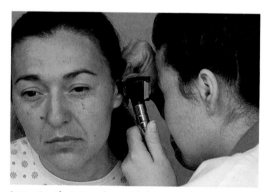

Inspecting the internal ear with the otoscope

6. EXAMINE THE ORAL CAVITY (Chap. 8).

   a. Inspect and palpate the outer structures of the oral cavity.

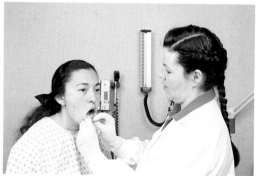

Palpating the lips

What To Observe and Record

- Ability to distinguish sounds varying in pitch and intensity
- Sound lateralization
- Perception of air conduction of sound vs. bone conduction

- Skin integrity
- Obstructions, foreign bodies
- Color, light reflection, landmarks, and configuration of the tympanic membrane

- Lips
- Jaw
- Temporomandibular joint
- Parotid glands

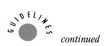
continued

Head-to-Toe Examination

Procedure

b. Inspect and palpate the inner structures of the oral cavity.

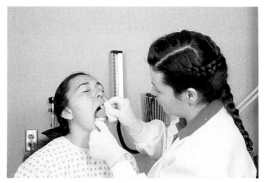

Inspecting the internal structures of the oral cavity

c. Test cranial nerves V, IX, and XII (Chap. 11).

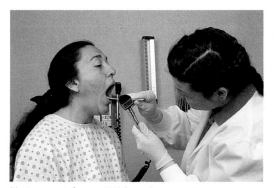

Testing cranial nerve IX (glossopharyngeal) by eliciting a gag reflex

7. EXAMINE THE NECK.

a. Inspect musculoskeletal structures.

b. Palpate the lymph nodes (Chap. 8).

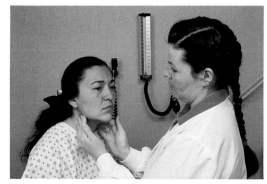

Palpating the cervical lymph nodes

What To Observe and Record

- Oral mucosa
- Tongue
- Inner cheek
- Hard and soft palates
- Oropharynx
- Uvula

- Motor responses

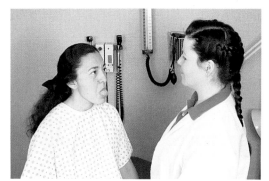

Testing cranial nerve XII (hypoglossal) by observing the tongue for symmetry and movements

- Alignment
- Symmetry
- Consistency
- Enlargement
- Nodules
- Tenderness

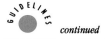

Head-to-Toe Examination

Procedure

What To Observe and Record

c. Inspect and palpate the thyroid gland (Chap. 8).

- Consistency
- Enlargement
- Nodules
- Tenderness

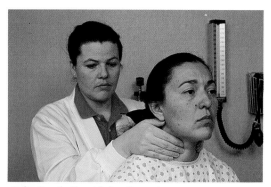

Palpating the thyroid gland

d. Test neck musculoskeletal function and cranial nerve XI.

- Muscle strength and tone
- Range of motion

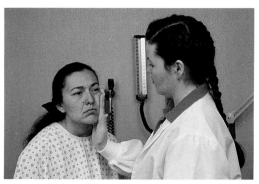

*Testing motor function of cranial nerve XI
(spinal accessory)*

e. Palpate and auscultate the carotid arteries.

- Pulsations
- Vascular sounds

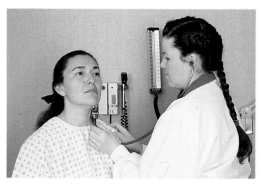

Auscultating the carotid artery

8. EXAMINE THE UPPER EXTREMITIES.

a. Inspect musculoskeletal structures, skin, and nails.

- Skin integrity
- Muscle mass
- Alignment and symmetry

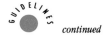
continued

Head-to-Toe Examination

Procedure

    b. Test musculoskeletal function.

What To Observe and Record

- Muscle strength and tone
- Range of motion

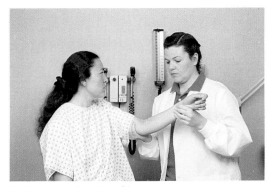

Testing range of motion of the upper extremity

    c. Palpate brachial and radial arteries.

- Pulsations

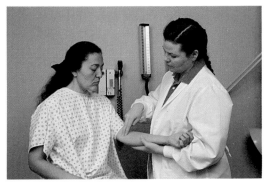

Palpating the brachial artery

    d. Test deep tendon reflexes.

- Motor response

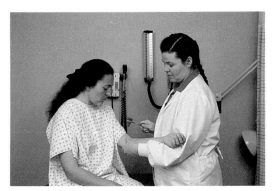

Testing the biceps deep tendon reflex

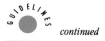

Head-to-Toe Examination

Procedure

9. EXAMINE THE ANTERIOR CHEST.

   a. Inspect and palpate the breasts and axillae (Chap. 15).

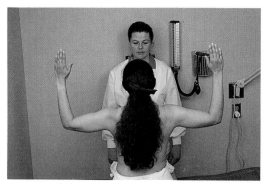

Inspecting the breasts

   b. Inspect, palpate, percuss, and auscultate the thorax (Chap. 10).

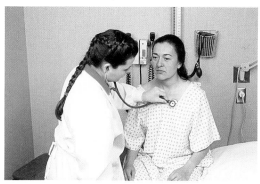

Auscultating the anterior chest

   c. Inspect, palpate, and auscultate the precordium (Chap. 10).

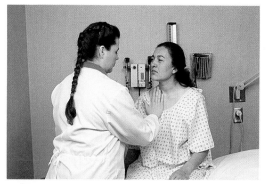

Palpating precordial landmarks

10. EXAMINE THE BACK.

   a. Inspect and test musculoskeletal structures.

What To Observe and Record

- Skin integrity
- Size, shape, and symmetry
- Consistency

- Skin integrity
- Ventilatory pattern
- Shape and symmetry
- Chest excursion
- Vibrations
- Percussion tones
- Breath sounds

- Pulsations
- Vibrations
- Heart sounds

- Spinal alignment
- Muscle tone
- Range of motion

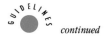

Head-to-Toe Examination

Procedure

  b. Perform fist percussion over the spine and kidneys.

What To Observe and Record

• Tenderness

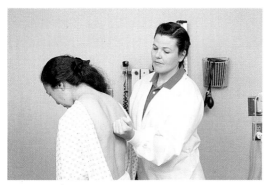

Percussing the spine

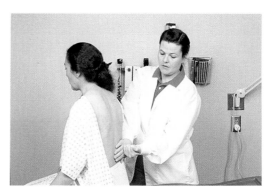

Percussing the kidney

  c. Inspect, palpate, percuss, and auscultate the posterior thorax.

• Same as anterior thorax

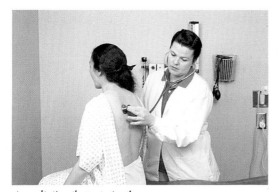

Auscultating the posterior thorax

Position client supine on the examining table or bed. Elevate the head 30 degrees to 60 degrees to inspect the neck veins. The examiner stands on the right side.

11. INSPECT THE NECK VEINS (Chap. 10).

• Jugular venous pulsations
• Central venous pressure

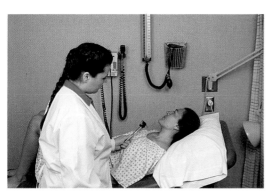

Inspecting neck veins

continued   ***Head-to-Toe Examination***

Procedure

12. EXAMINE THE ANTERIOR CHEST (as above, adding palpation of glandular breast tissue and precordial auscultation in the left lateral position).

What To Observe and Record

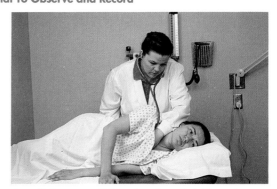
Auscultating precordial landmarks in the left lateral position

13. EXAMINE THE ABDOMEN.

   a. Inspect, auscultate, palpate, and percuss the four abdominal quadrants (Chap. 8).

- Contour and symmetry
- Skin integrity
- Bulges
- Bowel sounds
- Vascular sounds
- Muscle tone
- Masses
- Organ characteristics
- Percussion tones
- Tenderness

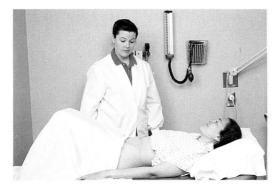
Inspecting the abdomen

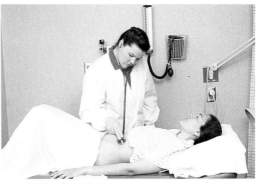
Auscultating the abdomen

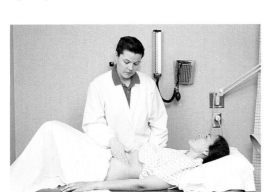
Palpating the abdomen

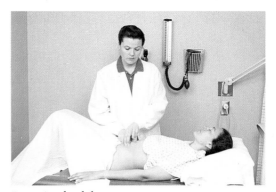
Percussing the abdomen

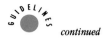 *continued*   ***Head-to-Toe Examination***

Procedure

    b. Palpate and percuss specific organs (liver, spleen, kidneys).

14. EXAMINE THE LOWER EXTREMITIES.

    a. Inspect musculoskeletal structures, skin, and toenails.

    b. Test musculoskeletal function.

    c. Palpate popliteal, posterior tibial, and pedal arteries.

What To Observe and Record

- Size
- Consistency
- Tenderness

- Skin integrity
- Muscle mass
- Alignment and symmetry
- Muscle strength and tone
- Range of motion
- Pulsations

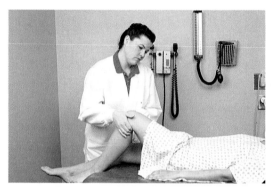

Palpating the popliteal pulse

    d. Test deep tendon reflexes and plantar reflex.

- Motor response

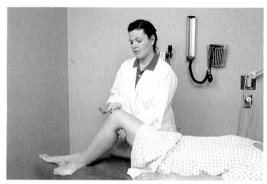

Testing the patellar deep tendon reflex

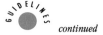

continued   ***Head-to-Toe Examination***

Procedure   **What To Observe and Record**

Position the female client in the lithotomy position with stirrups.

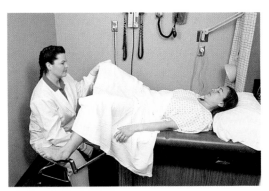

Positioning the client in the lithotomy position

15. EXAMINE THE GENITALS AND PELVIS (Chap. 15).

    a. Inspect the external genitals.

- Skin integrity
- Contour and symmetry
- Discharge

    b. Inspect the vagina and cervix.

- Skin integrity
- Masses
- Discharge

    c. Palpate the vagina, uterus, and adnexa.

- Muscle tone
- Position
- Size
- Consistency and masses

16. EXAMINE THE RECTUM (Chap. 9).

- Muscle tone
- Stool
- Tenderness
- Masses
- Bleeding, discharge

Assist the male client to a standing position.

17. EXAMINE THE EXTERNAL GENITALS (Chap. 15).

    a. Inspect and palpate the penis.

- Skin integrity
- Masses
- Discharge

    b. Inspect and palpate the scrotum.

- Skin integrity
- Size and shape
- Testicular descent and mobility
- Masses
- Tenderness

    c. Inspect and palpate for hernias.

- Bulges

18. EXAMINE THE RECTUM. (For male patients, different positions may be used and special attention is given to prostate palpation.)

Display 4–1
Modified Head-to-Toe Physical Examination Sequence for Infants and Children

Adults	*Infants and Children*
General survey	General survey
Vital signs	Skin
Hair, scalp, cranium	Heart sounds
Eyes and vision	Lung sounds
Ears and hearing	Head, scalp, cranium
Oral cavity	Eyes
Cranial nerves	Musculoskeletal system and reflexes
Thyroid gland	Abdomen
Neck veins	External genitals
Upper extremities	Ears
Nails	Oral cavity
Breasts	
Precordium	
Anterior thorax	
Abdomen	
Lower extremities	
Genitals and pelvis	
Anus and rectum	

Table 4–1. Body Systems Examination Focus for Four Major Body Systems

Body System	Examination Focus	Body System	Examination Focus
Neurologic	Mental status	Respiratory	Airway
	Cranial nerves		Breathing pattern
	Proprioception and cerebellar function		Chest—thoracic configuration, breath sounds, percussion tones, thoracic expansion, fremitus
	Peripheral nerve sensory functions (light touch, pain, temperature and pressure, vibration, joint position)		Skin color
	Cortical sensory functions (stereognosis, two-point discrimination, point location);	Renal	Skin—pigmentation, edema, uremic frost
			Abdomen—kidneys
	Muscle movement, strength, and tone		Genitalia
	Deep tendon reflexes		Rectum
Cardiovascular	Blood pressure		Pelvic structures (females) or prostate (males)
	Arterial and venous pulses		
	Heart sounds		
	Skin color, temperature, moisture, and edema		
	Capillary refill		

Display 4–2
Documentation of the Physical Examination

Patient Name: Jane Doe

General Survey: The patient is a 61-year-old female who appears 5 to 10 years older than her stated age. She is seated on the examining table, constantly shifting position and picking at the paper covering the table. There are no signs of respiratory distress or pain. She is alert but disoriented to time, person, and place and requires frequent orientation to the examination process. She is cooperative when given simple instructions, but her attention span is short. She is thin and well groomed but wears no cosmetics. Eye contact is minimal. She talks throughout the examination, with some phrases being unintelligible.

Vital Signs: BP 144/88 left arm seated; 142/88 left arm standing; 140/84 right arm seated; heart rate 90 and regular; respirations 16; otoscopic temperature 37.1.

Skin: Skin pink and dry; poor turgor; scattered lentigines over dorsal surfaces of the hands. Hair on head thick with some graying. Hair present on lower extremities.

Head: Normocephalic without evidence of trauma. Nontender to palpation; scalp smooth; facial features symmetric.

Eyes: Wears glasses; visual acuity with Snellen chart not assessed because patient unable to follow instructions. Able to read single words printed in phone book; unable to test peripheral vision due to lack of cooperation. EOMs intact; PERLA; eyelids symmetrical and without lesions; conjunctiva moist and pink; not injected. No discharge on palpation of lacrimal glands. Small opacity present on right lens. Fundoscopic exam reveals sharp discs bilaterally. A-V ratio 2:3 OU; fundus without lesions.

Ears: External ears not tender to palpation. Otoscopic exam reveals left ear impacted with dark brown cerumen. Unable to see left tympanic membrane. Right ear has small amount of soft yellow cerumen. Right tympanic membrane pearly gray and scarred. Landmarks visible. Rinne, BC > AC on left; AC > BC on right. Weber, lateralization to the left side.

Nose: Straight; no masses or drainage; patent bilaterally.

Sinuses: Facial and maxillary sinuses nontender.

Oral Cavity: Edentulous; no TMJ tenderness; oral mucosa pink, moist, and intact. No lesions seen or palpated on mucosa or tongue or beneath tongue. Tongue midline without fasiculations; gag reflex intact.

Neck: Full range of motion; trachea midline; no visible jugular pulsations when seated upright; carotids negative for bruits. Thyroid borders easily palpable with no palpable thyroid masses. Thyroid not enlarged. Old, well-healed linear scar from surgical incision noted on anterior neck beneath thyroid. No adenopathy.

Chest: Symmetric and effortless ventilatory pattern. Increased AP to lateral chest diameter. No visible or palpable masses. Breath sounds diminished at bases bilaterally with slight expiratory wheeze bilaterally. Upper lung fields auscultated for fine vesicular breath sounds. Fremitus not evaluated.

Breasts: Breasts symmetric, atrophic, skin intact. No visible masses or changes in breast shape with movement. No palpable masses; no nipple discharge; no palpable axillary or supraclavicular nodes.

Heart: No visible precordial pulsations. PMI not palpable. Auscultation reveals S1, S2, and Grade III/VI midsystolic murmur over Erb's point that does not radiate.

Vascular: No bruits heard over carotid, renal, femoral, or abdominal arteries. Peripheral pulses all 3+ with the exception of pedal pulses—1+ bilaterally. Mild varicosities noted in lower extremities; Homans' sign negative bilaterally.

Back: Marked kyphosis. No spinal tenderness.

(continued)

Display 4–2
Documentation of the Physical Examination (continued)

Abdomen:	Abdomen flat with slight pulsation noted over abdominal aorta. No visible or palpable masses. Well-healed linear surgical scar noted over right upper quadrant. Active bowel sounds in all quadrants. Percussion note is tympanic over all quadrants. Liver span 10 cm by percussion. Abdomen not tender to palpation.		without discharge. Bimanual exam reveals no tenderness or palpable masses. Uterus midline and mobile.
Rectal:	Atrophic skin tags present; anal sphincter tone intact. Hard stool in rectum—negative for occult blood. No masses palpable along rectal walls.	Lymphatics:	No palpable or tender nodes in cervical, axillary, supraclavicular, epitrochlear, or inguinal chains.
		Musculoskeletal:	Full range of motion to all extremities. Marked kyphosis; finger joints enlarged on both hands—nontender.
Genitals:	Wartlike lesion 1–2 cm noted on left vulvar surface. Parous cervix midline	Neurologic:	Orientation as previously noted. Long-term memory intact more than short-term memory. Cranial nerves intact. Gross sensory function intact. Gait unsteady. Unable to cooperate with cerebellar testing. DTRS symmetrical—2–3+.

Documenting the Head-to-Toe Physical Examination

The format for documenting the physical examination varies depending on such factors as the examiner's preferences and forms used for recording findings. General principles for documentation are discussed in Chapter 5. The example shown in Display 4-2 illustrates these principles and shows one way of recording physical examination findings. The use of abbreviations is acceptable, but it has been kept to a minimum in this example.

PHYSICAL EXAMINATION AND THE ASSESSMENT PROCESS

As you learned in Chapter 1, there is a vast difference between data collection and assessment. Whereas data collection is the process of obtaining uninterpreted information about a person (*e.g.,* body temperature, blood pressure, height and weight, lung sounds, skin color, bowel sounds), assessment includes analyzing the information and data in order to make judgments regarding the person's health status.

For this text, the approach to assessment is the framework of functional health patterns. Within this framework, the nurse analyzes collected data with a focus on how well the client functions within the 11 functional health patterns: health perception and health management; nutrition and metabolism; elimination; activity and exercise; cognition and perception; sleep and rest; self-concept; roles and relationships; sexuality and reproduction; coping and stress; and values and beliefs. This approach was chosen because it is pertinent to how nurses today must integrate and use the data they collect, that is, to focus on nursing diagnoses, level of wellness, patient strengths, and physiologic alterations as manifestations of human functioning.

There are other approaches to assessment, such as the body systems framework, in which the practitioner analyzes information and data according to the body systems, including the neurologic, cardiovascular, respiratory, gastrointestinal, genitourinary, endocrine, musculoskeletal, and integumentary systems. Physicians traditionally use the body systems approach in order to identify dysfunction and disease in the various body systems and to plan medical intervention. Nurses may also use this approach, especially when conducting a focused assessment of ill or injured patients.

Regardless of the physical examination sequence used to collect data, whether body systems or head-to-toe, the functional health patterns can be easily and comfortably used as the assessment framework. Tables 4-2, 4-3, and 4-4 demonstrate how data collected using both the body systems and head-to-toe sequences can correlate with the 11 functional health patterns.

Although assessment frameworks may differ, the techniques for collecting data and examining patients are similar for all nurses, physicians, and all other health care professionals. Nurses must learn to collect data and conduct physical examination of patients in an organized and systematic fashion and must devote special attention to interviewing and examining patients, as do physicians and other health care providers. In this text, the physical examinations are integrated within the 11 functional health patterns in order to emphasize the types of data required for the nurse to make judgments related to each area.

Table 4–2. Correlating Data Associated With Functional Health Areas With Body Systems

The following table lists the functional health areas and the corresponding body systems that are assessed to elicit data about the patient's functional status.

Functional Health Area	Body Systems
Health perception and health management	Examination of all body systems is pertinent. Inferences about a person's health management practices can be derived from assessment of all body systems.
Nutrition and metabolism	*Integumentary system:* Alterations in appearance of the skin, hair, and nails may indicate actual or potential alterations in nutrition.
	Gastrointestinal system: Physical or functional alterations of the oral cavity may interfere with the ingestion of nutrients or indicate nutritional problems; physical or functional alterations of the gastrointestinal tract may interfere with the ingestion of nutrients or indicate nutritional problems.
	Endocrine system: Thyroid gland alterations and disruption of hypothalamic temperature regulation may alter basal metabolism.
Elimination	*Gastrointestinal system:* Alterations in the lower gastrointestinal tract (anus and rectum) may contribute to problems with elimination.
	Neurologic system: Neurologic alterations may disrupt neural control of bowel or bladder elimination.
	Musculoskeletal system: Musculoskeletal alterations may interfere with bowel or bladder control.
	Reproductive and genitourinary system: Alterations in pelvic or genitourinary structures may interfere with bladder elimination or control.
	Integumentary system: Skin integrity may be threatened with bowel or bladder incontinence.
Activity and exercise	*Cardiovascular system:* The cardiovascular system assists with meeting oxygen requirements during activity and exercise.
	Pulmonary system: The pulmonary system assists with meeting oxygen requirements during activity and exercise.
	Musculoskeletal system: Alterations in the musculoskeletal system influence mobility and exercise.
	Neurologic system: Neurologic alterations may interfere with activity and exercise.
Cognition and perception	*Neurologic system:* Neurologic alterations may influence cognitive and perceptual functions.
	Sensory system: An intact and functioning sensory system, including the special senses and deep senses, is essential for perception.
Sleep and rest	Examination of all body systems is pertinent. Sleep disorders may be secondary to alterations in many body systems. Conversely, sleep disorders can result in body system alterations.
Self-concept	Body system alterations are evaluated to determine if they are related to threats to personal identity or body image.
Roles and relationships	Body systems usually are not evaluated to provide data about roles and relationships. Body system alterations that result in changes in life-style or daily activities, however, can threaten or disrupt usual roles and relationships.
Sexuality and reproduction	*Reproductive system:* Alterations in the development and physical status of reproductive structures (breasts, internal and external genitals) may contribute to altered patterns of sexuality or reproductive problems.
	Genitourinary system: Alterations in genitourinary structures may contribute to sexual dysfunction or reproductive problems.
Coping and stress tolerance	The physiologic effects of stress may be apparent by examining various body systems, especially the cardiovascular, respiratory, gastrointestinal, and integumentary systems. Alterations in the endocrine system may be associated with an altered response to stress.
Values and beliefs	Body systems usually are not evaluated to provide data about values and beliefs. Health beliefs can influence the way a person perceives body system functions, however.

Table 4–3. Correlating Data Associated With Functional Health Areas
With a Head-to-Toe Physical Examination

The following table shows how data collected by functional health areas interrelate with a head-to-toe
physical examination.

Head-to-Toe Physical Examination	Functional Health Area
General survey	General visual observation of a person may provide information about the level of functioning within each of the 11 functional health areas. Additionally, each component of the general survey may provide data specifically relevant to a particular pattern problem. *Health perception and health management:* The patient's general state of health and any obvious signs of distress will provide clues to his or her health perception and health management practices. *Nutrition and metabolism:* Survey height, weight, and general appearance as clues to nutritional status. Note the appearance of the skin, which may be altered with severe nutritional–metabolic problems. *Elimination:* Be alert for odors that may be associated with dysfunctional elimination patterns. Note impaired mobility or cognitive function that may contribute to elimination problems. *Activity and exercise:* Note any signs of distress related to activity and exercise. Observe the patient's posture, motor ability, and any physical deformities. *Cognition and perception:* Survey mental status, level of awareness, and the ability to communicate, which provide data about cognition and perception. *Sleep and rest:* Note facial expressions, affect, and behaviors that may be associated with sleep deprivation. *Self-concept and coping and stress tolerance:* Body language and behavior may provide clues to patient's self-concept and level of anxiety.
Anthropometric measurements	*Health perception and health management:* Body composition may reflect health management practices in relation to nutrition and exercise. *Nutrition and metabolism:* Anthropometric measurements are used to evaluate nutritional status and provide information about body tissues (viscera, skeletal muscle, and subcutaneous fat stores), which are altered during starvation or obesity.
Vital signs	*Health perception and health management:* Note whether the patient participates in blood pressure screening, a health management practice. *Nutrition and metabolism:* Alterations in the basal metabolic rate may be related to body temperature changes. *Activity and exercise:* Alterations in vital signs may suggest activity intolerance.
Hair, scalp, and cranium	*Nutrition and metabolism:* The appearance of the hair may be altered with severe nutritional–metabolic patterns.
Eyes and vision	*Cognition and perception:* Alterations in the eyes and visual acuity may interfere with visual sensation, perception, and cognition.
Ears and hearing	*Cognition and perception:* Alterations in the ears and hearing acuity may interfere with hearing sensation, perception, and cognitive functions.
Oral cavity	*Nutrition and metabolism:* Physical or functional alterations in the oral cavity may interfere with ingestion; alterations in the oral mucosa may be indicators of nutritional–metabolic problems.
Cranial nerves	*Cognition and perception:* Intact cranial nerve function is essential for a number of sensory–perceptual functions including eyesight, hearing, smell, touch, and taste.
Thyroid gland	*Nutrition and metabolism:* Thyroid alterations may affect basal metabolism.
Neck veins	*Activity and exercise:* The appearance of the neck veins may provide data about the cardiovascular system, whose function is essential for meeting oxygen requirements during activity.
Upper extremities	*Activity and exercise:* Observe the mobility of upper extremities and evaluate pulses to judge cardiovascular status.
Nails	*Nutrition and metabolism:* The appearance of the nails may be altered with severe nutritional–metabolic problems.
Breasts	*Health perception and health management:* Note whether the patient practices breast self-examination, a health screening practice.
Precordium and anterior thorax	*Activity and exercise:* The precordial examination provides data about the cardiovascular system; the anterior thorax examination provides data about the pulmonary system. Both systems are essential for meeting oxygen requirments during activity.
Posterior thorax	*Activity and exercise:* The posterior thorax examination provides data about the pulmonary system.
Abdomen	*Nutrition and metabolism:* Physical or functional alterations in abdominal organs may interfere with digestion, absorption, or metabolism. The appearance of the abdomen may be altered by nutritional problems. *Elimination:* Some abdominal examination alterations indicate elimination problems such as abdominal and bladder distention or bowel sound alterations.

(continued)

Table 4–3. Correlating Data Associated With Functional Health Areas
With a Head-to-Toe Physical Examination (continued)

The following table shows how data collected by functional health areas interrelate with a head-to-toe
physical examination.

Head-to-Toe Physical Examination	Functional Health Area
Lower extremities	*Activity and exercise:* Examination of the lower extremities may indicate the status of tissue oxygenation and level of motor function. Evaluate lower extremity pulses to judge cardiovascular status.
Genitals and pelvis	*Health perception and health management:* Note whether the patient participates in testicular self-examination, a health screening practice. Note whether the patient has routine pelvic examinations and PAP smears, health management screening examinations.
	Elimination: Pelvic structure alterations may contribute to problems with elimination.
Anus and rectum	*Health perception and health management:* The digital rectal examination is a health management screening practice for the detection of colorectal cancer.
	Elimination: Anal–rectal alterations may contribute to problems with elimination.

Table 4–4. Correlating a Body Systems Physical Examination With Functional Health Areas

Each body system can be affected by many areas of functional health. The following table lists the body
systems along with the most important functional health areas that are assessed to elicit data about that body
system.

Body System	Functional Health Areas	Body System	Functional Health Areas
Cardiovascular system	Activity and exercise	Musculoskeletal system	Elimination
	Coping and stress tolerance		Activity and exercise
Endocrine system	Nutrition and metabolism		Sleep and rest
	Coping and stress tolerance	Neurologic system	Elimination
Gastrointestinal system	Nutrition and metabolism		Activity and exercise
	Elimination		Cognition and perception
	Coping and stress tolerance	Pulmonary system	Sleep and rest
Genitourinary system	Elimination		Activity and exercise
	Sexuality and reproduction		Sleep and rest
	Coping and stress tolerance		Coping and stress tolerance
	Sleep and rest	Reproductive system	Elimination
Integumentary system	Nutrition and metabolism		Sexuality and reproduction
	Elimination	Sensory system	Cognition and perception
	Coping and stress tolerance		

Chapter 4 SUMMARY

This chapter focused on the following:
- The sequence used for performing a comprehensive physical examination
- Documentation of the physical examination
- The relevance of physical examination data to the overall assessment process

In preparing for the physical examination, consideration is given to the following:

- Preparation of equipment
- Client teaching
- The client's privacy
- Infection control measures
- Positioning of client and examiner

The comprehensive physical examination is conducted in a systematic manner, usually in a head-to-toe fashion or according to major body areas. Variations in this se-

quence may be necessary, especially when examining children.

Documentation of the physical exam may proceed using various formats, but general documentation principles should be kept in mind.

Physical examination is a method of data collection

and differs from assessment, which is the process of analyzing the data in order to make a clinical judgment. A variety of approaches and formats may be used for data analysis (assessment), including functional health patterns and body systems.

✸ CRITICAL THINKING

Physical examination is a process involving skill and analysis. Skill is required to conduct the examination and requires attention to technique, timing, and sequence. Analysis is required to make judgments about examination findings and requires knowledge, problem solving, and creativity.

Learning Exercises

1. Determine and specify how you would modify a head-to-toe examination sequence for an elderly woman confined to a wheelchair, who will remain seated in the wheelchair during most of the examination. The woman is hard of hearing and has left-sided weakness.

2. Plan and describe a sequence for examining the cardiovascular system for a healthy, ambulatory adult.

3. Review the physical examination documented in this chapter (Display 4-2). Using this data base, specify indicators for each of the functional health patterns listed below:
   Health perception and health management

   Nutrition and metabolism

   Elimination

   Activity and exercise

   Cognition and perception

   Sleep and rest

   Self-concept

BIBLIOGRAPHY

Centers for Disease Control. (1991). Recommendations for preventing transmission of human immunodeficiency virus and hepatitis B virus to patients during exposure-prone invasive procedures. *Morbidity and Mortality Weekly Report, 40.*

Fitzgerald, M.A. (1991). The physical exam. *RN, 54* (11), 34–39.

Gordon, M. (1987). *Nursing diagnosis: Process and application* (2nd ed.). New York: McGraw-Hill.

McConnell, W.E. (1990). Orderly assessment. *Emergency, 22* (10), 34–38.

Diagnostic Reasoning and Documentation

Assessment Terms

Diagnostic Reasoning
Cue
Data Base
Defining Characteristics
Indicators

North American Nursing Diagnosis
   Association (NANDA)
NANDA Taxonomy
Objective Data
Subjective Data
SOAP

DIAGNOSTIC REASONING

Health assessment begins with data collection, but it is not complete until the data are analyzed and conclusions are drawn. Data analysis is a process that requires specialized knowledge, skill, and judgment. In health care, this process is commonly referred to as *diagnostic reasoning*. Diagnostic reasoning requires skill in relation to the following:

- Recognizing significant data
- Organizing data so it has meaning
- Drawing a conclusion

Recognizing Significant Data

The diagnostic process begins with the nurse being able to recognize clinically significant information—that is, information that indicates normal or abnormal conditions or changes in the client's health condition and data that inform the nurse of the client's overall health status in relation to functional capacities.

Information collected during the assessment process provides *cues* to health status. A cue is a piece of information that influences decisions such as collecting more data or diagnosing a particular health problem. A cue may be a statement the client makes or a sign or behavior exhibited by the client. Cues are the "raw data" used to understand health problems and health status.

Jill Fuller and Jennifer Schaller-Ayers:
HEALTH ASSESSMENT: A NURSING APPROACH, Second Edition.
© 1990, 1994 by J. B. Lippincott Company.

1. BEGIN WITH AN ADEQUATE DATA BASE

It is important that the nurse collect enough information to give a thorough and complete picture of the client's health. An admission assessment, conducted when a nurse first meets the client, makes up the nursing *data base*. A nursing data base includes pertinent information about all 11 functional areas and becomes the basis for comparison when evaluating any changes in the person's condition. It is important for the nurse to use a systematic approach to acquiring a significant data base, so that important bits of information are not overlooked. Random collection of data is not advised because important data may be overlooked and, consequently, an important diagnosis missed entirely. Conducting a systematic head-to-toe physical examination that includes vital signs and inquiries regarding all 11 functional areas greatly increases the probability of obtaining a sufficient data base that tells the nurse all important problems, healthy behaviors, and sources of strength for each client.

The following scenario describes a situation in which the nurse initially overlooks an important and crucial piece of information regarding the client's health and well-being. This emphasizes the importance of a thorough assessment and a systematic method of obtaining an adequate data base to assure that all pertinent information is discovered.

Nurse: Aside from doing vital signs and asking a few questions from our hospital's admission form, I never really used to do what I would call a thorough nursing assessment. I tended to skip over the psychosocial parts and only listen to the heart and lungs. I was taking care of an elderly lady who had been very intoxicated on admission. She had been admitted with hypothermia after being found lying in a neighbor's yard. I kept coming out of her room saying, "Something's being missed here" or "Something's not right." I told another nurse about it and she said, "Well, did you ask her if something triggered her drinking" or "Did she have problems that were difficult to deal with?" I had never routinely assessed how people were coping or what type of problems they were facing outside the hospital. After talking with her, I found out that she had no prior history of alcohol abuse but that 2 days ago she had been notified that the drunk driver who had killed her husband 5 years ago in a hit-and-run accident had been released from prison. She talked about how difficult this was to deal with and how she was "falling apart." Now, rather than saying, "I think something's wrong," I do a thorough assessment so I can get a better idea of the patient's condition.

Conducting a systematic head-to-toe physical examination that includes vital signs and inquiring about all 11 functional areas increases the probability that you will have obtained sufficient data to indicate important problems, healthy behaviors, and sources of strength.

2. DRAW ON CLINICAL KNOWLEDGE AND EXPERIENCE

The type of data that you collect and begin to recognize as significant will be influenced by your own knowledge base. If you are a novice, you tend to rely on knowledge gained through study and other educational activities. On the other hand, if you are an experienced clinician, you draw more on what you know of clinical situations. You may even have developed an intuitive knowledge of clinical situations.

Nurses require knowledge about individuals and families and their responses to different health problems or life processes in order to make sound clinical judgments. For example, a nurse caring for postoperative patients will see what she expects to see based on knowledge stored in memory. Drawing on this stored knowledge and being able to anticipate the problems most commonly encountered in a particular context enable the nurse to focus on collecting and recognizing data that either confirm or rule out anticipated problems. Note how the nurse in the following example draws on her clinical knowledge when assessing the client.

Nurse: I knew that even though this man was only recovering from surgery under a local anesthetic that he was at risk for developing respiratory problems. His chart indicated that he had a long history of COPD, he was elderly, and he had the appearance of someone with longstanding COPD—he had the barrel chest, he was very thin, and he started to get short of breath with only minimal activity and even resorted to pursed-lip breathing. Then his wife told me that he had not taken his theophylline that morning because he was supposed to be NPO for surgery. Knowing what I did about the disease process, I decided I had better do more than just routine post-op vital signs, so I carefully listened to his lungs, observed his ventilatory effort, and skin color. I also assessed him more often than what was considered routine for a surgical outpatient. He had very little air exchange and was working very hard to breathe. I immediately notified the physician. If his man had been assessed "routinely," with no consideration of his underlying disease process, he may not have received the early and aggressive intervention he required.

Not having sufficient clinical background or theoretical knowledge may adversely affect the diagnostic reasoning process. If you have not had adequate education or experience and cannot rely on memory to supply the necessary knowledge about a particular client, especially in relation to pertinent physiologic, psychological, or developmental factors, you should consult appropriate references or knowledgeable colleagues.

Organizing Data for Meaning

The next step in the diagnostic process involves the ability to organize data so that patterns begin to emerge. Rarely is a sound diagnosis ever made on the basis of a single, isolated cue. The best diagnostic conclusions are usually based on interpreting patterns consisting of multiple cues.

1. GROUP TOGETHER RELATED DATA

As cues are perceived, note which cues seem to "fit" together and indicate a particular problem. Information is clustered in order to suggest certain diagnostic possibilities. For example, you may note that the client may (a) state that she is disappointed that her newborn baby is a girl, (b) leave the room as the baby begins to cry, (c) not make eye contact with her baby when she holds him, and (d) verbalize feelings of fatigue. Cues a, b, and c seem to be related because they are indicators of the mother's relationship with her baby. They should be grouped together for this reason. These cues match some of the characteristics associated with the nursing diagnosis, altered parenting. Grouping the cues together helps assure that the "match" was not made just on the basis of one cue, which may or may not be sufficient to assure a correct diagnosis.

2. ORGANIZE DATA BY USING A FRAMEWORK FOR COLLECTING AND RECORDING DATA

You already learned about the various frameworks for approaching data collection in Chapter 4. The reason one uses a particular framework is to help organize information to achieve a particular outcome. For example, if your goal is to formulate a medical diagnosis, a physiologic framework, such as the body systems approach, would be the logical choice because medical diagnoses are based on dysfunctions in body systems. If your goal is to arrive at a nursing diagnosis, however, you should use a framework that groups indicators of related nursing diagnoses. Collecting and recording information associated with each of the 11 functional health patterns can facilitate arriving at appropriate nursing diagnosis. For example, the nurse collects and records data associated with nutrition and metabolism, clusters findings that may indicate problems with nutrition and metabolism, and then checks the nursing diagnoses associated with nutrition and metabolism to see if any of the defining characteristics or "indicators" match those recorded.

Drawing a Conclusion

Once data are clustered, they should be interpreted and the conclusion that is drawn should be given a name. That name could represent a need or problem, a medical diagnosis, or a nursing diagnosis. Consider your conclusion tentative until you are certain that it is the best interpretation of the data. The diagnostic process should not be concluded until you are certain that your conclusion is valid. This involves considering all other possibilities and, often, collecting additional data to support your conclusions.

1. BECOME FAMILIAR WITH DIAGNOSTIC INDICATORS

A nursing diagnosis is formulated based on observing a cluster of cues, including those referred to as defining characteristics and related factors. To arrive at a diagnosis, the nurse must assure that there is a similarity or match between the information she has clustered and those known indicators for the diagnosis. The North American Nursing Diagnosis Association (NANDA) Taxonomy I Revised (1990) lists all the official nursing diagnoses with all the associated defining characteristics or "indicators" of each diagnosis. Nurses should be familiar with these defining characteristics, which can help them learn to cluster findings appropriately and recognize a match between those of a client and those listed in the NANDA Taxonomy for a certain diagnosis. This process of collection and organization occurs repeatedly during the diagnostic process.

Nurses do need to have knowledge of the signs and symptoms for various disease processes, but certainly for the professional nurse, emphasis should be centered on nursing diagnoses and defining characteristics.

An example of how the clustering of information can help lead to the appropriate nursing diagnosis is illustrated using the preceding example. The nurse assesses the functional area of roles and relationships and groups the following findings: (a) mother states she is disappointed her newborn is a girl, (b) mother leaves the room as the baby begins to cry, (c) mother does not make eye contact with her baby when holding her, and (d) mother verbalizes feelings of fatigue. Having knowledge of defining characteristics would help this nurse to associate her findings with several similar defining characteristics for the nursing diagnosis of Altered parenting (*i.e.,* lack of parental attachment behaviors; inappropriate visual, tactile and auditory stimulation; and verbalization of resentment towards the infant), thus helping her to make the appropriate diagnosis.

For the nursing diagnosis of Activity intolerance, the following defining characteristics are listed: verbal report of fatigue or weakness; abnormal heart rate or blood pressure response to activity; exertional discomfort or dyspnea; and electrocardiographic changes reflecting arrhythmias. The nurse must first observe some or all of these characteristics to make the diagnosis of Activity intolerance.

In addition to the general listings of defining characteristics, NANDA is working toward identifying critical defining characteristics or "critical indicators," which would be those signs and symptoms that *must be present* in order to formulate a particular nursing diagnosis.

2. TREAT YOUR CONCLUSIONS AS A WORKING HYPOTHESIS UNTIL YOU HAVE RULED OUT OTHER POSSIBILITIES

Initially, it is best to consider all diagnostic conclusions as tentative, like a hypothesis, until you effectively rule out competing possibilities. Resist the temptation to settle for the first diagnosis that comes to mind. Investigate further to determine whether or not your hypothesis is valid. Investigate by collecting additional data related to each cue on which your initial conclusion was based. For example, you may use the protocol for symptom analysis described in Chapter 3, or, if you have a cue related to elimination status, you may do a more exhaustive examination of the person's elimination pattern in order to better understand the nature of the problem. Consider the meaning of disconfirming data or data that have been uncovered that clearly do not support your hypothesis. Avoid the tendency to ignore disconfirming data just so that you can draw a conclusion and bring the process to closure.

3. EVALUATE YOUR CONCLUSION

Once you have investigated further and concluded that your final diagnosis is valid, consider again the quality of the match between the cues and the indicators for the diagnosis. Remember that even your final conclusion is, at best, a conjecture.

DOCUMENTATION
OF THE HEALTH ASSESSMENT

Assessment findings are documented for several reasons. They provide a written basis for the delivery and evaluation of health care; they serve as legal references that may be used in a court of law; and they substantiate financial expenditures for reimbursement purposes. Health assessment documentation should be based on the data collected and on the professional judgments resulting from the analysis of that data.

Subjective and Objective Data

For purposes of documentation, some practitioners make the distinction between objective and subjective data, although such a distinction may be untenable. Typically, *objective data* refer to data collected by means of the examiner's observations or measurements. The examiner observes the client through the senses of sight, hearing, touch, and smell. Because an outside observer has collected the data, it is referred to as objective. The implication is that it is free of bias. Examples of objective data, which may be referred to as signs, include blood pressure, height and weight, pulse rate, visual acuity, and body temperature. The client's laboratory reports, electrocardiogram results, x-ray reports, and other test results are also classified as objective data.

Subjective data refer to the perceptions of the client or significant others. Reports of pain, nausea, and dizziness are examples of subjective data. Subjective data may be referred to as symptoms.

Although an examiner may believe that he or she is an objective observer, often personal values or bias may influence the assessment process. Therefore, some of the data collected by the examiner may be subjective in that they are influenced by perceptions and feelings.

Documentation Principles

1. *Avoid inferences and judgments when recording subjective and objective data.* An inference is a statement about the unknown based on the examiner's observations. For example, *do not* write, "Oral examination reveals receding gum lines, food debris, and halitosis, *indicating poor oral hygiene.*"

   Avoid value-laden language or opinionated statements. For example, the following written statement is inappropriate: "Patient requests for pain medication are too frequent."

   Record professional inferences and judgments only after data have been collected and analyzed. Professional judgments may appear in the health record as nursing diagnoses, as problem statements in the problem-oriented record, or as the assessment component of a SOAP progress note (see following section, SOAP Progress Notes).

2. *Record findings rather than techniques.* Avoid a detailed discussion of how the data were obtained. For example, *do not* write, "The otoscopic examination was conducted by inserting the speculum after pulling the auricle upward and backward. Once the tympanic membrane was visualized, it was noted to be pearly gray with a light reflex." This entry is time-consuming to write and read and may discourage careful reading of the examiner's findings.

3. *Record the client's perceptions.* The client's perceptions are significant because they reveal what the individual knows about his or her health status. The client's responses to any problems or concerns and expectations in relation to health care are also significant.

4. *Write concisely and efficiently.* Avoid redundancy, which obscures important data and makes the record time-consuming to read. Examples of redundant statements include "Visible by inspection," "Heard on auscultation," "Bilaterally symmetric." It is also considered redundant to write, "The client . . . ," because the client is always the subject of the record.

   Summarize and condense the client's statements whenever possible. For example, *do not* record verbatim the client's 5-minute explanation of chest pain, but rather, write, "Substernal chest pain occurred three times today, with each episode lasting 5 minutes and relieved by sublingual nitroglycerin. Pain pressure-like without radiation. No shortness of breath, nausea, diaphoresis, palpitations or lightheadedness during pain."

   Avoid superfluous data. For example, *do not* write, "Able to drive car to work. Drives a red convertible."

5. *Record the relevant details.* All relevant data should be recorded, including both positive and negative findings that contribute to the diagnosis. Record data that are pertinent to ruling out a particular diagnosis. For example, data such as decreased mobility (walking) and dyspnea may suggest the diagnosis Self-care deficit. But if the client demonstrates the ability to carry out independently all activities of daily living in spite of these factors, the diagnosis may be ruled out.

   Also, record normal findings when abnormal findings might be expected. For example, normal heart sounds and the absence of ankle edema in patients with congestive heart failure should be duly noted.

6. *Describe normal findings.* Assessment findings should always be documented in specific, descriptive terms. Although findings that deviate from normal usually pose few problems, normal findings are somewhat difficult to describe. Terms such as *normal, within normal limits,* or *negative* are not sufficient because they do not describe your observations as much as reflect your judgment. In order to justify such a judgment, you must document your observations. Describe normal findings in terms of what you observe and note through inspection, palpation, percussion, and auscultation. Rather than writing "lung sounds normal," you should write "lungs clear to auscultation and percussion."

   An exception to the practice of thoroughly describing normal findings may be noted with the documentation method of "charting by exception." If you are charting by exception, only abnormal findings are addressed by the examiner in a chart entry (see also Chap. 21).

7. *Organize and format the data in a logical fashion.* As with all types of health care documentation, record information systematically. Generally, record the health history before the physical examination findings. Printed forms provided by the health care agency, such as admission forms and flowsheets, may organize the data base with headings and space for the recording of specific data. If a printed form is not used, create headings to promote organization and thoroughness.

Health assessment data may be logically organized in different ways by different health care providers. For example, physicians organize assessment data in relation to illness and symptoms (chief complaint, history of the present illness), past medical history, and body systems (review of systems). Nurses may organize assessment data in relation to human responses and functional abilities so that data relevant to nursing diagnoses are collected.

Finally, health assessment data relating to the client's present condition and health history should be organized in chronologic order to facilitate easy retrieval and understanding. Record present concerns or problems chronologically, beginning with the time of onset. List past surgeries or hospitalizations in reverse order, from most recent to the first. For each entry, specify the date, event, and significant consequences.

8. *Use appropriate grammar and punctuation.* Complete sentences should have subjects and verbs. Phrases may be used in place of complete sentences if you carefully consider the punctuation. Commas, dashes, periods, and semicolons give specific indications of how words relate to each other. Correct spelling as well as correct use of abbreviations are expected in a professional record.

SOAP Progress Notes

Assessment data and professional judgments may be documented in the form of a SOAP progress note. SOAP is an acronym for the following categories of information:

S = Subjective Data. This part of the SOAP entry documents the client's perceptions of the problem. Subjective data may be recorded as a direct quote, such as, "My mouth hurts." You may summarize or paraphrase the client's perceptions, such as, "States he is worried about surviving heart surgery." The latter approach may be used to condense a lengthy discussion about fears related to surgery.

O = Objective Data. This part of the SOAP entry documents your observations and factual information, such as physical examination findings and laboratory data. Examples include, "Crying following wife's visit," "Ulcerated lesion ½ cm in diameter on mucosa inside left cheek," and "White blood cell count 15,000."

A = Assessment. You should make a judgment about health status based on the client's signs and symptoms and record the judgment. This statement should usually be

more than a label of the problem and should represent nursing analysis and synthesis of assessment findings. Documentation may include possible etiologic factors, problem course, pertinent prognostic indicators, if known, and the client's response to therapy, such as the following: "Altered oral mucosa related to mechanical trauma from oral suction catheter; no longer requires oral suctioning and can maintain own oral hygiene; no signs of infection such as redness or drainage; should heal spontaneously as long as hygiene and nutrition are maintained."

P = Plan. The plan is not a health assessment documentation per se, but rather a brief statement of the therapeutic plan for problem resolution. The statement may also include additional measures to augment diagnosis and the health teaching plan. For example, "Assist with repositioning every 2 hours. Reevaluate effectiveness of turning schedule by inspecting pressure points with each position change. Modify turning frequency if indicated. Instruct patient regarding (1) the importance of position changes and (2) how to shift weight with the aid of overhead trapeze."

Narrative-Style Documentation

Health assessment data may also be recorded in a narrative style on the chart. Various logical, organizational approaches are acceptable. For example, narrative charting may be organized to reflect the application of the nursing process. In such a case, all narrative assessment data should be recorded and then followed by the problem statement, interventions, and the client's response. This narrative approach is similar to the SOAP format.

Another organizational approach involves arranging the findings according to body systems. For example, you may record observations in relation to each of the following systems:

Neurologic
Cardiovascular
Respiratory
Gastrointestinal
Genitourinary
Endocrine
Musculoskeletal
Integumentary

Similarly, data may be organized to reflect major areas of functional status and abilities, such as the following:

Health perception and health management
Nutrition and metabolism
Elimination
Activity and exercise
Cognition and perception
Sleep and rest
Self-concept
Roles and relationships
Sexuality and reproduction
Coping and stress tolerance
Values and beliefs

See the accompanying sample data base (Display 5-1) for this functional approach. Once the subjective and objective

(Text continues on pg. 62)

Display 5–1
Sample Health Assessment Data Base: Functional Approach

Demographic Data

Mr. Arnold K., 956 Cedar Lane, Mann City
46 years old, steel plant worker (welder)

Referral

Required annual physical for work.

Current Medications

1. Acetominophen or aspirin for headaches (occasional use)
2. Dihydroxy aluminum sodium carbonate (Rolaid) tablets for indigestion (2 to 3 times/month)
3. Clonidine hydrochloride (Catapres) prescribed for hypertension; does not know dosage and does not take as prescribed

Past Medical-Surgical History

1. Hypertension—diagnosed 1 year ago during routine physical; has not had routine blood pressure measurements since.
2. Fractured right wrist in industrial accident, 1984; treated with cast; healed with no residual problems.
3. Hemorrhoidectomy, 1982; recovery uncomplicated; no recurrence of hemorrhoids.

Health Perception and Health Management

Views self as healthy. Greatest concern is that present examination may reveal something is wrong with him. Being healthy means "not having to go to the doctor and not having to take any pills." Engages in no scheduled health screening activities except annual physical required by employer. Comprehensive health insurance provided by employer. Clonidine was prescribed 1 year ago for hypertension but he states he only takes it when he feels his BP is high—"when I get headaches." Reasons for not taking Catapres: "I don't like pills"; "I don't think my blood pressure is high"; cost. No regular blood pressure screening.

Illness and Injury Risk Factors

1. Family health history (see diagram at right).
2. Exposure to health and safety risks: Does not smoke cigarettes, drink alcohol, or use illegal drugs; has been exposed to asbestos through work; no pulmonary function testing to date; result of chest x-ray 1 year ago was normal (verified by record).
3. Safety measures: Wears safety glasses at work and while doing yard work; wears seatbelt on freeways or rural highways but not for city driving. Wears helmet for dirt biking and requires same of children.

Objective Data

BP 144/88 (LA)
BP 140/90 (LA—repeated 10 minutes after first measurement)

Nutrition and Metabolism

Sees self as 20 pounds overweight because of sedentary life-style and "love of food." Views weight gain as "part of life" and has no desire to reduce. Good appetite, likes most foods, no food allergies, no special diet, and no problems with eating. Wife does shopping and cooking. Eats out once per week.

Sample Diet

- Breakfast—Black coffee, 2 doughnuts, orange juice
- AM break at work—coffee, sweet roll
- Lunch—Ham and cheese sandwich, soda, potato chips, fruit
- Dinner—chicken, steak, or hamburger; cooked vegetable; potato with butter and sour cream; cookies or pudding
- Evening snacks—Chips or cookies; milk before retiring

Objective Data

Height: 6'0" Weight: 230 lbs.
Ideal weight (large frame): 168–192 lbs.

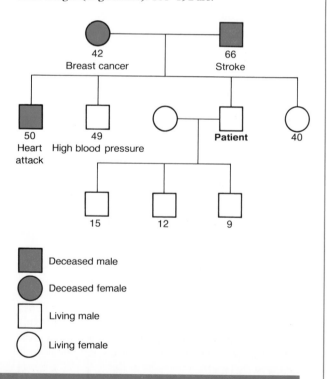

Deceased male

Deceased female

Living male

Living female

(continued)

Triceps skinfold: 17.5 mm
Skin: Intact; no lesions except for old scars from minor trauma.
Oral cavity: Moist oral mucosa. No lesions.
Cranial nerves IX, X, XII intact.

Elimination

- Urinary: No problems with voiding. Has never had hesitancy, burning, or urgency.
- Bowel: Usually has daily bowel movement after breakfast.
- Occasional constipation (once per month) when regular schedule is disrupted. Takes magnesium hydroxide (Milk of Magnesia) for constipation—"If I let it go, I think my hemorrhoids would be back." Currently no problems with hemorrhoids. Result of stool test for occult blood was negative 1 year ago; no gross blood noted in stools.

Objective Data

Rectal exam: No masses or tenderness. Prostate without enlargement or nodules, firm. Soft brown stool, negative for occult blood.

Activity and Exercise

Drives to work. Occasionally heavy lifting but otherwise little exertion required for work activities. Engages in yard work nightly after work (spring and summer) to maintain garden. Other leisure activities—fishing from boat once per week; watching TV; dirt bike riding with family once per week; camping; spectator sports. No regular exercise—views camping, fishing, and biking as exercise.
    Self-care: Independent in all ADLs.
    Denies any cardiovascular or musculoskeletal symptoms in relation to activity—no chest pain, dyspna, leg, joint, or back pain.

Objective Data

Musculoskeletal system: Full range of motion; muscle strength 3 on 5-point scale. Steady gait. No observed deficits in general mobility. No joint deformities.
Cardiovascular system: Regular heart rhythm. Pulse 88. Clear S_1 and S_2—no extra heart sounds or murmurs. No dependent edema. PMI 5th ICS at the MCL.
Respiratory system: Equal and full chest expansion. Lungs resonant. Breath sounds clear without adventitious sounds.

Cognition and Perception

Trade school graduate. Learns easily by "seeing something done and then doing it."

Special senses: Wears reading glasses; last eye exam 4 years ago; not sure if he was tested for glaucoma. No problems with hearing or other senses.
Frontal headaches every 2 to 3 months; takes aspirin or acetaminophen (Tylenol) and if unrelieved takes clonidine (Catapres) "since it might be my blood pressure."

Objective Data

Eyes: Vision 20/30 (OD) and 20/40 (OS); reads telephone print with reading glasses. Full peripheral vision by confrontation. PERRLA. Conjunctiva pink and moist; cornea and lens clear. No AV nicking, fundal lesions, or fundal edema.

Sleep and Rest

Usually sleeps 6 to 7 hours per night (10:30 PM–5:30 AM); stays up later and sleeps in on weekends. No problems falling asleep or maintaining sleep. Sleeps in king-size bed with wife. Presleep activities include watching television news and saying prayers.

Self-Concept

Views self as needing to be in control of own life and family's emotional and financial security. Wants to be strong and healthy for his family—"I feel like I'd be letting them down if I got sick." States he is a good husband and father, and dependable, skilled worker. Mostly positive about self and life. Describes self as religious.

Objective Data

Relaxed during interview except when questioned about medications and blood pressure. Well-groomed with greasy hands and fingernails from working with engines. Maintains eye contact.

Roles and Relationships

Family: Wife and children healthy and family relationships close and happy. Three sons—ages 15, 12, 9. Family goes camping and biking every weekend during summer. Takes sons deer hunting with friends every fall. States sons are "good boys" and active in church and sports. Family discusses social issues and uses religious concepts to guide life. States he would worry more about his sons if they weren't active in church activities. Wife works part time as receptionist.
Social: Socializes with other church members. Family-style get-togethers with friends once every 2 to 3 weeks. All close friends are part of this group. Compatible with coworkers but minimal interaction outside work.

(continued)

Display 5–1
Sample Health Assessment Data Base: Functional Approach (continued)

Work: Enjoys work but worries that it is "a young man's job" and he may have trouble with physical demands in a few years. Is being considered for foreman position but not pursuing aggressively—"The job looks like too much trouble—I make enough money to support my family." Belongs to labor union "because it goes with the territory." Not active in union affairs.

Sexuality and Reproduction

Reports no problems with sexual relationship but states BP medication affected his sexual performance. No problems when not taking medication. Three sons. States that commitment, monogamy, and "obeying God" are important for sexual fulfillment.

Coping and Stress Tolerance

Feels greatest stressor is worrying about work—feels that health or age may unexpectedly threaten ability to work. Concerned about potential loss of income because "I don't have much money stored away even though I make good wages." Work-related pension considered helpful but not adequate to maintain current life-style. States he has done little to resolve this problem except "worry about it."

Values and Beliefs

Family and religion most important to him. Describes self as "born again Christian." Attends church regularly with family except during summer when camping. Family Bible studies conducted weekly. Believes that persons with dissimilar beliefs need to "be saved" but generally avoids people with different beliefs. Describes social and political views as conservative. Believes strongly in after-life, which gives him a sense of peace and satisfaction.

Cues	*Inferences*
Does not take clonidine hydrocholoride (Catapres) as prescribed	Does not understand pathogenesis and treatment of high blood pressure
Weight reduction not desired	Clonidine not taken because it causes sexual problems
Clonidine affects sexual performance	The diagnosis of high blood pressure is contrary to healthy image of self
Describes self as healthy	
Describes health as not taking pills	
Concerned that physical disability will affect work role	Finds the diagnosis of hypertension threatening
Clonidine too expensive	Noncompliance with therapy is financially related

---

data have been collected, cues are clustered and inferences are made about the client's health strengths, risks, and problems. Some examiners find it helpful to cluster the cues revealed by each functional area of assessment. Organizing cues in this manner may help you recognize meaningful patterns associated with a particular set of cues. Using the sample data base in Display 5-1, you may evaluate one of the client's functional areas (health perception–health management) in this manner.

The cues and inferences suggest noncompliance related to negative side effects of the prescribed treatment. You should collect additional data to establish whether the client

- Desires to comply with recommended treatment or alternative treatments
- Understands the pathogenesis of hypertension
- Understands the treatment of hypertension
- Understands the link between obesity and hypertension

Additionally, you should consult with the client's physician to determine whether the prescribed medication is still indicated and whether alternative therapy is possible. Not until all such aspects have been explored can you state the nursing diagnosis with certainty and devise a treatment plan.

Chapter 5 SUMMARY

Diagnostic reasoning is a method for formulating judgments about the client's condition based on the data gathered. It is an intellectual process enabling you to make informed, professional judgments rather than value judgments. Diagnostic reasoning involves

- Recognizing significant data

- Organizing data so they have meaning.
- Drawing a conclusion

Documentation of health assessment data is similar in many respects to other types of documentation in the health record. Health assessment documentation focuses on recording objective and subjective data and the conclusions you draw from analyzing the data. Recording formats vary across settings, but data are usually organized

to facilitate easy retrieval and diagnostic reasoning. SOAP progress notes may be used to present the health assessment data base.

✳ CRITICAL THINKING

Diagnostic reasoning refers to the cognitive processes involved in clinical judgment. The clinician should strive to develop diagnostic skills with the same level of attention that would be used to develop the psychomotor skills required for a physical examination.

Learning Exercises

1. Specify and describe the cognitive processes involved in making a clinical diagnosis.

2. Explain how you would guard against drawing premature conclusions during the health assessment process.

3. You are revising the documentation system for the student health clinic. Develop some overall goals you would like to consider as you develop a system for documenting health assessment findings.

BIBLIOGRAPHY

Carnevali, D.L., et al. (1984). *Diagnostic reasoning in nursing.* Philadelphia: J.B. Lippincott.

Carnevali, D.L., & Thomas, M.D. (1993). *Diagnostic reasoning and treatment decision making in nursing.* Philadelphia: J.B. Lippincott.

Field, P. (1987). The impact of nursing theory on the clinical decision making process. *Journal of Advanced Nursing, 12* (5), 559–562.

Fitzmaurice, J.B. (1987). Nurses' use of cues in the clinical judgment of activity tolerance. In A.M. McLane (Ed.). *Classification of nursing diagnoses: Proceedings of the seventh conference.* St. Louis: C.V. Mosby.

Gordon, M. (1987). *Nursing diagnosis: Process and application* (2nd ed.). New York: McGraw-Hill.

Gruber, M. (1989). The power of certainty . . . pattern recognition. *American Journal of Nursing, 89* (4), 502–503.

Hammond, K.R., Kelly, K.J., Scheider, R.J., & Vancini, M. (1966). Clinical inference in nursing: Analyzing cognitive tasks representative of nursing problems. *Nursing Research, 15,* 134.

Henning, M. (1991). Comparison of nursing diagnostic statements using a functional health pattern and health history/body systems format. In R.M. Carroll-Johnson (Ed.). *Classification of nursing diagnoses: Proceedings of the ninth conference.* Philadelphia: J.B. Lippincott.

Jacoby, M.K., & Adams, D.J. (1981). Teaching assessment of client functioning. *Nursing Outlook, 29* (4), 248–250.

Morrissey, R.M. (1988). Documentation: If you haven't written it, you haven't done it. *Nursing Clinics of North America, 23* (2), 363–371.

Newell, A., & Simon, H. (1972). *Human problem solving.* Englewood Cliffs, NJ: Prentice-Hall.

North American Nursing Diagnosis Association. (1990). *Taxonomy I revised 1990 with official nursing diagnoses.* St. Louis: NANDA.

Padrick, K.P., et al. (1987). Hypothesis evaluation: A component of diagnostic reasoning. In A.M. McLane (Ed.). *Classification of nursing diagnoses: Proceedings of the seventh conference.* St. Louis: C.V. Mosby.

Putzier, D.J., et al. (1985). Diagnostic reasoning in critical care. *Heart and Lung, 14* (5), 430–437.

Rew, L. (1988). Intuition in decision making. *Image: Nursing Scholarship, 20* (3), 150–154.

Rhodes, A.M. (1986). Principles of documentation. *Maternal-Child Nursing Journal, 11* (6), 381.

Rossi, L. (1987). Organizing data for nursing diagnosis using functional health patterns. In McLane A.M. (Ed.). *Classification of nursing diagnoses: Proceedings of the seventh conference.* St. Louis: C.V. Mosby.

Tanner, C.A. (1982). Instruction in the diagnostic process: An experimental study. In M.J. Kim & D. Moritz (Eds.). *Classification of nursing diagnoses: Proceedings of the third and fourth national conferences.* New York: McGraw-Hill.

Tillis, M.S. (1986). What do you say when you can't say normal. *Nursing Success Today, 3* (6), 29–30.

Weed, L.L. (1970). *Medical records, medical evaluation, and patient care.* Chicago: Year Book Medical Publishers.

Westfall, U.E., Tanner, C.A., Putzier, D.J., & Padrick, K. (1987). Errors committed by nurses and nursing students in the diagnostic reasoning process. In A.M. McLane (Ed.). *Classification of nursing diagnoses: Proceedings of the seventh conference.* St. Louis: C.V. Mosby.

Wurzbach, M.E. (1991). Judgment under conditions of uncertainty. *Nursing Forum, 26* (3), 27–34.

Chapter 6

Assessing Vital Signs

Examination Guidelines

Assessment Terms

Vital Signs (Cardinal Signs)
Apical Pulse
Pulse Rate
Pulse Rhythm
Tachycardia
Bradycardia
Pulse Deficit

Respiration
Ventilation
Ventilatory Rate
Korotkoff Sounds
Systolic Blood Pressure
Diastolic Blood Pressure

INTRODUCTORY OVERVIEW

Vital signs, also called *cardinal signs,* include pulse, respiratory rate, blood pressure, and body temperature. Assessing vital signs provides a quick overview of a person's physiologic status. Vital signs also provide cues to the intensity of other human responses such as pain, anxiety, fear, and activity intolerance. Nurses routinely evaluate vital signs in order to monitor physical status. Vital sign data should be compared to the person's baseline values and interpreted according to health history, medical diagnosis, medication history, and laboratory results.

When and how frequently vital signs are assessed is determined by standards of practice and the client's physical status. For example, for a postoperative patient who is still lethargic from general anesthesia, vital signs should be taken every 15 minutes. Two days later, when the patient is fully ambulatory, vital signs may be assessed every 6 hours or when a change occurs in the person's overall appearance. Patients in acute care settings often are subject to routine monitoring of vital signs such as once every hour, every 4 hours, or every 8 hours depending on their health status. Vital signs are typically measured before conducting the physical examination of the person.

Pulse, respiratory rate, and blood pressure are influenced by diverse factors such as emotions and exercise. Therefore, every attempt should be made to measure vital signs when the person is calm and at rest. A person who reports to the clinic for blood pressure screening after climbing several flights of stairs should be seated and rested before blood pressure is taken. Vital sign values that are inconsistent with the person's baseline values should be double checked before therapeutic decisions are made.

Assessment Focus

Assessment of vital signs includes measurement of the following:

- Pulse rate and rhythm
- Respiratory rate and pattern
- Blood pressure
- Body temperature

If deviations from normal are detected, the nurse must determine whether or not additional assessment or intervention is indicated. First, you should evaluate deviations from normal in light of the person's baseline vital signs. For example, a blood pressure of 90/60 may deviate from the normal range for systolic blood pressure, but this value may represent the person's usual blood pressure and therefore be considered normal for that individual. Second, you should evaluate any deviations from normal in light of the person's overall physical status. For example, a blood pressure of 90/60 accompanied by cold, clammy skin, rapid heart rate, and decreased level of consciousness is significant and indicates a state of shock. In this case, a life-threatening situation exists and immediate intervention is required.

If deviations from normal pulse, respirations, and blood pressure are noted and if such deviations do not represent the person's baseline vital signs, additional assessment of the person should focus on the status of vital body systems, especially the cardiovascular system, the respiratory system, and neurologic system. Altered vital signs may be the first indication of life-threatening pathology involving these systems.

Deviations in body temperature, although significant and potentially life-threatening, do not usually indicate critical situations. However, additional assessment of vital body systems is still indicated to make this type of determination.

Nursing Diagnoses

Vital signs indicate the overall status of a number of body systems and human responses. Therefore, assessment of vital signs provides cues to the following nursing diagnoses:

Hypothermia
Hyperthermia
Ineffective thermoregulation
Dysreflexia
Fluid volume excess
Fluid volume deficit
Altered tissue perfusion
Decreased cardiac output
Ineffective airway clearance
Ineffective breathing pattern
Activity intolerance
Pain
Anxiety

ARTERIAL PULSE ASSESSMENT

Anatomy and Physiology Overview

The arteries are strong, compliant vessels that carry oxygenated blood away from the heart to peripheral tissues. The elastic properties of the arterial walls cause the arteries to stretch during systole and recoil during diastole. The result is a palpable arterial pulse. The arterial pulse not only reflects the status of the arterial vasculature, it also provides an index of heart function. When vital signs are assessed, the pulse is evaluated primarily to determine heart rate and rhythm. However, the pulse may also be evaluated to determine vessel patency, the state of the arterial wall, and the contour and amplitude of the pulse. Related examination techniques are discussed in Chapter 10.

PULSE RATE

The pulse rate refers to the number of pulse beats counted in 1 minute. In most cases, pulse rate is equal to heart rate. However, if pulse rate is evaluated by palpating a peripheral pulse site, and the arterial pressure wave is not propagated to the peripheral site because of vascular disease or impaired heart contractility, heart rate may be faster than pulse rate.

Normal adult pulse rate ranges from 60 to 100 beats/minute. *Tachycardia* refers to a pulse rate greater than 100 beats/minute; *bradycardia* is a pulse rate less than 60 beats/minute. Normal pulse rates vary among people. Children and infants generally have faster rates than adults (Table 6-1). Women have slightly faster rates than men, and elderly persons may have slightly faster rates than middle-aged adults.

Pulse rate is primarily determined by the automaticity rate of the sinoatrial (SA) node. The SA node is the normal cardiac pacemaker that spontaneously discharges at a rate of 60 to 100 times/minute.

Pulse rate is also influenced by autonomic nervous system activity, which, in turn, is influenced by the central nervous system and baroreceptor reflexes.

In the presence of psychophysiologic stressors, such as trauma, infection, fever, fear, pain, and anxiety, pulse rate may increase.

Other factors that influence pulse rate include oxygen and carbon dioxide levels in the blood, fluid and electrolyte status, drugs, exercise, and acid–base status. If you detect an alteration in pulse rate, you should investigate possible causes.

PULSE RHYTHM

Pulse rhythm refers to the time intervals between pulse beats. Normally, the pulse has a regular rhythm—in other words, an equal interval between each beat. Some irregular pulse rhythms, or dysrhythmias, are benign. For example, sinus dysrhythmia, commonly noted in children and adolescents, is characterized by a slightly increased pulse rate on inspiration and decreased pulse rate on expiration. Other dysrhythmias may indicate serious cardiac dysfunction and should be further evaluated by electrocardiogram (ECG).

Table 6–1. Vital Signs: Normal Range According to Age

| Age | Resting Pulse Rate* (beats/minute) | Ventilatory Rate (breaths/minute) | Blood Pressure | | Body Temperature† |
			Systolic† (mm Hg)	Diastolic (mm Hg)	
Newborn	120–170 Mean: 145	30–50	80±16 30–60 flush	46±16	35.9°–36.7°C (96.6°F–98.0°F) axillary
1 year	80–160 Mean: 120	20–40	96±30	66±25	36.2°–37.8°C (97.2°F–100.0°F) rectal
3 years	80–130 Mean: 106	20–30	100±25	67±23	>37.2°C (99.0°F) rectal
6 years	75–115	16–22	100±15	56±8	>37.0°C (98.6°F) oral
8 years	70–110	16–22	105±16	57±9	>37.0°C (98.6°F)
10 years	70–110	16–20	111±17	58±10	>37.0°C (98.6°F)
16 years	60–100	14–20	118±20	65±10	>36.7°C (98.1°F) oral
Adult	60–100	16–20	100–140	60–90	>36.7°C (98.1°F)
Elderly	60–100	16–20	Maximum 160	Same as adult	>36.0°C (96.8°F) oral

After age 12, a boy's average pulse is 5 beats/minute slower than a girl's.
†Temperatures are subject to circadian rhythms in all age groups.
‡Boys age 12 to 17 have slightly systolic blood pressure than do girls.

Physical Examination

The Arterial Pulse

General Principles

For purposes of vital sign assessment, an arterial pulse is examined by auscultation or palpation to determine pulse rate and rhythm. Arterial pulses may also be examined to evaluate blood flow, arterial wall elasticity, and vessel patency. An examination of this nature is not required when eliciting vital signs but would be indicated during a comprehensive evaluation of the cardiovascular system (see Chap. 10, "Cardiovascular System").

Pulse Sites

Peripheral pulses can be palpated at areas where large arteries are close to the skin surface. Palpable pulses include the carotid, brachial, radial, femoral, popliteal, posterior tibial, and dorsalis pedis. The apical pulse may be palpated or auscultated over the heart apex as the left ventricle distends and recoils during systole and diastole. Because the radial or apical pulse sites are so accessible, they are most commonly used during vital sign assessment. An apical pulse is considered more accurate than a radial pulse if conditions exist that interfere with the transmission of the pulse to the periphery (*e.g.,* low cardiac output, atherosclerosis).

Equipment

- Watch or clock with a second hand
- Stethoscope (if pulse rate and rhythm are determined by auscultation)

Examination and Documentation Focus

- Pulse rate
- Pulse rhythm

Examination Guidelines   *Pulse*

Procedure

1. LOCATE THE RADIAL PULSE.

    a. Place the pads of your first, second, and third fingers over the radial artery pulse point on the inner wrist surface over the radius.

    b. Press your fingers firmly against the artery and slowly release pressure until the pulse is palpable.

Clinical Significance

The thumb should not be used to locate the client's pulse because it has its own pulse.

Pressing too hard obliterates the pulse.

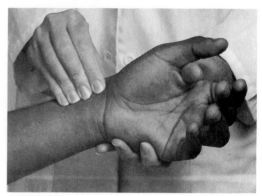

Radial pulse palpation

2. COUNT THE PULSE RATE.

    Use a watch with a second hand to count the pulse rate. If the pulse is regular, count for 30 seconds and multiply by 2. If irregular, count for a full minute and then evaluate the apical pulse, which may be more accurate.

Normal Findings
Pulse rate 60–100 beats/minute in adults (see also Table 6-1).

Deviations from Normal
A pulse rate less than 60/minute may be considered normal in persons who participate in regular aerobic exercise.

A pulse rate greater than 100/minute may be considered a normal response to exercise.

3. EVALUATE PULSE RHYTHM.

    Note the pulse rhythm while palpating the radial pulse.

Normal Findings
Regular rhythm

Deviations from Normal
Irregular rhythm; indicates cardiac dysrhythmias

4. LOCATE THE APICAL PULSE.

    In adults, the apical pulse is normally found at the fifth left intercostal space just medial to the midclavicular line. Palpate or auscultate the pulse with the stethoscope. Place the diaphragm of the stethoscope over the pulse site.

5. COUNT THE APICAL PULSE RATE.

    Use a watch with a second hand and count the pulse for 1 full minute.

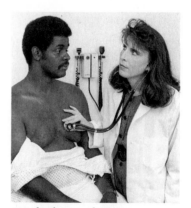

Apical pulse auscultation

6. IDENTIFY A PULSE DEFICIT (optional).

    a. Listen to the apical pulse while simultaneously palpating the radial pulse.

    b. Two nurses may simultaneously count the apical and radial pulses and record the difference to quantify the pulse deficit.

7. EVALUATE THE PULSE RHYTHM.

    Note pulse rhythm while listening to the apical pulse.

A pulse deficit exists if the apical rate is greater than the radial rate. Pulse deficits may occur with dysrhythmias such as atrial fibrillation, or in severe heart failure when some heart contractions are too weak to propagate the arterial pressure wave to peripheral pulse sites. A pulse deficit may also indicate vascular disease.

Documenting Pulse

Record the pulse rate and rhythm, indicating which pulse site was used. Pulse rate and other vital signs are typically recorded on flowsheets or presented graphically in the record so that trends are easily identified. If the pulse rhythm is irregular, describe your findings in greater detail. Note also whether the pulse felt thready (weak) or strong.

NDx

Nursing Diagnoses Related to Pulse Assessment

A person with deviations from normal pulse rate, rhythm, and quality should be further evaluated for signs and symptoms of the following nursing diagnoses: Decreased cardiac output, Fluid volume deficit or excess, Altered tissue perfusion, and Activity intolerance. An increased pulse rate may also be an indicator of pain or anxiety.

Clinical Problems Related to Pulse Assessment

Pulse rate and rhythm alterations can indicate a number of pathologic conditions, including some that may be life-threatening. Pathology of the cardiovascular, respiratory, and neurologic systems can all affect the quality of the arterial pulse.

RESPIRATORY RATE AND PATTERN ASSESSMENT

Anatomy and Physiology Overview

Respiration is the exchange of oxygen and carbon dioxide between the atmosphere and the cells of the body. The process of respiration includes *ventilation,* or air movement in and out of the lungs. *Breathing,* the alternate inspiration and expiration of air into and out of the lungs, is controlled by the respiratory center in the brain stem. The pons regulates respiratory rhythm, and the medulla controls respiratory rate and depth, which are affected by the carbon dioxide, hydrogen ion, and oxygen concentrations in the blood and body tissues.

Inspiration and expiration occur because of pressure changes within the lungs. Inspiratory pressure changes result primarily from muscle contraction, involving the diaphragm and external intercostal muscles. Expiration occurs passively as the muscles relax. Lung expansion is also influenced by lung and thoracic compliance (see Chap. 10). Evaluation of the respiratory system is further discussed in Chapter 10.

Physical Examination   *Respiratory Rate and Pattern*

General Principles   The respiratory rate and pattern may be observed visually by watching the person's chest rise and fall during inspiration and expiration. The examiner may also feel the chest movements by placing his or her hand over the chest.

Equipment   • Watch or clock with a second hand

Examination and Documentation Focus   • Respiratory (ventilatory) rate
• Respiratory (ventilatory) pattern

Examination Guidelines   *Respiratory Rate and Pattern*

Procedure

1. MINIMIZE INTERFERENCE.

    a. Evaulate respiratory rate while keeping your fingers on the radial pulse site, as if you are still evaluating the pulse.

    b. Alternatively, if the client is sleeping, you may count respiratory rate before assessing other vital signs.

    c. If the person appears to be holding his or her breath, a slight tap on the leg or shoulder may stimulate normal breathing.

2. OBSERVE THE VENTILATORY MOVEMENTS.

    a. You may either visualize or feel the person's respiratory movements. Visual observation involves watching the chest rise and fall. Tactile observation involves placing a hand on the chest to feel it rise and fall.

    b. Note also the work of breathing and the use of accessory muscles.

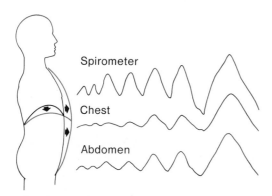

Normal breathing pattern: Inspiration is associated with downward movement of the diaphragm and outward movement of the chest and abdomen.

3. COUNT THE VENTILATORY (RESPIRATORY) RATE.

    Using a watch with a second hand, count the number of times the chest rises and falls in 30 seconds, and multiply by 2. If the respiratory rate is very slow or irregular, count for 1 full minute instead of 30 seconds.

4. DESCRIBE THE VENTILATORY PATTERN.

    Note the rhythm, depth, and pattern of the respirations.

Clinical Significance

If the person is aware that you are counting the respiratory rate, the ventilatory pattern may be altered.

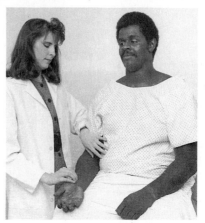

Tactile observation of the ventilatory rate

Respirations should be quiet and appear effortless. The chest and abdomen should move in a synchronous pattern.

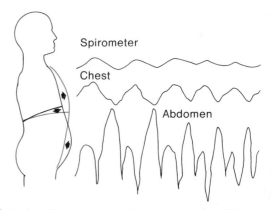

Ineffective breathing pattern: Asynchronous movement of the chest and abdomen. On inspiration, the abdomen moves inward while the chest moves outward.

Normal adult ventilatory rate: 12 to 20 breaths/minute at rest.

See "Ventilatory Patterns," Display 6-1.

Documenting Respiratory Rate and Pattern

Record the respiratory rate, indicating the number of breaths per minute. Respiratory rate and other vital signs are typically recorded on flowsheets or presented graphically in the record so that trends are easily identified. The descriptive terms shown in Display 6-1 may be used to document various ventilatory patterns.

NDx

Nursing Diagnoses Related to Respiratory Rate and Pattern Assessment

A person with deviations from normal respiratory rates and patterns should be further evaluated for signs and symptoms associated with the following nursing diagnoses: Ineffective airway clearance, ineffective breathing pattern, and activity intolerance. An increased ventilatory rate may also be an indicator of pain or anxiety.

Clinical Problems Related to Respiratory Rate and Pattern Assessment

Alterations in respiratory rate and pattern can indicate a number of pathologic conditions, including some that may be life-threatening. Altered respiratory rates and patterns may be noted in patients with brain stem disorders, respiratory muscle dysfunction, or altered lung compliance.

ARTERIAL BLOOD PRESSURE ASSESSMENT

Anatomy and Physiology Overview

Physiologically, blood pressure is the product of cardiac output and peripheral vascular resistance. Blood pressure changes may indicate variations in cardiac output, peripheral arteriolar resistance, artery distensibility, amount of blood in the system, and blood viscosity.

Elastic properties of the arterial walls allow the arteries to stretch during systole and recoil during diastole. In addition to providing a palpable arterial pulse, this arterial activity accounts for the physiologic principle behind blood pressure measurement. *Systolic* blood pressure represents the maximum arterial pressure at the peak of systole, and *diastolic* blood pressure represents the lowest level of arterial pressure at the end of diastole. The difference between the systolic and diastolic blood pressures is the pulse pressure.

Blood pressure may be measured directly, with invasive arterial catheters connected to pressure-transducer systems, or indirectly, with a sphygmomanometer. Only the indirect method is discussed here.

Korotkoff Sounds. During indirect blood pressure measurement, a stethoscope is used to auscultate *Korotkoff sounds*. Korotkoff sounds reflect changes in blood flow through the artery as sphygmomanometer cuff pressure is released and the artery goes from a state of complete occlusion to maximum patency. Korotkoff sounds are generated as normal laminar blood flow is disrupted by cuff pressure, and resulting turbulent flow creates vessel wall vibrations. There are five distinct sound phases (Fig 6-1):

Phase I sounds are the first sounds heard as the sphygmomanometer cuff pressure is released. The point at which sounds are first audible represents the systolic blood pressure. The sounds can be heard as clear tapping that gradually increases in intensity for a brief period, generated by rapid distension of the artery wall as the blood suddenly rushes into the previously collapsed artery. Sound intensity is related to the force of the blood flow.

Phase II sounds have a murmur-like or swishing quality. Murmurs represent turbulent blood flow and subsequent vessel wall vibration, created as blood flows from the relatively narrowed artery, caused by cuff inflation, to the wider artery lumen distal to the cuff.

Phase III sounds are clear, tapping sounds similar to phase I sounds, but more intense. Increased sound pitch and volume distinguish phase II from phase III sounds.

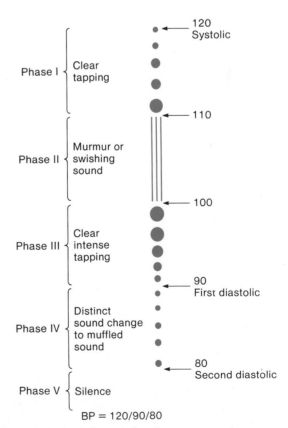

Figure 6-1. Korotkoff sounds: five phases.

Display 6–1
Ventilatory Patterns

Normal Ventilatory Pattern

- 12 to 20 breaths per minute
- Average tidal volume 350–500 mL (adults)
- Regular, occasional sigh breath
- Inspiration to expiration (I:E) ratio 1:2

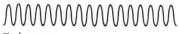

Normal ventilatory pattern

Tachypnea

- Rapid rate (>20 breaths per minute)
- Shallow—small tidal volume with each breath
- May be associated with CO_2 retention
- Regular rhythm
- I:E ratio approaches 1:1

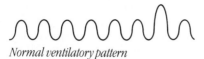

Tachypnea

Hyperventilation

(Also called *central neurogenic hyperventilation* if secondary to lower midbrain or upper pons lesions, or *Kussmaul's breathing* when secondary to diabetic coma.)

- Rapid rate
- Deep—large tidal volumes
- May be associated with CO_2 loss
- Usually regular
- I:E ratio approaches 1:1

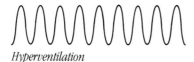

Hyperventilation

Bradypnea

- Slow rate (<12 breaths per minute)
- Tidal volumes vary depending on the cause
- Regular
- I:E ratio 1:2

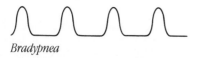

Bradypnea

Cheyne-Stokes Respiration

- Variable rate
- Apneic periods alternate with hyperventilation
- Depth of each breath varies in a cyclical pattern: shallow before and after apnea, deep with hyperventilation
- Regular-irregular—crescendo-decrescendo pattern

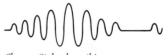

Cheyne-Stokes breathing

Apnea

- Complete cessation of breathing
- May be of a temporary nature

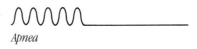

Apnea

Biot's Breathing (Ataxia)

- Variable rate
- Apnea alternates with breathing periods
- Depth variable—predominantly shallow
- Unpredictable irregularity

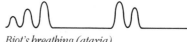

Biot's breathing (ataxia)

Obstructive Breathing

- Noted with obstructive pulmonary disease
- Rate increases as air trapping occurs
- Becomes shallower with air trapping
- Longer expiratory phase

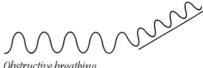

Obstructive breathing

During phase III, blood flow occurs during systole, but cuff pressure remains high enough to collapse the vessel during diastole.

Phase IV sounds are different from the previous sounds in their muffled quality. The first diastolic sound occurs when the sound changes from a tapping to a muffled sound, and represents the diastolic blood pressure.

Phase V occurs when the sounds cannot be heard because normal laminar blood flow has been restored. The second diastolic sound occurs when the muffled sound can no longer be heard.

Auscultatory Gap. Occasionally, if the person is hypertensive, no sounds will be heard between the systolic and diastolic pressures. This silence is called the auscultatory gap and may last for 10 to 20 mm Hg. The auscultatory gap, if not detected, represents a possible source of error in blood pressure measurement because phase III sounds may be mistaken for phase I sounds.

Blood Pressure Ranges. Normal blood pressure ranges for adults are 100 to 140 mm Hg systolic and 60 to 90 mm Hg diastolic (Table 6-1). Blood pressure readings consistently greater than 140/90 in adults may indicate hypertension. Few guidelines are available for the lower limits of hypertension in children.

Factors Affecting Arterial Blood Pressure. An abnormal blood pressure should be investigated to determine contributing factors. Arterial blood pressure is affected by the following factors:

Cardiac output
Heart rate
Systemic vascular resistance
Arterial elasticity
Blood volume
Blood viscosity
Age
Body surface area
Exercise
Emotions

Physical Examination | *Blood Pressure*

General Principles

Blood pressure may be measured by a number of methods: indirectly, by palpating an arterial pulse distal to a blood pressure cuff; indirectly, by auscultating Korotkoff sounds distal to a blood pressure cuff; or directly, by means of a catheter placed in an artery. A complete cardiovascular examination requires blood pressure evaluation on both arms.

Equipment

Stethoscope and Doppler Probe

Korotkoff sounds can be detected by listening over a pulse site distal to the blood pressure cuff. Usually, the sounds can be heard by placing the diaphragm of the stethoscope over the pulse site. If it is difficult to hear the sounds, use the bell (Korotkoff sounds are low frequency). If you still cannot hear the Korotkoff sounds, place a Doppler probe over the artery. You can also palpate the artery in the same manner as taking a pulse. Inflate the cuff, and record the point at which the first beat is palpated during cuff deflation as the systolic blood pressure. The diastolic pressure cannot be determined by palpation.

Sphygmomanometer

The term *sphygmomanometer* refers to the blood pressure cuff, connecting tubes, air pump, and pressure manometer (Fig. 6-2).

Blood Pressure Cuff. Korotkoff sounds are generated when arterial flow properties are altered by inflation of the blood pressure cuff. The cuff has an air-distensible bladder and is covered with cloth. A rubber tube connects the air bladder to a hand-held rubber air pump used to inflate the cuff. Another rubber tube attaches to the manometer and indicates air pressure within the cuff. The entire cuff can be wrapped around the extremity and secured with Velcro or hooks.

For accurate measurement, the cuff should be wide enough to cover two thirds of the upper arm or upper thigh and long enough to completely encircle the extremity. For the average adult arm, a 12- to 14-cm wide cuff should be sufficient. For the arm of the obese adult or when the pressure is taken at the thigh, use an 18- to 20-cm wide cuff. Small cuffs are available for children. If the cuff is too small, an abnormally high blood pressure reading may result. Similarly, if the cuff is too large, the blood pressure may be underestimated.

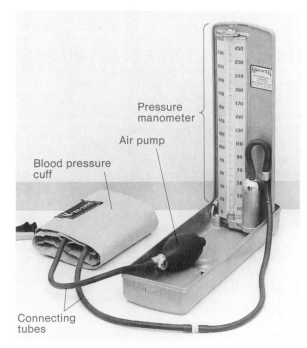

Figure 6–2. Sphygmomanometer.

Pressure Manometer. The pressure manometer is the instrument that displays cuff pressure in millimeters of mercury (mm Hg), an indirect reading of the client's blood pressure. There are two types of pressure manometers: the aneroid instrument, which uses a needle that points to numbers on a calibrated dial, and the mercury manometer, which uses the height of a mercury column in a glass tube to indicate the pressure. The mercury manometer is read by looking at the mercury column meniscus at eye level and reading the corresponding number. Mercury manometers are more accurate simply because they do not require calibration. Aneroid manometers are calibrated against mercury manometers by using a Y connector between the two manometers.

Positioning the Client

The client may be standing, seated, or supine during blood pressure measurement. An orthostatic or standing blood pressure should be evaluated by first measuring the pressure while the person is supine and then while he or she is sitting and standing. If the orthostatic value is significantly lower (>30 mm Hg), orthostatic hypotension is indicated and may point to excessive volume depletion, prolonged immobility, or neurologic disease.

The extremity that is being used for blood pressure measurement should be positioned at a level equal to or lower than the heart to avoid a false low reading. If the arm is used for measuring blood pressure, the forearm should be in a relaxed position (*e.g.,* resting on a tabletop). Alternatively, the person's forearm can be placed over your forearm.

Repeating the Procedure

Occasionally, you may deflate the cuff too rapidly, or there may be another reason to question the accuracy of the blood pressure reading. In such a case you should repeat the blood pressure measurement. Before rechecking the pressure, completely deflate the cuff and wait for 1 minute, allowing for normal blood flow to return and ensuring that Korotkoff sounds are generated from a baseline flow state.

Noninvasive Electronic Measurement

Electronic devices are available for continuous noninvasive, indirect blood pressure monitoring. A blood pressure cuff is applied to the client's arm, but the rubber connecting tubes attach to an electronic monitoring and inflation device rather than to a hand-held pump and manometer.

Examination Guidelines   *Blood Pressure Measurement*

Procedure

1. APPLY THE BLOOD PRESSURE CUFF.

   Caution: Never apply a blood pressure cuff to an extremity where a hemodialysis access device such as a shunt or AV fistula is in place.

   a. *Upper arm:* Wrap the completely deflated blood pressure cuff snugly and smoothly around the client's bare, upper arm. The bottom of the cuff should be approximately 1 inch above the antecubital space (closer in infants), and the center of the air bladder should be directly above the brachial artery.

   b. *Leg:* Wrap the blood pressure cuff around the thigh with the bottom of the cuff 1 inch above the knee. The remainder of the procedure for blood pressure measurement in the leg is similar to that for arm blood pressure measurement except that Korotkoff sounds should be auscultated over the popliteal artery.

2. ESTIMATE THE SYSTOLIC BLOOD PRESSURE BY PALPATION (optional after baseline established).

   a. Palpate the radial artery with the fingertips of your nondominant hand.

   b. Inflate the cuff while simultaneously palpating the artery. Close the valve on the air pump by turning it clockwise between the thumb and first finger of your dominant hand, and then squeeze the bulb.

   c. Note the point on the manometer at which the radial artery pulsation is no longer palpable.

   d. Inflate the cuff 20 mm Hg above this point when measuring the auscultated blood pressure.

Clinical Significance

Repeated occlusion of the device may contribute to clotting and limit the life-span of the device.

Inaccurate cuff placement may result in inaccurate BP measurement.

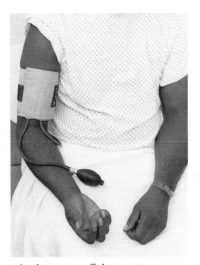

Blood pressure cuff placement

The systolic blood pressure values read 10 to 20 mm Hg higher in the leg than in the arm.

This method prevents measurement errors that might occur by not inflating the cuff high enough, or errors caused by the presence of an auscultatory gap. This step may be omitted if you are familiar with the client's usual blood pressure.

This provides a rough estimate of the systolic pressure.

GUIDELINES *continued*

Blood Pressure Measurement

Procedure

Clinical Significance

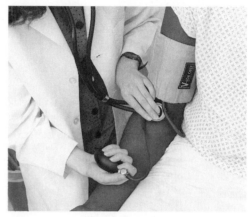

Blood pressure measurement: Stethoscope placement

3. AUSCULTATE THE BLOOD PRESSURE.

   a. Find the brachial artery by palpation. Place the diaphragm or the bell of the stethoscope over the brachial artery site.

   b. Inflate the cuff. Close the valve on the air pump by turning it clockwise between the thumb and first finger of your dominant hand, and then squeeze the bulb.

   Inflate the cuff until the manometer reading is 20 mm Hg above the client's usual systolic value.

   c. Slowly deflate the cuff while auscultating the brachial artery. Deflate the cuff at a rate of 2 to 3 mm Hg per second by turning the air pump valve counterclockwise.

   Rapid deflation results in inaccurate readings.

   d. Note the Korotkoff sounds and manometer readings. As the cuff is deflated, note the manometer reading when the first Korotkoff sound is heard. This is the systolic blood pressure. Read the first diastolic pressure at the point when the sounds become muffled. Read the second diastolic pressure at the point when the sound disappears completely. Finish deflating the cuff and remove, unless a second measurement is necessary. Wait 1 minute before reinflating.

   Read the manometer at eye level to avoid error.

4. REPEAT THE PROCEDURE ON THE OPPOSITE EXTREMITY (initial examination only).

   Check the blood pressure in the other arm and note any differences. Take subsequent blood pressure readings on the arm with the higher pressure.

   A 5- to 10-mm Hg difference is normal.

   Greater pressure differences may indicate coarctation of the aorta, aortic aneurysm, or impaired blood flow to the upper arm arteries.

NDx

Documenting Blood Pressure

The American Heart Association recommends that three blood pressure readings be recorded: the systolic, first diastolic, and second diastolic pressures. The recording would appear as follows: 130/82/26. Despite this recommendation, many health care providers record only the systolic and first diastolic readings, such as 112/70.

Record the blood pressure, indicating the extremity used and the client's position in order to make accurate comparisons. For example, "RA sit" indicates the use of the right arm with the person in the sitting position. Blood pressure, as well as other vital signs, is typically recorded on flowsheets or presented graphically in the record so that trends are easily identified.

Nursing Diagnoses Related to Blood Pressure Measurement

A person with deviations from normal blood pressure should be further evaluated for signs and symptoms associated with the following nursing diagnoses: Decreased cardiac output, Fluid volume deficit or excess, Altered tissue perfusion, and Activity intolerance. An increased blood pressure may also be an indicator of pain or anxiety.

If a person has a medical diagnosis of hypertension, those nursing diagnoses that are associated with management of a complex and chronic disease should also be considered, including Noncompliance and Altered health maintenance.

Clinical Problems Related to Blood Pressure Measurement

Hypertension

Hypertension is an intermittent or sustained elevation of systolic or diastolic blood pressure. Adults are diagnosed as having hypertension when the diastolic blood pressure is observed to be greater than 90 mm Hg or higher on at least two consecutive clinical assessments, or when the systolic blood pressure is greater than 140 mm Hg on at least two consecutive visits. Persons with hypertensive disease may have combined systolic and diastolic hypertension or isolated systolic hypertension.

Primary (essential) hypertension affects about 90% of all hypertensive individuals and occurs when there is no known cause for the elevated blood pressure. Secondary hypertension refers to elevated blood pressure that is related to some other underlying disease, such as renal failure or arteriosclerosis.

Risk factors for the development of primary hypertension include the following: family history of hypertension, advancing age, male gender, black race, obesity, high sodium intake, diabetes mellitus, cigarette smoking, and excessive alcohol intake.

Orthostatic (Postural) Hypotension

Orthostatic (postural) hypotension is a drop in both systolic and diastolic blood pressure when a person moves to an upright or standing position. For example, if the person has his or her blood pressure recorded as 138/88 while in a seated position and the value is recorded as 100/60 after standing, orthostatic hypotension exists. Additional observations may be noted as the person assumes an upright position, including dizziness, blurring or loss of vision, and fainting.

Orthostatic hypotension is associated with dehydration or volume depletion, antihypertensive medications, and prolonged immobility.

BODY TEMPERATURE ASSESSMENT

Anatomy and Physiology Overview

Temperature regulation is one of the body's homeostatic mechanisms. In healthy states, core body temperature remains relatively constant with minor fluctuations ($\pm$ 0.5°C), despite changes in environmental temperature, internal production of heat energy, and exercise. Body temperature is closely related to basal metabolism. As basal metabolic activities increase, such as through the activity of skeletal muscles or the processing of nutrients in the liver, body heat increases. Without a regulating mechanism, the core body temperature would rise, eventually reaching a febrile or hyperpyretic state.

HYPOTHALAMIC CONTROL

Each species has a genetically determined "set point," which represents the optimal core body temperature for maintaining normal physiologic activities. In humans, this set point is approximately 37°C (98.6°F), with slight variation in response to circadian rhythms and the menstrual cycle (Fig. 6-3). Normal occurrences, such as food ingestion, bathing, emotions, and exercise, generate body heat, causing an increase in core body temperature. The hypothalamus senses such temperature changes as deviations from the set point and initiates mechanisms to restore equilibrium. The fact that body temperature normally varies only 0.5°C to 1.0°C (1°F or 2°F) in a 24-hour period indicates that hypothalamic temperature regulating mechanisms are rapid and efficient.

Mechanisms for restoring body heat to normal include the following:

- *Sweating.* Sweating allows heat to escape from the body through evaporation.
- *Vasodilation.* Heat can escape the body by conduction and radiation when the blood vessels dilate.
- *Vasoconstriction.* Blood vessels can constrict and shunt blood to the body core preserving body heat.
- *Shivering.* Shivering generates body heat.
- *Hormone production.* An increase in thyroid hormone will increase body heat.

HYPOTHALAMIC INFLUENCES

The hypothalamic thermostat is reset under certain conditions, such as infection. Substances released from leukocytes, called *pyrogens,* may cause an increase in body temperature to as high as 40°C (104°F) by interfering with temperature-lowering mechanisms in the hypothalamus. Controversy exists about the physiologic significance of such temperature elevation. It may represent an increase in the basal metabolic rate, which is essential for the body to fight invading organisms. On the other hand, an increased temperature and basal metabolic rate leads to increased oxygen consumption in the body, which may be detrimental. Oxygen requirements increase 10% for every 1°C temperature increase. Fever may cause convulsions in young children, and tissue in the brain and other organs may be damaged as enzyme activity and transport processes are adversely affected by high temperatures. For these reasons, high temperatures associated with infections are generally considered pathologic.

BODY TEMPERATURE VARIABLES

Core body temperature normally varies according to age, time of day, activity, and menstrual cycle phase (Table 6-1).

Age. The hypothalamic regulating center is not fully developed in infants and young children. This fact may account for their greater body temperature fluctuations. Because infants are unable to shiver, they are especially susceptible to lowered core temperatures. Infants must rely on their supply of "brown fat," rich in energy-producing

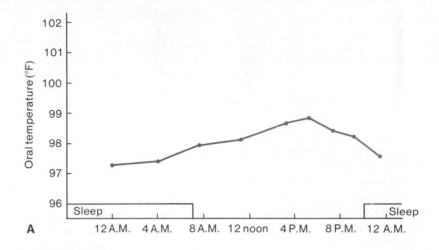

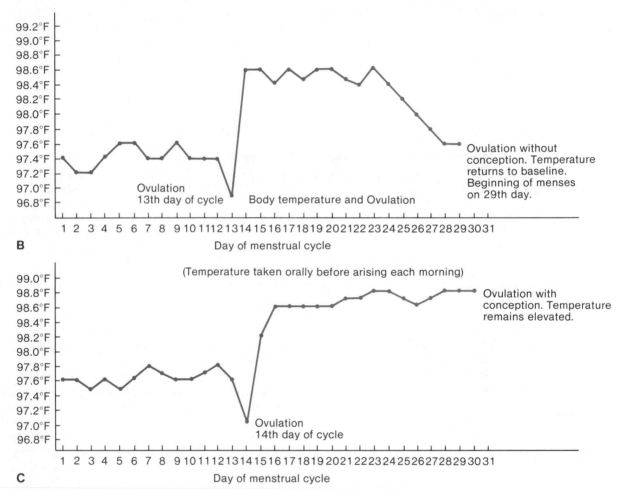

Figure 6–3. Body temperature variations. (**A**) Circadian variations. Note body temperature lowering during sleep. (**B** and **C**) Menstrual cycle and variations. Body temperature drops before ovulation and increases above the woman's baseline after ovulation.

mitochondria, for heat production. Brown fat atrophies after infancy when shivering mechanisms have developed.

Elderly persons adapt slowly to changes in body temperature. Their response to an increase in body heat is slower because the number of functioning sweat glands decreases with age. An elderly person may feel cold when the environmental temperature is low because blood supply to the skin is diminished. Although vasoconstriction is a normal reaction to low environmental temperatures, a diminished capillary supply to the skin will accentuate a cold feeling.

Activity and Time of Day. Generally, core body temperature is lower during sleep than during waking activity and reaches its lowest point, or basal body temperature (BBT), just before a person awakens (Fig. 6-3). Body tem-

perature fluctuates 0.5°C to 1.0°C (1°F or 2°F) over a 24-hour period, and is highest in late afternoon or early evening. For those who sleep during the day and work at night, this pattern changes, depending on the sleep cycle. The daily variation in body temperature is consistent with the body's metabolic rate, which also decreases during sleep. ~basal body temp.

Progesterone. The BBT fluctuates in women according to the phase of the menstrual cycle. Following ovulation, progesterone secretion increases and causes a rise in BBT for 1 to 3 days. Thereafter, the BBT decreases as progesterone secretion also decreases. Infertility evaluation may involve BBT assessment, as do some methods of birth control.

Physical Examination   *Body Temperature*

Equipment

Body temperature is determined by reading the measurement registered on a glass thermometer or an electronic thermometer, or on a monitor associated with a thermistor, such as on the tip of a thermodilution pulmonary artery catheter or Foley catheter. For an accurate reading, these instruments must be used and read correctly.

Electronic thermometers are more accurate and are preferred over glass thermometers. Electronic thermometers also afford less chance of cross-contamination because of the disposable probe covers.

Site Selection and Interpretation

Body temperature may be measured at different sites, such as the mouth, the rectum, the tympanic membrane, and the axillae. Rectal and tympanic membrane measurements are considered most accurate. The rectal site or tympanic membrane should be used in children under the age of 6 or for anyone who is confused, prone to seizure activity, comatose, or intubated (*e.g.,* endotracheally, nasogastrically). Some authorities recommend that rectal thermometers not be inserted in children less than 2 years of age because of the risk of rectal perforation. The rectal method is also contraindicated following abdominoperineal resection or hemorrhoidectomy, and in persons with cardiac illness, because rectal stimulation could lead to Valsalva maneuvers.

The oral method can be used in clients who are alert, cooperative, and over 6 years of age. The client should be able to breathe through the nose and should be without oral pathology or recent oral surgery.

The axillary method is considered least accurate but is preferred for infants because it is safer than other methods.

Temperatures differ depending on measurement site. For example, rectal temperatures are usually 0.4°C (0.7°F) higher than oral temperatures, whereas axillary temperatures are 0.6°C (1°F) lower than oral temperatures. You should take into account the person's physiologic status as well as the time of day when interpreting temperatures.

Accuracy

For accurate temperature measurement, the thermometer must be inserted properly and left in place for the required length of time. Numerous studies confirm that the optimal time for keeping oral glass thermometers in place is 8 minutes. However, this time period should be increased (or the temperature reading postponed) if a hot or cold beverage was ingested immediately before the thermometer was placed in the mouth. Contrary to popular belief, oxygen administration by mask should not affect the accuracy of the reading. Electronic thermometer readings require much less time, often less than 10 seconds. Rectal glass thermometers may be left in place for 3 minutes. Nurses have conducted clinical research studies to identify and evaluate factors affecting temperature measurement accuracy (see the Research Highlight at the end of this chapter).

Examination and Documentation Focus

• Body temperature value

Examination Guidelines *Measuring Temperature with Mercury Thermometers*

Procedure	Clinical Significance

Procedure

1. PREPARATION:
   a. Choose the type of thermometer to use. Use an "oral" thermometer for oral or axillary measurements and a "rectal" thermometer for rectal measurements.
   b. If you are taking the temperature orally, ask the person about recent ingestion of hot or cold beverages. Wait about 10 minutes before taking the temperature if hot or cold beverages were ingested.
   c. Cleanse the thermometer. If the thermometer is stored in disinfectant solution, wipe off the disinfectant with a tissue or rinse under cold water. Wipe from the distal end to the bulb end holding the thermometer by the distal end.
   d. Shake down the thermometer to 35°C (95°F) or below. Hold the thermometer between your thumb and first finger at the distal end and shake downward by snapping the wrist.

2. MEASUREMENT: ORAL TEMPERATURE
   a. Ask the person to open his or her mouth. Place the thermometer bulb in the right or left sublingual pocket (on either side of the frenulum), and instruct the person to close the mouth and hold the thermometer in place between the lips.

Clinical Significance

The mercury thermometer may be used for any site but the distinctions are made to prevent cross-use and cross-contamination. Rectal thermometers are often designated with red on the blunt end.

Hot or cold substances can alter the temperature of mouth tissues.

Unpleasant-tasting solutions should be removed before inserting.

Be careful not to break the thermometer by shaking it too close to a hard surface (desk, tabletop).

The large blood vessels in this area reflect core body heat.

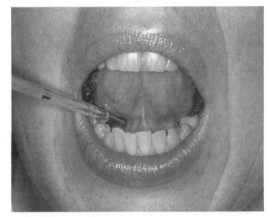

Oral temperature measurement: thermometer placement

b. Leave the thermometer in place for 4 to 11 minutes. Use this time to measure other vital signs.
c. Remove the thermometer and wipe away any secretions with tissue from end to bulb. Hold the thermometer at eye level and read at the end of the mercury column.
d. Wash in soapy water, then rinse and return to disinfectant solution or protective case after shaking down again.

The optimal placement time is 8 minutes (see Research Highlight at the end of this chapter), but often the peak temperature registers after 4 or 5 minutes.

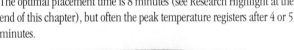
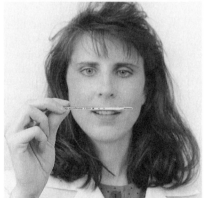

Reading the glass thermometer

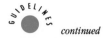

continued

Measuring Temperature with Mercury Thermometers

Procedure

3. MEASUREMENT: AXILLARY TEMPERATURE

   a. Remove the person's clothing, exposing the arm and shoulder. Dry the axilla with a towel.

   b. Place the bulb in the center of the axilla. Fold the arm across the person's chest to keep the thermometer in place.

   c. Leave the thermometer in place for 10 minutes.

   d. Read and cleanse as you would an oral thermometer.

   e. Axillary temperatures usually register one degree lower than oral temperatures.

Clinical Significance

Moisture should be removed from the skin to prevent a lower temperature reading through evaporation.

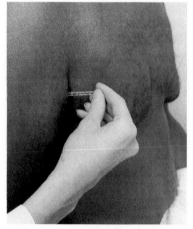

Axillary temperature measurement:
thermometer placement

4. MEASUREMENT: RECTAL TEMPERATURE

   a. Lubricate the thermometer before inserting.

   b. Apply clean gloves.

   c. Place the person on the side with the knees slightly flexed. Expose the anus by lifting the buttocks. Insert the thermometer into the rectum. Point the thermometer toward the person's umbilicus, guiding it along the rectal wall. Insert the thermometer approximately 1 inch into the rectum.

   d. Hold the thermometer in place for 3 minutes.

   e. Read and cleanse the rectal thermometer as you would an oral thermometer.

   f. Rectal temperatures usually read 1 degree higher than oral temperatures.

Never force or insert the thermometer into feces. Injury may result from improper placement.

Examination Guidelines   *Measuring Temperature with Electronic Thermometers*

Procedure

1. PREPARATION:

   a. Obtain the electronic thermometer from the battery-charging unit. Cover the metal probe with a disposable plastic cover according to the manufacturer's instructions.

   b. Inquire about ingestion of hot or cold substances as you would when using oral mercury thermometers.

2. TEMPERATURE MEASUREMENT:

   a. Proceed to take the temperature as you would using a mercury thermometer by inserting the plastic-covered probe into the appropriate body area.

   b. *Tympanic temperature:* Place tympanic probe in the ear canal so as to seal the opening.

   c. At the sound of the tone, note temperature reading, remove probe, and discard probe cover in the waste basket.

   d. Return thermometer to base unit.

Clinical Significance

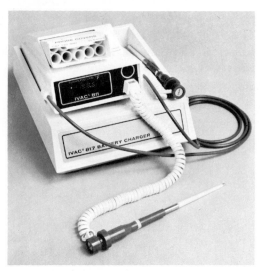

Electronic thermometer

The blood vessels in the tympanic membrane reflect core body temperature.

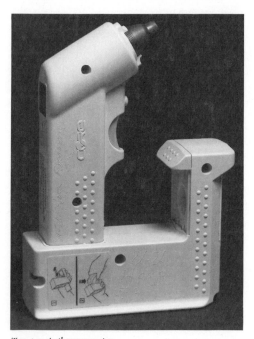

Tympanic thermometer

Documenting Body Temperature

Record the body temperature indicating the site used for temperature measurement. For example, (O) indicates oral, (AX) indicates axillary, and (R) indicates rectal. Temperature and other vital signs are typically recorded on flowsheets or presented graphically in the record so that trends are easily identified.

NDx

Nursing Diagnoses Related to Body Temperature Assessment

Hypothermia

Hypothermia occurs when body temperature registers between 25°C and 35°C (77°F to 95°F). Often, the temperature will not even register on the thermometer. Hypothermia occurs secondary to prolonged exposure to cold or administration of large volumes of unwarmed blood products. It may be induced for therapeutic purposes, such as total body cooling during heart surgery.

Physical signs of severe hypothermia include changes in the skin and cardiovascular system that are induced by cold injury. Prolonged cold causes damage to the capillary endothelium, resulting in "leaky" capillaries. When the patient is rewarmed, edema may occur as the plasma moves from the capillaries into the interstitial space. Such edema may occur in early postoperative periods following cardiopulmonary bypass surgery, during which the body temperature was lowered. The skin is usually cool to the touch, and excessive fluid shifts contribute to hypotension. The heart and respiratory rates may be severely decreased, and the person may be lethargic or unconscious. Severe hypothermia may not result in shivering, because in such cases this compensatory mechanism fails.

Frostbite is localized hypothermia, usually affecting exposed skin such as ears, fingers, or toes. Vascular injury caused by the cold may be so intense that vessel occlusion may be followed by ischemia. The initial vascular damage usually causes the affected part to appear red, changing to white as vessel occlusion progresses.

Hyperthermia

Hyperthermia, or hyperpyrexia, is an excessively high core body temperature, exceeding 39°C (102.2°F). Hyperthermia occurs secondary to hypothalamus damage, which may be caused by intracranial surgery, stroke, or traumatic head injury, or by the release of endogenous pyrogens from cells associated with inflammation and bacteria. Endogenous pyrogens reset the thermostat in the hypothalamus to a higher level. Consequently, higher body temperatures will be perceived as normal by the hypothalamus. In other words, a new equilibrium, defined as *fever,* will occur.

Fever Levels

Three phases of fever related to thermostat alteration have been identified. Each phase involves different assessment findings (Fig. 6-4).

Phase I occurs when the hypothalamic thermostat has been reset to a higher level. The body responds with heat-generating mechanisms as the core temperature rises from 37°C (98.6°F) to 40°C (104°F). The patient may assume a knee-chest position in an attempt to conserve body heat. Shivering may occur as the body attempts to generate necessary heat. The skin may be pale and cool to the touch, secondary to the conserving vasoconstriction.

Phase II occurs with the core temperature reaches the new thermostatic level. The body acts to protect this temperature with the usual hypothalamic mechanisms. Excessive cooling will cause shivering, and excessive temperature increases will result in cutaneous vasodilation and sweat gland secretion.

Phase III is often referred to as "breaking" the fever. Endogenous pyrogen production ceases, and the stimulus for a higher thermostat setting is removed. As the hypothalamic set point returns to its prefever level, hypothalamic-mediated cooling mechanisms lower body temperature. Severe diaphoresis, or diffuse perspiration, may occur as the sweat glands work to cool the body by evaporation. Placing the patient in a cooler environment or removing clothing will also help cool the body.

Some diseases show characteristic fever patterns that may be related to different patterns of endogenous pyrogen production. A sustained fever may accompany infectious diseases such as typhoid, for instance. In hyperthermia, relapsing fever alternates with periods of normal temperatures. Such a pattern may also be observed in patients with syphilis and malaria. A single daily fever spike, or remittent fever, is common in septicemic patients, whose temperatures rarely return to normal. An intermittent fever is usually characterized by diurnal variations of peaks and troughs. The patient's temperature may be high in the late afternoon and subnormal in the early morning. This pattern may occur with certain pyrogenic infections.

Clinical Problems Related to Body Temperature Assessment

Body temperature alterations may be noted with a number of pathologic conditions. Hypothermia may be observed in persons with acute illnesses, including congestive heart failure, uremia, diabetes mellitus, drug overdose, respiratory failure, and hypoglycemia. The mechanism appears to be a failure of thermoregulation. Hyperthermia may be observed in persons with infectious diseases, central nervous system pathology, and heat stroke. Malignant hyperthermia is an inherited disorder characterized by a rapid increase in temperature following the administration of inhaled anesthetic agents or muscle relaxants. Malignant hyperthermia is life-threatening and represents a medical emergency.

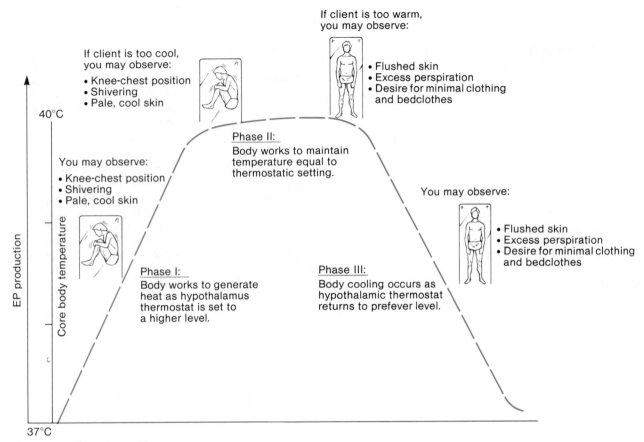

Figure 6–4. Three phases of fever.

$\overset{Chapter}{6}$ SUMMARY

Vital sign assessment may be implemented as a general evaluation of a person's physical status. Vital signs include the following:
- Arterial pulse (rate and rhythm)
- Ventilatory rate and pattern
- Arterial blood pressure
- Body temperature

Measurement procedures have been established to increase the accuracy of vital sign assessment. The vital signs are interpreted in relation to age-related norms and the person's physiologic status.

Alterations in vital signs may provide cues to the following nursing diagnoses:

Hypothermia
Hyperthermia
Ineffective thermoregulation
Dysreflexia
Fluid volume excess
Fluid volume deficit
Decreased cardiac output
Ineffective airway clearance
Ineffective breathing pattern
Activity intolerance
Pain
Anxiety

RESEARCH *Hi*GHLIGHT

"What is the most accurate method for body temperature evaluation?"

Measuring a client's vital signs, such as pulse, respiratory rate, and temperature, was one of the earliest assessment techniques incorporated into nursing practice. Because nurses suspected that many factors could influence accurate body temperature measurement, nurse researchers have investigated recommended procedures. During the past 20 years, numerous published studies explored factors affecting body temperature measurement.

How long should the oral glass thermometer remain in place?

Nichols and her colleagues conducted several controlled studies to determine optimal placement time for oral glass mercury thermometers.[1-3] The researchers found that, contrary to traditional practice, which recommended reading the thermometer after 2 to 4 minutes, optimal placement time, or the time required for 90% of the subjects' thermometers to reach maximal readings, was 8 minutes.

Advances in technology have resulted in widespread use of electronic oral thermometers designed to guarantee adequate placement time. Therefore, Nichols' studies may not seem important to modern nursing practice. In the early 1970s, however, Ketefian designed a study to evaluate whether nurses used these research findings in practice.[4] She studied Nichols' results because temperature measurement was a common nursing practice; because the recommended 8-minute placement time had been confirmed by studies replicating Nichols'; and because the findings had been widely published for at least 5 years. Of the 87 registered nurses whose practice Ketefian studied, only one knew the recommended placement time for glass mercury thermometers. Ketefian concluded that staff nurses either were unaware of research literature or did not know how to utilize research findings.

Which site should be used for temperature measurement?

A team headed by Nichols compared the temperature readings obtained at oral, axillary, and rectal sites, and concluded that rectal temperature measurements are most accurate.[1] Other researchers, concerned that rectal thermometers may cause inadvertent injury to infants,[5,6] compared the use of the three sites in infants. They concluded that axillary temperature measurements can be accurately as well as safely obtained in infants. Other studies, on intubated adult patients following coronary artery bypass surgery, concluded that oral temperature readings are not significantly different from rectal temperature readings as long as the nurse uses proper procedures.[7]

Other factors affecting accuracy

The ingestion of hot or cold fluids can affect the accuracy of oral temperature readings unless the patient waits at least 15 minutes after ingestion before having the temperature measured.[8] Oxygen administration by nasal cannula does not significantly affect temperature; however, administration by cool or heated aerosal mist may alter readings.[9] More studies are needed to clarify whether this difference is clinically significant.

REFERENCES

1. Nichols, G.A. et al. (1966). Oral, axillary, and rectal temperature determinations and relationships. *Nursing Research, 15,* 307-310.
2. Nichols, G.A., & Verhonick, P.J. (1967). Time and temperature. *American Journal of Nursing, 67,* 2304-2306.
3. Nichols, G.A., & Kucha, D.H. (1972). Taking adult temperatures: Oral measurements. *American Journal of Nursing, 72,* 1090-1093.
4. Ketefian, S. (1975). Application of selected nursing research findings in nursing practice. *Nursing Research, 24,* 89-92.
5. Eoff, M. J., Meier, R., & Miller, C. (1974). Temperature measurement in infants. *Nursing Research, 23,* 457-460.
6. Schiffman, R. (1982). Temperature monitoring in the neonate: A comparison of axillary and rectal temperatures. *Nursing Research, 31,* 274-277.
7. Cashion, A., & Cason, C. (1984). Accuracy of oral temperatures in intubated patients. *DCCN, 3,* 343-350.
8. Forster, B., Adler, D., & Davis, M. (1970). Duration of effects of drinking iced water on oral temperature. *Nursing Research, 19,* 167-180.
9. Yonkman, C. (1982). Cool and heated aerosol and the measurement of oral temperature. *Nursing Research, 31,* 354-357.

✳ CRITICAL THINKING

You are conducting a routine physical examination of a 40-year-old male who is obese and in poor cardiovascular condition. He has just been seated in the examination room and appears out of breath and perspiring. The physical examination begins with the measurement of his vital signs.

Learning Exercises

1. Determine and discuss any additional background information about this patient that would be useful as you evaluate his vital signs.

2. Propose and discuss several alternative explanations for an elevated blood pressure in this patient.

3. Specify how you would minimize error when measuring this patient's blood pressure.

4. Explain how you would further evaluate hyperventilation in this patient.

5. You are unable to locate this patient's radial pulse. Identify and explain your next actions.

BIBLIOGRAPHY

American Heart Association. (1980). *Recommendations for human blood pressure determination by sphygmomanometers.* Pub. No. 70-019-B, 80-100M. Dallas: American Heart Association.

Cooper, K.M. (1992). Measuring blood pressure the right way. *Nursing 92, 22* (4), 75.

Erikson, R. (1980). Oral temperature differences in relation to thermometer and technique. *Nursing Research, 29,* 157–164.

Guyton, A.C. (1991). *Textbook of medical physiology* (8th ed.). Philadelphia: W.B. Saunders.

Hahn, W.K., et al. (1989). Blood pressure norms for healthy young adults: Relation to sex, age, and reported parental hypertension. *Research in Nursing and Health, 12* (1), 53–56.

Henneman, E.A. et al. (1989). Intricacies of blood pressure measurement: Reexamining in rituals. *Heart and Lung, 18* (3), 263–273.

Hill, M.N. (1980). Hypertension: What can go wrong when you measure blood pressure. *American Journal of Nursing, 80* (5), 942–945.

US Department of Health and Human Services Report of the Second Task Force on Blood Pressure Control in Children. (1987). Bethesda, MD: National Institutes of Health.

US Department of Health and Human Services Report of the Joint National Committee on Detection, Evaluation, and Treatment of High Blood Pressure. (1988). Bethesda, MD: National Institutes of Health.

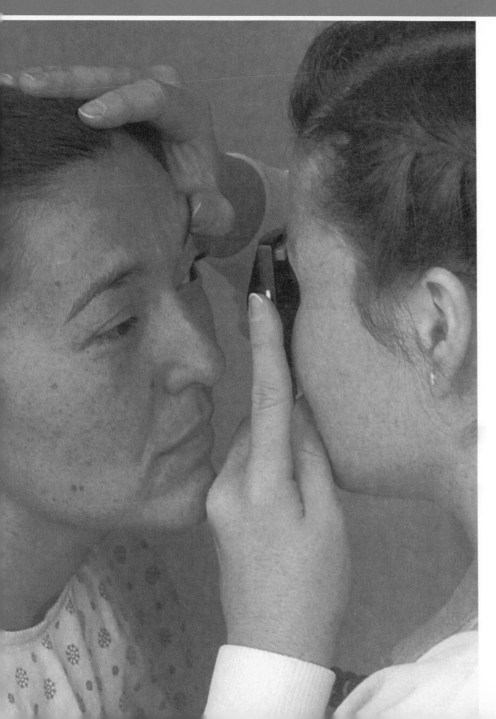

Unit II

Health Assessment of Human Function

Chapter 7

Assessing Health Perception and Health Management

Assessment Terms

Health Maintenance

Health Promotion

Disease Prevention

  Primary Prevention

  Secondary Prevention

  Tertiary Prevention

Risk Factors

Adherence Behavior

Screening

Breast Self-Examination

Testicular Self-Examination

Environmental Safety

INTRODUCTORY OVERVIEW

Traditionally, nurses have recognized a responsibility to promote and protect health rather than merely to treat illness. Florence Nightingale identified two types of nursing: health nursing and illness nursing. In its 1980 Social Policy Statement, the American Nurses' Association states that nurses are responsible for maintaining and managing clients' routine health practices during wellness as well as during illness. However, health promotion and protection depend on how people perceive health and their ability to manage health-related activities. To assist people in maintaining optimal health, it is important to identify their health perceptions, health practices, and preventive practices.

Assessment Focus

Assessing a client's health perceptions and health management abilities involves conducting a general inspection of the person's appearance, evaluating health habits and self-examination techniques, and comparing data in the health history with observations. It also includes identifying safety hazards or health threats in the person's home and immediate environment.

Factors to assess include the following:

- The client's definition of health
- The value the client places on health
- The client's existing level of health and the optimum level possible
- Risk factors that might disrupt health
- The client's ability to perform self-care and self-examination skills for self management.

Jill Fuller and Jennifer Schaller-Ayers:
HEALTH ASSESSMENT: A NURSING APPROACH, Second Edition.
© 1990, 1994 by J. B. Lippincott Company.

Suggested methods for collecting this type of data are listed in the accompanying display. The data you obtain should be analyzed in connection with cultural, psychosocial, developmental, and physiologic influences on health and related preventive practices.

Thorough assessment of health perception and health management behavior will help you identify and understand the client's strengths and risks, and enable you to plan with the client appropriate nursing services.

Nursing Diagnoses

Nursing diagnoses associated with health perception and health management include the following:

High risk for aspiration
Altered health maintenance
Health-seeking behaviors
High risk for infection
High risk for injury
Noncompliance (specify)
High risk for poisoning
Altered protection
High risk for suffocation
High risk for trauma

Dysfunctions in health perception and health management may be related to other health problems. Nursing diagnoses related to health perception and health management include the following:

Impaired adjustment
Altered family processes
Altered growth and development
Impaired home maintenance/management
Ineffective individual or family coping
Knowledge deficit (specify)
Self-care deficit (specify)
Spiritual distress
Altered thought process

KNOWLEDGE BASE FOR ASSESSMENT

Assessment of health perception and health management is based on understanding such concepts as health maintenance, promoting health, disease prevention, self-directed behavior, adherence behavior, risk factors, potential for injury, and environmental safety.

Maintaining Health

Health maintenance refers to activities that assist a person to maintain a satisfactory level of health and includes responsible behavior such as taking prescribed medications, exercising regularly, managing stress, and eating a balanced diet. Without responsible management, health cannot be maintained for an extended time.

Promoting Health

Health promotion includes activities that assist a person to develop internal and external resources to maintain or enhance physical, psychological, and social well being. Such activities are not usually directed at any particular disease or condition but seek to enhance general well being. Health promotion involves self-assessment, professional assessment, and health screening. Self-assessments can be performed by any individual at home (*e.g.*, breast self-examination for women and testicular self-examination for men to detect any signs of cancer). Many self-assessment tools are available to instruct individuals on how to conduct these self-examinations; these are often available in brochures distributed by hospitals and clinics or in books available at a general book store or library. For example, brochures published by the American Cancer Society ("Breast Self-Examination" and "Testicular Self-Examination"); *The New Our Bodies Our Selves* (The Boston Women's Health Book Collection, 1992); *50 Simple Things You Can Do To Save Your Life* (Faculty of the UCLA School of Public Health, 1991); and *Readers Digest: The Good Health Fact Book* (Shuher, 1992).

Professional health assessment and health screenings are conducted by health professionals usually in a local clinic, hospitals, or schools. Occasionally, organizations or corporations may sponsor special health screenings (*i.e.*, blood pressure measurement, blood cholesterol levels, glaucoma testing) at various convenient locations such as a shopping mall or community center or in a special mobile unit. These special promotional screenings are usually announced by the local media and are a good opportunity for people to obtain a health screening either free or at a minimal charge at a convenient location.

Health promotion has two levels of intervention: individual and populations. Individual health promotion is associated with personal life-style choices within the social setting such as physical activity and fitness, tobacco/drug/alcohol use, and family planning. Promoting health at the population level (known as health protection) is associated with environmental and regulatory measures designed to protect large population groups. Examples of health protection interventions are occupational safety and health regulations, fluoridation of public water, and safe street/playground designs.

Nurses in settings other than public health departments have been involved in health promotion and protection activities such as tobacco cessation programs, lobbying for automobile restraint laws, parenting and child birth preparation classes, and stress-management programs. Computer programs have been developed to identify health risks and health promotion activities of individuals; these programs are available to health professionals and the public. Two computer health risk appraisals are the "Lifestyle Assessment Questionnaire" (available from National Wellness Institute, Inc., 1988) and "The Healthier People Health Risk Appraisal" (available from The Carter Center of Emory University, 1989).

Assessment Focus Health Perception and Health Management

Assessment Goal	*Data Collection Methods*
1. Identify the person's definition of health.	*Interview* • Health perception: How does the person define health? Does this definition influence health practices?
2. Evaluate the person's willingness or ability to engage in health-promoting activities.	*Interview* • Health perception • Factors influencing health and health management: Do culture and personal beliefs influence the way the person defines and manages health? What factors influence adherence behavior? • Preventive health screenig activities: Does the person value participation in health screening? *Observation* • Statements about health and behaviors: Is there congruence between what the person says and does about health?
3. Determine the person's current health status.	*Interview* • Comprehensive health history: What are the person's strengths, risk factors, and problems related to optimal health? *Physical Examination* • Complete head-to-toe physical examination: What inferences can be made about the person's health on the basis of physical examination findings? • Evaluate physical findings in relation to established indicators of physical health. Are the person's anthropometric measurement, blood pressure, and results of laboratory tests within recommended ranges?
4. Identify risk factors that might disrupt the person's health and safety.	*Interview* • Identity risk factors that might be modified. *Health Screening Tests and Physical Examination* • Have risk factors for illness or injury been identified? • Breast examination and testicular examination: Are there abnormal findings? Is additional evaluation needed? *Observation* • Are there potentially injurious substances or hazards in the persons's environment?
5. Evaluate the person's ability to perform self-examination for health management.	*Observation* • Can the person perform and interpret the results of self-examination such as breast self-examination, testicular self-examination, blood glucose testing, blood pressure measurement, pulse and temperature measurements? *Physical Examination* • Breast examination: Can you validate the client's self-examination finding? • Testicular examination: Can you validate the client's findings?

Preventing Diseases

Health care providers have traditionally advocated the prevention of disease or illnesses by screening presumably healthy people. The concept of the annual physical examination was initially endorsed by the American Medical Association in the 1920s. In 1903 Lillian Wald demonstrated in the first school nurse project that nurses were effective in reducing the number of sick school days through early detection and treatment of health problems, control of contagious diseases, and health teaching. With the entry of school nurses, school records document that 98% of children previously excluded from school for health reasons were attending classes (Stahnope and Lancaster, 1992). Today, preventive health screening activities are divided into three levels: primary, secondary, and tertiary prevention.

Primary prevention refers to practices that prevent disease and injury from occurring. Examples of strategies include immunizations, car-seat restraints, and proper dental hygiene. Individual life-style behaviors can also be in this category; for example, reducing risk of developing hypertension by diet management, weight control, exercise program, and avoiding tobacco products. Clearly, primary prevention is the most cost-efficient approach to health management.

Secondary prevention includes measures to detect possible health programs at an early stage of development. Screening programs help to detect conditions in the early stage of pathology to help the person to get early treatment that will either rid the client of the condition or for chronic conditions to minimize or control the effects. Examples of such screening include hypertension, scoliosis, colorectal cancer, developmental problems of children (Denver Development Screening Tests), diabetes (blood glucose tests), and cystic fibrosis and amniocentesis (chromosomal testing).

When establishing screening clinics, tests or measurements should be appropriate for the target group. Screening for sickle cell anemia, which usually affects people of African heritage, would not be appropriate in a neighborhood of Vietnam immigrants. Similarly, if a target population worked from 8 AM to 5 PM week days, a screening clinic would be most efficient in the evenings or weekends. The availability of appropriate referrals and counseling for individuals with positive or abnormal findings is essential and ethically mandated.

Tertiary prevention includes activities that promote maximum health *after* disability has occurred. Such activities may be carried out through self-help groups such as Alcoholics Anonymous and Reach for Recovery (a program to help postmastectomy patients). Nurses direct or co-direct programs such as cardiac rehabilitation and diabetic self-care programs.

Self-Directed Behavior

A client's level of health should be the result of individual choice based on genetic predisposition, knowledge, and the amount of energy he or she is willing to expend on health behaviors. The ability of the person to knowledgeably choose a life-style and maintain that life-style is dependent upon the person's internal and external resources. The individual's choice may not always be consistent with health knowledge and health professional values. For example, some people continue to use tobacco products in spite of information about hazards to health. However, if a person who uses tobacco is willing to eat properly, exercise regularly, and limit the amount of tobacco, then that person's health, although compromised by tobacco use, is enhanced by other conscious health-promoting behaviors.

Adherence Behavior

People have always based decisions about their health and health care upon beliefs and available knowledge and resources. People determine when and to what extent a health professional should be consulted for health issues. Today, there is also an emphasis on containing health care costs, and individuals are encouraged to assume more responsibility to contain costs and maintain their health. Concurrently, people are changing their attitudes about health care, the relationship with health providers, and participation in movements for consumer rights and self-care. More information about health, health options, and alternative health practices is available to the public.

Adherence to prescribed health regimens is believed to help contain health costs. Conditions that increase the likelihood of people adhering to prescribed health regimens include the following:

- Participation in formulating the health regimen
- Informed agreement to the health regimen
- Knowledge of the problem or risk factor(s)
- Knowledge of available options and consequences
- Motivation
- History of past success with health regimens
- Practical and noncomplex health regimen

Setting goals with health care providers assists clients in adhering to health regimen. Short- and long-term goals are established, and target dates set for evaluating how close the person has come to achieving goals. In addition, when people make agreements with themselves, they have a vested interest in achievement. Because experiences affect motivation, a client who has been unable to adhere to previous health regimens is at greater risk for failure. Examine possible causes of failures such as noninvolvement in setting the health regimen and the cost of following the health regimen. Success increases motivation. Small, easily achievable goals in the early stages of a complex health regimen may prove to be very useful.

To increase adherence, health care regimens must be practical and as simple as possible. In numerous studies about medication adherence, researchers have overwhelmingly found that the more complex the regimen, the greater number of different medications, and the greater number of doses a day the less adherence to the regimen. Because of life-style and/or certain limitations (physical, cognitive, or environmental), adherence to some health regimens is improbable and inappropriate. When presenting options, consider the client's life-style and ability to follow through.

Risk Factors

Risk factors are attributes that intensify a person's probability of developing a particular disease or condition. Identifying risk factors that may compromise a person's health or life is essential for health maintenance. Some risk factors pose health risks for everyone (such as poor air quality), whereas other risk factors may affect only certain ethnic, occupational, or familial groups. The following features are characteristic of risk factors: they vary in intensity (some risks pose greater threat than others, such as drinking alcohol and driving), the possibility of jeopardizing health increases as the strength of the risk factor increases, and multiple risk factors may present a greater risk through risk factor interaction (Pender, 1987).

Risk factors may be classified according to genetics, age, biologic characteristics, personal habits, life-style, and environment (Display 7-1). Evaluating risk factors in relation to such categories may reveal a person's vulnerability to

---

Display 7–1
Risk Factor Classification

Genetic
- Sickle cell trait and sickle cell anemia
- Phenylketonuria
- Family incidence of genetically transmissible diseases: cystic fibrosis, Huntington's chorea, hemophilia, diabetes, heart disease

Age-Related
- Chronic disease in the elderly
- Sensory deficits in the elderly
- Acute illnesses in children
- Sensory-motor immaturity

Biological
- Elevated cholesterol level
- Elevated blood glucose level
- Altered immune status

Personal Habits
- Alcohol or drug abuse
- Tobacco use

Life Style
- Sedentary life-style
- Sun bathing
- Multiple sexual partners
- Low socioeconomic status

Environmental
- Proximity or exposure to toxic substances
- Hazardous working conditions
- Noise
- Substandard housing

---

disease or injury before the condition develops, and enables you to devise a health regimen with the client to reduce risks. Low socioeconomic status is a powerful risk factor; with poverty, the risk of developing and dying from chronic or preventable acute health problems increases dramatically. You should evaluate each identified risk factor to determine the degree to which the factor can be controlled through modification of health behaviors and referral to social agencies.

Potential for Injury

When assessing health and planning nursing care, consider the client's potential risk for injury. Injuries occur when a conflict exists between the individual and the external environment and may be influenced by the internal environment. Different age groups are at risk for different types of injuries (see Chaps. 19 and 20). Potential injuries include not only lacerations, abrasions, and fractures, but also poisoning, infection, emotional distress, and disability.

Assessing the external environment involves evaluating hazards that may exist in the home, school, or play area, at work, and in other surroundings. Assessment should also include identifying potential contaminants such as polluted water or air, or the presence of allergens, poisons, and toxic substances.

The internal environment refers to biologic, genetic, and personality features of the individual. Certain disease processes and conditions compromise the body's ability to protect itself from injury. Diabetes mellitus, for example,

complicates the body's attempt to recover from breaks in the skin's integrity. The HIV disease interferes with the body's ability to prevent and fight infections. Immature taste buds and curiosity limit children's ability to protect themselves from bad-tasting poisons. Finally, lack of sight hinders a blind person from avoiding harmful obstacles.

Environmental Safety

Many accidents and illnesses are preventable through protective measures. Assessing the external environment can reveal hazards and target environmental improvements that will prevent accidental injury. In addition, minimizing contamination of the environment is a primary prevention approach to acute and chronic illnesses and conditions.

THE HOME ENVIRONMENT

People of different ages are at risk for different hazards, even in the same environment. From infancy on, a person's environment enlarges to a peak size at some point in adulthood, and then with increasing age and infirmity the size of the environment may contract. The internal environment influences the potential for injury or illness associated with environmental hazards. For example, a person with airborne allergies is more susceptible to environmental factors such as plant pollens and animal dander.

Environmental risks in or around the home may include improperly stored household cleaning products, a nearby toxic waste disposal site, busy streets, a location near a high-traffic area such as an interstate highway (potential for lead poisoning), nearby smokestack industries, polluted or stagnant water, substandard housing, overcrowding, insects, rodents, lack of play areas, poor food storage facilities, and inadequate immunization of the home's occupants and contacts.

When assessing a home, anticipating possible hazards is important. For example, medications on the kitchen table may be safe for the 70-year-old grandmother, but not for her 2-year-old grandson. Assessment of the home environment for health promotion and injury prevention is focused on the following:

- The sanitation of the home
- Safety features, such as working smoke alarms and safety catches on cupboards
- Potential outdoor hazards, such as unfenced yards near busy streets, unfenced swimming pools, and uneven sidewalks
- Potential indoor hazards, such as poor lighting, drug storage in bathroom, and scatter rugs
- Neighborhood crime rate and crime precautions

Tools for Environmental Assessment. Evaluation tools, in the form of questionnaires or checklists, have been developed to assist nurses with environmental assessment. An age-related tool for evaluating the environment of children, known as Home Observation for Measurement of the Environment (HOME), has been used extensively by public health nurses (Caldwell, 1976). The following assessment areas for children from birth to 3 years are incorporated:

- Emotional and verbal responsibility of the parent
- Avoidance of restriction and punishment
- Organization of the physical and temporal environment
- Provision of appropriate play materials
- Parental involvement with the child
- Opportunities for variety in daily stimulation

Home safety assessment tools have also been developed for people with disabilities (Stanhope and Lancaster, 1988), and elders (Burnside, 1982). Hill and Smith (1985) have developed an assessment tool to evaluate the air, water, energy, safety, noise, light, and space in a person's environment. Pynoos and Gohen (1990) have developed a home safety guide that provides a room-to-room check list to identify potential hazards, suggestions of how to minimize or fix problems, and a resource guide for community assistance.

HEALTH CARE ENVIRONMENT

Nurses and other employees in health care agencies are responsible for providing a safe environment for clients and visitors. Many hospitals employ individuals, such as infection control nurses, to monitor safety conditions.

Obvious hazards, such as frayed electrical cords, water spills, and malfunctioning equipment, place both you and the client at risk for injury. To avoid injury to the client, you must consider his or her age, level of consciousness, and level of cognitive and physical capabilities.

When assessing safety, note the condition of all equipment prior to use. Electrical equipment is especially hazardous if a short exists in the system. However, safety means more than safe equipment. Safety includes protection from nosocomial infections, hazardous or infectious wastes, excessive noise levels, unnecessary radiation exposure, invasion of personal space, and proper disposal of needles and other sharp instruments.

Safety assessment should take into account age and individual needs. For example, a patient using oxygen should not be exposed to an open flame or tobacco smoking. A patient with a radium implant or infectious disease should be isolated to protect others. A confused person should not be left unsupervised. If a young child who can climb is left unattended in a crib, a safety net should be placed over the crib.

THE INTERVIEW
AND HEALTH HISTORY

You can obtain data related to a person's health perception and health management behavior in formal and informal interviews. Data collection may be organized in relation to the following factors:

- Health perception
- General information about factors influencing health management and adherence behavior
- Risk factors
- Preventive health screening activities

The interview to collect this information may be either brief or extensive, depending on time and focus. For any long-term or extensive health care, a comprehensive assessment of health maintenance behavior is necessary. Identifying risk factors as well as the person's ability to manage health behaviors and understand health is essential to achieve and maintain optimal health. You may use a structured interview guide to facilitate data collection (see the accompanying display).

Health Perception

Pender (1987) identifies a person's definition of health as one of the factors influencing health practices and related decision making. Gather this information by asking the person to describe his or her health status and the meaning of "being healthy" or "in good health." The following questions are examples:

How would you describe your health at this time?
What does it mean to you to be healthy?
How do you describe good health?
Compared to others your age, how is your health?

Identify any tendency of the client to underrate his or her health status, or perceptions that are incongruent with yours.

Interview Guide Health-Perception—Health-Management Pattern

A structured interview guide may be used to facilitate data collection. The headings provided on this screening interview form correlate with major interview areas discussed in the text and may be deleted when creating forms to record data in practice settings.

Health Perception

Client's description of health now and during last year _____

_____

Immediate health concerns _____

Influencing Factors: Health Management and Adherence Behavior

What factors make it difficult to follow health advice? _____

_____

What factors support health management activities? _____

_____

What do you do on your own to stay healthy? _____

Risk Factors

Family Incidence of:

_____ Cardiovascular disease
_____ Hypertension
_____ Cancer
_____ Diabetes mellitus
_____ Psychiatric illness
_____ Abuse or violence
_____ Drug or alcohol abuse
_____ Genetic disorders
_____ Other (specify): _____

_____

Health Habits

Do you smoke/use tobacco? _____ If yes, estimated pack-years* _____
Alcohol use (frequency, amount, type) _____
Drug use (prescribed, over-the-counter) _____

Dietary consumption of fat/salt/sugar _____

_____

Environmental Risk Factors

Do you use seat belts or child restraints? _____
Is home child-proofed? (If appropriate, determine measures taken) _____

Any factors in the home or at work that could cause falls or accidents? _____

Are there any other factors you can identify that could potentially threaten your health or cause injury? _____

Preventive Health Screening Activities

Self-examinations (breast, testicular, blood pressure): Indicate frequency and perceived problems _____

_____

Last professional examination (dental, pelvic, rectal, vision, hearing, complete physical) _____

_____

Last laboratory or other diagnostic testing (ECG, CBC, cholesterol, occult blood, Pap, chest x-ray) _____

_____

Pack-years = packs/day × number of smoking years. Example: 2 packs/day × 10 smoking years = 20 pack-years.

Factors Influencing Health Management and Adherence Behavior

Other client factors identified as influencing health management include the following:

- A positive attitude about good health (people who value health are generally more active in their own health management)
- Perceived control (people who believe health is related to personal practices rather than fate are more apt to actively manage health)
- A desire for competence
- Self-awareness
- Self-esteem
- Perceived benefits of health-promoting behaviors

Additional factors that influence a person's health perception and health management include age, gender, cultural background, emotions, socioeconomic status, experiences, situational factors, and knowledge and understanding of health-related matters.

Age. Age may have a significant impact upon how people view their own health status and what should be done to maintain or improve that status. For example, a 70-year-old woman with arthritis, diabetes, and hypertension may consider herself healthy, whereas a 20-year-old with the same disorders may feel unhealthy.

Gender. Men and women differ in the degree to which they use traditional health care services in the United States. Regardless of age, women visit a health care provider significantly more often than men. Additionally, women are the primary "health care brokers" of the family; 70% of the time, women determine which family members seek primary health care and when. Women working outside of the home, however, tend to use fewer health care services than other women (Triolo, 1987).

Cultural Background. Cultural beliefs and practices have a definite influence on health, but assuming that a person from a particular group practices specific beliefs may be erroneous. Cultural beliefs may influence a person's definition of health and illness, perceptions of health control, and health activity expectations. In the United States, nontraditional health care providers include curanderos (Hispanics), folk healers/practitioners, medicine men and women (Native Americans), lay midwives, acupuncturists, and spiritual healers.

Being aware of the client's cultural beliefs and practices will help you plan realistic health management behaviors. For example, encouraging an orthodox Jewish woman to drink milk to prevent calcium loss between meals as opposed to with meals will be more successful. Likewise encouraging a vegetarian to eat more leafy green vegetables will be more effective than suggesting liver to prevent anemia. Suggestions that conflict with cultural values have little chance of success and may create conflict between you and the client.

Emotions. Emotions such as embarrassment, fear, and denial may also influence health maintenance behavior. For example, a woman with a family history of breast cancer may fear the disease to the extent that she will not do a breast self-examination (BSE) or, to the other extreme, performs daily BSE.

Socioeconomic Factors. Income and means of purchasing health care also influence client behaviors. In the United States, health care is usually paid for by the individual or insurance, or a combination of both. A client who has insufficient income and/or no health insurance, and is ineligible for public subsidized insurance (Medicare or Medicaid) has very limited options for health care and may be unable to follow health recommendations. Frequently, prescriptions are not filled because of cost. Additionally, a person may refuse a referral to a health facility, even if at low cost, if his or her experiences there have been negative.

Situational Factors. Evaluating the client's health perception and management in terms of situational factors is particularly important. For example, if you discover that the client has not had weekly blood pressure measurement, as recommended, for the last month, you might decide upon a nursing diagnosis of Noncompliance. Further investigation might reveal that the person lives alone in a rural area, does not drive, and is 6 miles to the nearest public clinic for blood pressure measurement. Alternatives could be found that would allow the client to follow the recommendation (e.g., home monitoring equipment, weekly visits from a home health nurse, and arranging transportation to the public clinic). This example illustrates the importance of exploring the client's individual situation before making a recommendation.

Knowledge. Limited knowledge may affect a person's motivation or performance. A person who is unaware of free or sliding-scale clinics may unnecessarily neglect professional health care because of cost. Lack of knowledge about particular illnesses and prescribed medication or treatments may influence health management. Often elders confuse symptoms of health problems with those of "old age." When you assess the client's knowledge base, you may discover discrepancies between what the client knows and does. For example, people know that car-seat restraints save lives, but many do not "buckle up."

As you continue the interview, ask questions to elicit data on the factors that influence health behaviors. For example, the following questions may be appropriate:

Tell me how your personal beliefs influence your health practices.
Who makes decisions about your health care?
Some people believe that good health is a matter of fate. What do you think of this?
What makes it difficult to follow health advice?
What makes it easier to follow health advice?

Evaluate the person's knowledge base by asking for descriptions of any illnesses, including perceived cause, prescribed medication, and treatments. Determine if the person knows safety principles for managing medications.

Risk Factors

Illness and injury risk factors should be identified so that appropriate primary and secondary preventive activities may be implemented. For example people who are older, African–Americans, and have a family history of hypertension have an increased risk of developing hypertension and should be screened on a regular basis. Teaching about diet and exercise should also be included. Risk factors associated with selected dysfunctions or problems are shown in Display 7-2.

During the interview, make observations related to risk factors and elicit a relevant family history. Ask about the incidence in blood relatives of cardiovascular disorders (stroke, myocardial infarction, coronary artery disease), hypertension, cancer, diabetes, and genetic disorders. A useful technique is to ask the person to describe the health status or cause of death of children, siblings, parents, and grandparents. While collecting this data, diagram a genogram (Figure 7-1).

Ask additional questions relating to habits and environment to reveal other possible risk factors. Note tobacco behavior, use of automobile restraints, drug or alcohol use, dietary patterns, sexual activity patterns, stressors, and the nature of work and leisure activities. Inquire about immunization status; preschool children, adults, and elders are most likely to have deficiencies. A risk in one area may increase risks in other areas. If a child lives in a house where tobacco products are used, he or she has a higher risk of developing bronchitis, this risk is increased if the child's respiratory system is compromised.

Knowledge of health risks allows people to make conscious efforts to reduce risks, thereby enabling them to maintain health and prevent disability. Most people realize that some activities, such as driving after excessive alcohol intake, do not promote health. On a limited basis, such ac-

---

Display 7–2
Risk Factors Associated with Common Dysfunctions or Problems

Some risk factors may be modified, whereas others, such as age gender and ethnicity cannot. The former may be the focus of nursing intervention.

Atherosclerotic Heart Disease

- Positive family history
- Increasing age
- Male sex
- Hypertension
- Elevated serum lipid levels
- Tobacco use
- Carbohydrate intolerance
- Diet high in calories, fats, cholesterol, refined sugars, and salts
- Obesity
- Type A personality

Hypertension

- Positive family history
- Increasing age
- African heritage
- Pregnancy
- Oral contraceptive use
- Obesity
- Diabetes mellitus
- Labile blood pressure (readings alternate between normotensive and hypertensive ranges)
- Tobacco use
- Heavy alcohol consumption

Abuse or Violence

- Crisis situations
- Dysfunctional family relationships (incest, abuse)
- Drug or alcohol abuse
- Threatened self-esteem

Infection

- Chronic disease states
- Altered immune status or function
- Altered skin or mucous membrane integrity
- Medications: antibiotics, antifungals, antivirals, steroids, immunosuppressants, insulin
- Therapeutic modalities: surgery, radiation, hyperalimentation, dialysis, invasive lines or procedures
- Contact with nosocomial agents
- Trauma
- Malnutrition
- Stress
- Prolonged immobility
- Thermal injuries
- Warm, dark, moist environments (skinfolds, under dressings)

Trauma

- Physical alterations affecting judgment, coordination, sensory function, mobility, or level of consciousness
- Medications causing sedation or hypotension
- Use of alcohol
- Lack of use of automobile restraints, hardhats, motorcycle or bicycle helmets
- Unsafe household
- Stress
- Fire hazards
- Improper footwear

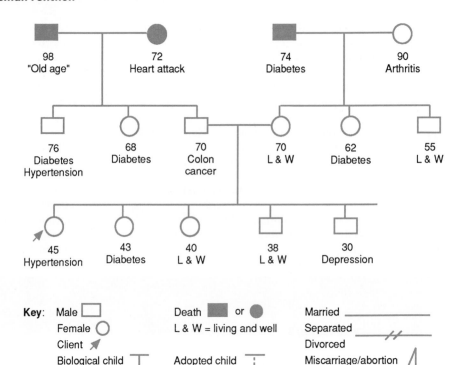

Figure 7–1. Genogram, 3 generations.

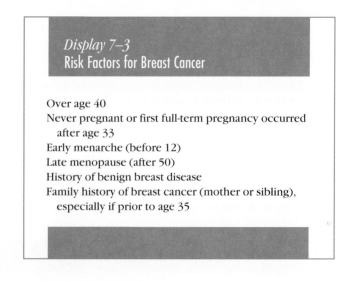

tivities may not cause disease, disability, or death, but the risk increases as the frequency of the activity increases. On the other hand, a person may engage in unprotected sexual intercourse on one occasion or drive under the influence of alcohol just one time, only to suffer the most undesirable results.

Identifying risks is appropriate throughout life and may even begin before conception through genetic counseling.

Preventive Health Screening Activities

During the interview, determine how extensively a person participates in preventive health screening activities and evaluate the frequency in relation to current recommendations. Annual screening for every common disease or condition is no longer considered cost-effective or necessary. Screening recommendations vary depending on the person's age and identified risk factors. You should also consider factors that might influence a person's participation, such as personal beliefs, knowledge of health maintenance services, confusion about scientific evidence and recommendation, and inability to procure third-party payment for screening programs. Evaluate the person's immunization, which influences the prevention of infectious diseases. Be alert to changing recommendations; for example, in the last few years immunization recommendations have been rapidly changing. Health screening is recommended for a number of illnesses and conditions, which are discussed in the following sections.

BREAST CANCER

Early detection and treatment of breast cancer significantly affects mortality. Breast cancer is first in the number of new cases and is the second leading cause of cancer death in women in the United States. The occurrence of breast cancer increases with age, and it is almost eight times more common in women aged 75 to 80 than in those aged 35 to 40. See Display 7-3 for risk factors. Determine the person's knowledge and practice with respect to the following currently recommended screening modalities for breast cancer.

- Breast self-examination monthly for women over age 20 years
- Breast examination by health professional every 3 years for those 20 to 40 years and annually for those over 40
- Baseline mammogram for women between 35 and 39 years; mammogram every 1 to 2 years (depending on

Display 7–3
Risk Factors for Breast Cancer

Over age 40
Never pregnant or first full-term pregnancy occurred after age 33
Early menarche (before 12)
Late menopause (after 50)
History of benign breast disease
Family history of breast cancer (mother or sibling), especially if prior to age 35

risks and baseline findings) for women 40 to 49; mammogram annually from 50 years on

- For women at high risk (close relative with diagnosed premenopausal breast cancer), yearly mammogram and examination by health professional beginning at 35 years

TESTICULAR CANCER

Young men aged 15 to 34 years are at greatest risk for developing testicular cancer. Approximately 3 of every 100,000 men in the United States develop testicular cancer yearly. Testicular cancer represents about 1% of all cancers, but it is the most common cancer of adolescent and young men. Most men have never heard of the need for regular testicular examinations. Detected early, testicular cancer has nearly a 100% cure rate; however, screening for testicular cancer is often neglected (Wilson, 1991). The following screening activities are recommended by the American Cancer Society:

- Testicular self-examination monthly for men beginning with puberty
- Testicular examination by a health professional annually beginning with puberty
- Special attention paid to those at high risk (see Display 7-4)

COLORECTAL CANCER

Colorectal cancer affects both men and women, and the incidence increases with advancing age. Those at highest risk include people with a personal or family history of colorectal polyps, inflammatory bowel disease, and those who routinely ingest a high-fat/low-fiber diet. Those at higher risk may require more intensive screening. Mortality is significantly lowered through programs of early detection, which include the following:

- Digital rectal examination by a health professional, annually from age 40 years
- Stool guaiac (occult blood) testing annually from age 50

Display 7–4
Risk Factors for Testicular Cancer

Between the ages of 15 and 34
Partially to totally undescended testicle
History of maternal use of diethylstilbestrol or oral contraceptives during first trimester
History of cryptorchidism, inguinal hernia, Klinefelter's syndrome, atrophy of testes, and hermaphroditism

---

- Sigmoidoscopy every 3 to 5 years following two negative test results obtained 1 year apart for persons over age 50

CERVICAL CANCER

The American Cancer Society's cervical cancer screening recommendation for sexually active women under 65 years is a Pap smear every 3 years after two initial negative Pap smear results obtained 1 year apart. Women at increased risk for cervical cancer require annual screening. Increased risk is associated with multiple sexual partners, first sexual intercourse at an early age, and previous abnormal Pap smear results.

PROSTATE CANCER

One of every 11 men will develop prostate cancer in their lifetime. Over 80% of all prostate cancer is diagnosed in men over age 65 years. The American Cancer Society recommends yearly digital rectal examination of the prostate beginning at age 40 years. The mortality rate of prostatic cancer is 50% greater in African–American men than in white men (Wilson, 1991).

HEART DISEASE

Coronary artery disease may develop without symptoms. The disease may be undetected until a major problem develops, such as myocardial infarction or cardiac dysrhythmia. Screening efforts focus on risk factor identification and life-style modification. Electrocardiograms are not recommended for routine screening of heart disease in healthy individuals.

- *Tobacco:* Every 3 to 6 years, evaluate tobacco behavior (including use of chewing tobacco and snuff). Determine pack-year history, and the desire to stop using tobacco.
- *Hypertension:* Screen healthy persons aged 20 to 40 years every 3 to 5 years; aged 40 to 60 every 2 years; and annually after age 60. Screen high-risk persons more frequently (African-Americans, obese persons, and those with family history of hypertension). Children can be hypertensive.
- *Hypercholesterolemia:* Obtain a baseline serum cholesterol and blood lipid measurement at 20 years and every 6 years thereafter. Persons with elevated baseline values or those with a family history of hypercholesterolemia should be screened more frequently.
- *Obesity:* Although the person may recognize obesity without the aid of a health professional, it is helpful to determine if body weight is 20% greater than ideal at least every 3 to 4 years.

DIABETES MELLITUS

Diabetes affects over 10 million people in the United States; approximately one half of these people have not been diagnosed. Although diabetes is a leading cause of death, it also increase one's risk for other conditions, such as heart and renal diseases and blindness. At about age 40, individuals should be screened on a regular basis for diabetes. African–Americans, Hispanics, and Native Americans have a higher risk of developing adult-onset, non–insulin-dependent diabetes.

OTHER RECOMMENDED SCREENINGS

Other screenings recommended for children include developmental testing, vision and hearing, speech, and scoliosis. Hearing and vision screenings are also recommended as people age, usually beginning between 35 and 40 years.

DIAGNOSTIC STUDIES

A complete health perception and health management assessment includes consideration of laboratory values, x-rays, and test results, including cholesterol level, blood glucose, Pap smear, stool guaiac, mammogram, prostate-specific antigen, blood pressure measurement, tuberculous skin test, vision, hearing, scoliosis, and developmental testing. The type of screening test used for any complete assessment is dependent upon age (developmental tests are performed on children), gender (mammograms for women), and ethnic origin (blood glucose screening may begin at an earlier age with ethnic high-risk groups, and sickle cell anemia screening would be performed only on people of African heritage). Many of the diagnostic studies performed for health maintenance are not for diagnosing illnesses or conditions but to alert the health provider to potential problems and the need for a diagnostic work-up. For example, a single elevated blood pressure reading would not indicate hypertension but would indicate that after three elevated measurements the individual should be referred to a physician or nurse practitioner for further evaluation. The single elevated blood pressure should alert the nurse to consider the need for further evaluation of the nutrition–metabolic function and the activity–exercise pattern or the coping–stress tolerance function. Display 7-5 contains a schedule of diagnostic screening tests for adults (see Chaps. 19 and 20 for the schedule for children and elders).

Elevated *cholesterol serum levels* are associated with increased risk for cardiovascular disease. Generally, people in the United States ingest a high-fat diet that, in many individuals increases cholesterol levels. Reducing total fat to less than 30% and animal fat and tropical oils (*i.e.,* palm, coconut) to 10% or less of total dietary intake will keep cholesterol levels below 160 for most people.

Blood glucose levels are indicative of a balance between foods ingested, insulin production and activity, and exercise/metabolic rate. Glucose is essential for energy production and life. If the body production of insulin is insufficient or ineffective, then blood glucose increases. A person with an elevated blood glucose level should be referred for diagnostic testing, such as a glucose tolerance test.

Display 7–5
Schedule for Routine Diagnostic Screening Tests

Vision	Visual acuity every 1–5 yers, glaucoma every 3 years beginning at age 35
Hearing	Gross screening yearly, acuity every 3–5 years beginning at age 35
General Physical Assessment	Every 3–5 years including height, weight and nutrition
Blood Pressure	Every 2–3 years
Dental	Every 6–12 months
Urinanalysis	Every 5–10 years
Blood	
Cholesterol	Every 5 years unless high risk, then more frequently
Glucose	Every 10 years unless high risk, then more frequently
Hematocrit	Women every 3–5 years; men every 5–10 years
Stool Guaiac	Yearly after age 35
Sigmoidoscopy	For colon cancer every 5 years beginning at age 50
EKG	Baseline at age 40 and then as indicated
Tuberculosis	Establish base line during adult years
Women only	
Cervix	Pap smear every 3 years after two successive normal reports
Breasts	BSE monthly with professional evaluation every 1–2 years; mammogram—baseline prior to age 39, then every 1–2 years
Men only	
Testicles	TSE monthly with professional evaluation every 1–2 years during high-risk years
Prostate	The routine use of PSA blood test for screening is controversial. Digital rectal examination every 1–2 years after age 50, earlier if high risk

---

Blood glucose measurement can also be used to monitor the health maintenance of an individual with diabetes mellitus. An elevated or low blood glucose reading may indicate that the individual is having difficulty in managing diabetes.

A *mammogram* is a soft-tissue x-ray of the breasts that is

utilized to detect abnormalities such as cysts and cancerous tumors. Cancerous tumors can be identified through mammograms before they can be palpated.

Prostate-specific antigen is a blood test used to identify nonpalpable prostate cancer. The prostate-specific antigen is produced exclusively by the prostate, and the blood antigen level increases with prostate cancer. The use of this test as a routine screening tool is controversial, as there are many false-positive results. Additionally, it is not known if the use of this test will decrease prostate cancer mortality; therefore, the cost–benefit ratio of this screening tool is questionable (Roetzheim and Herold, 1992).

Tuberculin skin tests are used to identify those individuals who have been exposed to and have developed antibodies toward the tuberculosis bacillus. Purified tuberculosis protein is injected into the interdermus. The test is considered positive if the area of reaction is greater than 10 mm if under age 35, or greater than 15 mm if aged 35 or over (CDC, 1990). A person with a positive test should be referred for a chest x-ray and follow up. Once a person has had a positive tuberculosis bacillus skin test, it should not be repeated.

Blood pressure measurement and its significance are discussed in Chapter 10. Blood pressure measurement can be used for screening or to monitor health management of people with known hypertension. *Vision and hearing testing* are discussed in Chapters 11, 19, and 20. *Scoliosis* testing and implications are discussed in Chapter 10. *Developmental testing* is discussed in Chapter 18. *Stool guaiac* is discussed in Chapter 9. To monitor health management of individuals with known health problems, other diagnostic tests may be used, such as urine drug screens for individuals with chemical dependency problems, and blood drug levels for individuals on drugs with narrow therapeutic ranges, such as digoxin, antibiotics, and antipsychotic drugs.

NURSING OBSERVATIONS RELATED TO HEALTH PERCEPTIONS AND HEALTH MANAGEMENT

Examination Focus

The primary goals of the observations related to health perception and health management are to (1) identify visible evidence of the client's health perceptions and health management behavior, (2) validate data obtained during the interview, and (3) identify problems with health management. This information is analyzed to formulate nursing diagnoses and to identify possible problems of health management and ways health can be promoted through better management.

In order to evaluate health perception and health management functions, it is necessary to analyze the data obtained from the following:

- Observation and physical examination from other functional areas
- General appearance
- Mental status
- Body structure
- Self-examination techniques
- Environment

The individual's health perception and health management skills impact all other functional abilities and health status. Therefore, information from other assessment areas can provide cues to health misinformation, conflict between health beliefs and traditional health practices, and problem or potential problems in health management.

General appearance and body structure can provide cues as to how the individual is managing health. Also, one can make some judgments regarding the validity of interview data. Mental status is useful in determining the individual's ability to manage health as well as to learn new knowledge and behaviors regarding health and health management.

Data from Other Functional Areas

Physical examination data may indicate possible problems with health management practices and safety. For example, a person with limited vision may have difficulty distinguishing different medications or may be unaware of environmental hazards. Noting the person's limited vision should prompt you to consider other nursing diagnoses, such as High risk for injury and Altered health maintenance.

Physical examination data also serve to identify other assessment needs. Evaluation of blood pressure and nutrition and integumentary and activity assessment all provide data regarding how effectively an individual is managing a healthy life style. You may use examination data to detect and monitor health problems not classified as nursing diagnoses such as diabetes mellitus and hypertension. In such cases, you would make referrals to other health care providers for medical care, while monitoring the individual's ability to manage a medical regimen.

During a complete health assessment, other cues regarding health perception and management may become available as you are performing different examinations. For example, asking an elderly client about a swollen knee joint while examining the musculoskeletal system may reveal that she mistakenly believes that arthritis is a normal part of aging. You may also discover that she has not sought medical care for her knee and that she takes eight aspirin tablets a day that she forgot about when asked about medications during the interview.

For a well individual, the entire physical assessment may be considered to be a diagnostic screening examination. The purposes of such an assessment would be to identify potential problems and risks and to improve or maintain health status through better health maintenance and education.

Nursing Observations   *Health Perception and Health Management*

General Principles

Health perception and health management are assessed through observation and the analysis of data from other assessment areas. If the individual has or is at risk for a health problem, assess how the individual is managing the regimen prescribed to control or prevent the problem. Assessment of how the individual maintains or improves health status is also considered.

Equipment

No special equipment is needed unless the client is using a piece of equipment for self-examination. For example, if a person is using blood pressure equipment or a blood glucose monitor at home, you should assess the accuracy of measurement and the client's skill in using the equipment.

Preparation for Assessment

Privacy should be assured during the assessment, and adequate lighting should be available. If a spouse, parent, or other person routinely performs an assessment on the client, then that person should also be included during assessment of self-examination skills, if the client is agreeable.

Examination and Documentation Focus

- *Perceptions of health:* Observe for overt signs of health.
- *Maintenance of health:* Observe general appearance, body structure, mental status, and gross mobility.
- *Risk factors:* Observe for risk factors such as ethnicity, tobacco use, and occupation.
- *Assessment of self-examination skills:* All self-examinations performed by the client should be assessed for knowledge and skill, including breast and testicular self-examination.
- Assess environment for possible hazards when possible.

Examination Guidelines   *Health Perception and Health Management*

Procedure

1. OBSERVE CLIENT FOR OVERALL HEALTH STATUS.
   a. Does the person appear healthy or sick?
   b. Does your opinion of client's health status (from poor to excellent) agree with the client's perception?

2. OBSERVE FOR PROPER HEALTH MAINTENANCE.
   a. Observe client's general appearance, including overall appearance, hygiene, body odor, fit of clothing, condition of nails, hair, obvious dental caries, and missing teeth.

   Avoid making quick judgments or assumptions at first glance and try to verify your assumptions by confirming with the client. For example, ask the client what he or she was doing just prior to coming to the hospital.

   b. Observe body structure.

   Observe and chart body height and weight, noting the following:
   Is weight appropriate for height?
   Are body parts in proportion to body size and age?
   Are there any gross deformities or missing extremities?
   Does muscle tone correlate with reported activity?

   c. Observe and evaluate client's mental status.

   If accuracy of health history is in question, verify information from relative or friend. The client's permission may be necessary. Note the following:

Clinical Significance

Verifying client's perceptions with yours provides valuable information (*i.e.,* whether the client minimizes or exaggerates health problems). Many clients rate their health status as comparable with that of the health professional's.

Proper dress and grooming can provide insight into client's self-esteem and ability to manage self-care needs for health.

Deviations from Normal

Any deviations from normal should be followed up with the appropriate examination, for example, an adult with ammonia smell should alert you to possible urinary incontinence, or a fruity breath smell may indicate diabetes mellitus.

Clinical observations should validate the client's health history.

Deviations from Normal

Any abnormal findings should be evaluated further and the risks for injury or illness considered.

An alert, logical mental status is helpful in managing health care. The mental status of a client is important in determining the amount of assistance needed to assume independence in self health care. Some clients are totally independent, others are totally dependent on others for health care, but most people fall somewhere between those extremes.

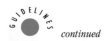 *continued*

Health Perception and Health Management

Procedure

Has health history been logical?

Do judgments about health or health care seem rational?

What is client's affect? Are there mood swings?

Are there any signs of distress?

How easy is it to establish a relationship with the client?

d. Observe gross mobility.

Note any indications of potential interference of health maintenance activities.

3. OBSERVE FOR OBVIOUS RISK FACTORS, INCLUDING THE FOLLOWING:

Obesity, racial/ethnic heritage that predispose to certain diseases or conditions, risky occupations or activities, educational status.

See Displays 7-1 and 7-2 regarding specific risk factors.

Be careful not to form judgments without validation from client.

4. OBSERVE SELF-EXAMINATION TECHNIQUES FOR ANY SELF-EXAMINATIONS PERFORMED (*i.e.,* blood pressure check, testicular self-examination, breast self-examination, or blood glucose test).

See Displays, "Breast Self-Examination" and "Testicular Self-Examination."

Clinical Significance

Deviations from Normal

Any unusual or unexpected finding should alert the nurse to the need for more extensive mental status assessment.

Ability to perform such tasks as going to the store to purchase food or necessities, preparing food or opening medication containers, and going to the toilet to avoid incontinence greatly impact the client's ability to effectively carry out health maintenance.

Deviations from Normal

Unsteady gait, arthritic hands, poor coordination, unpurposeful movements (such as tics, tremors, and limb jerks)

The identification of risk is of primary importance if health is to be maintained and risks minimized. People of certain ethnic heritage are at a higher risk for certain diseases or conditions, although changes in life-style or eating habits can reduce these added risks. Type of clothing can often indicate if a person engages in an occupation or activity that poses an occupational health risk (*i.e.,* someone working with toxic substances or a construction worker). Educational level can often influence how well an individual can read and comprehend health care instructions or medication instructions.

If a client does take the time and energy to perform self-examinations, it is important that he or she does them properly and is assured that findings are accurate. The vertical strip pattern method of breast self-examination has been shown to be a method in which women cover more breast tissue than other methods (Murali & Crabtree, 1992). See Chapter 15 for breast examination techniques.

Testicular Self-Examination

Screening Recommendations

Monthly testicular self-examination (TSE) is recommended by the American Cancer Society for early detection and cure of testicular cancer.

Characteristics of Testicular Tumors

An established testicular tumor is palpable as an irregular, nontender, fixed mass. A dragging sensation or heaviness may be reported. Nearby lymph node enlargement is rarely noted because the scrotal lymphatics drain deep within the abdominal cavity.

Procedure

1. TSE is performed as a 3-minute examination, preferably after a warm bath or shower when the scrotal skin is relaxed and easy to manipulate.

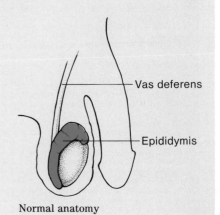

Normal anatomy

continued

Health Perception and Health Management

Testicular Self-Examination (continued)

2. Examine each testicle along a horizontal plane by rolling the skin between the thumb and forefinger of each hand (*A*).
3. Repeat the procedure by feeling for lumps or other abnormalities along the vertical plane (B). Perform this examination on each testis. It is normal to find one testis larger than the other. Any hard lumps or nodules should be reported to a health professional. See Chapter 14 for examination guidelines for health professionals.

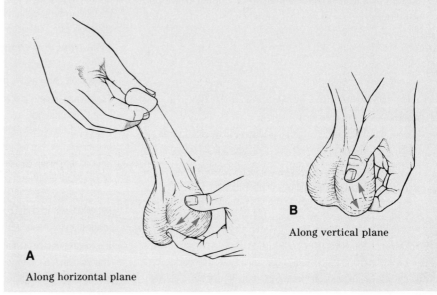

B

Along vertical plane

A

Along horizontal plane

Breast Self-Examination

Screening Recommendations

The American Cancer Society recommends monthly BSE for women over age 20. About 90% of all breast lumps are found by women or their significant others.

Procedure

1. Examine the breasts in the tub or shower when skin is wet and hands move easily over breast tissue (*A, B*). Use the right hand to examine the left breast as you raise the left arm over the head to expose more breast tissue.

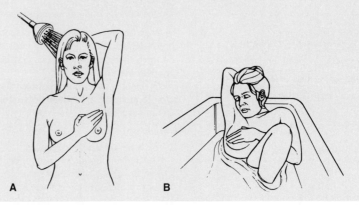

A   **B**

(continued)

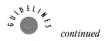

Health Perception and Health Management

Procedure   **Clinical Significance**

Breast Self-Examination (continued)

2. Examine the breast in front of a mirror to detect unusual contours or changes in the skin appearance, such as puckering, dimpling, or retraction of the nipple. Note the appearance of the breasts in three different positions: arms at the sides (*C*), arms over the head (*D*), and hands on the hips while flexing the chest muscles (*E*).

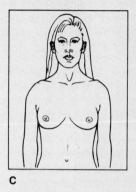
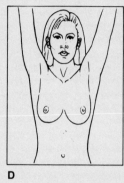
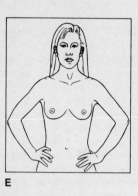

C   D   E

3. Examine the breast lying down. Place a small pillow or blanket under your shoulder on the side being examined, to expose more breast tissue (*F*). Use the right hand to examine the left breast. Be thorough, proceeding in a circular pattern from the center of the breast outward. Feel the breast tissues that extend to the armpit. Squeeze the nipple to detect any discharge (*G*). Any hard lumps, clear or bloody nipple discharge, or skin changes should be reported to a health professional.

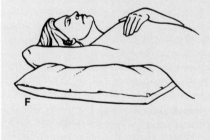

F

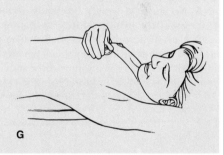

G

Observe these self-examination techniques just prior to examination of that body part.

If technique or findings are inappropriate, instruct the client in proper techniques or help client to identify problems.

Common Improper Techniques

Blood pressure measurement: cuff may be inappropriately placed, deflating the cuff too quickly

Breast self-examination: using insufficient finger pressure; using finger tips rather than finger pads; neglecting to cover the total breast tissue, particularly near axilla

Testicular self-examination: performing exam while scrotum is not relaxed, neglecting to assess proximal area, not using enough pressure

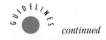 *continued*

Health Perception and Health Management

Procedure

5. ASSESS THE ENVIRONMENT.

   When possible, assess the environment for hazards and potential hazards. Consider the client's capabilities and how the environment either enhances or detracts from maintaining health.

Clinical Significance

Environmental concerns will vary depending on the age of the client and the client's specific capabilities, *i.e.,* side rails may not pose a problem for an alert hospitalized person, but confused elders often try to crawl over side rails, causing falls.

Potential Hospital Hazards

Fluid spills, frayed electrical cords, smoking in bed, loose sharp instruments such as needles, tubes inadequately secured, damaged equipment, inadequate lighting, inadequate handwashing by providers

Potential Home Hazards

Children: toxic substances within child's reach and access, peeling paint (lead poisoning), windows not properly secured, uncovered electrical outlets, inappropriate toys—small pieces cause choking, nonsecured play area, swimming pools, matches, stairs, water temperatures too hot causing scalding, malfunctioning or absent smoke detectors

Elders: frayed electrical cords, space heaters—fire hazard, smoking in bed, scatter rugs, lack of fire alarms and smoke detectors, gas stoves, poor lighting, unlevel sidewalk, unstable furniture, slippery bathtub, cluttered walkways and stairs

Documenting Examination Findings

A normal examination finding may be documented as follows:

S: No current health problems—believes in good-to-excellent health; history of hypertension controlled with Tenormin, 50 mg daily; rides stationary bicycle 30 minutes four to six times per week; eats food from all food groups and has three meals per day; avoids salt and high-cholesterol foods. Last tetanus immunization 9 years ago. Performs monthly BSE—no abnormal findings. Last Pap smear 2 years ago—normal. No specific questions or concerns.

O: Height 5′ 6″, weight 120 lb, Blood pressure 124/76, pulse 72. Weight appears proportional for height. Hygiene adequate. Dress appropriate. Uses correct technique for BSE. Normal findings confirmed.

A: Health maintenance is appropriate.

P: To continue with monthly BSE. Return in 1 year for tetanus–diphtheria immunization, baseline mammogram, and cervical Pap smear.

Abnormal examination findings may be documented as follows:

S: Moans when repositioned. No other data.

O: Thirty-two year old man, post-traumatic head injury—125 days. Eyes closed most of time. Nasogastric feeding tube in place, continuous feeding. Tracheostomy. History of aspiration pneumonia. Lungs clear in all fields.

A: High risk for aspiration related to feeding tube, tracheostomy, and past history.

P: Keep head of bed elevated to 30 degrees. Verify position of nasogastric tube every 4 hours. Check gastric residual every 4 hours; if more than 50 cc, stop feeding for 30 minutes and recheck. Assess lung fields every 4 hours. Suction as necessary.

S: Taking one pink pill three times a day for blood pressure, one blue pill twice a day, one iron pill a day, one water pill twice a day, metamucil at bedtime, one yellow pill at bedtime for nerves, and arthritis medicine four times a day. Uses two pharmacies. Not sure what all pills are for and having difficulty remembering to take medications, unaware of any side effects.

O: Blood pressure 152/90, pulse 54, pale. Walks with cane, gait steady. Dress appropriate for weather. Able to provide adequate health history and 48-hour recall of food intake and activities. Unable to accurately recall what medications taken in last 24 hours—numerous "I think I took" responses.

A: Health maintenance altered related to insufficient knowledge of medications. Difficulty managing medication regimen evidenced by elevated blood pressure.

P: Encourage use of one pharmacy—for pharmacist to monitor prescription drugs for possible duplication/contraindication.

   Return tomorrow (if possible, home visit may be more appropriate) with all prescription and over-the-counter medications.

   Together develop a written schedule for medications

and initiate teaching on purpose, effect, side effects, and untoward effects for each medication.

Evaluate schedule for medications for degree of complexity and likelihood of adherence. If potential problem exists, contact physician and discuss findings.

NDx

Nursing Diagnoses Related to Health Perception and Health Maintenance

High Risk for Aspiration

The diagnosis High risk for aspiration is utilized for the individual who is at risk for secretions, fluids, or solid objects entering tracheobronchial passages. This diagnosis is useful for individuals with altered consciousness, structural defects (such as cleft palate), and neurologic (such as cerebral palsy) and gastrointestinal disorders. Individuals with swallowing disorders may also be at risk for aspiration; however, if the goal is to improve swallowing, then the diagnosis Impaired swallowing (Chap. 8) should be used. See the diagnosis High risk for injury in this section.

History

The risk for aspiration may be increased in the following circumstances:

Premature infants, infants with cleft palate, and children from ages 1 to 3 are at high risk. Food items commonly aspirated by children include nuts, candy, and popcorn. Nonfood items frequently aspirated include small toys or pieces and balloons.

Elders with poor dentition are at high risk because of reduced salivation and inability to chew food completely.

The presence of some illnesses or conditions, such as parkinsonism, cerebrovascular accident, suppressed gag or cough reflex, dementias, post–head injury, and tracheoesophageal fistula, can place the individual at a high risk for aspiration. Also, tracheostomies, gastrointestinal tubes, enteral feedings, trauma or surgery to the mouth or neck, and anesthesia increase a person's risk for aspiration.

Any condition that increases intragastric pressure, such as decreased motility and delayed gastric emptying, also places the individual at higher risk of aspiration. Examples of these conditions include pregnancy, obesity, intestinal obstruction, and gastrointestinal outlet syndrome.

Any time the diagnosis Impaired swallowing is used, the diagnosis of High risk for aspiration should be considered. Additionally, a history of previous aspiration places the individual at risk for aspiration.

Physical Examination Findings

Physical examination findings from the other functional patterns, such as nutrition (Chap. 8), should alert the nurse to the diagnosis of High risk for aspiration. Examination findings such as the absence of gag reflex, poor dentition, presence of a tracheostomy, or prematurity in a newborn are all examples of findings from other assessment areas that are used to make the diagnosis of High risk for aspiration.

Altered Health Maintenance

Altered health maintenance is an actual or potential interruption in health because of an unhealthy life-style or knowledge deficiency of how to manage a disease or condition. The NANDA Diagnosis Review Committee is considering changing this diagnosis to Health management (Fitzpatrick 1991).

History

The ability to maintain health may be compromised under the following circumstances:

- Reports of unhealthy life-style or habits such as tobacco use, excessive caloric intake, substance abuse, excessive exposure to the sun, and unprotected nonmonogamous sexual intercourse
- Reports of difficulty with managing medication or performing health care regimens such as managing colostomy, foot, or wound care
- Reports of difficulty in ability to perform activities of daily living such as bathing and meal preparation (may also consider other diagnoses such as Activity intolerance and Self-care deficits)

In addition, any new diagnosis or skill required of an individual places that person at risk for Potential altered health maintenance. The individual may not process sufficient knowledge or skill to manage a new health care regimen.

Physical Examination

The physical examination may reveal cues to altered health maintenance such as poor hygiene, early tooth loss or teeth in poor repair, nonhealing wounds, obesity, and blood pressure or blood glucose level remaining elevated despite prescribed regimen.

Physical examination findings to support the diagnosis Altered health maintenance often come from other examination areas such as integumentary system, the cardiovascular system, and cognitive status. The nurse should consider the diagnosis Altered health maintenance any time the individual is not responding as expected or is given a new diagnosis, prescription, or activity to perform.

Health-Seeking Behaviors

The diagnosis Health-seeking behaviors is closely related to Health maintenance. With the diagnosis Health-seeking behavior, however, the individual is actively seeking to improve his or her level of wellness through a change in health habits or the environment. This diagnosis is wellness-focused, whereas Altered health maintenance is illness/condition-focused.

History

The desire to enhance one's level of wellness is evidenced in the history by the following:

- Expressing a desire for health promotion
- Voicing a desire to gain greater control of own health, concern of environmental effects on health, and unfa-

miliarity with health promotion resources in community.

Physical Examination Findings

Generally, there are no physical examination findings for this diagnosis; however, be alert while doing examination of other areas to the patients voicing any concerns about health promotion.

High Risk for Infection

The diagnosis of High risk for infection involves a situation in which the individual is at risk for an opportunistic agent or pathogen to invade the body and cause a localized infection or generalized illness.

History

Situations or conditions that place the individual at high risk would include the following:

- Reports of altered immune response related to such factors as altered production of leukocytes, altered T-cell production, and altered circulation
- History of illnesses and conditions such as HIV disease (AIDS), diabetes mellitus, cancer, hematologic disorders, respiratory disorders, and alcoholism
- Newborns, infants, and elders are at high risk owing to either immature immune systems or diminished immune responses. These groups, especially elders and children under age 2, are at high risk owing to incomplete immunization status.
- Situational factors that increase risk include prolonged immobility, trauma, malnutrition, use of tobacco products in the home, unsafe sexual intercourse, hospitalization, and exposure to infectious agents.

Physical Examination Findings

As with other diagnoses in this category, physical examination findings from other patterns are used to confirm the diagnosis of High risk for infection. For example, any break in the integumentary system increases the risk of infection. Any laboratory blood findings that document an altered white blood cell count also place the individual at increased risk. Finding the presence of any infectious process in the body increases the risk for additional infections.

High Risk for Injury

The diagnosis of High risk for injury is employed when the individual is at risk for harm because of factors such as age, lack of knowledge of hazards, or perceptual/physiologic defect. Lynda Carpenito (1992) suggests that the diagnosis High risk for injury is used when the nurse is providing on-site protection and not teaching about prevention in the home; in the home situation, the diagnosis Altered health maintenance related to insufficient knowledge of safety precautions may be more correct. The diagnosis High risk for injury actually has four subcategories: aspiration, poisoning, suffocation, and trauma. These subcategories can be isolated so that the nurse can focus on only that aspect of potential for harm. Many times an individual who is at risk for aspiration may also be at risk for suffocation. Therefore, the subcategories can be handled separately or to-

gether in the general diagnosis of High risk for injury. For clarity, each of these diagnoses is treated separately.

History

The risk for injury may be increased by the following factors:

- History of accidents, especially accidents requiring medical attention
- Environmental hazards such as busy streets, substandard housing, unsafe sidewalks, gas leaks, and non-functioning/absent fire–smoke alarms
- Any factor that can impair mobility, such as activity intolerance, syncope, arthritis, paralysis, multiple sclerosis, and seizures
- Age is a significant factor for specific types of risks. For example, infants are at high risk for suffocation, poisoning, and burns. Elders are at high risk for drug toxicity, bone fractures, and falls.

Physical Examination Findings

Physical examination findings from other functional examinations are utilized to confirm the diagnosis High risk for injury. The presence of scars and bruises indicates a history of injury. Findings such as orthostatic hypotension, syncope, seizures, impaired vision, hearing loss, poor memory, unsteady ambulation, confusion, or tissue hypoxia should alert the nurse of the need to implement strategies to prevent potential injury to the individual.

Noncompliance (Specify)

Noncompliance occurs when the individual desires to adhere to a health regimen or health advice but is prevented from doing so by factors that impede adherence. To be noncompliant, the individual must have agreed through informed consent to follow the regimen or advice. Strategies used by the nurse are to reduce or eliminate the barriers the client has encountered in attempting to comply. There are other reasons people may not follow health-related advice, and in such cases, the nursing diagnosis of Noncompliance does not apply. If the person lacks the knowledge for compliance, then the diagnosis should be Knowledge deficit. If the individual has made an informed, autonomous decision *not* to adhere to the regimen or health advice, a more appropriate diagnosis might be Altered health maintenance. For example, if a person knows that smoking·is hazardous to one's health and refuses to quit, the diagnosis of Noncompliance would not apply because that person has never agreed to try to stop smoking. Noncompliance assumes that the person desires to comply but is prevented from doing so by other factors.

History

Factors that influence an individual's ability to comply with health advice or health regimen include the following:

- Socioeconomic status influences the ability to purchase medications and foods for special diets.
- Individuals with a past history of Noncompliance are more likely to be noncompliant than others who have complied.

- The person has insufficient knowledge regarding the advice, regimen, or health problem or inability to read directions.
- Complex, long-term regimens make it more difficult to maintain compliance.
- Lack of resources, such as transportation, nearby pharmacy, and family support, hinder compliance.

Physical Examination Findings

Findings from other assessment areas are used to support the diagnosis of Noncompliance (*e.g.,* the persistence or progression of symptoms that should have been controlled or eliminated with treatment prescribed, or the occurrence of undesired outcomes, such as pregnancy for a person with a prescription for oral contraceptives). Other findings, such as confusion, impaired vision, decreased hand dexterity, and physical signs or laboratory findings of drug toxicity, can alert the nurse to problems the individual may have in attempting to follow the advise of health care providers.

High Risk for Poisoning

High risk for poisoning involves the potential for an individual to be exposed to or to ingest drugs or toxic substances. This diagnosis is one of the four subcategories of the diagnosis High risk for injury.

History

Factors that increase an individual's risk for poisoning include the following:

- Age: The very young and very old are more susceptible to drug toxicity, even when drugs are given within the normal dose range. Many drugs that elders take have a very narrow therapeutic range and a high risk of toxic side effects.
- History of past poisoning, especially if drugs were involved
- Impaired judgment either because of maturational level or cognitive impairments such as occur with Alzheimer's disease
- Hazardous working/living environment, such as working with chemicals and pesticides and the presence of poisonous house plants

Physical Examination Findings

Most of the data used to confirm the diagnosis High risk for poisoning is from data collected during the interview. Physical examination findings such as reduced renal and liver function (especially in elders), confusion, visual impairments, and the inability to read prescription labels all contribute to increase an individual's risk for poisoning. Occupational health and public health nurses have the ability to assess living and working conditions of clients. The observation of unsafe handling of toxic chemicals, the presence of poisonous house plants, or unsafe storage of chemicals and medications may also alert the nurse to the potential for poisoning.

Altered Protection

The diagnosis Altered protection is used to describe the situation in which the individual has a decreased ability or is unable to protect the self from internal or external threats such as injury or illness. The goal of this diagnosis is to protect the client from the threats. The nurse may wish to consider the diagnoses of High risk for infection and High risk for injury before selecting this diagnosis.

History

The ability to protect oneself from harm may be impaired by the following:

- An impaired immune system, impaired healing, altered blood clotting, maladaptive stress, neurosensory alterations, and autoimmune disorders
- Weakness, fatigue, immobility, skin breakdown, confusion, inadequate nutrition, substance abuse
- Being very young, very old, or having a debilitating disease such as parkinsonism

Physical Examination Findings

Examination findings for this diagnosis comes from other examination areas such as the integumentary system and lymphatic system. The presence of reddened areas on the skin in an immobile patient should alert the nurse that the patient's skin needs to be protected. Laboratory findings that indicate an altered immune system or prolonged bleeding time also are evidence for added precautionary protection.

High Risk for Suffocation

The diagnosis High risk for suffocation involves the potential a person has for smothering and asphyxiating. It is a subcategory of the diagnosis High risk for injury.

History

Identification of individuals at an increased risk of suffocation include the following factors:

- Age: The very young and the very elderly, especially those who are frail, are at increased risk of suffocating from pillows and other soft items.
- Immobility, diminished vasovagal reflex, and reduced level of consciousness/unconsciousness
- Use of enteral feedings or unsupervised bottle of feeding of infants

Physical Examination Findings

Any time a person has been assessed as having a reduced level of consciousness, either from drugs, alcohol, or trauma, the risk for suffocation increases. The presence of a nasogastric feeding tube interferes with the gag and cough reflexes. A reduction in these reflexes increases the risk of reflux and aspiration, which, if large enough, can cause suffocation. Findings such as the inability to roll over or turn one's head also increase the client's risk for suffocation.

High Risk for Trauma

The diagnosis High risk for trauma is used in the situation in which an individual is at great risk for accidental tissue injury. Such injury can be the result of burns, puncture wounds, wounds from gun shot and blunt instruments, and fractures. This diagnosis is a subcategory of the diagnosis High risk for injury.

History

An individual's risk for trauma may be increased by these factors:

- Age: Different age groups are at risk for different types of trauma. For example, children are at risk for trauma from fire, traffic accidents, drownings, and falls. Adolescents are at risk for trauma from automobile and sports accidents, and guns. Elders are at risk for trauma from fire and falls.
- A history of trauma injuries
- Tobacco smoking in the home
- Participation in activities such as contact sports, use of sensory-altering drugs, operation of mechanical equipment, and employment in high-risk occupations such as police and firefighters

Physical Examination Findings

Physical evidence such as scars and bruises in varying stages of healing should alert the nurse to the potential for the diagnosis High risk for trauma. Other examination findings such as unsteady gait, confusion, syncope, impaired vision, hearing loss, or evidence of environmental hazards would increase the individual's risk for trauma. A positive sign of previous trauma that is poorly explained may be evidence of physical abuse, especially in children, women, and elders. The nurse should explore the possibility of the diagnosis High risk for violence for the possible perpetrator of the abuse.

Clinical Problems Related to Health Perception and Health Maintenance

The focus of this health pattern is to prevent problems from occurring by identifying potential risks and barriers to the maintenance and promotion of health. The goal of the nurse is to assist the client to reduce risks, maintain or promote health, or protect the client from harm. Therefore, clinical problems in other areas create clinical problems in the health perception–health management pattern.

ASSESSMENT PROFILE

• •

Nancy, aged 40, a single mother of three children, has enrolled in a health maintenance organization for health care. The children (Paul, age 16; Nicole, age 14; and Cassie, age 16 months) and Nancy have come into the clinic for an initial evaluation.

Nancy believed that all her family was healthy, and she desired to maintain or improve health status because it was difficult for her to stay home from her job as a sales clerk when any of the children were sick. She reports that the older children eat breakfast and lunch at school, and Cassie has these meals at a day-care center. On nonschool days, Paul and Nicole share the responsibility for meal preparation and care of Cassie. Nancy tries to have the family eat their evening meal together. All immunizations are current, except Nancy has not had a tetanus–diphtheria booster in 15 years. Nancy is unaware of any tobacco or alcohol use in her family.

Nancy is sure her children engage in adequate exercise, as the two older children are in after-school sports. She has no exercise program of her own because she is on her feet all day and too tired when she comes home. Cassie always is placed in a car-seat restraint, and the rest of the family uses car restraints most of the time. Except for multivitamins, no one takes medication regularly; occasionally, over-the-counter drugs such as cough syrups, acetaminophen, and aspirin are used. All medications are kept in the medicine cabinet in the bathroom. Nancy has ipecac syrup.

Nancy is unaware of any genetic, cardiac, or cancer-related family history, although her mother has diabetes.

The family lives in a three-bedroom apartment on the ground level. Nancy reports that there is sufficient living space and a playground in the complex. In talking with Nancy and the older children individually, the following was discovered: Nancy performs BSE less than once every 3 months and has had a baseline mammogram; Paul does not know anything about TSE and neither does Nancy; Nicole uses tampons for menses and replaces them once or twice a day. Both adolescents deny sexual activity and are familiar with contraceptive devices and risks of unprotected sexual intercourse. Cassie is just beginning to walk independently and climb furniture.

The nurse notes that family members appear healthy, their height and weight are proportional, there is no obvious bruising or old trauma, and they are well groomed. Nancy was attentive to all of her children and allowed the older children to respond to questions about their own health. All the children interacted well with each other and with Nancy.

Profile Analysis

This profile illustrates the type of information you can elicit by paying close attention to clients' health maintenance behaviors and using your own observation skills to make judgments about health management. Important factors to consider during this aspect of health assessment are as follows: Who is responsible for managing the health of the family? What cultural factors influence health-related behaviors? What biologic factors, such as genetic background, influence health? Are there environmental conditions that influence health and safety? The assessment of this family's health maintenance revealed an essentially healthy family engaged in numerous health-promoting behaviors. Even though the nurse's first impression was that this is a healthy family, she conducted the assessment process in a thorough and systematic manner. Optimal collaboration between the nurse and this family for purposes of health promotion could occur only after actual and unrecognized potentials for health promotion were identified.

Assessment Focus

The nurse recognized many cues reflecting the family's health perceptions and health management practices. The cues were organized as strengths or risk factors for the maintenance of health-promoting behaviors:

Strengths

- Nancy views the maintenance and improvement of health as important.
- Children eat three meals a day and have regular exercise.
- Cassie always uses car-seat restraint, and everyone else usually uses restraints.
- No tobacco or alcohol use is reported.
- Adolescents know safe-sex procedures.
- Nancy has had baseline mammogram (negative).
- Immunization status of children is current.
- All appear healthy.

Risks

- Nancy does not perform BSE monthly.
- Nancy's immunization status is deficient.
- Nancy is unaware of need for TSE for Paul.

- Paul does not know about or how to do TSE.
- Adolescents are at risk for sports-related injuries.
- Nicole uses tampons and does not change frequently enough to prevent toxic-shock syndrome.
- Cassie is at risk for age-related injuries and illnesses.
- Medications are stored incorrectly.

Possible Nursing Diagnoses

Based on the nursing assessment, the possible diagnoses include Altered health maintenance demonstrated by lack of knowledge regarding TSE, adult immunizations, medication storage, and inappropriate tampon use; High risk for injury related to age and sports activity; High risk for poisoning related to age (Cassie) and improper medication storage; Health-seeking behavior; and Noncompliance related to inconsistent use of car restraint and BSE practice (Nancy).

Additional Data Gathering and Analysis

The nurse decided to collect additional data about the BSE practices of Nancy and car restraint use of all but Cassie before making the diagnosis of Noncompliance. *Noncompliance* describes the behavior of clients who desire to comply with health-promoting activities but are prevented from complying for some reason. For example, noncompliance may occur if the person has experienced negative side effects from a particular treatment, has difficulty coping with the responsibility of health management, or is dissatisfied with the manner of treatment. Appropriate interventions involve removing these barriers to compliance.

The nurse collected additional data from Nancy and her children to rule out other possibilities. Follow-up evaluations were planned to support the family's health maintenance activities.

Chapter 7 Summary

Health perception and health management are evaluated to determine the following:
- The person's ability to maintain or improve health status
- Risk factors that may negatively affect health status
- The person's or family's knowledge base and ability to relate to health promotion and disease prevention.

When assessing health perception and health management activities, you should consider the following:
- Cultural influences on health status
- The level of responsibility for health maintenance the person is capable of assuming
- The person's cognitive ability and knowledge of health-related activities
- Adaption related to age and health status that might be necessary for health management
- The value the person places on health

Before diagnosing a person as noncompliant, assess for knowledge deficits and the person's willingness or ability to be compliant. The following information sources are used during assessment:

The Client Interview
- Health perception
- General information on factors influencing health management and adherence behavior
- Risk factors
- Preventive health screening activities

Nursing Observations
- General appearance, including dress, and speech patterns
- Body structure, including height/weight proportions

- Mental status: Is the person capable of managing health and how much assistance would be needed?
- Validation of disease/condition detection skills: BSE, TSE
- Assessment of environment for possible hazards to health

Assessment of health perception and health management can be considered as a synthesis of all examinations. The nurse uses data from all assessment areas to make decisions on risks, potential problems, and how an individual is managing health problems. Knowing what risks the individual has and the type of assistance a client needs to manage health status will assist the nurse and client in their collaboration on a care plan that will maintain or enhance health status.

Assessment of health perception and health management is based on principles and examination techniques that enable the nurse to identify defining characteristics for the following nursing diagnoses:
  High risk for aspiration
  Altered health maintenance

  Health-seeking behaviors
  High risk for infection
  High risk for injury
  Noncompliance (specify)
  High risk for poisoning
  Altered protection
  High risk for suffocation
  High risk for trauma

Related nursing diagnoses that may be identified include the following:
  Impaired adjustment
  Altered family processes
  Altered growth and development
  Impaired home maintenance management
  Ineffective individual and family coping
  Knowledge deficit (specify)
  Self-care deficit (specify)
  Spiritual distress (distress of the human spirit)
  Altered thought process

RESEARCH *Hi*GHLIGHT

A majority of young men have been unaware of the recommendation of the American Cancer Society for testicular self-examination (TSE). What can nurses do to increase knowledge about testicular cancer (TC) and TSE and encourage regular TSE practice?

Testicular cancer in early stages has no symptoms. In later stages when metastasis has occurred, vague feelings of discomfort may be the only symptom. When TC is diagnosed, metastasis has already occurred in 88% of cases (Reno, 1988).

From a research study, Reno concluded that nurses need to provide information to young adolescents on TC and TSE as well as the benefits of practicing TSE regularly. Of the 126 men sampled from a rural Midwest college, only 12 reported practicing TSE. Of those who practiced TSE, only one felt very confident that he was performing the examination correctly.

None of the 114 nonpractitioners knew of TSE, or had any one ever shown them how to perform TSE. One hundred of these men said they would perform TSE if given the information. On the knowledge test of TC and TSE, out of a possible 9 points, the average score for the 12 practitioners was 3.58; for the 114 nonpractitioners the score was 1.87. Both are considered very low.

What significance does this study have for health assessment?

Assessing a client's knowledge of and skills in performing self-examinations for health protection is essential. Many individuals would be willing to consider self-examinations if they knew about the practice. Health assessment is an ideal time to assess a person's knowledge and skill. An opportune time to teach TSE would be while performing a testicular examination and allowing the client to repeat the examination.

Can the study's findings be applied to practice?

Reno's findings have been supported by many studies, for example, Rudolf and Quinn (1988) and Millon-Underwood and Sanders (1991). In an educational program, one study documented that 63% of the men previously unaware of TSE did perform TSE at least once after instruction. Lack of knowledge of TSE and TC may be greater in African-American men, who account for 25% of new cases of TC.

Nurses need to consider how to get information to adolescent males prior to their high-risk years. Providing consultation or doing actual courses in high schools, church groups, parent groups, and boys' organizations may be one way to reach adolescents and their parents. The knowledge base of parents of TSE is unknown.

REFERENCE

Reno, D. (1988). Men's knowledge and health beliefs about testicular cancer and testicular self-examination. *Cancer Nursing,* 11(2), 112-117.

☀ CRITICAL THINKING

You are completing a well baby check on a 6-month-old infant. Both parents are present. The mother believes that well baby checks are an important preventive health practice. The father believes that well baby checks are unnecessary and were designed to generate income for health practitioners. He also believes that immunizations are potentially harmful because he read about babies who died after receiving them.

Learning Exercises

1. Explain how a more thorough assessment of the parents' health perceptions will assist you in planning care for this family.

2. Determine and discuss what you would do when a person's health beliefs conflict with your own. For example, this father may not believe in immunizing his child because of the belief that immunizations are harmful; you disagree with his opinion.

3. Describe how you would display acceptance of each parent's beliefs.

4. As you ask the father more about his health beliefs, the parents start to argue. Describe how you would respond.

BIBLIOGRAPHY

American Cancer Society. (1984). *Breast self-examination and the nurse.* 73-50M-Rev. 3/85-No. 3408-PE.

American Cancer Society. (1978). *Facts on testicular cancer.* 78-500M-2/78-No. 2645-LE.

American Cancer Society. (1975). *How to examine your breasts.* 75-1R-6MM-5/77-No. 2088-LE.

American Nurses' Association. (1980). *Nursing: A social policy statement.* Kansas City. American Nurses' Association.

Burnside, I. (Ed.). (1988). *Nursing and the aged* (3rd ed.). St. Louis: C.V. Mosby.

Carpenito, L.J. (1993). *Nursing diagnosis: Application to clinical practice* (5th ed.). Philadelphia: J.B. Lippincott.

Caldwell, B. (1976). *Home observation measurement of the environment.* Little Rock: University of Arkansas Center for Child Development and Education.

Department of Health and Human Services. (1991). *Healthy people 2000: National Health Promotion and Disease Prevention Objectives.* US Government Printing Office: DHHS Publication No (PHS) 91-50212.

Hill, J. & Smith, N. (1989). *Self-care nursing* (2nd ed.). Norwalk, CT: Appleton-Century-Crofts.

Horgan, P.A. (1987). Health status perceptions affect health-related behaviors. *Journal of Gerontological Nursing, 13* (12), 30–35.

Kieckhafer, G.M. (1987). Testing self-perception of health theory to predict health promotion and illness management behavior in children with asthma. *Journal of Pediatric Nursing,* 381–391.

Lechtenstein, R.L. & Thomas, J.W. (1987). A comparison of self-reported measures of perceived health and functional health in an elderly population. *Journal of Community Health, 12* (4), 213–230.

Lee, H. & Frenn, M.D. (1986). The use of nursing diagnoses for health promotion in community practice. *Nursing Clinics of North America, 22* (4), 981–986.

Lenchan, A.A. (1988). Identification of self-care behaviors in the elderly: A nursing assessment tool. *Journal of Professional Nursing, 4* (4), 285–288.

Lindberg, S.C. (1987). Adult preventive health screening: 1987 update. *Nurse Practitioner 12* (5), 19–41.

Martaus, T.M. (1986). The health-seeking process of Mexican-American migrant farm workers. *Home Healthcare Nurse, 4* (5), 32–38.

Melnyk, K. (1988). Barriers: A critical review of recent literature. *Nursing Research, 37* (4), 192–201.

Millon-Underwood, S., & Sanders, E. (1991). Testicular self-examination among African–American men. *Journal of National Black Nurses Association, 5* (1), 18–28.

Murali, M.E., & Crabtree, K. (1992). Comparison of two breast self-examination techniques. *Cancer Nursing, 15* (4), 276–282.

Pender, N. (1987). *Health promotion in nursing practice* (2nd ed.). Norwalk, CT: Appleton-Century-Crofts.

Petersen-Martin, J. & Cattrell, R.R. (1987). Self-concept and health behavior. *Health Education 18* (5), 6–9.

Redeker, N.S. (1988). Health beliefs and adherence in chronic illness. *Image: Journal of Nursing Scholarship, 20* (1), 31–35.

Reno, D.R. (1988). Men's knowledge and health beliefs about testicular cancer and testicular self-examination. *Cancer Nursing 11* (2), 112–117.

Rudolf, A., et al. (1987). Breast physical examination: Its value in early cancer detection. *Cancer Nursing 10* (2), 100–106.

Rudolph, V.M., & Quinn, K. (1988). The practice of TSE among college men: Effectiveness of an educational program. *Oncology Nursing Forum, 15* (1), 45–48.

Segovia, J. (1981). The association between self-assessed health status and individual health practices. *Canadian Journal of Public Health, 80* (1), 32–37.

Standhope, M., & Lancaster, J. (1992). *Community health nursing: Process and practice for promoting health* (3rd ed). St Louis: C.V. Mosby.

Triolo, P.K. (1987). Marketing women's health care. *Journal of Nursing Administration, 17* (11), 9–14.

Tynan, C. et al. (1987). Home health hazard assessment. *Journal of Gerontological Nursing, 13* (10), 25–28, 44–45.

Wilson, P. (1991). Testicular, prostate and penile cancers in primary care settings: The importance of early detection. *Nurse Practitioner, 16* (11), 18–26.

Assessing Nutrition and Metabolism

Examination Guidelines

Anthropometric Measurement

Skin

Decubitus Ulcers

Wounds

Hair

Nails

Jaw and Oral Cavity

Abdomen

Evaluating Abdominal Fluid

Thyroid Gland

Lymphatic System

Assessment Terms

24-Hour Diet Recall

Food Diary

Calorie Count

Nitrogen Balance

Anthropometrics

Midarm Circumference

Triceps Skinfold

Midarm Muscle Circumference

Atrophy

Hypertrophy

Cachexia

Pallor

Jaundice

Cyanosis

Erythema

Skin Turgor

Edema

Primary Lesion

Secondary Lesion

Vascular Lesion

Decubitus Ulcer

Primary Intention

Secondary Intention

Spooning

Clubbing

Capillary Refill Time

Peristaltic Rush

Venous Hum

Ballottement

Hypoactive Bowel Sounds

Hyperactive Bowel Sounds

Borborygmi

INTRODUCTORY OVERVIEW

Assessment of nutritional and metabolic status is focused on (1) the amount of food and fluids consumed in relation to metabolic needs and (2) the degree to which the body demonstrates that the ingested nutrients are adequately used. When evaluating a person's level of nutritional function, it is important to consider the entire nutritional pattern. The fact that a person's nutritional intake amounts to 2200 kilocalories (kcal) per/day does not in itself describe a pattern or provide information about the influence of physiologic alterations on nutrition. The amount of calories ingested daily (2200 kcal/day) must be analyzed in relation to the individual's metabolic needs. For example, someone who has a wound that is healing will need more caloric intake than usual.

Jill Fuller and Jennifer Schaller-Ayers:
HEALTH ASSESSMENT: A NURSING APPROACH, Second Edition.
© 1990, 1994 by J. B. Lippincott Company.

The assessment of nutritional patterns and metabolic functions also helps identify risk factors for potential problems related to ingestion, digestion, absorption, transport, and metabolism. Each nutritional process requires the integrated function of a number of organs, tissues, and cells. For example, the apparently simple act of swallowing requires an intact nervous system, coordination of tongue and pharynx, and functioning oropharynx structures.

You must also consider and evaluate any indirect signs and symptoms of nutritional–metabolic dysfunction. For example, certain changes in the skin, hair, and nails may occur in some nutritional–metabolic disorders, and you should duly note them during the assessment process. Gross indicators of altered metabolism should also be considered during assessment of nutrition and metabolism. For example, signs and symptoms of infection, such as fever and lymphatic system alterations, are significant because metabolic needs generally increase with infection. Thyroid alterations are also significant because thyroid hormones play a major role in regulating metabolism.

Assessment Focus

The methods used to obtain data pertaining to nutrition and metabolism include interviewing; obtaining anthropometric measurements; conducting a physical examination of the skin, hair, nails, mouth, abdomen, thyroid, and lymphatic system; and reviewing the results of relevant laboratory tests, diagnostic procedures, and dietary intake records.

The condition of the skin, mucous membranes, hair, and nails is an indication of nutritional status. Examination of the mouth and abdomen may provide data about nutritional processes such as ingestion, digestion, and absorption. The thyroid gland is examined with consideration of its role in metabolism, lymphatic alterations are noted, and any effects on nutrition or metabolism are identified.

The factors to assess in evaluating nutrition and metabolism include:

General appearance
Pattern of food and fluid intake
Understanding of a balanced diet
Cultural and psychosocial factors affecting diet
Metabolic state
Physiologic alternations associated with nutritional dysfunction
Physical indicators of malnutrition

Suggested methods for obtaining this information are presented in the Assessment Focus display.

Nursing Diagnoses

Assessment of nutrition and metabolism provides cues used to diagnose the following nutritional problems:

Altered nutrition: More than body requirements
Altered nutrition: Less than body requirements
Altered nutrition: Potential for more than body requirements

Feeding self-care deficit
Fluid volume excess
Fluid volume deficit
High risk for fluid volume deficit

The following problems associated with altered nutrition are also identified:

Altered growth and development
Impaired tissue integrity
Altered oral mucous membrane
Impaired skin integrity
High risk for impaired skin integrity
High risk for infection
Impaired swallowing

KNOWLEDGE BASE FOR ASSESSMENT

Assessment of nutrition includes an evaluation of diet in relation to nutritional requirements. Nutritional processes, including ingestion, digestion, absorption, transport, and metabolism, also are evaluated.

Nutritional Requirements

A balanced diet is one in which an individual's needs are met, but not exceeded, in relation to the following:

- *Energy requirements (calories).* For healthy adults with light activity levels, the recommended daily dietary allowances of calories has been estimated as 2800 calories for men and 2000 calories for women (see also Appendix A, for "Recommended Daily Calorie Intake"). Energy requirements may change dramatically with illness. For example, sepsis may increase energy requirements by 25%, and major burns may double caloric needs. Consider factors that contribute to increased energy demands, including pregnancy, stress, fever, and infection, when evaluating energy requirements.
- *Protein requirements (nitrogen).* Adults require 45 g to 56 g of protein per day (see Appendix B, "Recommended Daily Dietary Allowances"). Protein requirements will be higher in situations associated with increased nitrogen loss, including postoperative states, sepsis, skeletal trauma or severe burns, and steroid ingestion.
- *Fat requirements.* Fat provides a concentrated energy source. American diets are rarely deficient in fat, with the average American consuming 90 g to 100 g of fat per day. Fat consumption is curtailed when weight loss is desired. Fats may be infused peripherally when ingestion is impaired.
- *Vitamin and mineral requirements.* Recommended intake of vitamins and minerals is presented in Appendix B, "Recommended Daily Dietary Allowances." Major injuries or stress may increase the requirements for vitamin C, niacin, thiamine, and riboflavin.

Assessment Focus **Nutrition and Metabolism**

Assessment Goal	*Data Collection Methods*
1. Considering the person's general appearance, identify findings associated with actual or potential alterations in nutrition.	*General Inspection* • Subcutaneous fat distribution: Too much or too little fat? • Skeletal muscle mass: Muscle wasting? • Skin, hair, and nails: Integument changes associated with malnutrition?
2. Identify the person's typical food and fluid intake pattern.	*Interview* • Food intake: What is a typical daily diet? • Fluid intake: What types and amounts of fluids are consumed? *Review Dietary Records* • 24-hour diet recall: What is the usual dietary pattern? • Calorie count records: What is the amount of kilocalories ingested? • Food diary: What are typical eating patterns and habits? *Observation* • Food and fluid intake: What is ingested or refused at meals or between meals?
3. Evaluate the person's metabolic status.	*Interview and Observe* • Food and fluid intake: Sufficient or excessive for metabolic needs? • Activity level: Effect on metabolic status? • Signs and symptoms of altered metabolic states: Are there findings indicating changes in metabolism? *Review of Medical Records* • Conditions that alter metabolism, for example, surgery, burns, fever, infection. • Medications that alter metabolism. *Review of Laboratory Tests* • Nitrogen balance measurements: Is the person in positive or negative nitrogen balance? *Physical Examination* • Thyroid examination: Are there abnormal findings? Could basal metabolism be affected? • Body temperature: Is there hypothermia or hyperthermia? Could this be associated with decreased or increased metabolic rates? • Lymphatic system: Are there findings suggesting infection or malignancy? Could metabolic needs be increased?
4. Evaluate diet adequacy in relation to nutrient balance and metabolic needs.	*Review and Evaluate Dietary Records* • Food composition: Does the diet meet accepted standards for recommended daily allowances of nutrients? • Kilocalorie intake: Appropriate for metabolic needs and maintenance of ideal weight?
5. Identify cultural, psychological, and sociological factors that influence food and fluid consumption.	*Interview and Observe* • Psychological influences on consumption: Stress, self-concept, depression, boredom. • Cultural influences on consumption: Food customs, beliefs, food preferences. • Sociological influences on consumption: Income, meal preparation, significant others.
6. Identify physical alterations that affect nutritional processes.	*Interview* • Symptoms of pertinent physiologic alterations: Do symptoms suggest conditions known to affect nutritional status? *Physical Examination* • Oral cavity examination: Are there physical or functional alterations of the oral cavity interfering with ingestion? • Abdominal examination: Are there physical or functional alterations of abdominal organs interfering with digestion, absorption, or metabolism? *Stool Examination* • Stool character: Does the stool indicate problems with intestinal absorption?

(continued)

Assessment Focus Nutrition and Metabolism (continued)

Assessment Goal	Data Collection Methods
7. Identify physical changes associated with malnutrition.	*Physical Examination* • Anthropometric measurements: Are height, weight, muscle circumference, and skinfold thicknesses altered? Do the alterations suggest malnutrition? • Skin examination: Are there integument changes resulting from malnutrition? • Abdominal examination: Are there abdominal alterations resulting from malnutrition?

Selection of data collection methods is influenced by the patient's status, the depth of the assessment, and the nurse's skill and expertise. During screening evaluations, fewer methods may be used.

Nutritional Processes

Nutritional status is influenced by all the processes involved in nutrient intake and use: ingestion, digestion, absorption, transport, and metabolism. Each process requires integrated anatomic and physiologic function. Physical examination techniques provide cues to functional status.

Ingestion involves the process of taking nutrients into the gastrointestinal tract. Under normal conditions, this process involves all activities that lead to placing food in the mouth. Significant influences include habits, culture, socioeconomic status, ability to prepare food, and satiety.

Digestion refers to breakdown of ingested nutrients in the gastrointestinal tract to forms that can be absorbed by the body. It involves a number of mechanical acts and chemical reactions. Digestion begins in the mouth with the mechanical act of chewing and enzymatic breakdown of starch by substances in the saliva. The bolus of food is then swallowed, enters the esophagus, and is propelled into the stomach by peristalsis. Digestion continues as the stomach muscles further churn and compress the food bolus. At the same time, numerous chemical reactions occur in the stomach to break down nutrients into small particles for absorption. As the food enters the small intestine, secretions from the pancreas, liver, and gallbladder, as well as the intestinal walls, complete the digestive process so that the nutrients may be absorbed through the walls of the small intestine.

Absorption involves the passage of digested food substances from the gastrointestinal tract to the blood or lymphatic circulation. The blood is then channeled to the liver, where metabolic processes occur.

Transport refers to the movement of nutrients across cell membranes. Transport problems are usually detected by laboratory screening. In a person with diabetes mellitus, for example, glucose is prevented from entering the cells and serum blood sugar levels may be characteristically high.

Metabolism is the final process of nutrition. Metabolism consists of the processes that produce and use energy within body cells. The production and use of energy in the cell is a complex process that begins when the cell is fueled by nutrients. Ultimately, however, energy use must be matched by energy production to achieve optimal health.

In the human body, energy is used in two major ways: to maintain essential life processes, such as breathing, nervous system function, and blood circulation, and to support "nonessential" life activities such as running, working, thinking, and dealing with stress. Additionally, some energy is expended for nutritional processes such as digestion and absorption.

The amount of energy required for essential life processes is referred to as the basal metabolism or basal metabolic rate (BMR). The BMR is measured when the body is physically, metabolically, and emotionally at rest, and is usually expressed in kilocalories per hour (kcal/hour). Surprisingly, a large number of kilocalories are required to maintain basal metabolic activities. For example, someone whose total energy needs are 2000 kcal/day may use as many as 1400 of these kilocalories for basal metabolism.

Metabolic processes are referred to as anabolic or catabolic. *Anabolism* is a constructive metabolic state in which ingested raw materials are converted to cell-building substances. *Catabolism* is a destructive metabolic process in that tissues or other substances such as glycogen are broken down to generate energy or heat.

Optimal metabolic function is characterized by a balance between anabolic and catabolic processes. Factors other than the amount and type of nutrients ingested daily may affect this balance and should be considered when assessing nutritional–metabolic status. Activity levels, hormonal imbalances, environmental temperature, stress, and illness may significantly influence the metabolic state.

THE HEALTH HISTORY

The assessment of nutrition and metabolic functions begins by obtaining a history of the individual's pattern of food and fluid consumption. Metabolic needs are evaluated by noting the person's activity level as well as other conditions that influence energy requirements. Factors that influence food and fluid consumption and use, including socioeconomic status, physical, psychological, and cognitive processes, are also identified.

Data obtained by eliciting a history pertaining to nutrition and metabolism should help you make judgments about the following:

• *Dietary intake.* The person's typical daily diet. Are nutritional requirements inadequate, adequate, or exceeded?

- *Factors that influence diet.* Personal preferences, eating patterns, cultural and psychological factors that affect diet.
- *Metabolic needs.* Has the basal metabolism been altered and in what way? Are metabolic needs being met?
- *Nutrition knowledge.* How well does the person understand nutritional concepts? Can learning needs be identified?
- *Factors related to nutritional problems.* Are there weight problems, food allergies, or problems with nutritional processes? Has poor nutrition contributed to other health problems? Have other health problems interfered with nutrition?

The Interview Guide shown in the accompanying display may be used to direct the collection of appropriate data. Begin the interview by asking general questions about height and weight, including the person's perceptions of weight. Then proceed with the diet history.

A screening interview may be appropriate if no nutritional–metabolic problems are obvious, as would be the case if the person's weight appears proportional to height, and the skin, hair, and nails have a healthy appearance. A screening interview is based on questions about food and fluid intake as reflected in the usual number of meals and snacks eaten daily and the amount of fluid ingested; the degree of activity engaged in daily; and whether there has been any weight change in the last 6 months or any discomfort associated with eating or digestion, such as nausea, vomiting, or swallowing difficulties.

If the screening interview reveals a possible or actual nutritional problem, or if general inspection clearly indicates a problem, as may be evident if the person appears to be emaciated, you can conduct a more comprehensive and lengthy interview, as indicated in the interview guide. Of course, you can initiate a comprehensive interview even if the person appears to have no nutritional problems. If the person values good nutritional practices as a means of promoting healthy living, then you can evaluate the soundness of the diet by means of a detailed interview, dietary recall, and analysis.

Dietary Intake

The simplest way to determine dietary intake is to ask the person to describe a typical day's diet, including fluids and snacks. It may be difficult to obtain an accurate depiction of the diet with this approach because one day may not be representative of the typical diet. Moreover, people may forget the types and amounts of food eaten or they may be hesitant to reveal their eating patterns. Food diaries may be helpful, but you should remember that recording may influence people to alter their usual diet habits.

A number of methods can be used to determine dietary intake, including the 24-hour diet recall, food frequency questionnaires, food diaries, and calorie counts. For any method, the examiner compares the information about the types and amounts of food ingested with established standards of sound nutrition (such as recommended daily allowances; see Appendix B) to make judgments about the adequacy or inadequacy of the diet.

24-Hour Diet Recall. Ask the person to list all the foods and fluids consumed during the last 24 hours. If the person has a reliable memory and the last 24-hour period was typical, then this method is a quick and easy way to evaluate the quality of the diet. This method is not as reliable if the person has a poor memory or if typical dietary patterns have been altered, as might occur with hospitalization.

Food Frequency Questionnaire. In this method, the person is provided with forms having checklists. Using the checklist, the person indicates the types and amounts of foods ingested over a period of time, such as a week or a month. This method readily indicates dietary practices such as "eats meat" or "eats meat 4 days a week." The food frequency questionnaire is of limited value if the person has memory problems.

Food Diary. A food diary may provide the most accurate record of dietary intake provided there is time to collect data in this manner and the person is motivated to keep the diary. A food diary involves recording every food and fluid ingested immediately after consumption for several days. A 3-day diary is usually adequate if the 3 days reflect typical patterns. In addition to recording food types and amounts, the person is asked to record circumstances, including where the food was eaten and with whom. This type of information provides additional insight into eating habits and patterns. Accurate measurements are important when keeping the food diary. You can assist the person by displaying examples of different serving sizes. For example, you may show the person 8-, 12-, and 15-ounce glasses or a 6-ounce versus a 10-ounce serving of chicken. An example of a form that might be used in keeping a food diary is shown in Display 8-1.

Calorie Count. The calorie count is usually initiated by a nutritionist to determine the exact number of calories ingested. Its primary use is to prescribe diets and supplements containing adequate calories. This method requires recording all food ingested in a day, but unlike a food diary, time and other circumstances are not described.

Factors That Influence Diet

Ask the person to describe food preferences and dislikes. You can also ask the person how his or her culture and religious beliefs influence eating habits. The American culture emphasizes a varied and abundant diet. Persons from other cultures may follow a more restricted diet even after assimilation into this culture. Certain religions provide explicit dietary guidelines, and this, too, may influence food preferences. Nonreligious beliefs may also influence eating habits, as is the case with many vegetarians.

Determine whether or not economic factors play a role in the types of foods purchased. Ascertain whether or not the person can afford to purchase milk products or fresh fruits and vegetables.

Inquire about who purchases and prepares the food. Determine whether or not facilities for food storage and preparation are adequate.

(Text continues on pg. 122)

Interview Guide Nutrition and Metabolism

General Information

Current weight _____
Current height _____
How the person feels about present weight _____
Weight three months ago _____
Easy to gain/lose weight? _____

Diet and Food/Fluid Intake

Any special diet, vitamins, or dietary supplements _____
Reason for special diet, vitamins, supplements _____
Typical daily diet:
  Breakfast _____
  Lunch _____
  Supper _____
  Snacks _____

Factors that Influence Diet

Food preferences _____
Food dislikes _____
Ethnic/cultural influences on diet _____
Religious dietary practices _____
Regional influences on diet _____
Reaction to stress (eat or drink more? less?) _____
Number of people at home _____ Who shops for food? _____
Who cooks? _____ Prepares meals? _____
Food preparation storage facilities _____
Income adequate for food needs? _____ Food stamps? _____

Metabolic Needs

Activity—occupation, exercise type and frequency, usual daily activities _____
_____

Nutrition Knowledge

Name basic food groups _____
Name foods high in calories _____
Name foods high/low in fats _____
Name foods with low nutritional value _____
How the person could improve present diet _____

Factors Related to Nutritional Problems

Current medical diagnosis _____
Previous hospitalizations/surgeries _____
Length of present hospitalization (if applicable) _____

Any of the following problems?	yes	no
Indigestion	—	—
Nausea/vomiting	—	—
Sore mouth	—	—
Swallowing difficulty	—	—
Chewing problems	—	—
Problems feeding self	—	—
Constipation	—	—
Diarrhea	—	—
Abdominal pain	—	—
Skin problems	—	—
Infections	—	—
Ulcers	—	—
Diabetes mellitus	—	—

(continued)

Interview Guide **Nutrition and Metabolism (continued)**

Factors Related to Nutritional Problems (continued)

	yes	no
Renal disease	——	——
Cancer	——	——
Hypertension	——	——
Heart disease	——	——
Lung disease	——	——
Endocrine disease	——	——
Other (pancreas, gallbladder, liver, autoimmune disorders)	——	——

Medication/Drug History

	yes	no
Chemotherapy	——	——
Antacids	——	——
Steroids	——	——
Immunosuppressants	——	——
Anticonvulsants	——	——
Oral contraceptives	——	——
Alcohol	——	——
Caffeine	——	——
Nicotine	——	——

Display 8–1
Food Diary: Dietary Recall Form

Name:

Age:

Height (inches):

Weight (lb):

Ideal Weight (lb):

Directions: Use this form to keep a 3-day record of what you eat and drink, including between-meal snacks. Write down the preparation method (baked, broiled, fried, etc.) and what, if anything, you added to the food (butter, margarine, salad dressing, sugar, etc.). Write down the circumstances at the time you ate (party, watching TV, bored, depressed, regular family meal, etc.). Use a different form for each day.

Time/Place	Food and Preparation Method	Amount	Circumstances

Table 8-1. Serum Indicators of Malnutrition

Indicator	Normal Range	Moderately Malnourished	Severely Malnourished
Albumin (g/dL)	4.5–5.5	2.8–3.5	<2.8
Transferrin (mg/dL)	150–250	160–180	<160
Total lymphocyte count (number/L)	>1550	1000–1500	<1000

Metabolic Needs

Inquire about the person's activity level and medical history in order to make judgments about energy requirements. The more active person generally requires more calories than an inactive person to support metabolism. Note any physiologic alterations that may alter the metabolic rate. For example, if the person has an infection or is septic, note that a hypermetabolic state exists and that metabolic needs are greater. The person might require the administration of protein and nonprotein calories in combination with vitamins, minerals, and fatty acids to maintain a positive nitrogen balance. Other common conditions that are associated with a depletion of the body's energy stores and predispose the person to an increased metabolic rate include burns, trauma, major surgery, major wounds, hyperthyroidism, and malignancies.

Nutrition Knowledge

Ask the person to name the four basic food groups. You can also assess knowledge by asking the person to name some foods high in calories, foods with limited nutritional value, and so on. Ask the person, "If there was one thing you would do to improve your diet, what would it be?" The response to these questions should indicate teaching/learning needs and obvious misconceptions about nutrition.

Factors Related to Nutritional Problems

A number of factors are associated with or known to contribute to nutritional problems. For example, persons receiving cancer therapy may experience dramatic appetite suppression. Persons with poorly fitted dentures may have limited dietary options because they will have difficulty ingesting foods such as fruits and meats. The health history should include consideration of these and other factors that are shown in the interview guide. A number of these factors are considered part of the person's medical history (e.g., illnesses and medications). Some practitioners choose to obtain a medical history during the opening moments of the assessment interview before proceeding to inquiries about specific health patterns (e.g., nutrition and metabolism). If this information was previously disclosed, it is not necessary to ask for it again. However, you should reevaluate this information in light of its significance to nutrition and metabolic functions.

Factors that may be associated with nutritional problems include many illnesses that carry a risk of affecting nutri-

tion. Many illnesses interfere with the basic nutritional processes of ingestion, digestion, and absorption. During the interview, be alert to reports of nausea, abdominal pain, and other symptoms associated with nutritional problems.

Drugs can alter both nutritional and metabolic states. Chemotherapeutic agents such as antibiotics and antineoplastic drugs can induce nausea and vomiting and can further compromise nutritional processes by suppressing the appetite, causing sores in the mouth, and altering taste. Drugs that induce a hypermetabolic state include steroids and immunosuppressants, which can potentiate catabolic processes and thus increase the body's energy requirements. Anticonvulsants, oral contraceptives, and corticosteroids interfere with vitamin metabolism. Alcohol interferes with the metabolism of B vitamins and, if abused, may lead to protein–calorie malnutrition and liver disease. Drug dosage and the duration of drug therapy should be determined when asking about drugs that may affect the nutritional–metabolic status.

DIAGNOSTIC STUDIES

A complete nutritional assessment includes consideration of laboratory values, including serum albumin, serum transferrin, total lymphocyte count, and urine urea nitrogen. The urine urea nitrogen is used to make judgments about nitrogen balance.

Albumin and *transferrin* are proteins found in the serum. Serum levels of these proteins are decreased when the diet is deficient in protein (Table 8-1). A decrease in albumin (*hypoalbuminemia*) causes the serum osmotic pressure to decrease so that fluid escapes to the interstitium and causes edema. Therefore, a person with malnutrition from a protein-deficient diet may develop an enlarged abdomen as fluid moves out of the blood vessels and into the abdomen.

A decrease in the *total lymphocyte count* may also indicate protein malnutrition (see Table 8-1). Lymphocytes are proteins, and maintenance of normal levels requires normal protein stores in the body. A decrease in total lymphocyte count predisposes the person to greater risk for infection because lymphocytes are an essential component of the body's immune system.

Nitrogen balance is an indicator of protein metabolism and provides a measure of metabolic rate. Clinically, nitrogen balance is used to determine whether or not protein needs are being met adequately. For optimal nutrition, the goal is +2 to +4 g positive nitrogen balance. The calculation to determine nitrogen balance is as follows:

Nitrogen balance = Nitrogen in − Nitrogen out

in which *nitrogen in* = protein intake in grams for a 24-hour period × 0.16, and *nitrogen out* = measured value for 24-hour urine urea nitrogen in grams plus 4 g of nitrogen lost through feces.

Positive nitrogen balance occurs when more nitrogen is consumed than excreted. The body's metabolic demands are exceeded, indicating an anabolic state. A positive nitrogen balance normally is noted in growing children and during pregnancy.

Negative nitrogen balance occurs when nitrogen intake is less than output. This represents a catabolic state and is associated with loss of protein in the form of muscle and other tissue. In such a case, metabolic demands are not met.

THE PHYSICAL EXAMINATION

Examination Focus

The primary goals of the physical examination in relation to nutrition and metabolism are (1) to determine the status of the nutritional processes of ingestion, digestion, absorption, transport, and metabolism, and (2) to identify signs of altered nutrition. This information is analyzed to formulate nursing diagnoses and to identify or monitor possible physiologic alterations noted during the examination, such as an ileus or intestinal obstruction.

In order to evaluate nutritional and metabolic functions, a physical examination is conducted with emphasis on the following:

- General appearance
- Anthropometric measurements
- Skin, hair, and nails
- Oral cavity
- Abdomen
- Thyroid gland
- Lymphatic system

Additionally, the body temperature is evaluated as an indicator of metabolic needs.

Anthropometric measurements include height, weight, midarm muscle circumference, and triceps skinfold. These measurements provide data about fat and muscle and serve as indicators of nutritional status.

Examination of the skin, hair, and nails provides data about general nutritional status and the supply of nutrients to these tissues. The appearance of the skin, hair, and nails may be altered in the presence of severe nutritional–metabolic problems. Wound healing also should be evaluated because normal wound healing can be an indicator of nutritional and metabolic function. For a complete discussion, refer to the section on physical examination of the skin, hair, and nails.

The oral cavity is examined to determine its functional status relative to the nutritional processes of ingestion and digestion. For example, persons with poor dentition, including few or deteriorating teeth, may have difficulty ingesting certain foods. The status of the oral mucosa is important because the condition of this tissue can indicate nutritional status or a condition contributing to altered nu-

trition. For example, the person with stomatitis may have difficulty with food intake. Stomatitis is a severe and painful inflammation of the oral mucosa that may be caused by infection, irritants, trauma, or drugs.

During a nutritional–metabolic assessment, the abdomen is examined to evaluate digestive structures such as the stomach, liver, bowel, and related functions. Examination of the thyroid gland is relevant because it secretes hormones that control the metabolic rate. The lymphatic system is examined to identify pathology associated with metabolic alterations such as infection or malignancy.

General Appearance

The overall nutritional status of a person is reflected by general appearance. A visual inspection readily reveals weight, muscle mass status, and skin appearance. Nutritional problems that are evident on general inspection are usually long standing rather than in an early stage of development. For example, a 5-pound weight loss may not be detectable on inspection, but a 20-pound weight loss that gives the person a gaunt, emaciated appearance will be obvious and represents a more established nutritional problem. Similarly, the initial changes in the appearance of the skin associated with certain vitamin deficiencies will not be evident on general inspection, whereas a severe and sustained nutrient deficit will cause visible changes, such as the dryness and cracking of the skin around the mouth associated with riboflavin deficiency.

For nutritional assessment, the general survey is directed at evaluating the following physical features:

- Subcutaneous fat distribution
- Skeletal muscle mass
- Skin integrity

Subcutaneous Fat Distribution

Fat is adipose tissue distributed throughout the body; it is found beneath the skin, embedded in the muscles and liver, and packed around the kidneys. A certain amount of fat is essential for health. Fat is an energy source, and it provides protection as well as insulation from temperature extremes. For example, fat around the kidneys protects these organs from injuries. It is impossible, however, to evaluate the fat surrounding organs by simple inspection.

Subcutaneous fat that accumulates directly under the skin is visible by inspection. It is especially prevalent around the waist, upper thighs, and triceps. These areas should be inspected visually to evaluate fat distribution. More accurate evaluation of the subcutaneous fat may be accomplished through anthropometric techniques. Variations in the distribution of subcutaneous fat may be noted in different stages of growth and development and in certain dysfunctional nutritional–metabolic states. In general, men and women differ in the amount of body fat. A healthy man's body weight is 15% to 16% fat; a woman's body weight is 19% to 22% fat.

Age. Fat distribution changes throughout the life span. In a healthy infant, accumulations of subcutaneous fat result in a slightly protuberant abdomen as well as chubby cheeks, arms, and legs. As an infant develops, the waist slims and muscle begins to replace some of the subcutaneous fat. In later life, fat again tends to accumulate in the subcutaneous tissue as muscles atrophy, and is often apparent on inspection.

Malnutrition. Excessive food and fluid ingestion leads to obesity as fat accumulates in the adipose tissue. In women, fat also tends to accumulate in the buttocks. If careful inspection reveals fat accumulation only in certain body areas, other causes may be indicated. For example, in Cushing's syndrome, an endocrine disease characterized by excessive glucocorticoid secretion, fat accumulations occur in the trunk portion of the body, whereas the arms and legs remain relatively thin.

Severe protein deficiencies can lead to fluid accumulation in the abdomen and subcutaneous compartments. In starvation states, abdominal enlargement, called *ascites,* and swelling of the extremities occur secondary to fluid shifts in the body, not as a result of fat accumulation. Protein plays many important roles in the body, such as exerting an oncotic pressure, which pulls fluid into the bloodstream. In protein deficiencies, oncotic pressure loss causes fluid to leave the vascular spaces and enter those body areas with higher oncotic pressures, such as the abdominal cavity and subcutaneous tissues. Ascites occurs in the protein starvation disease kwashiorkor, which may develop in weeks and may be observed in critical hospitalized patients who are not fed. Kwashiorkor also occurs in children who live in areas of the world where starvation is widespread. Usually, the disease develops after breast-feeding is discontinued and the child loses a protein source. The body responds to an acute starvation state by catabolizing protein for energy, which quickly depletes the lean body mass. The fluid shifts result in a protuberant abdomen.

In starvation states that are not accompanied by ascites, fat depletion may be easily observed in the waist, arms, and legs.

Skeletal Muscle Mass

The status of body protein is evaluated by inspecting the skeletal muscles or voluntary muscles used primarily for movement. The skeletal muscles also represent a backup source of energy for basal metabolic processes. If a person limits or stops ingesting food, the body will break down fat for energy. In an acute starvation state, protein rather than fat may be broken down, or muscle protein will be broken down for energy after body fat has been depleted. In either case, the muscles lose mass.

The contour and mass of the skeletal muscle are noted by inspecting the face, chest, abdomen, back, hands, arms, legs, and feet. Although muscle mass can be evaluated by inspection, anthropometric measurements are more accurate. Variations in the appearance of the skeletal muscle mass are associated with activity level and nutritional status.

Activity Level. Skeletal muscle mass may enlarge secondary to an increase in activity or muscle use. A person who lifts weights may have large chest and arm muscles,

whereas someone who walks long distances regularly may have well-developed calf muscles. Such an increase in muscle mass, or *hypertrophy,* occurs secondary to an increase in the size of existing muscle cells rather than from an increase in the overall number of muscle cells. Hypertrophied muscles are distinguished from fat accumulation by location and appearance.

Conversely, unused muscles will decrease in size, a condition called *atrophy.* People on long-term bed rest may develop atrophied muscles, which appear small and wasted. Usually the muscles in the arms and legs are most obviously affected.

Nutritional Status. Starvation states may result in depletion of skeletal muscle mass as muscle protein is used for energy. It is important to distinguish carefully between muscle wasting due to malnutrition and muscle atrophy related to disuse. Wasting of the muscles of the temporal areas, the dorsum of the hands, and the spine is usually indicative of poor nutrition or protein depletion. With advancing age, the appearance of skeletal muscle mass is a less reliable indicator of overall nutritional status. For example, in elderly clients, the muscles on the backs of the hands and other areas often atrophy despite good nutritional status.

People with muscle and fat depletion may have *cachexia,* a syndrome characterized by weight loss, muscle wasting, subcutaneous fat depletion, weakness, and anemia. Cachexia, also referred to as marasmus, is a starvation state that results from kilocalorie deprivation, in contrast to kwashiorkor, which results from protein deprivation. The cachexic client looks like a "walking skeleton," while the victim of kwashiorkor has a plump appearance.

Associated Body System Alterations

Malnutrition involving either an excess or deficit of nutrients affects many body systems, including the gastrointestinal and musculoskeletal systems as well as the cardiovascular, respiratory, and neurologic systems. The physical examination skills presented in this chapter emphasize techniques to evaluate the gastrointestinal system. The anthropometric techniques provide guidelines for evaluating part of the musculoskeletal system. The examination techniques for the cardiovascular, respiratory, and neurologic systems are discussed more fully in Chapters 10 and 11. However, a brief discussion of the relationship of each of these systems to nutritional or metabolic function is included here.

THE CARDIOVASCULAR SYSTEM

Obesity affects the cardiovascular system and is believed to be a primary risk factor for coronary artery disease. However, the cardiovascular manifestations related to obesity vary greatly among people. Moreover, cardiovascular changes associated with obesity, such as elevated diastolic blood pressure and varicose veins, may occur in people who are not overweight. In overweight people, the increase in diastolic blood pressure may be secondary to the higher intake of dietary fats accompanying obesity. Varicose veins form because the leg muscles are infiltrated with fat and do not contract effectively to return lower-extremity blood to the heart. Pooling of blood in the legs leads to varicosities.

A long-term calorie deficiency may affect the cardiovascular system, resulting in an overall reduction of heart size and a subsequent lowered cardiac output. In an undernourished person, physical examination may reveal abnormally low blood pressure, low energy levels, and weakness.

Thiamine deficiency may result in an increase in the heart size and a sustained increase in heart rate. The nurse should check for signs of high-output cardiac failure such as warm extremities and a widened pulse pressure.

THE RESPIRATORY SYSTEM

In obese people, fat that accumulates in and around the chest may restrict chest movement and compromise pulmonary function. Pickwickian syndrome, which results from respiratory compromise secondary to extreme obesity, is characterized by somnolence and hypoventilation.

THE NEUROLOGIC SYSTEM

Vitamin B deficiencies may be related to abnormal neurologic findings, as follows:

Clinical Finding	*Possible Deficiency*
Confabulation, disorientation	Thiamine
Decreased position and vibratory sense, ataxia	Vitamin B_{12}, thiamine
Decreased tendon reflexes, slowed relaxation phase	Thiamine
Ophthalmoplegia	Thiamine
Weakness, parasthesias, decreased fine tactile sensation	Vitamin B_{12}, pyridoxine, thiamine

Because B vitamins are interrelated and occur together in many foods, the clinical findings listed here will often appear in combination in a client with a B vitamin deficiency. However, if one clinical finding predominates, a specific B vitamin deficiency should be explored.

Physical Examination

Anthropometrics

Anthropometrics is a method of measuring the human body and assessing nutritional status as well as growth and development. Measuring weight, midarm muscle circumference, and skinfold thickness provides information about three body tissues altered during starvation or obesity: visceral proteins, skeletal muscle, and subcutaneous fat stores. In children under 3 years of age, head circumference and height are often measured as well. Growth retardation indicated by these measurements may be a sign of poor nutritional status.

A person's anthropometric measurements are compared to average standards for his or her age group and sex. Although taking anthropometric measurements is relatively easy to learn, practice is essential for precise measurement. Anthropometric measurements are most meaningful when they are obtained serially so that trends can be identified. You should routinely obtain or review anthropometric data on patients who are at risk for protein–calorie malnutrition during hospitalization.

General Principles Anthropometric measurements used to evaluate nutritional status include weight, midarm circumference, and triceps skinfold. Height, wrist circumference, and midarm muscle circumference are also used to complete the evaluation of nutritional status.

Equipment
- Metric tape measure
- Beam balance scale
- Calipers

Frame Size Standardized weight tables recommend ideal body weight ranges on the basis of height, sex, and frame size (small, medium, and large). The ratio of height to wrist circumference is used to estimate frame size:

Height (cm)/Wrist Circumference (cm)		*Frame Size*
Men	Women	
>10.4	>11	Small
9.6–10.4	10.1–11	Medium
<9.6	<10.1	Large

Measure wrist circumference in centimeters by placing a flexible tape around the wrist where it bends at the styloid process.

Examination Guidelines *Anthropometric Measurement*

Procedure

1. HEIGHT.

   a. Instruct the person to stand erect, without shoes, against a wall to which a measuring tape has been affixed. Be sure the feet are together and the heels, buttocks, shoulders, and head are touching the wall.

   b. Record the height in centimeters.

   c. If the person cannot stand, position supine with body fully extended and measure height from heels to top of head with a tape measure.

2. WEIGHT.

   a. Obtain weight from a beam balance scale after the person has voided. Bed scales may be used for immobile patients.

   b. Standardize the procedure as much as possible. Serial weights, such as daily weights in hospital settings, are obtained at the same time each day with the patient wearing the same amount of clothing.

   c. Record the weight in kilograms.

   d. Interpret the body weight. Consult a standardized height and weight table, such as the one found in Appendix B at the back of the book.

3. MIDARM CIRCUMFERENCE (MAC; in cm).

   a. To measure MAC, determine the midpoint on the person's nondominant arm. With the arm in a relaxed position, palpate the acromial process at the top of the humerus. Sliding your fingers across the clavicle helps locate this landmark. Place a tape measure between the acrominal process and the olecranon process or elbow and mark the midpoint on the arm.

Clinical Significance

Height is used to estimate ideal body weight and to interpret other data. Using the rod on a balance scale to measure height is less accurate than a tape but more accurate than asking the client.

Metric measurements are used to determine other values derived from height, for example, frame size and body surface area.

Body weight greater than 10% above or below the ideal range for height and frame is associated with nutritional dysfunction.

Beam balance scales are more accurate than bathroom scales.

A consistent method of weighing increases accuracy, especially in a setting with multiple care-givers.

Metric weights are used for other calculations such as drug dosages and body surface area.

Reflects both muscle mass and fat. MAC is used to calculate midarm muscle circumference.

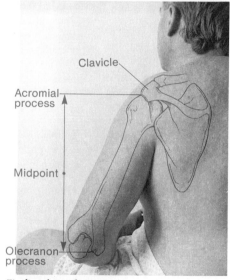

Finding the midpoint

continued

Anthropometric Measurement

Procedure

b. Next, instruct the person to let the arm hang loosely at the side. Place a tape measure around the person's arm at the midpoint and record the measurement in centimeters.

c. Interpret the MAC. MAC decreases with undernutrition and increases with an increase in fat (obesity) or muscle (hypertrophy). Undernutrition may be indicated by a measurement below the 90% reference:

Clinical Significance

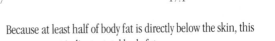

Midarm
circumference

Midarm circumference measurement

Adult MAC (cm)	Standard Reference	90% of Standard Reference Moderately Malnourished	60% of Standard Reference Severely Malnourished
Men	29.3	26.3	17.6
Women	28.5	25.7	17.1

4. TRICEPS SKINFOLD (TSF; in mm).

a. Obtain the measurement on the nondominant arm using plastic or precision metal calipers.

b. Find the midpoint of the arm using the method described for MAC measurement.

c. With the arm hanging loosely at the side, grasp a fold of skin at the midpoint on the posterior aspect of the arm. Apply the caliper and take a reading after waiting for 3 seconds. Repeat the procedure three times.

Because at least half of body fat is directly below the skin, this measurement indicates total body fat.

Metal calipers can be calibrated, making them more accurate.

TSF is measured at the midpoint mark.

Measuring triceps skinfold requires practice. A common error is measuring underlying muscle as well as fat. To avoid such an error, grasp the fold of skin and ask the person to flex the arm muscle. If you feel the contraction, you have probably grasped muscle as well as fat. In this case, release the skin and try again.

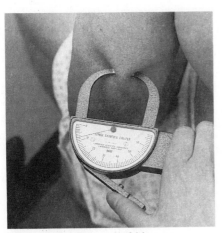

Measurement of triceps skinfold

Anthropometric Measurement

Procedure   **Clinical Significance**

d. Interpret the TSF. Fat stores decrease because of long-term undernutrition and successful weight loss. Obesity increases fat stores. Standard values are used to make clinical judgments:

Adult TSF (mm)	Standard Reference	90% of Standard Reference Moderately Malnourished	60% of Standard Reference Severely Malnourished
Men	12.5	11.3	7.5
Women	16.5	14.9	9.9

5. MIDARM MUSCLE CIRCUMFERENCE (MAMC; in cm).   Reflects skeletal muscle mass status.

   a. Calculate MAMC by using the following equation: MAC and TSF must be measured to derive the MAMC.

$$\text{MAMC} = \text{MAC (cm)} - [0.314 \times \text{TSF (mm)}]$$

b. Interpret the MAMC. MAMC decreases with undernutrition and increases with obesity and muscle hypertrophy. The severe muscle wasting of protein-calorie malnutrition is indicated by a MAMC of less than 15.2 cm in men and less than 13.9 cm in women:

Adult MAMC (cm)	Standard Reference	90% of Standard Reference Moderately Malnourished	60% of Standard Reference Severely Malnourished
Men	25.3	22.8	15.2
Women	23.2	20.9	13.9

Documenting Anthropometric Measurements

Record anthropometric measurements indicating the value obtained for each measurement as well as the number being used as the standard reference for midarm circumference (MAC), triceps skinfold (TSF), and midarm muscle circumference (MAMC). Indicate what percentage of the standard reference the value obtained represents. For example, the following measurements were recorded following the examination of a moderately undernourished woman:

MAC (cm) = 23 cm; 81% of standard
Standard = 28.5 cm

TSF (mm) = 12.87 mm; 78% of standard
Standard = 16.5 mm

MAMC (cm) = 18.96; 81% of standard
Standard = 23.2

Height: 170 cm
Weight: 46 kg

Nursing Diagnoses Related to Anthropometric Assessment

Anthropometric measurements may be used as indicators for the following nursing diagnoses: Altered nutrition: Less than body requirements; Altered nutrition: More than body requirements.

Altered Nutrition: Less than Body Requirements

The following defining characteristics or physical signs associated with the diagnosis of Altered nutrition: Less than body requirements are determined by anthropometric assessment:

- Body weight 10% to 20% below ideal for height and frame
- Decreased triceps skinfold (less than 60% of standard measurement)
- Decreased midarm circumference (less than 60% of standard measurement)
- Decreased midarm muscle circumference (less than 60% of standard measurement)

Altered Nutrition: More than Body Requirements

The following defining characteristics for the nursing diagnosis Altered nutrition: More than body requirements are determined by anthropometric assessment:

- Body weight 10% above ideal for height and frame (overweight)
- Body weight 20% above ideal for height and frame (obese)
- Triceps skinfold greater than 15 mm in men and 25 mm in women

Anthropometric measurements may be used to provide an objective evaluation of the effectiveness of weight loss programs in the overweight client.

INTEGUMENTARY SYSTEM: SKIN, HAIR, AND NAILS

Anatomy and Physiology Overview

The skin is composed of three layers: the epidermis, the dermis, and the subcutaneous tissue. Hair, nails, sweat glands, and sebaceous glands are considered appendages of the skin. Examining the integument requires knowledge of the normal anatomy and function of these structures. Figure 8-1 depicts a cross-sectional view of the skin.

Epidermis. The epidermis consists of several avascular or bloodless layers. The thin outermost layer, called the stratum corneum or horny layer, is composed of dead cells, which are flattened and keratinized. Keratin is a strong protein that is formed in an epidermal layer beneath the stratum corneum. Keratinization occurs as epidermal cells lose their nuclei and become flattened while they push to the outermost skin surface. The epidermis functions as a barrier; it protects the skin from invasion by foreign substances, prevents fluid and electrolyte loss, and aids in temperature regulation.

Normally, an equilibrium exists between keratin cell production and cell sloughing; this equilibrium gives the skin a smooth texture. When the equilibrium is disrupted, skin appearance will change. When sloughing is slower than keratin cell production, the skin may appear rough and thick. When keratin cell production decreases, the skin may lose its softness and suppleness because keratin retains water. When the sloughing rate exceeds keratin cell production, the skin may appear thin and eroded because the barrier function of the skin is compromised. Keratinized cells will lose water when they are exposed to a dry environment, giving the skin a chapped appearance.

Several distinct living epidermal layers are found beneath the stratum corneum. The deepest layer, the stratum germinativum, is significant because this is where epithelial cells are renewed in growth and repair processes. In addition, the stratum germinativum contains melanocytes, cells that produce the pigment melanin, which is responsible for skin color.

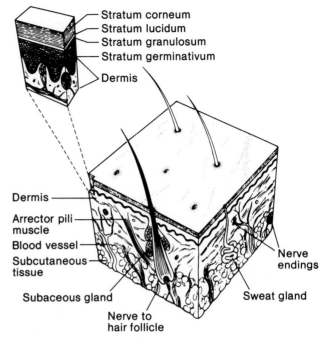

Figure 8–1. Cross-sectional view of the skin.

The production and accumulation of melanin varies with race, age, and exposure to ultraviolet light. All races have roughly the same number of melanocytes. In darkly pigmented races, however, the melanocytes are more active and produce more melanin. Exposing the skin to sunlight will stimulate melanin production, resulting in a tan appearance. Aging affects melanin production because the total number of functioning melanocytes decreases. In elderly people, however, local accumulation of melanin can be observed, especially on the backs of the hands.

Dermis. The dermis contains connective tissue and blood vessels. Connective tissue is composed largely of the proteins collagen and elastin. Collagen, a fibrous protein, helps strengthen the skin and provides a supporting framework for blood vessels and nerve endings. Elastin provides flexibility, protection, and storage of water and electrolytes. Wrinkling of the skin is associated with elastin degeneration and subcutaneous fat loss.

Blood vessels in the dermis provide nutrients for both the dermis and the avascular epidermis. The vessels must remain patent or the skin will die from lack of oxygen. A decubitus ulcer or pressure sore forms when such vessels are occluded by pressure. Blood flow through the dermal vessels can affect skin color. For example, cutaneous vasoconstriction, which occurs with shock or exposure to cold, may cause the skin to become pale or mottled. Vasodilation, which often occurs with fever or emotions such as embarrassment, may cause the skin to become flushed or bright red. Redness may also occur in a localized area when capillary congestion results from acute inflammation.

Subcutaneous Tissue. The subcutaneous tissue or hypodermis is composed of connective tissue infiltrated with fat. Blood and lymph vessels, nerves, and glands are also located in the hypodermis. The subcutaneous layer varies in thickness throughout the body. For example, this tissue is usually thicker in the abdominal area, upper arm, and thigh, and is virtually absent in other areas such as the eyelids. Subcutaneous tissue functions as a calorie reserve, heat source, insulator, and shock absorber.

Appendages. The skin appendages result from invaginations of the epidermis into the dermis. *Hair* is a skin appendage composed of the protein keratin. The visible portion of the hair is the hair shaft, which is embedded in the hair follicle beneath the skin's surface. Sebaceous glands, attached to the hair follicles, secrete oil. Tiny muscles associated with the glands constrict when stimulated, which causes the hair to stand out and small indentations to be noted on the surrounding skin ("goose bumps")

Generally, the appearance and distribution of hair varies with age, sex, and genetic background. This pattern, however, may be altered in nutritional and metabolic disorders such as starvation and hypothyroidism. Two types of hair, vellus and terminal, are distributed over the entire body except the palms of the hands, the soles of the feet, and parts of the genitals. Vellus hair, finely textured and not readily visible, includes the short hairs often observed on the faces of women. Terminal hair, generally coarser and with a longer shaft, includes scalp hair, pubic hair, and leg hair. Hair is constantly being formed and shed; the scalp loses from 20 to 100 hairs per day.

Nails are also composed of keratin. Low water content and high sulfur content contribute to nail hardness. The nail surface, called the plate, is derived from the nail matrix, which is not visible. The first part of the nail plate to form is the lunula, the half-moon–shaped portion at the nail base. The lunula is the only part of the nail plate that will not blanch when pressure is applied. Blanching is secondary to occlusion of the rich capillary network underlying the nail plate. The two types of skin surrounding the nail, the hyponychium and the eponychium, are susceptible to nail disease.

Similar to the hair, the nails are constantly renewed. Nail growth and shape depends on adequate nutrient and oxygen supplies. Under normal conditions, a fingernail can completely regenerate in 170 days.

Two types of *sweat glands* are located in the skin: eccrine and apocrine. The apocrine glands, found mainly in hairy areas such as the axillae and the groin, develop after puberty. The odor of perspiration is related to a bacterial breakdown of secretions from the apocrine glands. The eccrine glands are widely distributed and secrete sweat. Such secretory activity is important in regulation of body temperature.

Physical Examination   ## Skin, Hair, and Nails

General Principles

Assess the skin, hair, and nails by inspection and palpation. Further assess any detected abnormalities by interviewing the person and inquiring how long the abnormality has been present; whether any associated pain or discomfort is present; what exacerbates or relieves the finding; and what other pathology or disease may be involved. Wound healing, whether from injury or surgery, can be an indicator of a person's nutritional and metabolic status. Wounds should be monitored and assessed for normal healing.

Equipment

- Metric ruler for measuring skin lesions
- Gloves for skin palpation if body fluid precautions are indicated

Exposure and Lighting

Expose skin crevices and pressure points where lesions such as pressure sores may be in early stages of formation. Uncover wounds to assess healing, and note any excessive drainage, provided such a practice is not contraindicated. A good source of lighting will ensure thorough and effective skin examination. Good lighting is especially important for accurately assessing skin color because color changes are often subtle.

Thoroughness

Examine the skin and hair thoroughly from the head to the toes, and evaluate vulnerable areas. For example, if you are examining an immobilized patient for signs of skin breakdown, focus on inspecting the skin overlying body pressure points, which are areas at highest risk for breakdown and pressure sores (decubitus ulcers). In addition to the bony prominences of the occiput, scapulae, sacrum, greater trochanters, and heels, other pressure points to be examined include those areas in which the skin is in contact with tubes used for treatment, including the nares (nasogastric tube), lips (endotracheal tube), or ears (oxygen cannula tubing). Also, examine the skin underneath tape, restraints, skin folds, and pendulous breasts, where moisture is easily trapped and may contribute to skin breakdown or the growth of microorganisms.

Comparisons Compare the left and right sides of the body whenever an abnormal integumentary finding is detected. For example, if the left foot feels cold and clammy, check the right foot for similar signs. Is an abnormal appearance in one nail plate evident in all of the nail plates? Does a rash appear on one arm but not the other?

Examination and Documentation Focus
- *Skin:* Color and pigmentation, moisture, temperature, texture and thickness, turgor and mobility, hygiene, lesions (particularly decubitus ulcers for bedridden persons) and healing of any wounds
- *Hair:* Color and pigmentation, quantity, texture, distribution, hygiene
- *Nails:* Shape and configuration, color, lesions

Examination Guidelines *Skin*

Procedure

1. SURVEY THE SKIN TO EVALUATE COLOR AND PIGMENTATION.

2. SURVEY AND PALPATE THE SKIN TO EVALUATE MOISTURE.

Clinical Significance

Normal Findings

Lighter-pigmented races: Skin color will appear ivory to pink with possible olive or yellow overtones. Exposed areas are usually darker in color than nonexposed areas.

Darker-pigmented races: Skin color will appear tan to dark brown. The lips may have a bluish hue in people of Mediterranean descent. Blacks may have a blue or reddish hue to lips and mucous membranes.

Hyperpigmentation such as freckles on face and arms is common in light-skinned people.

Yellow skin may be associated with callusing or, when confined to a specific area, pigment retention.

Deviations from Normal Skin

Skin color deviations suggest compromises in metabolism, circulation or oxygenation.

Pallor: Paleness; usually generalized if abnormal. Reflects decreased oxyhemoglobin concentration.

Jaundice: Yellow cast; usually generalized if abnormal; secondary to impaired bilirubin metabolism. In a black person, jaundice is difficult to observe on the skin but can be detected by inspecting the sclera of the eyes for yellow discoloration. However, it is important to distinguish sclera yellowing from pigment accumulation in the sclera, which appears more concentrated.

Cyanosis: Bluish cast. Observe the distribution of cyanosis. Cyanosis of the mucous membranes and around the mouth (circumoral) is called central cyanosis and indicates an excessive amount of circulating deoxygenated hemoglobin (approximately 5 gm/2100 mL before detectable by inspection). Cyanosis that involves the extremities and lips is called peripheral cyanosis and indicates reduced peripheral blood flow.

Erythema: Redness; when confined, reflects a local inflammatory response. Widespread erythema is associated with systemic vasodilation or polycythemia.

Normal Findings

Normal skin is dry to touch, but moisture may accumulate in skin folds. A slightly warm, moist feeling is noted if the person is in a warm environment or is exercising and perspiring to cool the body. Anxiety may cause sweaty palms and perspiration in the axillae and on the forehead and scalp.

GUIDELINES   *continued*   *Skin*

Procedure

3. PALPATE THE SKIN TO DETERMINE TEMPERATURE.

4. SURVEY AND PALPATE THE SKIN TO EVALUATE TEXTURE AND THICKNESS

5. EVALUATE SKIN TUGOR BY LIFTING A FOLD OF SKIN BETWEEN YOUR THUMB AND FOREFINGER.

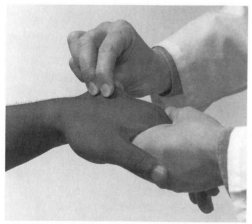

Evaluating skin turgor

6. SURVEY GENERAL HYGIENE OF THE SKIN.

Make note of infestations, irritating body secretions, or secretions with potential for disrupting skin integrity.

7. EXAMINE THE SKIN FOR THE PRESENCE OF EDEMA (SWELLING).

a. Survey dependent body parts. In bedridden persons, survey the lower extremities or sacrum.

Clinical Significance

Deviations from Normal

Dryness, sweating, or oiliness may be abnormal but are not always clinically significant. Determine whether these conditions are widespread or confined to certain areas. Diaphoresis (profuse sweating) can occur in shock states. Abnormally dry skin may indicate dehydration.

Normal Findings

The skin should feel warm. Cool skin temperatures may also be normal if coolness is accompanied by a dry skin surface.

Deviations from Normal

Local increases in skin temperature accompany acute inflammation. Decreased skin temperature is noted with vasoconstriction or arterial insufficiency.

Normal Findings

Unexposed skin is smooth, whereas exposed skin may be rough, especially on the feet and hands. Skin thickness varies; the epidermis covering the eyelids and ears may be 1/50 inch thick, whereas the epidermis over the soles of the feet may be as thick as 1/4 inch.

Deviations from Normal

Note very thin skin that may be friable, easily broken, or disrupted in integrity. Very rough skin may also be abnormal.

Normal Findings

Skin is elastic and rapidly returns to original shape when grasped between thumb and forefinger.

Deviations from Normal

Poor skin turgor is demonstrated if the skin is slow to resume its original shape when pinched. Loss of turgor occurs with dehydration or as a normal aging process.

Normal Findings

Hygienic practices associated with the skin, such as frequency of bathing, vary widely depending on the individual's cultural and social practices and physiologic needs. Health skin usually is clean.

Deviations from Normal

Edema or swelling occurs as a result of excess fluid in the tissues. Causes include increased capillary hydrostatic pressure, which occurs from renal disease or congestive heart failure, and decreased capillary oncotic pressure, which occurs from protein deficits. In addition, edema may result from tumors or injuries that obstruct lymphatic drainage channels.

Edema in dependent body parts can be a sign of heart failure.

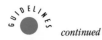 *continued*   *Skin*

Procedure

b. Press on edematous skin with your thumb or forefinger.

c. Quantify the extent of edema (grading edema) by gently pressing the edematous area with your thumb or fingers for up to 5 seconds. Note: The method of grading edema is somewhat subjective and reported findings may vary between examiners. Nevertheless, grading edema is a common clinical practice. Serial examinations by the same examiner are most reliable. (See display, Grading Edema.)

8. EXAMINE THE SKIN FOR PRESENCE OF LESIONS.

a. Note any distinguishing characteristics of the lesion: color, texture, and general appearance.

b. Note size of lesion(s). You may want to measure the diameter with a metric ruler.

c. Note patterns of distribution for lesions.

Clinical Significance

For detailed descriptions of the types of skin lesions, see displays: Primary and Secondary Skin Lesions and Vascular Skin Lesions.

Some skin disorders are recognized according to distribution patterns over the body as well as on the basis of primary lesions. (See display, Distribution Patterns for Skin Disorders.)

Grading Edema

1+ Pitting Edema

- Slight indentation (2 mm)
- Normal contours
- Associated with interstitial fluid volume 30% above normal

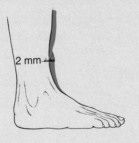

2+ Pitting Edema

- Deeper pit after pressing (4 mm)
- Lasts longer than 1+
- Fairly normal contour

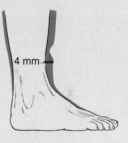

3+ Pitting Edema

- Deep pit (6 mm)
- Remains several seconds after pressing
- Skin swelling obvious by general inspection

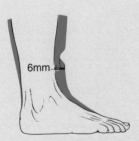

4+ Pitting Edema

- Deep pit (8 mm)
- Remains for a prolonged time after pressing, possibly minutes
- Frank swelling

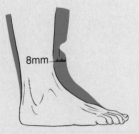

Brawny Edema

- Fluid can no longer be displaced secondary to excessive interstitial fluid accumulation
- No pitting
- Tissue palpates as firm or hard
- Skin surface shiny, warm, moist

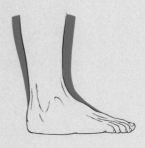

(continued)

Primary Skin Lesions

Primary skin lesions are original lesions arising from previously normal skin. Secondary lesions can originate from primary lesions.

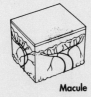

Macule, Patch

- *Macule:* <1 cm, circumscribed border
- *Patch:* >1 cm, may have irregular border
- Flat, nonpalpable skin color change (color may be brown, white, tan, purple, red)

Examples:

Freckles, flat moles, petechia, rubella, vitiligo, port wine stains, ecchymosis

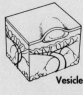

Vesicle, Bulla

- *Vesicle:* <0.5 cm
- *Bulla:* >0.5 cm
- Circumscribed, elevated, palpable mass containing serous fluid

Examples:

Vesicles: Herpes simplex/zoster, chickenpox, poison ivy, second degree burn (blister)

Bulla: Pemphigus, contact dermatitis, large burn blisters, poison ivy, bullous impetigo

Papule, Plaque

- *Papule:* <0.5 cm
- *Plaque:* >0.5 cm
- Elevated, palpable, solid mass
- Circumscribed border
- Plaque may be coalesced papules with flat top

Examples:

Papules: Elevated nevi, warts, lichen planus

Plaques: Psoriasis, actinic keratosis

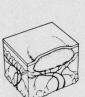

Wheal

- Elevated mass with transient borders
- Often irregular
- Size, color varies
- Caused by movement of serous fluid into the dermis
- Does not contain free fluid in a cavity as, for example, a vesicle

Examples:

Urticaria (hives), insect bites

Nodule, Tumor

- *Nodule:* 0.5–2 cm
- *Tumor:* >1–2 cm
- Elevated, palpable, solid mass
- Extends deeper into the dermis than a papule
- Nodules circumscribed
- Tumors do not always have sharp borders

Examples:

Nodules: Lipoma, squamous cell carcinoma, poorly absorbed injection, dermatofibroma

Tumors: Larger lipoma, carcinoma

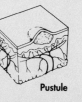

Pustule

- Pus-filled vesicle or bulla

Examples:

Acne, impetigo, furuncles, carbuncles

Cyst

- Encapsulated fluid-filled or semisolid mass
- In the subcutaneous tissue or dermis

Examples:

Sebaceous cyst, epidermoid cyst

Secondary Skin Lesions

Secondary skin lesions result from changes in primary lesions.

Erosion

- Loss of superficial epidermis
- Does not extend to dermis
- Depressed, moist area

Examples:
Ruptured vesicles, scratch marks

Erosion

Ulcer

- Skin loss extending past epidermis
- Necrotic tissue loss
- Bleeding and scarring possible

Examples:
Stasis ulcer of venous insufficiency, decubitus ulcer

Ulcer

Fissure

- Linear crack in the skin
- May extend to dermis

Examples:
Chapped lips or hands, athlete's foot

Fissure

Scales

- Flakes secondary to desquamated, dead epithelium
- Flakes may adhere to skin surface
- Color varies (silvery, white)
- Texture varies (thick, fine)

Examples:
Dandruff, psoriasis, dry skin, pityriasis rosea

Scales

Crust

- Dried residue of serum, blood or pus on skin surface
- Large adherent crust is a scab

Examples:
Residue left following vesicle rupture: impetigo, herpes, eczema

Crust

Scar (Cicatrix)

- Skin mark left after healing of a wound or lesion
- Represents replacement by connective tissue of the injured tissue
- Young scars: red or purple
- Mature scars: white or glistening

Examples:
Healed wound or surgical incision

Scar

Keloid

- Hypertrophied scar tissue
- Secondary to excessive collagen formation during healing
- Elevated, irregular, red
- Greater incidence in blacks

Example:
Keloid of ear piercing or surgical incision

Keloid

Atrophy

- Thin, dry, transparent appearance of epidermis
- Loss of surface markings
- Secondary to loss of collagen and elastin
- Underlying vessels may be visible

Example:
Aged skin, arterial insufficiency

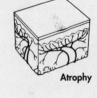
Atrophy

Lichenification

- Thickening and roughening of the skin
- Accentuated skin markings
- May be secondary to repeated rubbing, irritation, scratching

Example:
Contact dermatitis

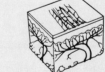
Lichenification

Vascular Skin Lesions

Petechia (*pl.* petechiae)

- Round red or purple macule
- Small: 1–2 mm
- Secondary to blood extravasation
- Associated with bleeding tendencies or emboli to skin

Petechiae

Ecchymosis (*pl.* ecchymoses)

- Round or irregular macular lesion
- Larger than petechia
- Color varies and changes: black, yellow, and green hues
- Secondary to blood extravasation
- Associated with trauma, bleeding tendencies

Ecchymoses

Cherry Angioma

- Papular and round
- Red or purple
- Noted on trunk, extremities
- May blanch with pressure
- Normal age-related skin alteration
- Usually not clinically significant

Cherry angioma

Spider Angioma

- Red, arteriole lesion
- Central body with radiating branches
- Noted on face, neck, arms, trunk
- Rare below the waist
- May blanch with pressure
- Associated with liver disease, pregnancy, vitamin B deficiency

Spider angioma

Telangiectasis (Venous Star)

- Shape varies: spider-like or linear
- Color bluish or red
- Does not blanch when pressure is applied
- Noted on legs, anterior chest
- Secondary to superficial dilation of venous vessels and capillaries
- Associated with increased venous pressure states (varicosities)

Telengiectasis

Distribution Patterns for Skin Disorders

A number of skin disorders are recognized according to distribution patterns over the body as well as on the basis of the primary lesion.

Adult Atopic Eczema

Lesions noted especially on the flexor surfaces of the body.

Lesions: Erythema, papules, vesicles, pustules, crusts

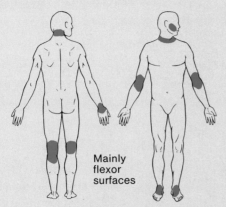

Mainly flexor surfaces

Adult atopic eczema

Psoriasis

Lesions noted especially on the extensor surfaces of the body.

Lesions: Pink or red based, topped with silvery scales; may be confluent (merged together)

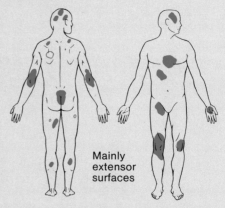

Mainly extensor surfaces

Psoriasis

Distribution Patterns for Skin Disorders (continued)

Seborrheic Dermatitis

Lesions noted especially on the scalp, nasolabial folds, and axillary, interscapular, sternal, and genitocrural regions.

Lesions: Rounded, irregular, or circular, covered with yellowish or brownish gray greasy scales

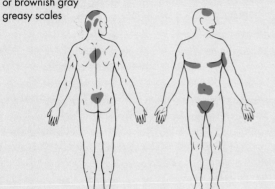

Seborrheic dermatitis

Acne Vulgaris

Noted especially on face, neck, chest, and back.

Lesions: Papules, comedones, pustules

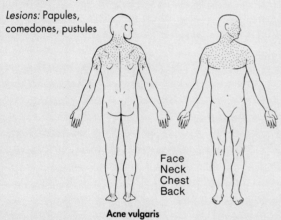

Face
Neck
Chest
Back

Acne vulgaris

Lichen Planus

Found primarily on extremities.

Lesions: Papules and scaly patches; associated with severe itching

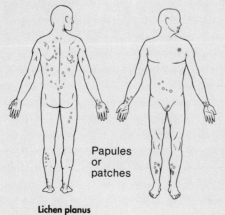

Papules
or
patches

Lichen planus

Contact Dermatitis

Affects surfaces in contact with the irritating agent. Diagram depicts contact dermatitis from contact with cosmetics, lotions, earrings.

Lesions: Erythema, papules, vesicles, pustules, crusts

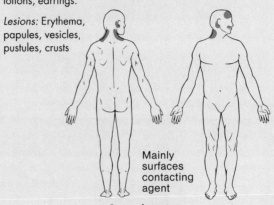

Mainly
surfaces
contacting
agent

Contact dermatitus

Herpes Zoster (Shingles)

Distribution is along cutaneous nerve tracts, almost always unilateral.
Lesions: Painful vesicles

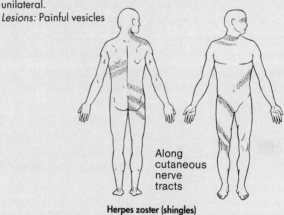

Along
cutaneous
nerve
tracts

Herpes zoster (shingles)

Pityriasis Rosea

Distributed mainly over the trunk; rare on the face.

Lesions: Macular lesions covered with scales; centers eventually clear, leaving elevated reddish rings with pale centers (ringworm-like)

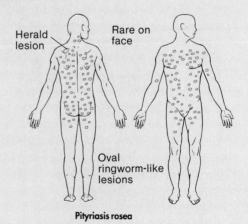

Herald
lesion

Rare on
face

Oval
ringworm-like
lesions

Pityriasis rosea

Examination Guidelines *Decubitus Ulcers*

Procedure

1. IDENTIFY DECUBITUS ULCERS (PRESSURE SORES).

   Carefully examine pressure points and skin over bony prominences.

2. STAGE DECUBITUS ULCERS BASED ON THE EXTENT OF DAMAGE TO SKIN LAYERS AND STRUCTURES BENEATH THE SKIN.

Clinical Significance

Decubitus ulcers are skin lesions resulting from prolonged pressure. Pressure deprives the skin of oxygen, an essential nutrient, and results in changes in skin appearance and integrity. (See display, Stages of Decubitus Ulcers.)

Stages of Decubitus Ulcers

Stage I

- Blood stasis in underlying tissues (hyperemia)
- Not relieved by massage or pressure relief
- Reddened skin color
- Warm to touch

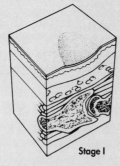

Stage I

Stage II

- Epidermal tissue loss
- May be damage to the dermis
- Moist and depressed skin erosion

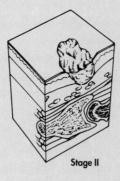

Stage II

Stage III

- Full-thickness skin loss
- Dermal ulceration may extend to the subcutaneous layer
- Serosanguineous or purulent drainage common

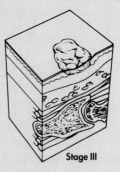

Stage III

Stage IV

- Full-thickness skin destruction
- Ulceration into deeper tissue structures (fascia, connective tissue, muscle, bone)

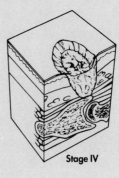

Stage IV

Examination Guidelines   *Wounds*

Procedure

1. REVIEW THE PERSON'S HISTORY AND NOTE THE PRESENCE OF THE FOLLOWING FACTORS AFFECTING WOUND HEALING.

   a. Nutritional Status

   b. Adipose tissue

   c. Oxygenation and blood supply

   d. Age

   e. Diabetes mellitus

   f. Medications
   g. Radiation therapy
   h. Infection

2. EVALUATE WOUNDS HEALING BY PRIMARY INTENTION.

   a. Note the history of the wound and determine phase of healing: inflammatory phase, proliferative phase, or maturation phase. (See display, Stages of Primary Intention Wound Healing.)

Clinical Significance

A number of factors may contribute to impaired wound healing.

Wound healing requires a diet high in protein. Vitamins A and C, and zinc are also required.

Fat tissue has fewer blood vessels, which may result in reduced oxygen delivery to the healing wound and delay healing. Adipose tissue may be more difficult to suture.

Arterial and venous insufficiency and anemia are associated with impaired wound healing.

Normal immune functions decline with increasing age; healing open wounds takes longer in the elderly.

Hemoglobin molecules in diabetics have a greater affinity for oxygen, which inhibits ready release to the wound. Hyperglycemia is associated with decreased phagocytic activity by leukocytes.

Steroids inhibit inflammation and delay healing.

Inhibits cell division.

Infection associated with wound contamination (foreign bodies, bacterial invasion) or host factors (immunosuppression) delays wound healing.

Primary or first intention wound healing occurs when there is minimal tissue loss and wound edges are closely approximated. Example: surgical wounds.

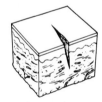

Wound healing by primary intention

Stages of Primary Intention Wound Healing

Inflammatory Phase (1–4 days)

Inflammatory Process
- Blood vessel dilation
- Increased vascular permeability

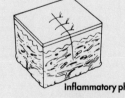

Inflammatory phase

Normal Findings
- Redness
- Swelling
- Warm to touch
- Approximation of wound edges

Deviations from Normal
- Swelling causing separation at the suture line
- Active bleeding
- Suppuration (pus formation)
- Hematoma

(continued)

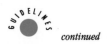

continued

Wounds

Stages of Primary Intention Wound Healing (continued)

Proliferative Phase (5–20 days)

Proliferative Processes
- Collagen synthesis
- Collagen cross-linking, increases tensile strength of the wound.

Increased collagen deposition in wound

Proliferative phase

Normal Findings
- Decreased swelling
- Decreased redness
- Approximation of wound edges even after suture removal

Deviations from Normal
- Pain
- Redness
- Swelling

- Increased white blood cell count
- Fever, especially with late afternoon or evening temperature spike
- Serosanguineous drainage
- Dehiscence (disruption of wound layers)
- Evisceration (protrusion of viscera through the incisional area)

Maturation Phase (21 days to Years)

Remodeling Processes
- Collagen synthesis and lysis
- Tissue contraction

Normal Findings
- Continual fading of scar color

Deviations from Normal
- Keloid formation

Procedure

b. Inspect the wound, noting skin color, swelling, and wound edges.

3. EVALUATE WOUNDS HEALING BY SECONDARY INTENTION.
   a. Note the history of the wound and determine phase of healing: inflammatory phase, proliferative phase, or maturation phase. (See display, Stages of Secondary Intention Wound Healing.)
   b. Inspect the wound, noting skin color, swelling, wound bed, and wound exudate.

Clinical Significance

Clinical findings will vary depending on the phase of healing. Different complications may occur at different stages of wound healing.

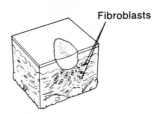

Fibroblasts

Wound healing by secondary intention

Secondary intention wound healing occurs in wounds with excessive tissue loss and suppuration (pus). Wound edges become approximated by adhesion of two granulating surfaces.

Clinical findings will vary depending on the phase of healing. Different complications may occur at different stages of wound healing.

Stages of Secondary Intention Wound Healing

Inflammatory Phase (1–4 days or longer)

Inflammation is prolonged in contaminated wounds. Purulent drainage indicates contamination and infection. The wound must be clean (debrided) before healing can occur.

Normal Findings

- Redness
- Swelling
- Moist, serous exudate in wound bed

Deviations from Normal

- White or yellow wound bed
- Purulent exudate
- Active bleeding

Proliferative Phase (5–20 days)

Proliferative Processes

- Skin repair by epithelial cell migration
- Connective tissue repair by formation of granulation tissue

Granulation Tissue

- Fibroblasts that synthesize collagen
- Newly formed capillary buds that transport nutrients and oxygen
- Phagocytic cells (monocytes, lymphocytes)

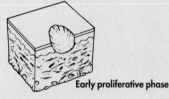

Early proliferative phase

Early Proliferative Phase:

Normal Findings

- Bright, shiny, beefy-red tissue in wound bed (color of healthy granulation tissue)

Deviations from Normal

- Dull or pale pink, yellow, or white wound bed
- Dry wound bed

Late Proliferative Phase

Normal Findings

- Progressive increase in the quantity of wound granulation tissue
- Moist, serous exudate in wound bed (needed for easy migration of epithelial cells)
- Healing ridge (represents movement of epithelial cells toward wound center)
- Progressive contraction of the wound

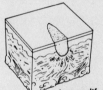

Late proliferative phase

Deviations from Normal

- Decrease in the quantity of granulation tissue
- Suppuration
- Dehiscence
- Evisceration
- Fistula formation

Maturation Phase (21 days to years)

Normal Findings

- Continual fading of scar color
- Decrease in scar size

Deviations from Normal

- Keloid formation

Examination Guidelines *Hair*

Procedure

1. INSPECT THE HAIR TO EVALUATE COLOR AND PIGMENTATION.

2. NOTE THE QUANTITY OF HAIR. PULL GENTLY AT A FEW STRANDS TO DETERMINE IF IT COMES OUT EASILY.

3. MOVE A FEW STRANDS OF HAIR BETWEEN YOUR THUMB AND FOREFINGER TO EVALUATE TEXTURE.

4. SURVEY GENERAL HYGIENE OF THE HAIR AND SCALP.

   Grasp handfuls of hair and pull it gently away from the scalp to better visualize the hair shaft and skin. Inspect carefully at the back of the head and neck.

Clinical Significance

Normal Findings

Normal hair color is largely influenced by genetic makeup and age. Natural hair colors include black, brown, red, and yellow. Pigment distribution is uniform in the hair shaft. Gray hair occurs secondary to loss of melanocytes and represents normal aging. Cosmetic alteration of healthy hair is a common practice in many cultures.

Deviations from Normal

Alterations in color and pigmentation may indicate nutrition alterations. Flag sign: Transverse depigmentation of the hair indicating nutrient deficiency, especially of copper and protein.

Normal Findings

Hair quantity generally increases after puberty in both males and females and decreases with age. Body hair quantity may vary greatly among healthy persons of both sexes.

Male balding that occurs as anterior regression of the hairline is a genetic tendency and is considered normal.

Deviations from Normal

Easy pluckability and sparse hair may be noted with protein deficiencies. Loss of hair may also occur with anemia, heavy metal poisoning, and hypopituitarism.

Normal Findings

Normal hair texture may be coarse or silky. Dark-skinned people tend to have coarser hair, whereas light-skinned people will probably have fine or silky hair.

Deviations from Normal

Very coarse hair is associated with hypothyroidism. Very fine hair is associated with hyperthyroidism.

Normal Findings

Healthy hair and scalp will have a shiny appearance and will be free from lice infestations and nits (louse eggs).

Deviations from Normal

Flakiness, sores, and infestations are considered abnormal. Lice infestations may be more readily observed in these areas.

Examination Guidelines *Nails*

Procedure

1. OBSERVE THE SHAPE AND CONFIGURATION OF THE NAIL.

Normal angle
160 degrees

Normal angle

Clinical Significance

Normal Findings

Dorsal nail surface: slightly convex. Nail thickness: 0.3 to 0.65 mm. Angle at the nail base, at the skin–nail interface, is normally 160 degrees.

continued

Nails

Procedure	Clinical Significance

Clinical Significance

Deviations from Normal

Abnormal nail shape may indicate malnutrition.

Spooning: Concave nail plates; associated with iron deficiency anemia.

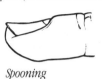

Spooning

Estimate the angle at the base of the nail where the skin and nail interface.

Clubbing: The angle at the base of the nail where the skin and nail interface is greater than 160 degrees. Clubbing is associated with congenital heart disease and pulmonary pathology. See the display, Nail Abnormalities, for other abnormalities and possible causes.

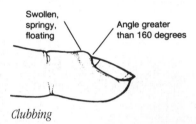

Swollen, springy, floating

Angle greater than 160 degrees

Clubbing

Nail Abnormalities

Onychorrhexis

- Brittle, fragile, uneven nail edge
- Associated with malnutrition, overhydration, thyrotoxicosis, chemical damage, radiation, aging

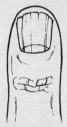

Onychorrhexis

Onychauxis

- Nail hypertrophy
- Associated with trauma, aging, fungal infections

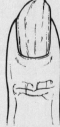

Onychauxis

Splinter Hemorrhages

- Blood streaks
- Associated with heart disease, hypertension, rheumatoid arthritis, neoplasms, trauma

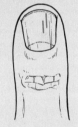

Splinter hemorrhage

Subungual Hematoma

- Blood clot
- Associated with trauma

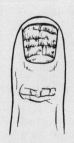

Subungual hematoma

Beau's Lines

- Transverse furrows in nail plate
- Associated with malnutrition, severe illness

Beau's lines

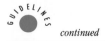

continued   ***Nails***

Procedure

2. NOTE THE COLOR OF THE NAILS.

3. SQUEEZE THE NAIL BETWEEN THE THUMB AND THE FOREFINGER
   TO DETERMINE CAPILLARY REFILL TIME.

   When pressure is released, the nail will appear white (blanching). The
   number of seconds that elapse before the nail bed returns to its baseline
   color is the capillary refill time.

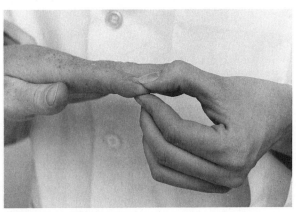

Determining capillary refill time

4. EXAMINE THE NAILS FOR PRESENCE OF LESIONS OR OTHER
   ABNORMALITIES.

Clinical Significance

Normal Findings
Uniform with the exception of color difference between lunula and the rest
of the nail. Nails appear pink in whites and may have a bluish hue in
dark-skinned people.

Deviations from Normal
Nail lesions may alter the color of the nail plate.
Cyanosis: Bluish discoloration of the nail bed; associated with pulmonary
pathology.

Normal Findings
Normal capillary refill time is less than 3 seconds.

Deviations from Normal
Capillary refill time greater than 3 seconds indicates poor tissue perfusion.

See display, Nail Abnormalities.

Documenting Integumentary Examination Findings

Describe the characteristics of any skin or nail lesions. Document the size of any lesions in the patient's record so that
any changes may be monitored. It may be helpful to draw
simple diagrams of any significant lesions and place them
in the patient's record with accompanying dimensions.

Example 1: Normal Skin
Ms. J, aged 67, was recovering from a concussion following
a motor vehicle accident. The patient was lethargic but
arousable, and she had remained in bed for the 24 hours
since hospital admission. Skin examination was conducted
as part of a routine head-to-toe examination. Examination

results were normal and recorded in the progress notes as
follows:

> Skin pale flesh color, warm, and dry without lesions; no erythema
> over pressure points; no prolonged tenting when pinched, and no
> sacral or other types of dependent edema observed.

These findings may also be recorded in a problem-oriented
format as follows:

S: Patient noncommunicative. Family reports no previ-
    ous skin problems and describes past health as excel-
    lent.
O: Immobile and requires total nursing care. Skin pink,
    warm, and dry without lesions; no erythema over
    pressure points; no prolonged tenting when pinched
    and no sacral or other types of dependent edema ob-
    served.
A: No skin alterations but remains at risk for decubitus
    ulcer formation while immobile.

P: Continue to examine skin. Turn and reposition q2h; increase to q1h if skin erythema noted over pressure points; pressure-relief mattress. Monitor nutritional and hydration status.

Example 2: Decubitus Ulcer

Mr. B, aged 88, was confined to bed following a massive cerebral vascular accident 6 months ago. He had developed a sacral decubitus ulcer that the nurses examined daily. Examination findings were charted as follows:

Sacral ulcer 5 × 6 cm; epidermal surface disrupted and dermis exposed. Wound bed reddened without drainage; small yellow patch (0.5 × 0.5 cm) noted in center of ulcer.

These findings may also be recorded in a problem-oriented format as follows:

S: Nothing to report
O: Sacral ulcer 5 cm by 6 cm; epidermal surface disrupted and dermis exposed. Wound bed reddened without drainage; small yellow patch (0.5 × 0.5 cm) noted in center of ulcer.
A: Stage II decubitus ulcer. No change in examination findings for last 2 days; no granulation tissue.
P: Continue current treatment plan as per patient care plan.

Example 3: Normal Hair

A.J., aged 6, was examined by the school nurse during a pediculosis (lice) screening program. Special attention was given to the condition of the scalp and hair. Examination findings were recorded as follows:

Hair thick, shiny, and clean. Scalp and hair shafts show no signs of flaking, redness, or infestation.

Example 4: Severe Malnutrition

G.H., aged 17, was hospitalized for treatment of severe anorexia nervosa. She was 60% below her ideal body weight. Her physical appearance had been altered as a result of malnutrition. The appearance of her hair was documented as follows:

Hair is thin and coarse. Areas of depigmentation noted in transverse distribution. Hair pulls out easily with minimal tugging. Scalp skin flaky but without redness.

Example 5: Healthy Nails

The appearance of the nails is described with attention to shape and configuration, color, and lesions. Consider the following, for example:

Nail plates smooth, uniform pinkish color, convex, and without lesions. Nail bed–skin angle 160 degrees. Capillary refill less than 3 seconds.

Example 6: Clubbing

Mr. K.K., aged 68, had a long history of chronic obstructive pulmonary disease secondary to a 40-pack year history of cigarette smoking. Manifestations of chronic hypoxia were evident during the examination of the nails and findings were recorded as follows:

Nail beds dusky-cyanotic color. Capillary refill 3 seconds. All nails have increased nail bed–skin angle of approximately 190 degrees.

NDx

Nursing Diagnoses Related to Integumentary Assessment

Impaired Skin Integrity

The nursing diagnosis of Impaired skin integrity may be applied to a person whose skin is adversely altered. The indicators of impaired skin integrity include disruption of skin surface, destruction of skin layers, and invasion of body structures. The examination guidelines in this chapter related to skin can help to identify impaired skin integrity and further evaluate any alterations. This requires identifying possible etiologies for impaired skin integrity, including environmental and mechanical factors, immobility, moisture, nutritional or metabolic problems, and circulatory problems.

Clinical Problems Related to Integumentary Assessment

Metabolic and Endocrine Pathology

Diabetes Mellitus. People with diabetes mellitus are prone to chronic skin infections with skin ulceration, especially if the disease is poorly controlled. Such infections may occur because diabetes alters immunity and peripheral circulation. Candidal (yeast) infections are common and usually occur below the breasts, between fingers and toes, in the axilla, and in female genitals, producing erythema, swelling, pain, and itching.

Ulceration and infection may occur in the feet, where circulation is often impaired. The nurse should carefully inspect the feet for redness, swelling, and pain and report such signs of inflammation to a physician.

Shin spots (brownish, rounded, painless atrophic lesions) may be observed on the pretibial area of the adult with diabetes.

Some poorly controlled diabetics may develop xanthomas, small round lesions resembling slightly elevated, soft plaques, on the lower legs or ankles.

Liver Disease. Many types of pathologic processes can affect the liver, and skin alterations may vary depending on the specific pathology. Jaundice is a common finding in most types of liver disease. Edema may also occur, and may be generalized or limited to the abdomen as protein metabolism and fluid dynamics of the liver are impaired.

Excessive alcohol consumption is a common cause of liver pathology. In clients with this problem, the skin examination may reveal palmar erythema, spider nevi over the upper chest, and skin changes associated with vitamin deficiencies. (Spider nevi are vascular skin lesions caused by capillary dilation and congestion.)

Liver pathology may interfere with estrogen metabolism. High serum levels of estrogen may cause skin changes, including gynecomastia (as increased deposition of fat in breast tissue) and pectoral alopecia (hair loss).

Renal Disease. Skin alterations observed with renal failure may be secondary to hematologic alterations caused by renal dysfunction. Pallor may be observed secondary to anemia. Purpura, a sign associated with platelet dysfunction, is caused by hemorrhage into the skin. The hemorrhage appears as a dark purple to brownish yellow macular lesion.

Some skin changes occur because the kidney can no longer metabolize or excrete certain substances. A yellow skin discoloration may occur secondary to pigment retention; it differs from jaundice in that the discoloration is not always generalized and does not affect the appearance of mucous membranes. Pigment retention may occur in the sclera and should not be confused with jaundice. Impaired metabolism may cause urate crystals to precipitate through the skin, causing a frosted appearance (uremic frost). Generalized edema may occur secondary to impaired protein metabolism and fluid retention.

Cancer. Different types of skin cancer are associated with various lesions. Cancers occurring in body systems other than the integumentary system may also lead to changes in the appearance of the skin. If you observe cancerous lesions during skin assessment, refer the client to a physician.

Actinic keratosis is a premalignant skin lesion found on areas that have been exposed to the sun. Usually, the lesion appears as a small, scaly papule with underlying erythema; scales return if the lesion is scraped off. In most cases, the borders of the lesion are well circumscribed but may become indistinct when undergoing malignant transformation. Lesions commonly occur in fair-skinned, light-haired people.

Basal cell carcinoma is a malignant skin lesion that may occur in a fair-skinned person who has been chronically exposed to sunlight. The small papular lesion grows very slowly, reaching only 1 to 2 cm in diameter after 1 year. Lesion borders usually appear semitranslucent and waxy. Telangiectatic vessels may appear, and the center of the lesion may ulcerate and invade the underlying tissue.

Squamous cell carcinoma may develop from actinic keratoses. The lesion appears as a small, hard, conical nodule that rapidly grows and invades surrounding tissues. Ulcers with poorly defined, irregular borders accompany such rapid growth.

Malignant melanoma, the most lethal type of skin cancer, arises from a malignant transformation in the melanocytes and may, in the precancerous state, exist as a mole that develops into a lesion with more elevation, more pigmentation, and a tendency to bleed easily. Lesion borders become irregular, and pigmentation may be blue, purple, red, or black.

Several skin changes may be observed with cancers not originating in the integumentary system and often occur because the cancer has affected a specific body system. A person with lung cancer, for example, may develop cyanosis as the lung tissue is damaged, whereas a person with liver cancer may be jaundiced. Persons with acquired immunodeficiency syndrome (AIDS) may develop the macular, purplish skin lesions associated with Kaposi's sarcoma. Skin infections may occur because cancer usually affects the immune system. A person with cancer who is malnourished may develop skin changes associated with vitamin, mineral, and calorie depletion.

Finally, cancer treatment may alter skin integrity. Radiation therapy, for example, can cause hair loss, erythema, dryness, and blistering of the skin surface. Chemotherapeutic agents may also cause hair loss as well as dermatitis, skin color changes, nail bed hyperpigmentation, and oral mucosa skin damage.

Nutritional Impairment

Protein-Calorie Malnutrition. Changes in the hair are indicative of protein–calorie deficiencies. If the nurse can easily pull strands of hair from the scalp (easy pluckability), the person may have a protein deficiency. Alternating bands of dark and light hair (flag sign) may indicate a protein or copper deficiency. In general, protein–calorie malnutrition causes a dull, dry, sparse hair condition. Nail changes associated with protein–calorie malnutrition include a dull, lackluster appearance and transverse ridging across the nail plate.

With a protein deficiency such as kwashiorkor, the person's entire body may become dry, with the skin flaking off like old paint (flaky paint dermatosis). Flaky skin may be noted around the nose of clients with less severe protein malnutrition.

Vitamin-Mineral Deficiencies. In severe niacin deficiency (pellagra), the person's skin also flakes, but unlike flaky paint dermatosis, the condition is limited to sun-exposed areas. Flaking skin areas usually appear darker in color. Vitamin B_6 and riboflavin deficiencies cause cheilosis, a condition in which reddening and cracking occurs at the corners of the mouth. Vascular skin lesions may be noted with vitamin C and K deficiencies. Petechiae, especially around the hair follicles, are associated with vitamin C deficiency, whereas purpura occurs with a lack of vitamin K. Vitamin A deficiency is associated with hyperkeratosis, a condition in which hair follicles become plugged with excess keratin, causing rough skin.

Iron deficiencies may cause spooning of the fingernail plates, and copper and zinc deficiencies may cause hair thinning and pigmentation changes.

Fluid Imbalance

Fluid imbalances affect the skin's turgor or mobility and place the skin at high risk for further breakdown from associated circulatory and structural impairment.

Fluid Volume Excess. Fluid volume excess contributes to impairment of the skin integrity, especially if the skin develops edema.

Fluid Volume Deficit. Loss of skin turgor is usually noted in people with dehydration. Additional skin signs include increased skin temperature, flushing, dryness, and sunken eyeballs. In advanced dehydration states, the skin may appear wrinkled.

Impaired Oxygenation

Impaired oxygenation refers to a hypoxic state secondary to either a systemic disorder such as a cardiopulmonary system disease or a localized oxygen transport problem such as occurs with decubitus ulcers or peripheral vascular disease.

Cardiopulmonary Disease. Cardiopulmonary disease may result in the following skin changes: pallor, cyanosis, flushing of the face and extremities, and edema. Pallor results from the impaired circulation and decreased red blood cells that occur with anemia. Cyanosis indicates pulmonary dysfunction and subsequent impairment of the saturation of hemoglobin with oxygen. Flushing may occur from some types of chronic obstructive pulmonary diseases; in response to chronic hypoxia, the body produces more red blood cells (polycythemia), a condition that contributes to a flushed appearance. Excessive hydrostatic capillary pressure may cause edema.

Shock involves changes that include cold, clammy, pale skin. The lips may be cyanotic. Capillary refill time is greater than 3 seconds.

Peripheral Vascular Disease. Disease in the peripheral vascular system may occur in the venous or arterial vessels. It may be either chronic or acute; it will influence skin appearance accordingly.

Acute arterial occlusion may cause the skin to feel cold and appear mottled or pale. Skin changes may progress to bleb formation, skin necrosis, cyanosis, and gangrene. *Any such finding, in addition to loss of peripheral pulses, signals a medical emergency.*

Chronic arterial occlusion, which occurs with atherosclerosis, may result in atrophic skin changes, including hair loss in the involved area (usually a lower extremity) and skin thinning. Rubor is noted when the extremity is dependent, and blanching occurs with elevation. The affected extremity may be cool on palpation.

Chronic venous insufficiency usually affects the lower extremities, and ankle edema is common. Stasis ulcers may form as a result of fluid pressure on surface capillaries. Scar tissue from previously healed stasis ulcers is common. The skin surface appears thin, shiny, and atrophic. Skin color may be cyanotic, and brownish pigment may accumulate.

Infection and Infestations

Skin infections or infestations are identified according to the characteristics and distribution of the lesions. It is important to question the patient about how the lesion developed and any associated symptoms that might help to establish the diagnosis.

Bacterial Skin Infections. Impetigo, a common bacterial skin infection, is caused by staphylococci, streptococci, or both. The bacteria is transmitted by touch, and the infection commonly occurs on the face or other exposed body areas. The lesions may appear as macules, vesicles, or pustules that become crusted and rupture. A red base is found beneath denuded lesions. The patient should be questioned about symptoms of intense itching.

Folliculitis is an inflammation of the hair follicles caused by staphylococci. Pustules may be present at the surface of the hair follicle, and the hair shaft may be observed at the center of the pustule. This infection occurs most commonly on skin that has been shaved, on the buttocks, and on areas with hair follicles. Itching may accompany the infection.

Furuncles, boils, and carbuncles are deep-seated staphylococcal infections of hair follicles. A carbuncle is the coalescence of several furuncles. The lesion is pustular with a rounded, raised core that eventually opens, releasing ne-

crotic tissue and pus. Furuncles and boils commonly occur on the back of the neck and the buttocks.

Viral Skin Infections. Herpes is responsible for many common viral skin infections. Two types of herpes simplex viruses, HSV-1 and HSV-2, have been identified. The HSV-1 virus infects the oral mucosa, labia, eyes, and the skin overlying sensory nerve segments. The HSV-2 virus infects the genitals, anus, and oral mucosa by sexual transmission. Lesions associated with both virus types are small vesicles that eventually rupture and form crusts. Erythema and itching may precede vesicle formation.

Fungal Skin Infections. Monilial or candidal infections are caused by yeast-like fungi that are part of the normal skin flora. The most common sites where this normal flora may become pathogenic are the genital, anal, and axillary areas as well as beneath breasts and between fingers and toes. The lesions appear as bright red, eroded patches. Satellite vesicopustules may or may not be present. Whitish, curd-like secretions may be observed in the affected areas, especially on oral or vaginal mucous membranes. The person may report severe itching.

Tinea (ringworm) is a fungal infection that usually occurs on the groin, scalp, feet, or trunk. The lesions vary slightly in appearance, depending on site. Tinea capitis (scalp ringworm) appears as round, scaly gray patches that cause hair breakage and lead to small bald areas. Tinea corporis (body ringworm) appears as a group of lesions surrounded by a ring. Within the ring, scaling with central clearing occurs. Small vesicles may be noted at the border of the ring. Tinea cruris (groin ringworm), also known as "jock itch," appears as erythematous macules with sharp margins. The center of the macule is clear, but vesicles appear at the borders. Tinea pedis (foot ringworm), also known as "athlete's foot," occurs in the interdigital webs and soles of the feet. In the acute phase, a reddened macular rash appears and may be followed by fissuring and tissue maceration.

Common Infestations. Scabies is a parasitic infestation of the skin caused by *Sarcoptes scabiei,* or itch mite, which usually affects the hands, wrists, axillae, genitalia, and inner aspect of the thighs. The skin of the head and neck is rarely affected. Associated lesions include small papules, vesicles, and burrows that result after the mite enters the skin to lay eggs. Burrows appear as short, irregular marks that look like they were made by a sharp pencil.

Pediculosis (lice infestation) affects the scalp, body, and pubic hairs. The eggs (nits) are visible small, white particles. The skin underlying the infested area usually appears excoriated.

Noninfectious Inflammatory Processes

Contact dermatitis, a form of eczema, is an inflammatory skin condition caused by exposure to external factors (primary irritant contact dermatitis) or specific allergens in a sensitized person (allergic contact dermatitis). Causal agents include plant oils and pollens, soaps, detergents, industrial chemicals, and rubber. Lesions appear as erythematous macules that may form vesicles and crusts. The lesions are easily infected and then discharge a purulent exudate. Distribution depends on the location of the skin that contacts the causative agent. For example, the hands may be affected if the agent is a dishwashing detergent. Similarly, the face may be affected if a cosmetic is the causative agent.

THE JAW AND ORAL CAVITY
Anatomy and Physiology Overview

The body's gastrointestinal tract begins with the oral cavity, including the lips, salivary glands, tongue and taste buds, gingiva, teeth, hard and soft palates, uvula, tonsils, and pharynx. Except for the teeth, the visible structures of the oral cavity are covered by a mucous membrane referred to as the oral mucosa.

Oral Mucosa. The oral mucosa begins inside the lips and is composed of three layers: the epithelium, the lamina propria, and the submucosa (Fig. 8-2). The oral mucosa keeps the mouth hydrated, aids in digestion, and serves as both a mechanical and a chemical barrier to trauma and infectious organisms. The lips are covered by special skin called vermilion that forms a border between the integument and oral mucosa.

The epithelium, the surface layer of the mucosa, is separated from the lamina propria by a basement membrane. Epithelial cells undergo progressive differentiation as they migrate from the basement membrane to the outermost layer. Rapid cell growth and differentiation occur in the epithelium, and the epithelial surface is renewed every 7 to 14 days. The final differentiated state of cells varies throughout the oral cavity. For example, epithelial cells in the tongue evolve to form papillae that contain the taste buds, whereas lip and cheek epithelia differentiate into cells that secrete saliva.

The lamina propria consists mainly of fibrous connective tissue that extends into the epithelium. Blood vessels and nerve endings extend through the lamina propria.

The deepest layer of the oral mucosa, the submucosa, interfaces the mucous membranes and underlying structures, such as muscle and bone. The submucosa is thin over the roof of the mouth or palate, providing the ability to withstand mechanical stress, and is thicker in the lips, cheeks, and tongue, giving a soft appearance. Blood flow through the submucosa and lamina propria accounts for the pink color of the oral mucosa. Cyanosis may occur with hypoxemia, and erythema is common with inflammation.

Salivary Glands. A number of glands in or near the oral cavity secrete saliva, including the parotid glands located below each ear, the submandibular and the sublingual glands in the floor of the mouth, and the buccal glands in the epithelium of the lips and cheeks (Fig. 8-3). The opening of the parotid gland is opposite the second molar of the upper row of teeth and is marked by a small papilla called Stensen's duct. The submandibular gland openings, called Wharton's ducts, are located under the tongue at the base of the frenulum, the structure that attaches the lower tongue to the floor of the mouth. Each sublingual gland has about 20 ducts that open over the gland's surface at the base of the mouth.

Under normal circumstances, 1500 mL of saliva is produced in a 24-hour period. The production rate varies from 0.2 mL/min when the glands are at rest, to 4 mL/min during maximum activity. Saliva production is regulated by the salivatory nuclei located in the brain stem, which are stimulated by certain tastes, odors, and tactile sensations, and even by food thoughts. Excessive salivation may be associated with nausea because the salivatory nuclei and vomiting center are in close proximity in the brain.

Saliva gives the oral mucosa a moist and shiny appearance, cleanses the mucosa, and provides protection from bacterial infections in several ways. First, saliva pH (6.0–7.0) maintains a balanced environment for the mouth's normal bacterial flora. If this balance is disrupted, uncontrolled growth of one or several organisms may occur, possibly leading to infections. Second, substances within the saliva, such as lytic enzymes and the immunoglobulin secretory IgA, further inhibit bacterial growth. In addition to protection, saliva has an important digestive function: it contains enzymes that initiate starch breakdown.

Tongue and Taste Buds. The tongue is a muscular organ extending into the pharynx; it is infiltrated with fat, and contains many mucous and serous glands. Connected to the base of the mouth by the frenulum, the tongue functions in speech, food mixing, and swallowing.

The dorsal surface of the tongue is covered by papillae, which give the tongue a rough appearance. Large vallate papillae are located toward the back of the tongue, and taste buds are located on the papillae surfaces. Each taste bud is composed of 20 epithelial taste cells. Extending to the surface of the tongue from the taste cells are microvilli, projections that sense taste stimuli. Microvilli destruction may cause taste bud degeneration and a subsequent decrease or absence of taste sensation. Ebner's glands at the back of the tongue provide serous secretions that distribute substances over the taste buds. Taste sensations are conducted to the cerebral cortex by sensory divisions of cranial nerves VII (facial) and IX (glossopharyngeal). Epithelial taste cells undergo rapid synthesis and differentiation, and are highly vulnerable to chemotherapeutic agents, which destroy rapidly dividing cells.

Although all taste buds have some ability to distinguish sweet, sour, salty, and bitter taste sensations, these four sensations are associated with different areas of the tongue.

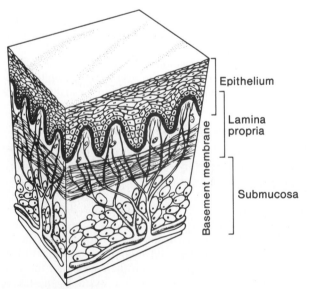

Figure 8–2. Cross section of the oral mucosa.

Epithelium

Lamina propria

Basement membrane

Submucosa

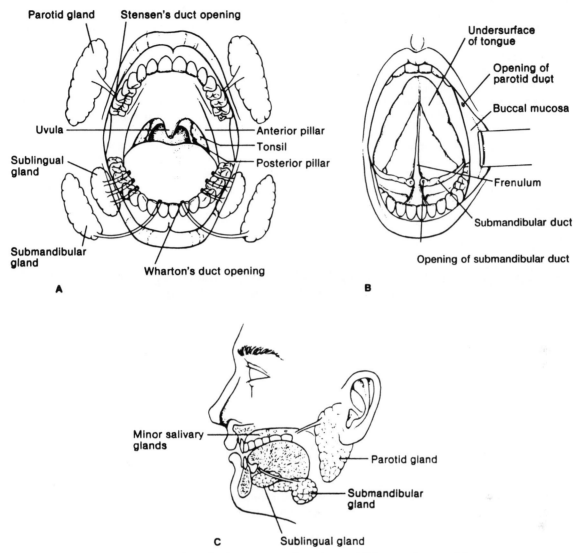

Figure 8–3. Salivary glands. (**A** and **B**) Gland openings into the oral cavity. (**C**) Anatomic location of the salivary glands.

For example, taste buds specialized to detect sweetness are located at the anterior tongue, whereas taste buds that detect bitterness are located at the posterior tongue. Sour taste buds are concentrated on the lateral surfaces, and salty tastes are detected over the tongue's entire surface.

Taste perception may decrease with age. Taste sensation is influenced by smell and may be diminished or absent when the olfactory sense is impaired.

The ventral surface of the tongue is smooth and shiny, and underlying veins are easily observed. Cranial nerve XII (hypoglossal) provides motor innervation to the tongue, allowing numerous muscular movements.

Gingiva and Teeth. The highly vascularized and innervated gingiva or gum is the oral mucosa surrounding the necks of the teeth that attaches to the maxilla and mandible. Lacking submucosal tissue, gingiva is tough and dense.

The names and locations of the 32 permanent teeth are shown in Figure 8-4. Teeth facilitate digestion by cutting, grinding, and mixing food in coordination with the jaw's

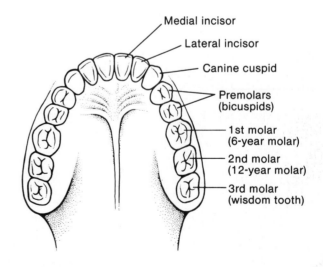

Figure 8–4. The permanent teeth.

mastication muscles, which are innervated by cranial nerves V (trigeminal) and VII (facial).

The exposed portion of the tooth, or crown, is covered by enamel, the hardest substance in the body. Nevertheless, enamel can be invaded by an adherent mass of bacteria and colorless, transparent debris called plaque.

Palate. In addition to forming the roof of the mouth, the palate separates the mouth from the oropharynx and is divided into the hard palate (anteriorly) and the soft palate (posteriorly). The hard palate assumes a convex configuration and is covered with a thick, pale mucous membrane. The soft palate, covered with a thin, red mucous membrane, extends to the uvula, the free-hanging structure at

the opening of the pharynx. The soft palate is flexible and changes shape when the mouth is relaxed; it moves upward during swallowing, closing the nasopharynx and pharynx and preventing food from being aspirated into the respiratory tract.

Oropharynx. The oropharynx lies between the soft palate and the epiglottis. The palatine tonsils, small masses of lymphoid tissue, are located on each side of the oropharynx beneath the pharyngopalatine arch behind the uvula. The epithelial tissue covering the tonsils invaginates to form surface indentations or crypts. Tonsils normally have the same color as surrounding mucous membranes.

Physical Examination   Jaw and Oral Cavity

General Principles

The oral cavity is examined by inspection and palpation. Palpate lesions with a gloved hand to determine the status of the underlying tissues. Cancerous lesions are often associated with underlying tissue hardness, which is secondary to tumor infiltration. Interview the client to obtain a history if you note oral cavity abnormalities.

Equipment

- Tongue blades
- Dental mirror
- Gauze pads (4″ × 4″)
- Gloves
- Penlight or flashlight

Exposure and Lighting

Use a flashlight or penlight to inspect the oral mucosa. Before the examination, ask the client to remove any dental prostheses. To facilitate inspection, displace the client's tongue with gauze or tongue blades and use a dental mirror.

Examinaton and Documentation Focus

- *Mucous membranes:* Color and pigmentation, moisture, texture, hygiene, lesions
- *Structural integrity:* Structural symmetry, tooth alignment, deformities
- *Functional ability:* Cranial nerves (IX [glossopharyngeal], X [vagus], XII [hypoglossal]); taste sensation; chewing; swallowing; speech

Examining the Oral Cavity of the Unconscious or Semiconscious Patient

An oral examination is relatively easy to perform when the patient is fully alert and cooperative. The person with a decreased level of consciousness, however, presents a special challenge. Because such a patient is at high risk for oral mucosa alterations, he or she should be examined frequently.

Often, semiconscious and unconscious people clench their jaws and resist opening thier mouths, especially after tactile stimulation of the lips or oral mucosa. Attempting to force the jaw open may be unsuccessful or harmful to the patient. The best approach is to wait until the person spontaneously opens the jaw and inspect as much of the oral mucosa as possible by shining a penlight into the mouth without touching the patient.

If spontaneous jaw opening does not occur, the mouth may be opened by using a chin-lift maneuver such as that used for opening an obstructed airway. Place the fingers of one hand under the patient's lower jaw while lifting the patient's chin forward to open the mouth. To perform a thorough inspection, place a hard plastic bite block between the patient's upper and lower teeth. Never place your fingers in the patient's mouth. When using a block, take precautions against unnecessary tissue trauma. Remove the block quickly, not forcefully, after the patient releases jaw pressure. A block should never compromise the patient's airway.

Be sure to assess for tissue trauma from tubes passing through the oral cavity, such as an endotracheal tube.

Examination Guidelines *Jaw and Oral Cavity*

Procedure

1. INSPECT AND PALPATE THE OUTER STRUCTURES OF THE ORAL CAVITY.

    a. Assess for malocclusion by asking the person to open and shut the jaw and expose the teeth. While the mouth is opened and closed, palpate the temporomandibular joint for tenderness and deviation.

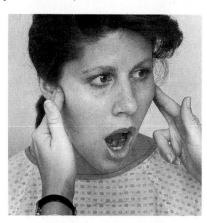

Temporomandibular joint palpation

    b. Inspect and palpate the skin over the parotid glands (anterior to the ear lobes) for symmetry and swelling.

    c. Inspect and palpate the lips.

2. EXAMINE THE DORSAL SURFACE OF THE TONGUE WHILE EVALUATING CRANIAL NERVES XII AND X.

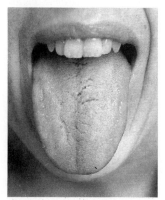

Dorsal surface of the tongue

    a. To inspect the dorsal tongue surface, ask the person to extend the tongue and say "ah."

Clinical Significance

Normal Findings

Upper and lower front teeth should align when the jaw is clenched.

Full range of voluntary motion to the mandibular joints exists; that is, the jaw can open and shut completely and the upper and lower jaws can move from side to side.

Deviations from Normal

Teeth may be missing or may deviate from normal alignment. The significance of such findings is determined by assessing functions such as chewing and talking. Missing teeth often have been replaced by partial or complete dentures, which should align with the surrounding teeth or jaw.

Deviation from Normal

Parotid gland enlargement, unilateral or bilateral.

Normal Finding

Lips are symmetric, although asymmetry is common and considered normal unless functional interference occurs.

Normal Finding

Taste buds give the posterior tongue a slightly rough texture.

Deviations from Normal

The appearance of the tongue mucosa is altered with malnutrition, inflammation, infection, and inflammatory states. During inflammatory states, the tongue forms a protective coating of a whitish cast; however, such a coating should not be confused with the white plaques that may adhere to the tongue as exudate from certain infections.

GUIDELINES *continued*   *Jaw and Oral Cavity*

Procedure

b. Note symmetry of the tongue and uvula when the tongue is protruded.

c. Inspect the soft palate when the person says "ah."

3. INSPECT THE HARD AND SOFT PALATES.

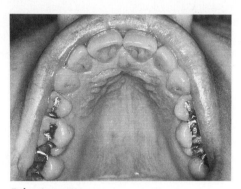

Palate inspection

Ask the person to tilt the head back with mouth open and examine the palate with a light or dental mirror.

4. EXAMINE THE OROPHARYNX, POSTERIOR TONGUE, AND UVULA.

a. If the person has difficulty holding the tongue flat, gently depress it with a tongue blade. Be careful not to initiate a gag reflex; to relax and reassure the person, explain the procedure.

b. Use a dental mirror to inspect the posterior pharynx and uvula.

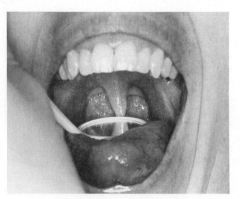

Inspection of posterior pharynx and uvula

Clinical Significance

Deviations from Normal

Loss of symmetry may indicate pathologic processes involving the nervous system. Tongue deviation as well as tremors indicate a problem with cranial nerve XII (hypoglossal).

Cranial nerve X (vagus) has one branch that innervates the soft palate.

Normal Finding

Normal nerve function is indicated by the soft palate's rising when the client says "ah."

Normal Findings

The anterior surface of the hard palate is corrugated. The palate is symmetric with no midline openings.

Structural abnormalities of the palate are often genetic.

Normal Finding

The oral mucosa of the tonsils is pink and moist, and may be characterized by crypts and indentations.

Deviation from Normal

Erythema restricted to the oropharynx usually represents a localized infection of that structure.

A gray oropharynx is a sign of diphtheria.

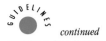

continued

Jaw and Oral Cavity

Procedure

   c. Elicit a gag reflex by touching the posterior wall of the pharynx with the tongue blade or dental mirror.

5. EXAMINE THE LIP AND CHEEK (BUCCAL) ORAL MUCOSA.

   a. Examine the underside of the lips and anterior surface of the gums by displacing the lips with fingers or gauze.

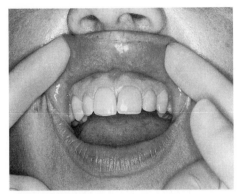

Lip displacement

   b. Examine the inner cheek by using a tongue blade or gloved finger to displace the cheek laterally and expose the surface.

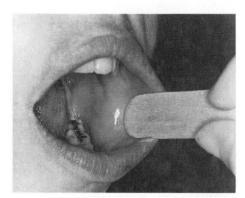

Inner cheek inspection: Using the tongue blade to expose the buccal mucosa

Clinical Significance

Normal Finding

Gagging with this manuever indicates normal function of cranial nerve IX (glossopharyngeal).

Normal Findings

Oral mucosa color inside the cheek (buccal mucosa) and lips may vary according to race. Blacks may have a slight blue undertone, and whites may have a pink or red undertone. In all races, the remaining oral mucosa appears pink, but variations in shade are normal depending on the thickness of mucosa layers. Although rare, hyperpigmentation may occur in dark- and light-skinned people as freckle-like macules inside the buccal mucosa.

The oral mucosa should appear moist secondary to saliva secretion, smooth, and free of lesions and exudates.

Deviations from Normal

Abnormal color changes include pallor (paleness or lack of color), cyanosis (bluish cast), erythema (redness), and gray mucous membranes. Any color changes are recorded in terms of location and distribution. Cyanosis usually indicates systemic hypoxemia and is distributed throughout the oral mucosa. Pallor reflects vasoconstriction of the vessels in the mucosa, which may occur with shock or before acute inflammatory states such as stomatitis, because the sympathetic nervous system is stimulated early. Stomatitis erythema is characterized by a sharp line of demarcation at the mucocutaneous border of the lips. Intensified pigmentation of the oral mucosa may be noted with Addison's disease.

Excessive dryness of the oral mucosa (xerostomia) occurs when salivary gland activity is arrested: Excessive moisture may be observed in early stages of inflammation.

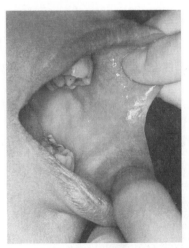

Inner cheek inspection: Using the fingers to expose the buccal mucosa

GUIDELINES *continued*   ***Jaw and Oral Cavity***

Procedure

6. EXAMINE THE LATERAL AND VENTRAL TONGUE SURFACES.

   a. Inspect the mucosa by displacing the tongue laterally.

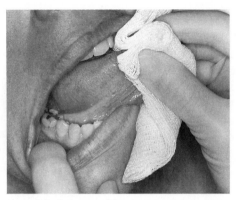

Lateral displacement of the tongue

   b. Then, ask the client to touch the hard palate with tongue tip, and examine the ventral surface. Palpate oral mucosa of the mouth floor with a gloved finger.

Clinical Significance

Oral lesions, including malignancies, may be hidden beneath the tongue. Accumulation of food and debris may indicate poor hygiene or impaired chewing or swallowing.

Oral Lesions and Conditions

Lip Vesicles

- Small lesions
- Occur singularly or in clusters
- Serous, fluid-filled masses

Example:
Herpes simplex

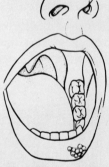

Lip vesicules

Lip Ulcers

- Necrotic loss of lip tissue

Examples:
The chancre that is the primary lesion of syphilis. A chancre ulcerates in the center and leaves a crusty residue. Pressure ulcer, such as those resulting from prolonged contact with tubes.

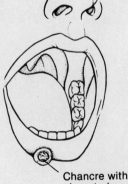

Chancre with ulcerated center

Lip ulcer

Mucocele

- Small, bluish, mucus-filled cyst
- Benign
- May be removed for cosmetic purposes

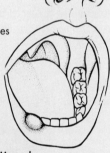

Mucocele

Cheilitis

- Inflammation and crust formation
- Lower lip most often affected
- May be chronic
- Cause often unknown

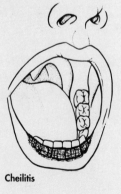

Cheilitis

(continued)

Oral Lesions and Conditions (continued)

Squamous Cell Carcinoma

- May appear as plaque, warty papule, or ulcer
- Nonhealing lesion
- Appers on lips or underside of tongue
- Most common form of oral cancer
- If not healed within 2 to 3 weeks, should be evaluated to rule out malignancy

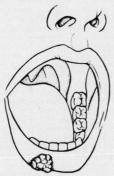

Squamous cell carcinoma

Fordyce Spots (Granules)

- Small yellow papules on oral mucosa
- Represent sebaceous glands
- Common benign lesion

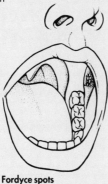

Fordyce spots

Aphthous Stomatitis (Canker Sore)

- Ulcerated lesion of oral mucosa
- Surrounded by white halo
- Tender
- Heals and recurs spontaneously
- May occur in groups

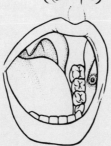

Canker sore

Torus Palatinus

- Nodular mass midline on the hard palate
- Benign
- Masses away from the midline may represent malignancies
- May not develop until adulthood

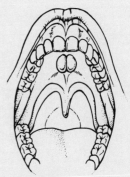

Torus palatinus

Glossitis

- Tongue becomes bright red, edematous, and smooth as papillae are lost
- Associated with stomatitis, malnutrition, chronic illness

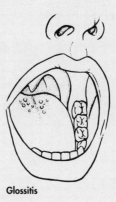

Glossitis

Hairy Tongue

- Hairy appearance secondary to papillae elongation
- Papillae dark brown or black
- Benign
- Associated with antibiotic therapy

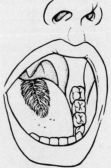

Hairy tongue

(continued)

Oral Lesions and Conditions (continued)

Leukoplakia

- Smooth, white, paint-like patch on the oral mucosa
- May represent a premalignant transformation of oral mucosa
- Associated with oral tobacco usage

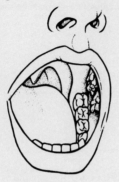

Leukoplakia

Stomatitis

- Inflammation of the oral cavity
- Mucosa, red, dry, edematous
- Predisposes oral mucosa to ulceration
- Red demarcation line may be noted at the vermilion border
- Associated with chemotherapeutic agents, dehydration, infectious agents, and radiation

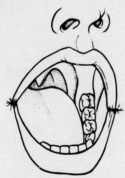

Stomatitis

Candida albicans (Yeast, Thrush, Moniliasis)

- Oral mucosa covered by white, curd-like patches
- Underlying mucosa may be bright red
- Associated with chronic illness, antibiotic therapy

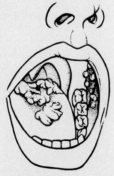

Candida albicans

Pseudomonas Infection

- Necrotic ulcers
- Dark brown central eschar
- Surrounded by erythematous ring

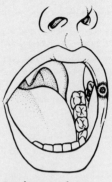

Pseudomonas infection

Streptococcal Pharyngitis

- Posterior pharynx bright red
- Tonsils, uvula, pillars may be swollen and covered with white or yellow exudate
- Definitive diagnosis requires throat culture
- Physical findings may vary

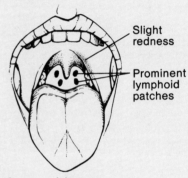

Slight redness

Prominent lymphoid patches

Streptococcal pharyngitis

Viral Pharyngitis

- Posterior pharynx red or normal in color
- Slight swelling of tonsils and uvula may occur
- Throat culture required to rule out streptococcal pharyngitis

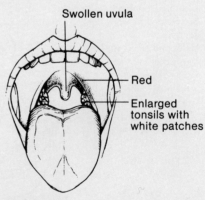

Swollen uvula

Red

Enlarged tonsils with white patches

Viral pharyngitis

Documenting Jaw and Oral Cavity Examination Findings

Example: Normal Jaw and Oral Cavity

The following was recorded after examining a 30-year-old woman:

> Temporomandibular joint palpated with jaw movement—no clicks, tenderness, or restricted range of motion. Parotids nonpalpable. Slight overbite but no associated impairment of chewing or talking. Tongue moist and shiny, and midline without tremor during protrusion. Gag reflex intact. Uvula and soft palate rises with "ah." Tonsils missing. No lesions seen or palpated on tongue, oral mucosa, or palate.

NDx

Nursing Diagnoses Related to Oral Cavity Assessment

Impaired Oral Mucous Membrane

Impaired oral mucous membrane is a state in which a person experiences disruptions in the oral cavity. During examination, you may recognize alterations as well as determine etiologies. Depending on the nature of the problem, you can then implement independent or collaborative treatment measures.

Poor Hygiene

Oral hygiene practices vary among individuals and are influenced by personal preference, sociocultural factors, and health status. Poor oral hygiene is reflected by the presence of both food debris and excessive plaque accumulation. Halitosis (bad breath) may not always indicate poor hygiene and may occur with systemic diseases.

Poor oral hygiene can contribute to or exacerbate most pathology to the oral cavity. Food debris may accumulate in the crevices between teeth. Excessive plaque buildup may be observed as a yellow or brown cast. Inadequate hygiene is a common cause of dental caries and peridontal disease. Both conditions may occur when excessive plaque accumulates on teeth and gingiva, destroying surfaces. Occasionally, peridontal disease and caries result despite good oral hygiene.

Peridontal disease (pyorrhea) is associated with plaque accumulation in dental pockets between gums and teeth. Such dental pockets enlarge as debris continues to accumulate. An inflammatory response is usually initiated; the gingiva appears swollen and red, and pus may be noted. Eventually, the gingiva recesses from the neck of the teeth, and teeth may loosen. Gingival tissue may become inflamed, and abscesses may form secondary to dental caries. Although you should screen the client for these oral mucosa lesions, regular dental examinations are essential.

Nutritional Impairment

Alterations in lip and oral mucosa may be caused by severe vitamin B and C deficiencies. For example, lack of B vitamins may result in reddened vermilion and cracks at the corners of the mouth (cheilosis). Vertical fissures may appear across the entire outer lip surface. In addition, the tongue may become swollen, bright red, and painful. Taste bud papillae may atrophy, and a smooth tongue surface may also occur. Painful ulcers (glossitis) may develop. In severe vitamin C deficiency (scurvy), the gingiva becomes spongy, bleeds easily, and recedes. The teeth may loosen and fall out.

Fluid Imbalance

The most common type of fluid imbalance that alters the oral mucosa is dehydration. Fluid deficits, which may be related to systemic factors or local assaults, cause red, dry oral mucosa. Saliva production decreases and saliva becomes more viscous.

Factors contributing to oral mucosa dehydration include inadequate hydration and actions of certain drugs, such as cholinergic blocking agents and antihistamines. A pattern of mouth breathing may decrease intravascular pressures, resulting in diminished blood flow to the oral mucosa that may contribute to dryness. Rapid respiratory rates lead to dehydration as the saliva is used to humidify inspired gases faster than saliva is produced. Oxygen administration, even with humidification devices, may cause additional oral cavity dryness.

Mechanical Trauma

Common sources of mechanical trauma include poorly fitting dentures, braces, endotracheal or nasogastric tubes, and oral cavity surgery. Improper suctioning and oral hygiene can also affect the oral mucosa. Assessing the surface of the oral mucosa that contacts prostheses or tubes is extremely important. The physical changes caused by trauma may vary depending on causes and associated infections of affected tissue. The classic signs of inflammation—redness, swelling, pain, heat, and functional impairment—are usually related to trauma.

Chemotherapeutic Agents

Anticholinergic agents and antihistamines may lead to oral mucosa dehydration, whereas antibiotics may upset microbial flora in the mouth. Chemotherapeutic agents used in cancer treatment are among the most damaging to the oral mucosa, and cause generalized stomatitis or oral cavity inflammation secondary to a lethal effect on rapidly dividing oral mucosal epithelial cells. The surface of the mucosa appears erythematous, dry, and edematous, and may be prone to ulceration. A bright red inflammatory demarcation line may be observed at the vermilion border.

Impaired Swallowing

Swallowing is a complex physiologic maneuver that occurs in three phases: oral, pharyngeal, and esophageal. Oral cavity assessment provides information about the oral phase of swallowing, which begins with placing the tongue against the hard palate. The larynx then elevates, and the tongue propels substances into the pharynx. Swallowing requires coordinated muscular movements of the tongue, which in turn depend on intact sensory and motor innervation. The pharyngeal phase of swallowing propels food or other substances from the mouth to the esophagus and is accomplished by contraction of the pharynx constrictor muscles. Normal function of these muscles is associated with a gag reflex.

Impaired swallowing may be indicated by food retention in the oral cavity, or coughing and choking while eating. The patient with impaired swallowing should be further evaluated to determine contributing factors such as neuromuscular alterations, mechanical obstruction, fatigue, decreased level of consciousness, and irritation of the oropharynx.

Clinical Problems Related to Oral Cavity Assessment

Metabolic and Endocrine Pathology

Diabetes Mellitus. Similar to the skin, the oral mucosa of patients with diabetes mellitus is susceptible to infection and ulceration because the disease alters circulation and immunity. After 10 to 15 years, a significant thickening of the vessels in the oral mucosa occurs. Impaired circulation may lead to ischemic ulcer formation in the mouth. Such lesions often heal slowly, and secondary infection is common.

Renal Disease. Severe renal disease, characterized by retention of ammonia in the body, can lead to oral mucosa impairment. Ammonia, secreted into the oral cavity through the saliva, is caustic and may cause gingival bleeding and buccal mucosa ulceration. The mouth may become dry (xerostomia), which further threatens the oral mucosa. The breath may have an ammonia odor (uremic breath), and the patient may report a metallic taste.

Cancer. Oral tumors may disrupt the patient's oral mucosa. Some systemic cancers, especially leukemia, also affect the oral cavity. Cancer treatments, including surgery, radiation, and chemotherapy, can further disrupt the oral mucosa.

Depending on the procedure, cancer surgery may disrupt the patient's oral mucosa by affecting self-care abilities or nutritional status, or by causing physical trauma.

Radiation therapy for head and neck cancers is related to death of rapidly dividing epithelial cells. The effects may be noted within 1 to 2 weeks after treatments have begun, and include inflamed mucosa, decreased saliva production, and diminished taste sensation.

THE ABDOMEN

Anatomy and Physiology Overview

Because the abdomen extends from the diaphragm to the pelvis, physical examination provides cues to the status of the gastrointestinal system and related processes such as digestion, secretion, absorption, and metabolism, as well as to the status of the genitourinary system. Certain vascular anomalies and inflammatory processes may also be detected during the abdominal examination. Although many abdominal organs are difficult to examine, some examina-

tion techniques provide indirect information about organ function. In the case of abnormal findings, abdominal examination should be augmented with diagnostic studies such as x-rays, ultrasound, endoscopic procedures, and laboratory tests.

ABDOMINAL ASSESSMENT LANDMARKS

Generally, the structures of the abdomen are not visible, but occasionally outlines of organs or structures may be observed in very thin clients. Likewise, abdominal structures are not easily palpated. The only structures that are normally palpable include the right edge of the liver at the right costal margin, the lower pole of the right kidney (in thin persons), the colon in the lower left quadrant, and rectus abdominal muscles in the midline, and aortic pulsations (in thin clients, especially women). A full and distended bladder is also palpable.

Because anatomic structures are not visible, a reference map of the abdomen is helpful. The four- and the nine-region maps are widely used (Fig. 8-5). These maps may be used to describe the location of abnormal physical examination findings and symptoms such as pain.

The four-region map, which divides the abdomen into four quadrants, is used commonly in clinical practice. An imaginary line extending from the xiphoid process to the symphysis pubis is crossed at the umbilicus by another line. The four regions are referred to as right and left upper quadrants and right and left lower quadrants. A knowledge of which abdominal organs are located in which quadrants is necessary for assessment findings to be meaningful.

The nine-region map is more specific. The numbers assigned to each of the nine regions are standard but may be confusing (see Fig. 8-5*B*). Midline regions are numbered first, and then numbers are assigned in a systematic manner to right and left areas, starting at the costal area and extending downward, as follows:

1: Epigastric
2: Umbilical
3: Suprapubic
4 & 5: Right and left hypochondriac
6 & 7: Right and left lumbar
8 & 9: Right and left inguinal

GASTROINTESTINAL MOTILITY

The esophagus, stomach, and small and large intestines are capable of peristalsis, a wave-like involuntary movement caused by contractions of the longitudinal and circular smooth muscles in the organ walls. Peristalsis depends on a functioning myoelectric complex and is influenced by the presence of food, diet composition, drugs, irritating substances such as bacteria and bile salts, and various hormones. Gastrointestinal tract distension, such as occurs from a food bolus, initiates a reflex muscular contraction of the area above and distal to the distension. Such contractions result in a progressive movement of food and fluids through the gastrointestinal tract. Although the mechanism is not clearly understood, peristalsis also occurs in fasting states to clear the gastrointestinal tract.

Peristaltic movements of the small intestine are more readily evaluated by a physical examination. A peristaltic

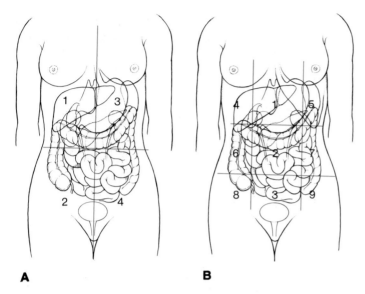

A   **B**

Figure 8–5. (A) Four-region abdominal map: (1) right upper quadrant, (2) right lower quadrant, (3) left upper quadrant, (4) left lower quadrant. **(B)** Nine-region abdominal map: (1) epigastric, (2) umbilical, (3) hypogastric (pubic), (4) right hypochondriac, (5) left hypochondriac, (6) right lumbar, (7) left lumbar, (8) right inguinal, (9) left inguinal.

"rush," or rapidly moving peristaltic wave, may be observed in a thin person by watching the surface of the abdomen. Peristaltic movements may also be evaluated by auscultating the abdomen. Created by peristaltic movements of fluid and air, bowel sounds are tinkling or gurgling sounds with a relatively high pitch and should be evaluated based on pattern and quality. Occasionally, such sounds can be heard without a stethoscope.

Because peristalsis is continual, bowel sounds should always be present, even during fasting. Sound frequency and intensity depend on the stage of digestion. Bowel sounds usually occur every 5 to 15 seconds and are more frequent 4 to 8 hours after a meal when intestinal contents are propelled over the ileocecal valve (right lower quandrant). Hypoactive or decreased bowel sounds, such as one every 2 minutes, may reflect an improperly functioning small intestine. Decreased peristalsis is associated with extensive handling of the bowel during surgery, severe hypokalemia, peritonitis, paralysis of the intestinal wall (paralytic ileus), and advanced intestinal obstruction.

Hyperactive or increased bowel sounds, such as every 3 seconds, may occur with diarrhea as intestinal contents are rapidly moved through the system, or in the early stages of intestinal obstruction, which causes distention of the bowel proximal to the obstruction. Distention stimulates an increase in the rate and force of peristalsis, which produces more frequent and higher-pitched bowel sounds (borborygmi).

THE PERITONEUM

The peritoneum is the double membrane that lines the abdominal cavity; it contains many blood vessels, lymphatic ducts, and nerves. The two layers, the visceral peritoneum and the parietal peritoneum, are separated by serous fluid. This thick membrane supports the abdominal organs, transports water and electrolytes from the abdominal cavity to the vasculature, and protects abdominal organs from infection and inflammation.

Early detection of peritoneal injuries is important because they can be life-threatening if peritoneal functions are impaired. After peritoneal injury, the bowel may be initially hyperactive, manifested by increased bowel sounds, as impaired transport mechanisms across the peritoneum retain substances and distend the bowel. Abdominal distention and rigidity also occur secondary to fluid accumulation in the retroperitoneal space. Because the peritoneum contains many nerves, the patient with peritoneal injury usually experiences severe pain. You may note rebound tenderness, which is pain elicited immediately after deep, quick palpation of the patient's abdomen.

VASCULATURE

Arterial blood is supplied to the abdomen by arterial branches from the abdominal aorta. One branch, the celiac artery, further divides into five major branches that supply blood to the stomach, spleen, gallbladder, pancreas, and duodenum. Another major branch, the superior mesenteric artery, supplies the jejunum, ileum, cecum, and ascending colon, and part of the transverse colon. The inferior mesenteric artery branches off the aorta to supply the transverse, descending, and sigmoid colon and rectum.

You may evaluate the abdominal aorta by inspection and palpation because of pulsations that may be seen and felt. If the patient has arterial obstructions affecting any of the abdominal vessels, you may find a bruit during auscultation.

The portal vein system collects blood from the entire gastrointestinal tract and delivers it to the liver. Portal vein hypertension, such as occurs with liver disease, may contribute to dramatic physical examination findings. Portal vein pressure is increased, causing congestion of blood. Consequently, collateral vessels develop to divert the flow from congested areas. The increased congestion often leads to spleen enlargement. In addition, increased pressures may force fluid out of the venous system. Ascites may be noted when fluid accumulates in the abdomen. Another consequence of portal hypertension is impaired delivery of important substances of digestion to the liver for further metabolism. Physical signs will depend on which metabolic process is affected. For example, vitamin K, a clotting factor, may not be optimally metabolized by the liver and may lead to a bleeding disorder.

Physical Examination   *Abdomen*

General Principles

The abdomen is examined in the following sequence: Inspect, auscultate, percuss, lightly palpate, and deeply palpate. Always auscultate the abdomen first, because percussion and palpation may alter the character of bowel sounds. Use the diaphragm of the stethoscope to auscultate high-pitched bowel sounds and the bell of the stethoscope to detect lower-pitched vascular sounds such as bruits, venous hums, and friction rubs.

Perform light palpation before deep palpation. Percussion and palpation may be combined; preferably, you should assess an organ completely by both methods before continuing. For example, percuss the liver borders, then palpate the liver.

Equipment

• Stethoscope
• Metric ruler or tape measure

Positioning, Preparation, and Exposure

Ask the person to assume a supine position with knees slightly flexed to help relax the abdominal muscles. Place a pillow beneath the head and knees for complete relaxation. Instruct the patient to place arms at the sides or across the chest. If the arms are over the head, the abdomen may tighten, making examination difficult. The person's bladder should be empty. Stand at the person's right side because many special examination techniques involve the liver and other right-side structures.

Because many patients may be apprehensive about the examination, explain the procedure to alleviate anxiety, and drape the chest and groin to ensure modesty. If the patient is ticklish or extremely anxious about the procedure, begin palpating the abdomen with the patient's hand under your hand.

Before initiating the examination, ask the patient if any abdominal areas are especially tender or painful. Such areas should be examined last, and the patient should be assured that existing discomfort will not be aggravated.

Keep the patient warm during the examination to avoid abdominal tensing. In addition, the examining room, your hands, and the stethoscope should be warm.

Measurements

Measure skin lesions on the abdomen with a metric ruler, and measure abdominal distention to monitor changes. Wrap a tape measure around the abdomen at the umbilicus or highest point, and then mark the exact area where the tape measure was placed on the skin for accurate successive measurements. Special techniques are available for measuring abdominal enlargement during pregnancy, and are discussed in Chapter 15. Measure the width of aortic pulsations if you suspect an aneurysm and if pulsations are visible.

Other Cues

Monitor the patient's facial expression and body language during the examination. Be especially sensitive to facial expressions of pain, tenderness, and anxiety. Try to determine what action precipitated a change in expression.

Examination and Documentation Focus

• *Inspection:* Contour, symmetry, masses, pulsations, peristalsis, skin integrity, respiratory movements
• *Auscultation:* Bowel sounds, vascular sounds
• *Percussion:* Tone, outline of abdominal organs
• *Palpation:* Muscle tone, organ characteristics, tenderness, masses, pulsations, fluid accumulation

Examination Guidelines   *Abdomen*

Procedure	Clinical Significance

Procedure

1. INSPECT THE OUTER ABDOMINAL SURFACE.

   a. Stand at the patient's right side with the abdomen exposed and note symmetry, masses, pulsations, skin integrity, and respiratory pattern. Ask the patient to cough to elicit previously unseen masses.

   b. Sit or stoop and view the abdomen tangentially to evaluate contour and peristaltic rushes.

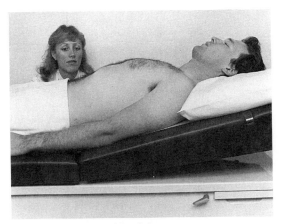

Tangential inspection of the abdomen

Clinical Significance

Normal Findings

Abdomen symmetric around the midline. No visible masses. Pulsation of the abdominal aorta at the midline and peristaltic rushes may be seen in thin people.

Deviations from Normal

No lesions should be present other than secondary lesions in the form of surgical scars. Although scars usually are not considered abnormal, the procedure that caused the scar and the related sequelae of abdominal adhesions should be considered.

Striae may be present if the skin has been stretched, as in pregnancy, obesity, abdominal tumors, and Cushing's disease.

Respirations are abdominal in men (the abdomen rises and falls with breathing).

Deviations from Normal

Visible abdominal masses: A mass that appears as a bulge when the person coughs or raises the head and shoulders may represent a hernia, an abnormal projection through the abdominal wall. Abdominal wall defects allow structures such as peritoneum, fat, bowel, or bladder to protrude. If the bulging is intermittent and appears only with coughing, the hernia is *reducible. Incarcerated hernias* always contain some abdominal contents. *Strangulated hernias* are so tightly constricted that the blood supply is cut off. Gangrene may result without surgical intervention.

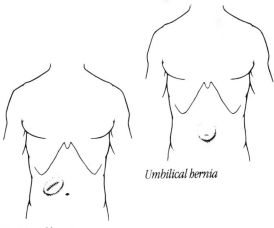

Umbilical hernia

Incisional hernia

GUIDELINES   *continued*   ***Abdomen***

Procedure	Clinical Significance

c. Identify altered abdominal contours.

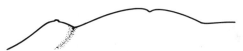

Generalized enlargement with umbilicus inverted

Gas distention, obesity

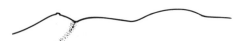

Distention over lower half

Ovarian mass, pregnancy, bladder distention

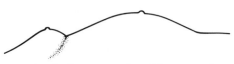

Generalized enlargement with umbilicus everted

Ascites, tumor, umbilical hernia

Scaphoid abdomen

Starvation, replacement of subcutaneous fat with muscle

2. AUSCULTATE THE ABDOMEN.

   a. Listen for bowel sounds using the diaphragm of the stethoscope. Listening to each quadrant is not necessary if pitch and frequency are normal. If bowel sounds are hypoactive or absent, listen for 1 or 2 minutes in each quadrant.

   Normal bowel sounds: High-pitched, "gurgling" sounds. Irregular frequency; range from 5 to 35/minute.

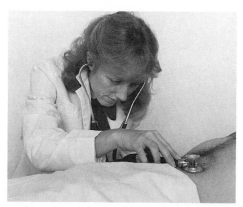

Abdominal auscultation: Listening for bowel sounds

GUIDELINES

continued

Abdomen

Procedure

b. Use the bell of the stethoscope to auscultate vascular sounds and friction rubs over the abdomen.

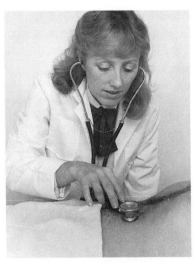

Abdominal auscultation: Listening for vascular sounds

Clinical Significance

Deviations from Normal

Vascular sounds (bruits and venous hums) are not normal findings. A friction rub indicates an inflammatory process.

A venous hum is a systolic bruit often heard when the liver is cirrhotic. Atherosclerosis of the renal and iliac arteries, and partial occulsion may cause bruits. Friction rubs may be heard over a damaged liver or spleen.

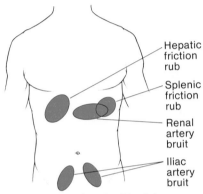

Hepatic friction rub

Splenic friction rub

Renal artery bruit

Iliac artery bruit

Auscultatory landmarks of the abdomen

3. PERCUSS THE FOUR ABDOMINAL QUADRANTS.

Systematically percuss the four quadrants of the abdomen to evaluate abnormal sounds.

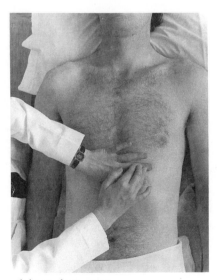

Abdominal percussion

Normal Findings

Tympany predominates, with dullness heard over solid organs and masses.

Deviations from Normal

Abdominal masses and fluid percuss as dull. Note the dullness of epigastric, ovarian, and uterine tumors that displace hollow, tympanic-sounding bowel.

continued

Abdomen

Procedure

4. PERCUSS THE LIVER.

   a. Percuss upper and lower liver borders at the midclavicular line, starting at a level below the umbilicus. A tympanic note indicates gas in the underlying bowel. As you percuss along the midclavicular line toward the head, the sound will become dull near the lower costal margin, the lower liver border.

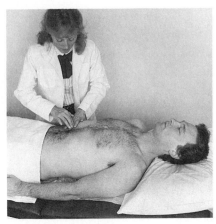

Percussing the lower liver border

Clinical Significance

Percussion is used to estimate liver span.

Normal liver span: 6 to 12 cm at the midclavicular line; 4 to 8 cm at the midsternal line.

Because liver span is related to lean body mass, men and taller people usually have greater spans than women and shorter people.

Deviations from Normal

The liver may be displaced downward if the diaphragm is low, which may occur in obstructive pulmonary diseases. However, liver span should not be affected.

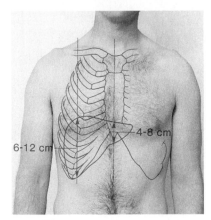

6-12 cm

4-8 cm

Normal liver span

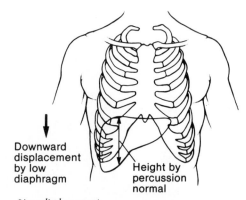

Downward
displacement
by low
diaphragm

Height by
percussion
normal

Liver displacement

GUIDELINES *continued*

Abdomen

Procedure

To locate the upper liver border, percuss along the midclavicular line at the upper thorax. A resonant percussion note indicates underlying lung tissue. The sound will become dull at the upper liver border.

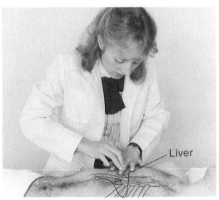

Abdominal percussion: Locating the upper liver border

b. To determine the span of the left side of the liver, percuss along the midsternal line. Begin at the umbilicus and move upward until you note dull sounds. Then percuss this line in the thorax and move down until you hear dullness again.

Clinical Significance

Percussion may be distorted in right lung consolidation, which may occur in right pleural effusion, pneumonia, or lung mass. Consequently, you may note dullness over the diseased lung, which could be mistaken for the liver border. Percussion may also be distorted when excessive gas is present in the bowel and may sound tympanic at the lower edge of the liver. In such cases, guard against overestimating liver size.

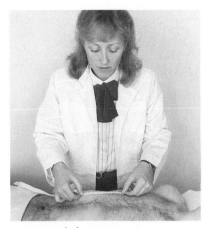

Measuring the liver span

Liver enlargement: The liver is usually enlarged in cases of cirrhosis, hepatitis, and venous congestion such as occurs with right heart failure.

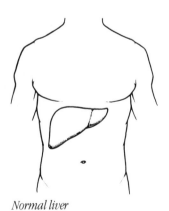

Normal liver

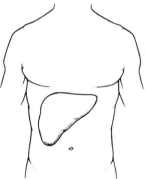

Liver enlargement

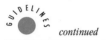

continued   ***Abdomen***

Procedure

5. PERCUSS THE STOMACH AND SPLEEN.

   a. The gastric air bubble in the stomach produces a tympanic percussion sound, which you can note by percussing at the left lower rib cage.

   b. Percuss splenic dullness at the area of the left 10th rib, posterior to the midaxillary line. This may be difficult to hear with the patient supine, but it may be easier with the patient lying midway between the supine and right lateral positions.

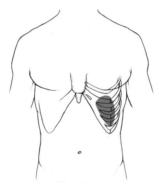

Location of the spleen

6. LIGHTLY PALPATE THE FOUR ABDOMINAL QUADRANTS.

   Lightly palpate by indenting the abdomen about 1 cm. Use smooth, circular movements with your finger pads, holding the fingers together. Systematically palpate each quadrant, noting any masses, muscle tenderness, or guarding. Monitor the client's facial expression. If the person is not relaxed, the entire abdomen may feel tense. Encourage the person to take slow, deep breaths and exhale with the mouth open. The abdomen should feel relaxed on exhalation.

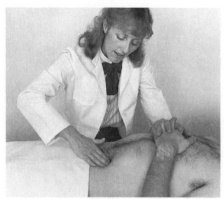

Light abdominal palpation

Clinical Significance

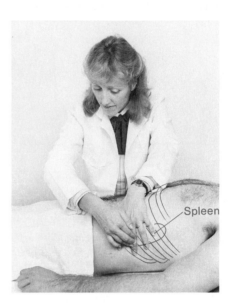

Normal Findings

Abdominal muscles may be palpable. They should feel relaxed on light palpation rather than tightly contracted or spastic. Muscle contraction may be noted with anxiety.

Rectus abdominus muscle: This muscle includes two large, midline muscles that extend from the xiphoid process to the symphysis pubis, tightly approximated at the abdominal midline. Occasionally, a separation of the rectus abdominal muscle can be observed, especially in obese or pregnant clients, by palpating the midline as the person raises the head. A midline ridge may occur with this maneuver, but it does not represent a significant problem.

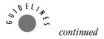
continued

Abdomen

Procedure

7. DEEPLY PALPATE THE FOUR ABDOMINAL QUADRANTS.

   a. Using the same hand position, deeply palpate the abdominal quadrants, but avoid jabbing movements. If depressing the abdomen is difficult, again try placing one hand over the other.

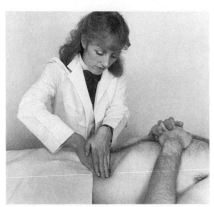
Deep abdominal palpation

   b. Check for rebound tenderness by depressing the abdomen and then quickly withdrawing your fingers.

8. PALPATE THE LIVER, SPLEEN, AND KIDNEY.

   a. Either of two techniques may be used to palpate the liver. First, instruct the client to do abdominal breathing. Then, place your left hand beneath the 11th and 12th ribs and pull the person slightly upward.

   Next, place your right hand lateral to the rectus muscle with your fingers pointing toward the ribs and palpate the liver edge, which is projected toward your upper hand as the person inhales.

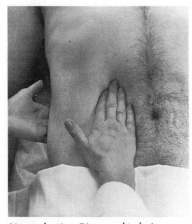
Liver palpation: Bimanual technique

Clinical Significance

Palpable masses: Masses should be further evaluated to determine size, shape, consistency, and mobility. Location should be described in reference to the abdominal wall. A mass may be inside the abdominal wall or deep within the abdominal cavity. While palpating the mass, ask the person to raise the head and shoulders. If the mass is still palpable, it is inside the abdominal wall. Muscle tenseness caused by raising the head will prevent you from palpating deep abdominal masses.

Abdominal structures commonly mistaken for masses include the aorta, rectus abdominus muscle, uterus, feces-filled colon, and sacral promontory (felt by deep palpation in very thin people). Stool is usually palpable as a tubular structure, as opposed to the rounded structure of an abnormal mass.

Tenderness: Although the abdomen is not normally tender to palpation, some people may complain of tenderness on deep palpation, especially over the abdominal aorta, the cecum (lower right quadrant), and the sigmoid colon (lower left quadrant).

Rebound tenderness may indicate inflammation of the peritoneum.

The liver may be impossible to feel by either method. Palpation is more easily performed on a very thin client or a client with an enlarged liver (hepatomegaly).

Normal Finding

Firm, smooth, nontender liver edge at or above the costal margin.

Deviations from normal: Enlargement, irregular or nodular edges; tenderness on palpation is associated with heart failure and hepatitis.

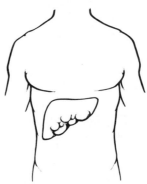
Nodular liver

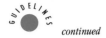
continued   ***Abdomen***

Procedure

Clinical Significance

b. Alternatively, you may use the hooking technique to palpate the liver. Stand at the client's right side facing the feet. Place both hands side by side at the lower liver border (previously determined by percussion). As the client inhales, press inward and pull upward toward the costal margin, feeling for the lower liver border.

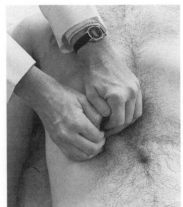
Liver palpation: Hooking technique

c. Palpate the spleen in the left upper quadrant. Remain on the client's right side and reach over the client, placing your left hand under the left costal margin. Gently pull the client upward with your right hand below the costal margin, and push upward to palpate. Deep breathing by the client may bring the spleen into line with your fingers.

Usually, the spleen must be enlarged to three times its normal size before it is palpable. Remember that palpation may further damage the spleen, especially if it is enlarged. Palpating the spleen is therefore not usually indicated, or is done very carefully by an experienced examiner.

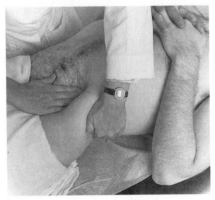
Palpating the spleen

An alternative technique is to repeat these movements with the client lying on the right side with knees flexed. This position moves the spleen slightly forward, making palpation easier.

d. The pole of the right kidney may be palpated in very thin people. The left kidney is difficult to detect on palpation. Place your upper hand at the costal margin with fingertips at the midclavicular line. Place your lower hand beneath the client. As the client inhales deeply, exert pressure to try to palpate the lower pole of the kidney. Palpation technique is identical for the left and right sides.

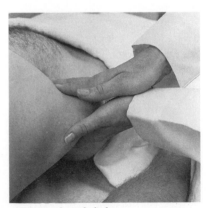
Palpating the right kidney

Examination Guidelines   *Evaluating Abdominal Fluid*

A distended abdomen may be further evaluated to differentiate edema fluid in the abdominal wall from ascites. Ascites is the accumulation of serous fluid in the abdominal cavity resulting from changes in vascular pressures. In starvation states, decreased intravascular protein will reduce plasma oncotic pressure, causing an outpouring of fluid into the abdominal cavity. In portal vein hypertension, increased hydrostatic pressure pushes fluid from the vessels into the abdominal cavity.

Procedure

1. PERCUSSION.

    a. Percuss the abdomen to detect fluid.

    b. Percuss for shifting dullness. Place the person in a lateral position and percuss the abdomen. Note any changes in the percussion notes with position changes. As ascites fluid gravitates to the dependent side, the area where you have percussed dullness also shifts. Shifting dullness is not usually observed with interstitial edema.

2. PALPATION.

    a. Palpate for a fluid wave. With the client lying supine, either the client or another person should place the lateral edge of his or her hand firmly along the abdominal midline to prevent impulse transmission through the subcutaneous fat. Then, tap one side of the abdomen, and feel and observe any movement to the opposite side of the abdomen. A positive fluid wave indicates ascites.

    b. *Ballottement* is a special palpatory technique used to identify a floating object in the abdomen.

    Place your fingers at a right angle to the client's abdomen and slightly depress the abdominal wall. While holding the abdomen in this position, note the rebound of a floating part against your fingers.

    Ballottement may also be done bimanually. Place one hand on the anterior surface of the lateral abdomen and the other hand under the client's back. Use your top hand to push the abdomen toward your lower hand. Again, note rebound of a floating object, this time with your lower hand.

Clinical Significance

Fluid in the abdomen or abdominal wall percusses as dullness.

Distinguishes ascites fluid, which is free-floating in the abdominal cavity and therefore gravity-dependent, from interstitial edema, which is more evenly distributed and less affected by gravity.

A large accumulation of free fluid within the abdomen is associated with a fluid wave.

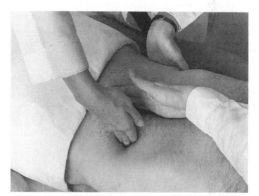

Evaluating abdominal fluid

With ascites, the patient's abdominal organs are actually floating in the abdomen. The pregnant uterus also represents a floating abdominal structure.

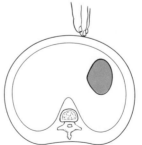

Single-handed ballottement

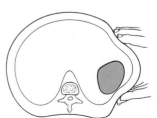

Bimanual ballottement

Documenting Abdominal Examination Findings

Example 1: Normal Abdomen

Mr. K, aged 55, had an abdominal examination as part of his routine annual health assessment. The examination results were normal and recorded as follows:

> Abdomen flat, symmetric, with well-developed musculature. No visible masses or pulsations; skin intact without lesions. Active bowel sounds heard over all quadrants. Liver span percussed 10 cm at midclavicular line. Nontender to light and deep palpation. No palpable masses.

The same examination may be summarized in a problem-oriented format:

S: Reports no dyspepsia, abdominal pain, or tenderness. No previous abdominal surgery.

O: Abdomen flat, symmetric, with well-developed masculature. No visible masses or pulsations; skin intact without lesions. Active bowel sounds heard over all quandrants. Liver span percussed 10 cm at midclavicular line. Nontender to light and deep palpation. No palpable masses.

A: Normal abdominal exam.

P: Follow up with routine exams.

Example 2: Abdominal Pain

Mr. H, aged 38, has been experiencing chronic, crampy abdominal pain. The abdominal examination findings are abnormal and recorded as follows:

> Abdominal inspection reveals no masses, skin lesions, pulsations; abdomen flat. Light palpation reveals diffuse tenderness, poorly localized but most pronounced in lower quadrant; no involuntary guarding, muscle rigidity, or rebound or referred pain.

The same examination may be summarized in a problem-oriented format:

S: Reports crampy lower abdominal pain relieved by bowel movements for past 6 months. States pain is exacerbated by stress. Bowel movements vary, with constipation alternating with diarrhea common. No gross blood noted in stools.

O: Abdominal inspection reveals no masses, skin lesions, pulsations; abdomen flat. Light palpation reveals diffuse tenderness, poorly localized but most pronounced in lower left quadrant; no involuntary guarding, muscle rigidity, or rebound or referred pain.

A: Symptoms suggest irritable colon syndrome. Need to rule out inflammatory bowel processes.

P: Test stool for occult blood. Evaluate diet and make appropriate recommendations regarding restriction of coffee, spicy foods, alcohol, and raw fruits and vegetables. Discuss relationship of stress and colon function. Follow-up examinations every 1 or 2 months until symptoms altered by life-style changes.

Nursing Diagnoses Related to Abdominal Assessment

Indicators for the following elimination problems may be noted during the abdominal exam:

Constipation
Diarrhea
Urinary retention

Although such diagnoses are thoroughly explored in Chapter 9, significant abdominal findings are included here because of the interrelationships of body systems.

Constipation

Constipation commonly causes gaseous distention of the abdomen. Gas accumulates and stretches the bowel walls, resulting in a tympanic abdomen. The contour becomes more rounded as distention progresses. The person may feel abdominal fullness and cramping. Peristaltic movements may decrease with constipation. Bowel sounds may be hypoactive.

Diarrhea

Diarrhea involves rapid movement of watery contents through the intestinal tract. Peristalsis increases, leading to two significant findings during the abdominal examination: the person may report cramping and abdominal pain, and the bowel sounds are usually more intense and frequent.

Urinary Retention

Urine retention in the bladder changes the normal abdominal contour. The area above the symphysis pubis may be distended. On palpation, bladder outlines may be evident, and the person may report tenderness. Percussion of a distended bladder results in dullness rather than tympany.

Clinical Problems Related to Abdominal Assessment

Inflammatory Processes

Although abdominal assessment can provide clues to the nature of inflammatory processes, a definitive diagnosis usually relies on additional information from endoscopic tests, x-ray examinations, and laboratory analyses. Nevertheless, nurses need a basis for evaluating signs and symptoms of inflammatory processes in the continual surveillance of the patient.

Stomach. Stomach inflammation occurs with gastritis and gastric ulcers. You may note epigastric tenderness and guarding to both light and deep palpation. Often, the person will report feelings of fullness and pressure in this area. Epigastric tenderness related to a gastric ulcer occurs more often when the stomach is empty, and is relieved by food or antacids. Gastric ulcer pain may be referred to the person's left subcostal region.

Epigastric tenderness and guarding may occur on palpation when the person has a duodenal ulcer. The pain is most intense 45 to 60 minutes after food ingestion or during the night. Such pain may radiate below the costal margins to the back. Occasionally, a unilateral spasm of the rectus abdominus muscle may be palpated over the duodenal bulb in the right upper quadrant. Antacids may help relieve the intensity of this pain.

Perforation of a gastrointestinal ulcer represents a life-threatening emergency. Initially, the person may experience an acute onset of abdominal pain often accompanied by nausea and vomiting. Several hours later, abdominal rigidity may occur as the abdominal muscles become spastic. Generalized rebound tenderness may occur, and bowel sounds may be absent because peritoneal inflammation inhibits intestinal motility.

Gallbladder. An inflamed gallbladder (cholecystitis) may cause pain in the epigastric or right upper quadrant area, usually precipitated by a large, fatty meal. The pain may be accompanied by nausea and vomiting. Guarding, rebound tenderness, and jaundice may be noted. A positive Murphy's sign, a sharp increase in pain with inspiration, may be elicited with acute cholecystitis: place your thumb below the right costal margin and ask the person to inhale deeply.

Appendix. Acute appendicitis may cause pain and tenderness in the right lower quadrant, which is aggravated by activity and coughing. The person can usually identify the area of maximal tenderness. You may note signs of peritoneal irritation, including muscle rigidity, rebound tenderness, and decreased bowel sounds. Psoas and obturator signs may be positive. The psoas sign is related to contact irritation of the iliopsoas muscle. Ask the person to assume a supine position and raise the right leg at the hip. Exert pressure on the person's thigh. Right lower abdominal pain with this maneuver constitutes a positive psoas sign. The obturator muscle may also be irritated by acute appendicitis. The obturator sign is positive when lower quadrant pain results from the following maneuver: Ask the person to flex the right leg at the hip and knee. Then, internally and externally, rotate the patient's leg at the ankle.

Diverticulum. Acute diverticulitis may cause tenderness in the lower left quadrant of the abdomen. The person may report cramping pain in this area, which is occasionally relieved by a bowel movement.

Obstructive Processes

Organic. An organic bowel obstruction may be caused by hernias, postoperative adhesions, neoplasms, foreign bodies, and intussusceptions.

Organic obstruction is associated with colicky abdominal pain and tenderness that becomes more intense as the obstruction develops. The abdomen becomes distended. Initially, peristalsis is increased as the muscles of the bowel contract in reaction to the increasing distension. You may note high-pitched, splashing bowel sounds (borborygmi), and you may observe peristaltic rushes across the abdominal surface. Eventually, bowel sounds cease and the abdomen is silent. Vomiting, constipation, and a shock-like state may occur.

Functional. A functional obstruction, also called paralytic ileus or adynamic ileus, is a neurogenic impairment of peristalsis. It may be precipitated by surgical handling of the bowel, peritoneal irritation, or acute illnesses. Functional obstruction causes continuous rather than colicky pain. The abdomen is usually distended, with minimal abdominal tenderness. Borborygmus is absent. Bowel sounds are hypoactive or absent, and vomiting is common.

THE THYROID GLAND

Anatomy and Physiology Overview

The thyroid gland, the largest endocrine gland in the body, is located in the anterior neck between the larynx and the trachea (Fig. 8-6). Two lobes are separated by a narrow band of tissue, or isthmus, which lies below the cricoid cartilage. The thyroid gland is a highly vascularized tissue, and has a rubbery texture on palpation.

Histologically, there are two distinct cell types in the thyroid gland that produce different hormones: the follicular cells produce triiodothyronine (T_3) and thyroxine (T_4), and the parafollicular cells (C cells) produce thyrocalcitonin. Two parathyroid glands are located on the posterior surface of each lobe of the thyroid gland and are not palpable.

The primary function of the thyroid gland is to control the metabolic rate with the hormones T_3 and T_4. Thyrocalcitonin has an effect on calcium metabolism. Hormone secretion is influenced by a negative feedback mechanism formed by the interrelationships among the hypothalamus,

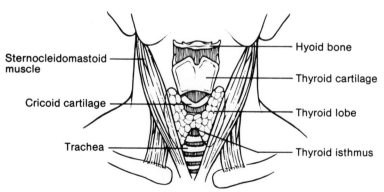

Sternocleidomastoid muscle

Cricoid cartilage

Trachea

Hyoid bone

Thyroid cartilage

Thyroid lobe

Thyroid isthmus

Figure 8-6. The thyroid gland.

the anterior pituitary, and the thyroid gland. Iodine, derived from bread, iodized salt, seafood, milk, and eggs, must enter the thyroid for the synthesis of T_3 and T_4. Daily iodine requirements range from 100 to 200 μg.

Triiodothyronine is the thyroid hormone responsible for most of the physiologic body activities. Although the thyroid secretes a greater amount of T_4, it is readily converted to T_3 in the periphery. Triiodothyronine affects most cells. It increases the basal metabolic rate, which results in increased oxygen consumption; increases chemical reaction rates; and increases heat production. In addition, T_3 stimu-

lates the metabolism of essential nutrients, including carbohydrates, fats, and proteins, and promotes human growth by acting synergistically with insulin and growth hormone. Because of the wide range of effects of this hormone, many body systems may be influenced by thyroid gland pathology. Therefore, in persons with thyroid disorders, assessment should include cardiovascular, gastrointestinal, neurologic, and integumentary (including hair and nails) systems. Changes may occur in these body systems even if physical examination of the thyroid gland reveals normal findings.

Physical Examination   *Thyroid Gland*

General Principles

The thyroid gland is examined by inspection and palpation. Auscultation is indicated if the gland is enlarged or if other findings, such as laboratory results or other physical examination findings, indicate altered thyroid function. Auscultate with the stethoscope bell to screen for a lower-pitched vascular bruit, the only type of abnormal vascular sound usually present.

Exposure and Lighting

For easier thyroid gland inspection, ask the person to swallow from a glass of water during the examination. As the person tilts the head back slightly and swallows, observe the anterior neck for any unusual bulges. Using tangential lighting may help you note any subtle changes in contour or symmetry.

Examination and Documentation Focus

- Size and shape
- Consistency
- Tenderness
- Occurrence of vascular sounds

Examination Guidelines   *Thyroid Gland*

Procedure

1. INSPECT THE AREA OF THE ANTERIOR NECK CONTAINING THE THYROID GLAND.
   a. Ask the person to hold the head and neck in a normal, relaxed position. Note any deviation or bulges in the trachea, as well as outlines of the thyroid and cricoid cartilages.

Clinical Significance

Normal Finding
The thyroid is usually too small to be observed by inspection.

Deviations from Normal
Goiter. Thyroid gland enlargement (goiter), caused by generalized hyperplasia of the thyroid gland, may be apparent on inspection. Goiters may be diffuse or slightly asymmetric, and may be softer in texture when palpated. Goiters indicate an iodine deficiency, goiterogenic substance ingestion, or thyroid inflammation.

continued

Thyroid Gland

Procedure

b. As the person extends the neck slightly and swallows water, note the upward, symmetrical movement of the trachea and other cartilage.

2. PALPATE THE THYROID (ANTERIOR APPROACH).

a. Stand facing the person, whose neck should be relaxed but held in slight extension to expose the underlying gland.

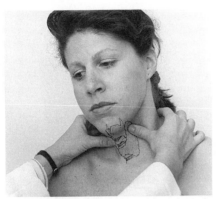

Lateral displacement of the thyroid: Anterior approach

b. Use the pads of your first and second fingers to locate the area of the thyroid isthmus directly below the cricoid cartilage. Ask the person to swallow, which causes the isthmus to rise. You will note a rubbery texture on palpation.

c. Next, move your hands laterally to palpate the thyroid lobes.

d. Then, place your fingers anterior to the large sternocleidomastoid muscle of the neck. Ask the person to swallow while you feel for any masses or bulges on the lateral lobes.

e. Palpate the left lobe of the thyroid. Ask the person to tilt the head slightly forward and to the right. Use your left thumb to displace the thyroid gland in a lateral left position while you palpate the left lobe with the thumb and fingers of your right hand. The lobe will be more palpable if you ask the client to swallow. Repeat the procedure for the right lobe.

Clinical Significance

The thyroid gland is attached to the trachea and rises with swallowing. Goiters may rise with swallowing.

Use either the anterior or posterior approach to palpate the thyroid. (The posterior approach may be easier to use.)

Overextension may tense the surrounding muscles, making palpation difficult.

Normal Findings

Size and shape: The thyroid glands weighs between 20 and 25 gm. The two lobes, which are connected by a central isthmus, give the gland a butterfly shape. The right lobe is slightly larger than the left. Each lobe is approximately 5 cm in length and 2 cm thick. Enlargement is associated with goiter.

Consistency: Lobe edges are slightly irregular and give the thyroid gland a rubbery texture on palpation. Hardened nodules or masses are not normal and can be easily distinguished from the usual texture. A single firm nodule may represent a benign cyst or a malignancy. Malignant nodules are often painless on palpation. Multiple nodules are found in some types of goiter. Conditions such as Hashimoto's disease and carcinoma cause the gland to become firm.

Tenderness: Palpation does not usually elicit tenderness, although the person may experience mild discomfort. Palpation tenderness reflects various forms of thyroiditis. Often, the pain will radiate to the ears.

continued   *Thyroid Gland*

Procedure

3. PALPATE THE THYROID (POSTERIOR APPROACH).

   a. Stand behind the person, who should be seated with the neck slightly flexed to relax the neck muscles.

   b. Rest your thumbs on the back of the person's neck and lightly place your fingers below the cricoid cartilage. Then palpate the middle isthmus as the person swallows some water.

   c. Ask the person to turn the head slightly to the side and palpate the lobes. Use your fingers on the opposite side to displace the gland in a lateral direction so that the fingers over the side being palpated can more readily feel the lobe. Ask the person to swallow as you examine the lobe. Repeat the procedure for the opposite side.

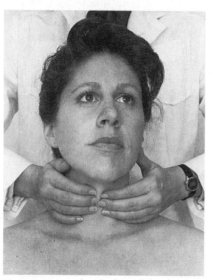

Posterior approach to the thyroid gland

Clinical Significance

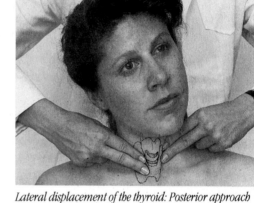

Lateral displacement of the thyroid: Posterior approach

4. AUSCULTATE THE THYROID (optional).

   Auscultate for bruits over each lobe, using the bell of the stethoscope.

Deviations from Normal

Vascular sounds may be auscultated in persons with hyperthyroidism. Blood flow through the vascular gland is accelerated, and increased turbulence generates a bruit. Occasionally, a bruit is accompanied by a palpable thrill.

Documenting Thyroid Examination Findings

A normal thyroid examination may be documented as follows:

> Thyroid palpated as symmetric without enlargement. Texture consistent with no masses, nodules, or tenderness.

An abnormal examination may be documented as follows:

> Thyroid palpated as symmetric without enlargement. Small, hard nodule observed on right lobe. No tenderness.

NDx

Nursing Diagnoses Related to Thyroid Assessment

Thyroid problems may contribute to a number of health problems treated by nurses. Persons with hypothyroidism are at increased risk for the following: Decreased cardiac output related to decreased metabolic rate, decreased cardiac conduction, atherosclerosis; Activity intolerance related to lethargy and fatigue, depressed neuromuscular status; and Altered nutrition: Less than body requirements related to decreased metabolic rate, poor appetite, and depressed gastrointestinal function.

Persons with hyperthyroidism are at increased risk for the following: Altered nutrition: Less than body requirements related to hypermetabolic state, increased fluid and calorie requirement, and fluid loss through diaphoresis; Impaired skin integrity related to extreme diaphoresis, fever, excessive restlessness, movement and tremor, and rapid weight loss; Altered thought processes related to insomnia, decreased attention span, and irritability; and Anxiety related to concern about disease and related treatments.

Clinical Problems Related to Thyroid Assessment

Thyroid dysfunction such as hypo- or hyperthyroidism may result in systemic clinical manifestations. Signs of *hypothyroidism* include the following:

Fatigue and lethargy
Weight gain
Cold hands and feet, cold intolerance
Memory impairment
Decreased peristalsis and constipation
Coarse, dry, scaling skin; dry, brittle hair
Menorrhagia or amenorrhea
Neurologic signs—polyneuropathy, cerebellar ataxia
Hypercholesterolemia
Enlarged heart
Hypotension
Slow speech; deep, hoarse voice

Signs of *hyperthyroidism* may include the following:

Nervousness, emotional lability, irritability, apprehension
Restlessness
Rapid pulse and palpitations
Hypertension
Heat intolerance, profuse perspiration, flushed skin
Fine tremor of hands
Constipation or diarrhea
Bulging eyes (exophthalmos)
Weight loss and emaciation
Goiter (in some cases)

THE LYMPHATIC SYSTEM

Anatomy and Physiology Overview

The lymphatic system is examined to detect abnormalities such as enlarged or tender lymph nodes, lymphedema, and lymphangitis. Lymph nodes consist of encapsulated lymphoid tissue that function as filters for lymphatic fluid. Su-

perficial lymph nodes are located in the head, neck, supraclavicular areas, breasts, axillae, epitrochlear areas, inguinal regions, and popliteal fossae (Fig. 8-7). They can be examined by palpation. Enlargement of the superficial lymph nodes may represent a benign deviation from normal, local infection, or neoplasm. Lymph nodes may be painful to palpation in association with acute inflammatory processes. *Lymphadenitis* refers to inflammation of the lymph nodes.

Lymphatic channels drain fluid from the body tissues to lymphatic vessels that empty into the bloodstream through the lymphatic ducts in the thorax. Obstruction of flow through lymphatic vessels results in movement of fluid from lymphatic vessels to the interstitial space. The tissue swelling is referred to as *lymphedema*.

Lymphangitis is an inflammatory process along the course of lymphatic vessel that is manifested by a red streak on the skin. It is caused by the spread of bacteria through the lymphatic vessel to the lymph node.

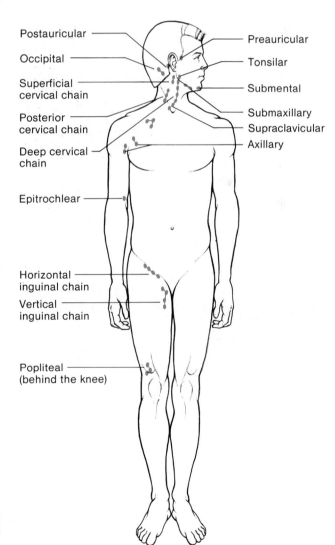

Figure 8–7. Distribution of lymph nodes.

Physical Examination   *Lymphatic System*

General Principles	The superficial lymph nodes are dispersed throughout the body. Therefore, examination of the lymphatic system may be incorporated into the head-to-toe physical examination. For example, lymph nodes of the neck are examined after the head; lymph nodes of the breast are evaluated during the breast examination. If abnormalities of the lymph nodes or lymphatic vessels are suspected, you should examine carefully the body area that drains toward the affected lymph node or vessel for signs of inflammation, infection, swelling, or injury.

The superficial lymphatic system is examined by inspection and palpation. Enlarged lymph nodes are detected more easily by light palpation than by deep palpation. Some variability is found among individuals in the number and location of lymph nodes in a particular area. Therefore, you should palpate the entire area where a lymphatic chain may be located. Encourage the person to report any tenderness experienced during palpation. |
| **Palpable Lymph Nodes** | Palpable lymph nodes should be distinguished from underlying tissue such as muscle. Unlike other surrounding tissue, an enlarged lymph node usually can be rolled up and down and side to side between the examiner's fingers.

Small palpable lymph nodes are common. Palpable nodes that are less than 1 cm wide, mobile, nontender, and discrete often are considered benign, but such findings still should be documented. You may detect a shotty node associated with frequent or chronic inflammation. A shotty node is enlarged over 1 cm, mobile, nontender, hard, and nodular. Malignancies may result in palpable lymph nodes that characteristically are nontender, nonmobile (fixed to underlying tissues), irregularly shaped, and firm, rubbery, or nodular. Such findings warrant further evaluation. |
| **Examination and Documentation Focus** | • *Inspection:* Location of any visible nodes, presence of swelling or red streaks
• *Palpation:* Palpable nodes are described in terms of location, size (millimeters or centimeters), consistency, discreteness, mobility, and tenderness. Determine when the palpable node was first noticed by the patient. |

Examination Guidelines   *Lymphatic System*

Procedure

Clinical Significance

1. INSPECT AND PALPATE THE LYMPHATICS OF THE HEAD AND NECK.

    a. Inspect the skin overlying the head and neck lymphatic chains for swelling, redness, or red streaks.

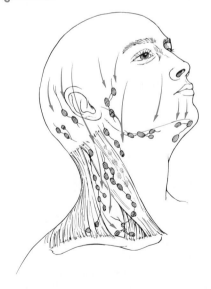

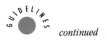

continued   *Lymphatic System*

Procedure

b. Palpate the lymphatics of the head and neck.

Right and left sides may be examined simultaneously as you palpate the lymphatic areas of the head and neck. Slight flexion of the head and turning the head away from the area being examined may be helpful. Systematically palpate the nodes of the head and neck using a sequence such as the following:

   (1) Preauricular (in front of the tragus of the ear)

   (2) Postauricular or mastoid (overlying the mastoid process)

   (3) Occipital or suboccipital (at the base of the skull)

   (4) Tonsilar (at the angle of the lower jaw)

   (5) Submaxillary (midway between the angle of the lower jaw and chin)

   (6) Submental (midline behind the tip of the chin)

   (7) Superficial cervical chain (over the sternocleidomastoid muscle)

   (8) Posterior cervical chain (anterior to the trapezius muscle)

   (9) Deep cervical chain (embedded in the sternocleidomastoid muscle). The deep cervical chain is difficult to palpate. Hook thumb and fingers around the sternocleidomastoid muscle and then palpate.

   (10) Supraclavicular (within the angle formed by the sternocleidomastoid muscle and clavicle)

2. INSPECT AND PALPATE THE LYMPHATICS OF THE BREAST, AXILLAE, AND SUPRACLAVICULAR AREA.

3. INSPECT AND PALPATE THE LYMPHATICS OF THE EPITROCHLEAR AREA.

The epitrochlear nodes are located just above the medial epicondyle of the humerus. To palpate for epitrochlear nodes, flex the patient's elbow 90 degrees and palpate above the epicondyle in the groove created by the biceps and triceps muscles.

Clinical Significance

Normal Findings

Superficial nodes are not palpable and not tender on palpation.

Deviations from Normal

Superficial nodes, less than 1 cm in diameter, may be normal in adults. Lymph nodes may be up to 3 cm in healthy children.

Infection: Lymph nodes may become enlarged, warm, and tender in head and throat infections. Enlarged postauricular lymph nodes may be noted in otitis media.

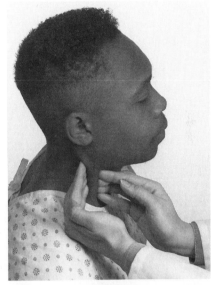

Palpation: Deep cervical chain

This is part of the routine breast and axillae examination. See Chapter 15, page 473.

Deviations from Normal

Enlargement and tenderness may be associated with infection of the ulnar aspect of the forearm and the fourth and fifth fingers.

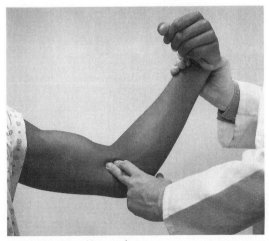

Palpation: Epitrochlear nodes

continued **Lymphatic System**

Procedure

4. INSPECT AND PALPATE THE LYMPHATICS OF THE INGUINAL REGION.

   The superficial inguinal lymph nodes may be palpated with the patient lying supine with the knees slightly flexed. Palpate for the horizontal superficial inguinal chain along the inguinal ligament. Palpate for the vertical superficial inguinal chain just medial to the femoral vein.

Clinical Significance

Enlargement and tenderness may be associated with infection of the lower abdominal and pelvic regions and lower extremities.

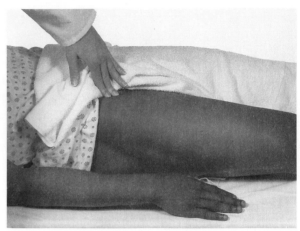

Palpation: Superficial inguinal lymph nodes

5. INSPECT AND PALPATE THE LYMPHATICS OF THE POPLITEAL FOSSA.

   Palpate for the popliteal nodes in the posterior fossa of the knee. Palpation is facilitated by placing the knee in a position of slight flexion.

Enlargement and tenderness may be associated with infection of the heel and foot.

Documenting Lymphatic Examination Findings

Example 1: Normal Superficial Lymphatics

Lymph nodes generally are not visible or palpable. In this case, the results of the examination may be documented in the following manner:

> No visible or palpable lymph nodes in the [specify body area or lymphatic chain]. No tenderness on palpation; no edema or skin color changes.

Example 2: Benign Palpable Lymph Node

Mary, aged 14, had a physical examination before participating in school sports. The examination of the superficial lymphatic chains of the neck was recorded as follows:

> No palpable neck nodes except right tonsilar node, 1.5 × 1.0 cm. Node is nontender, soft, and mobile with well-defined borders. Node has been palpable for several years and unchanged in size. History of frequent sore throat prior to age 8 years.

The same examination may be summarized in a problem-oriented format:

> S: Multiple sore throats prior to age 8 years. Right tonsi-lar nodes palpable for several years. Nontender, no changes in size.

> O: Palpable right tonsilar node, 1.5 × 1.0 cm. Node is nontender, soft, and mobile with well-defined borders.
> A: Palpable lymph node. Probably benign.
> P: Reevaluate yearly or if changes occur in this node or if other lymph nodes become palable.

Example 3: Generalized Lymphadenitis

Max, aged 24, has been tired lately and experiencing tenderness under his arms and in the groin area. He is a recovering intravenous drug user. The examination of the superficial lymphatic system was recorded as follows:

> Axillary lymph nodes palpable bilaterally. Nodes are tender, matted, nondiscrete, warm, soft, mobile, and irregularly shaped. Inguinal lymph nodes palpable bilaterally. Nodes are tender, matted, and warm. No other palpable lymph nodes.

The same examination may be summarized in a problem-oriented format:

> S: Tender groin and axillae for 1 month; increasing fatigue. Recovering intravenous drug user—no drug use past 5 years. Verbalizes fear of AIDS.
> O: Axillary lymph nodes palpable bilaterally. Nodes are tender, matted, nondiscrete, warm, soft, mobile, and irregularly shaped. Inguinal lymph nodes palpable bilaterally. Nodes are tender, matted, and warm. No other palpable lymph nodes. Abnormal lymphatic exam.

A: Abnormal lymphatic exam.
P: Laboratory blood tests, including HIV antibody as requested by physician. Discuss follow-up of lab results. Advise regarding sufficient rest, fluids, and nutrition.

NDx

Nursing Diagnoses Related to Lymphatic Assessment

A person with enlarged and painful lymph nodes (lymphadenitis) should be further evaluated for signs and symptoms of the following nursing diagnosis: Pain related to swelling and inflammation. Consider also the nursing diagnoses of Anxiety or Fear for persons undergoing evaluation

for ruling out malignant diseases as causes of lymph node alterations.

Clinical Problems Related to Lymphatic Assessment

An enlarged or tender lymph node can be associated with a number of disease entities. Localized lymphadenopathy may suggest a bacterial infection in an area draining into that lymphatic chain. Generalized lymphadenopathy is the presence of palpable lymph nodes in three or more lymph node chains. This condition may be associated with systemic infectious processes, lymphoma, leukemia, or collagen vascular disorders. Additional diagnostic evaluation is usually indicated and may include lymphatic biopsy.

ASSESSMENT PROFILE

•••

Mrs. Olsen was an 80-year-old widow who lived alone in an apartment building for elderly, low-income tenants. She was 5′4″, weighed 104 pounds, and appeared emaciated. For 8 months she had been enrolled in a portable meals program, which provided nutritional noonday meals Monday through Friday in the apartment complex dining area. Mrs. Olsen stated that she enjoyed conversing with her neighbors during meals. If she could not finish her entire portion, she took the leftovers home. Mrs. Olsen's daughter-in-law regularly brought groceries to the apartment, and on weekends Mrs. Olsen prepared her own meals: boullion soups and apple juice. Although she reported her appetite was good, she thought she did not eat as much as she had 10 years earlier and had noticed that her clothes were looser. Mrs. Olsen wore her upper and lower dentures only to eat. The physical examination revealed loose dentures with inflamed gingiva from denture contact. Oral mucosa was dry.

For this woman, an in-depth analysis of nutritional and metabolic functions was indicated. Further analysis of the data provided information about health strengths, additional risk factors for nutritional impairment, and etiologic factors for nutrition problems. Once such data were available, the nurse could make additional judgments about Mrs. Olsen's prognosis and treatment plan.

Profile Analysis

This chapter presents the concepts and skills used for comprehensive assessment of nutrition and metabolism. Comprehensive assessment, which involves extensive data collection, may not be required with all individuals. Even people who have actual or potential nutritional–metabolic dysfunctions may not require such detailed evaluation provided you know how to follow up on cues detected during the initial encounter with the client.

The initial encounter between the nurse and Mrs. Olsen was characterized by several significant cues indicating nutritional dysfunction. The nurse's observations of the client's emaciated appearance, ready access to nutritional meals, and altered oral mucosa prompted further investigation of specific aspects of the overall nutritional–metabolic pattern.

Identifying the Assessment Focus

One reason that home health nurses visit well elderly people such as Mrs. Olsen is to promote and maintain independent living status. Early problem detection and intervention is an important factor in maintaining independent living. Nurses focus patient assessment on abilities to manage tasks of daily living, especially in relation to mobility and safety, self-administration of medications, and nutrition.

General information about the patient group will influence your approach to nutritional assessment. For example, the nurse visiting Mrs. Olsen knew that elderly people living alone are at greater risk for malnutrition even if adequate food is available and there are no absorptive or utilization problems. Possible causes of nutritional problems included

- Food rejection secondary to lack of social stimuli for preparing proper meals, chronic disabling illness, or depression
- Unbalanced dietary intake
- Excessive caloric intake
- Mechanical eating problems

Based on such preencounter knowledge of nutritional risks in the elderly, the nurse made observations related to nutritional status during each home visit. Moreover, the nurse was sensitized to cues indicating possible nutritional dysfunction.

Possible Nursing Diagnoses

Based on visual inspection, the nurse judged Mrs. Olsen's body weight to be more than 10% below the ideal for her height and frame. This single cue activated the nursing diagnosis of Altered nutrition: Less than body requirements. The nurse's next task was to consider possible contributing factors and to collect data that would either support or rule out each possibility. The contributing factors that might explain other cues observed by the nurse included the following:

- Food rejection
  Cues: She did not eat all of the food offered. Even though food was provided for weekend meals, she did not prepare balanced meals.
- Unbalanced dietary intake
  Cues: Nutritionally poor weekend meals. Unfinished meals.
- Mechanical eating problems
  Cues: Client report of poor-fitting dentures. Evidence of oral trauma.

Additional Data Gathering and Analysis

Although additional data collection was focused on possible contributing factors suggested by the cues, the nurse also considered other contributing factors. For example, did the patient have an underlying pathologic process that impaired appetite and absorption? Even though the patient reported a "good appetite," the nurse wondered why she did not finish her prepared meal portions. She also wondered whether the patient understood nutritional principles or suffered from depression. Although she believed that poor dentition was the most probable contributing factor, the nurse decided to follow up on all such possibilities.

Subsequent data collection focused on interviewing the patient about food and fluid intake, psychosocial influ-ences, knowledge of nutrition, and related physiologic alterations. Additionally, the nurse examined the patient's oral cavity and measured height and weight. The nurse did not implement other examination methods used to assess the nutritional–metabolic pattern, such as thyroid examination, abdominal examination, and other anthropometric measurements, because data obtained by these methods were judged to be irrelevant to the diagnostic possibilities.

Final Nursing Diagnosis

Further data collection revealed that mealtime was associated with valued social interaction. Mrs. Olsen enjoyed eating with her neighbors but was self-conscious about her appearance and continued to wear ill-fitting dentures at mealtime to "keep from looking like a toothless old lady." Painful chewing prevented her from finishing meals. She did not seek professional care, believing that her dentures would never fit well. Moreover, she was worried about expenses associated with dental care. Mrs. Olsen expressed that she was apathetic about weekend meals that she had to prepare and eat alone. The resulting nursing diagnosis was Altered nutrition: Less than body requirements related to social isolation and ill-fitting dentures.

Finally, the data were analyzed to identify strengths that could help facilitate an optimal state of health. The nurse clustered the following cues as indicators of patient strengths:

- Remains alert and mobile
- Receives some nutritional meals
- Experiences mealtimes as social
- Receives groceries from family member
- Maintains good appetite

The patient strengths were considered when making a prognosis in relation to the problem and in planning subsequent interventions.

Chapter 8 SUMMARY

Nutritional–metabolic assessment focuses on analyzing
- The quality of the diet in relation to metabolic needs
- The degree to which the body demonstrates that the ingested nutrients are adequately used

Multiple data sources are used to evaluate nutrition and metabolism. The data base should consist of the following:

The Health History
- Dietary intake
- Factors that influence diet
- Metabolic needs
- Nutrition knowledge
- Factors related to nutritional problems

Physical Examination Findings
- General appearance
- Anthropometric measurements
- Integumentary system
- Oral cavity
- Abdomen
- Thyroid gland
- Lymphatic system

Reports from Laboratory Tests Pertaining to Nutritional Status
- Serum albumin
- Serum transferrin
- Total lymphocyte count
- Urine urea nitrogen
- Nitrogen balance (derived value)

Assessment of nutrition and metabolism provides cues to the following nursing diagnoses:
Altered nutrition: More than body requirements
Altered nutrition: Less than body requirements
Altered nutrition: Potential for more than body requirements

RESEARCH *Hi*GHLIGHT

What is the optimal way to identify clients at risk for Altered skin integrity?

Altered skin integrity is a nursing diagnosis that addresses actual and potential skin alterations. Although assessment techniques for evaluating actual skin integrity alterations are well defined, assessment techniques for identifying the client at risk for impaired skin integrity are not as clear.

*Concerned with preventing skin problems, nurses at a state psychiatric hospital developed and tested an assessment tool to identify clients at high risk for developing decubitus ulcers. Because clients in the researchers' long-term treatment unit were often elderly and sedentary, decubitus ulcers were occurring frequently. The nurses believed that a formal nursing assessment directed at identifying clients at high risk for skin breakdown would help establish effective preventive nursing treatment. They researched the literature and found a scale that could be used to assign a score to each client (see display). The higher the score, the greater the risk for skin breakdown. The research project involved several tasks: First, the assessment tool was evaluated for user consistency. Then, the tool was evaluated to determine if high scores were indicative of high risk for skin breakdown. Finally, the patients who had been assessed with the tool were tracked for assessment effectiveness. All evaluations were positive. Of all the assessed patients, more than half (60%) were found to be at high risk for skin breakdown. Before the study, 47% of these patients had decubitus ulcers. Nine months after the initial as-*sessment for impaired skin integrity, only 7% of the patients had decubitus ulcers.[1]

What significance does the study have for health assessment?

The study suggests that optimal assessment of potential problems requires a different approach than the assessment of actual problems. The approach involves identification of risk factors associated with the problem. Many types of data might be significant, and assessment tools may be constructed to aid the nurse in focused data collection.

Can the study's findings be applied to practice?

The nurse could use the assessment tool shown in the display with minimal risk to the client. However, this particular tool may not effectively identify clients at risk for decubitus ulcers who differ from the study group. For example, the tool may not effectively identify potential skin problems in critically ill newborn babies. Such studies should be repeated with different client groups to refine the accuracy and clinical usefulness of the assessment tool.

REFERENCE

1. Davenport, N., & McComb, M.D. (1984). Implementation of a nursing diagnosis to increase autonomy and accountability. In Kim, M.J. McFarland, G.K., & McLane, A.M. (Eds.). *Classification of nursing diagnoses: Proceedings of the fifth national conference.* St. Louis: C.V. Mosby.

Nursing Assessment Tool: Potential for Impaired Skin Integrity (*Adapted from Nursing Standards, Emmanual Hospital, Portland, Oregon*)

A General* Condition	B Mental State	C Activity	D Mobility	E Incontinence
___ 0 Good ___ 1 Fair ___ 2 Poor ___ 3 Bad	___ 0 Alert ___ 1 Confused ___ 2 Apathetic ___ 3 Stuporous ___ 4 Comatose	___ 0 Ambulates ___ 1 Walks with help ___ 2 Chair-fast ___ 3 In bed all day	___ 0 Full ___ 1 Slightly limited ___ 2 Moderately to very limited ___ 3 Immobile	___ 0 Continent ___ 1 Occasional (urine or stool) ___ 2 Usually (urine or stool) ___ 3 Incontinent of both urine and stool
_____ Score	_____ Score	_____ Score	_____ Score	_____ Score

_____ Total score[†]

Patient at high risk for skin impairment?   Yes _____

No _____

_____ / _____
R.N. Signature   Date

*This rating takes into account the patient's general state of health, especially hydration and nutrition and impaired peripheral circulation as indicated by color, temperature, and pulses.

[†]Total score of 5 or more mandates the nursing diagnosis High risk for impaired skin integrity.

Feeding self-care deficit
Fluid volume excess
Potential fluid volume deficit

The following problems associated with altered nutrition also are identified:
Altered growth and development
Impaired tissue integrity
Altered oral mucous membrane
Impaired skin integrity
Potential impaired skin integrity

Potential for infection
Impaired swallowing

Additionally, cues to the following clinical problems may be revealed in the process of generating the data base for nutrition and metabolism:
- Metastatic processes involving the skin, oral cavity, gastrointestinal tract and lymphatic system
- Inflammatory gastrointestinal processes
- Gastrointestinal obstruction

✳ CRITICAL THINKING

You are the nurse counseling a 65-year-old male who is receiving radiation therapy for rectal cancer on an outpatient basis. Nutritional problems are likely over the 6-week course of therapy. This is the patient's first week of therapy. A primary treatment goal is to design a plan to meet the patient's nutritional needs.

Learning Exercises

1. Select and describe the approach you would use to establish a useful data base pertaining to this patient's nutritional status. Explain how you would proceed if you had only 30 minutes to spend with the patient, and approximately 1/3 of that time would be used to answer questions and teach him about the overall treatment plan.

2. Specify how your nutrition data base would help you establish realistic treatment goals for this patient.

3. The patient is unable to maintain a food diary. Identify and describe alternative approaches for assessing his diet.

4. Explain how you would utilize laboratory values to evaluate the patient's nutritional status.

BIBLIOGRAPHY

Berecek, K. (1975). The etiology of decubitus ulcers. *Nursing Clinics of North America, 10,* 157.

Bryant, R. (1987). Wound repair: A review. *Enterostomal Therapy, 14* (6), 262–266, 268.

Bryant, R.A. (1992). *Acute and chronic wounds: Nursing management.* St. Louis: C.V. Mosby.

Curtas, S. (1989). Evaluation of nutritional status. *Nursing Clinics of North America, 24* (2), 301–303.

Cuzell, J.Z. (1988). The new RYB color code: Next time you assess an open wound, remember to protect red, lance yellow, and debride black. *American Journal of Nursing, 88* (10), 1342–1346.

Flory, C. (1992). Perfecting the art: Skin assessment. *RN, 55* (6), 22–27.

Gee, C.F. (1990). Nutrition and wound healing. *Nursing: The Journal of Clinical Practice, Education, and Management, 4* (18), 26–28.

Gray, D.P., & Smith, P. (1983). Nutritional assessment of the surgical patient: A nursing perspective. *Nutritional Support Services, 3* (9), 64–66.

Jacobs, B.B., & Jacobs, L.M. (1988). Anatomy of the abdomen. *Emergency Care Quarterly, 3* (4), 1–11.

Jacobs, B.B., & Jacobs, L.M. (1988). Assessment of the abdomen. *Emergency Care Quarterly, 3* (4), 12–21.

Leininger, M.M. (1988). Tanscultural eating patterns and nutrition: Transcultural nursing and anthropological perspectives. *Holistic Nursing Practice, 3* (1), 16–25.

Loogman, E.A. (1992). Nutritional assessment in nursing. *Gastroenterology Nursing, 14* (4), 189–194.

Mairis, E. (1992). An appetite for life: Assessing and meeting nutritional needs. *Professional Nursing, 7* (11), 732–737.

Neilley, L.K., & Darr Ellis, R.A. (1984). Nailing down a diagnosis. *Nurse Practice, 9* (5), 26–34.

O'Toole, M.T. (1990). Advanced assessment of the abdomen and gastrointestinal problems. *Nursing Clinics of North America, 25* (4), 771–776.

Young, M. (1988). Malnutrition and wound healing. *Heart and Lung, 17* (1), 60–69.

Chapter *9*

Assessing Elimination

Assessment Terms

Bowel Elimination
Urinary Elimination
Gastrocolic Reflex
Tenesmus
Ostomy
Pilonidal Cyst
Guaiac Test
Residual Volume
Bladder Capacity
Oliguria
Polyuria

Upper Motor Neuron (Reflex) Bladder
Lower Motor Neuron (Hypotonic;
   Atonic) Bladder
Frequency
Urgency
Nocturia
Enuresis
Dysuria
Hesitancy
Dribbling

INTRODUCTORY OVERVIEW

Eliminating body waste is a complex human function influenced by physiologic, psychological, environmental, and cultural factors. Therefore, assessing this important function involves more than analyzing or quantifying urine and stool specimens. It also includes analyzing structures involved in elimination, the person's responses to problems with elimination and identifying physiologic and psychological concerns that affect his or her self-esteem and physical well-being.

Assessment Focus

Elimination consists of bowel and urinary elimination. Data relevant to elimination functions is obtained by interviewing the person, examining body structures related to excretory function; and reviewing the results of stool and urine tests, diagnostic procedures related to excretory function, and pertinent laboratory tests.
   Assessment addresses the following points:

* The pattern of bowel and urinary elimination, including frequency and amount

- Self-care practices, knowledge, and perceptions of elimination
- Risk factors or conditions associated with altered elimination
- Physiologic, behavioral, and psychological responses to elimination problems

- Characteristics of specimens excreted from bowel or bladder
- Results of diagnostic tests relevant to elimination functions

The methods for collecting data for each of these areas are listed in the Assessment Focus display.

Assessment Focus **Elimination**

Assessment Goal	Data Collection Methods
1. Describe the person's bowel and urinary elimination pattern in terms of frequency, amount, and usual habits.	*Interview* • Usual voiding pattern • Usual defecation pattern • Usual elimination patterns following surgical alteration of the bowel or bladder (colostomy; ileal conduit): Has a typical pattern been established? Is it functional or dysfunctional? *Observation* • Urine and stool excretion pattern • Incidence of incontinence • Amount of urine or stool excreted • Frequency of urination or defecation • Relationship of bladder elimination to fluid intake
2. Evaluate the person's self-care practices and knowledge about elimination.	*Interview* • Are self-care measures related to bladder elimination practiced? Are there special learning needs? • Are self-care measures related to bowel elimination practiced? Are there special learning needs?
3. Identify risk factors or conditions associated with altered elimination patterns.	*Interview* • Are self-care practices related to bowel and bladder elimination safe and appropriate? • Do symptoms of altered bowel and urinary elimination suggest problems related to elimination? • Do dietary practices contribute to problems with elimination? *Physical Examination* • Are there ano-rectal abnormalities that may contribute to problems with elimination? • Are there pelvic structure abnormalities (Chap. 15) that may contribute to problems with elimination? • Are there gastrointestinal, neurologic, or musculoskeletal abnormalities that may contribute to problems with elimination?
4. Identify the person's physiologic, behavioral, and psychological responses to altered elimination patterns.	*Interview* • Has an elimination problem created special learning needs related to self-care? • Have problems with elimination altered self-concept (Chap. 13)? • Have problems with elimination affected sexuality (Chap. 15)? *Review of Laboratory Tests and Physical Examination* • Has fluid and electrolyte balance been disrupted as a result of diarrhea or diuresis? • Is skin integrity altered or at risk of being altered?
5. Differentiate various elimination problems.	*Stool and Urine Examination* • Does stool character suggest constipation? Diarrhea? Malabsorption? • Does urine character suggest infection? *Review of Diagnostic Tests* • Intravenous pyelogram: What do test results suggest about urinary system structures? • Cystometrogram: What do test results suggest about bladder function? • Electromyography: What do test results suggest about muscles involved in urination? • Barium enema, CT scan, and proctosigmoidoscopy: What do test results suggest about bowel structures?

Nursing Diagnoses

Assessment of elimination patterns provides cues to the following nursing diagnoses:

Constipation
Perceived constipation
Colonic constipation
Diarrhea
Bowel incontinence
Altered urinary elimination
Stress incontinence
Reflex incontinence
Urge incontinence
Functional incontinence
Total incontinence
Urinary retention

Other nursing diagnoses related to urinary and bowel problems include the following:

Body image disturbance
Fluid volume deficit
High risk for fluid volume deficit
Hoplessness
Ineffective coping
Self-care deficit (specify type)
Self-concept alteration
Self-esteem disturbance
Altered sexuality patterns
Impaired skin integrity
High risk for impaired skin integrity

KNOWLEDGE BASE FOR ASSESSMENT

Assessing elimination requires an understanding of the processes of bowel and urinary elimination. Each process has a physiologic basis that may be influenced by many factors, such as diet, age, activity, exercise, stress, drugs, and pathology.

Physiology of Bowel Elimination

The amount of feces evacuated from the bowel is related to the amount and composition of ingested food. Ingesting nutrients, however, is not essential for producing a bowel movement. Feces can form from the cellular residues desquamated from the intestinal tract lining, as well as from intestinal gland secretions, bacteria, blood and other substances. Under normal, nonfasting conditions, food residue (chyme) that passes through the ileocecal valve (the junction between the small and large intestines) contributes to total stool weight. At this point, most nutrients have been absorbed from the chyme; the bolus of food is further processed, with the semiliquid chyme being converted into solid feces that can be evacuated from the rectum. The formation and evacuation of feces are the result of the following normal colonic functions: fluid and electrolyte absorption, peristaltic contractions, and defecation (Fig. 9-1).

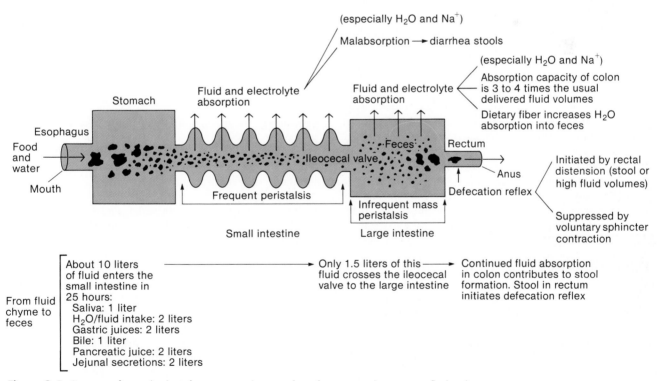

Figure 9–1. Summary of normal colonic functions contributing to feces formation and evacuation: fluid and electrolyte absorption, peristalsis, and defecation.

Absorption. Fluid and electrolyte absorption, a process of converting semiliquid chyme into a formed fecal mass, occurs across the mucosal surfaces of the ascending and transverse colon. Normally, the colon can absorb 90% of the water received from the small intestine. The daily capacity is about 6 L. Absorption occurs passively and is enhanced when segments of the colon contract. Circular muscles in the colon constrict around the lumen and divide the colon into segments, holding the chyme in contact with the absorptive surface. If the chyme remains in prolonged contact with the mucosal surface of the colon, too much water is absorbed and the stool may become hard and dry. On the other hand, if muscle tone is decreased and segmenting contractions do not occur, the chyme may trickle through the colon with little water being absorbed, resulting in liquid stools. Fibrous food portions, found in the colon because the body does not have the enzymes capable of breaking down fiber, are efficient water absorbers. High intake of dietary fiber, therefore, may cause stools to be softer secondary to increased water retention.

Peristalsis. Wavelike peristaltic movements propel the feces toward the sigmoid colon and rectum. Unlike the frequent peristaltic activity in the small intestine, peristalsis of the large intestine is relatively infrequent, with mass peristaltic movements occurring only two to four times daily. Mass peristalsis in the colon can be initiated by the gastrocolic reflex that occurs when food reaches the stomach, by bulk-forming agents such as fiber in the intestinal lumen, and by the stool in the rectum. Adding bulk to the diet causes the lumen of the colon to distend, which results in increased peristaltic activity to move feces through the colon. Usually parasympathetic nervous system discharge stimulates peristalsis in the colon, whereas sympathetic nervous system stimulation inhibits peristalsis. Prolonged stress may affect the autonomic nervous system and may result in bowel elimination problems, with alternating constipation and diarrhea.

Defecation. Defecation is the movement of feces out of the bowel. The defecation reflex is initiated when stool enters the rectum. Secondary to the defecation reflex, the internal and external anal sphincters relax, which allows the stool to be evacuated. The defecation reflex may be suppressed by voluntarily contracting the external anal sphincter. Obviously, the ability to suppress the defecation reflex is essential for bowel control, but continued suppression may have adverse effects. Eventually, this reflex may become weakened and the motor tone of the rectum more flaccid, contributing to constipation and fecal impaction.

Physiology of Urinary Elimination

Urinary elimination occurs when urine is excreted from the bladder. Urine production occurs in the nephrons of the kidneys. If no urine is produced, as in renal failure, a problem exists with urine production, not urinary elimination.

The process of emptying the urinary bladder may be called micturition, voiding, or urination, and is a reflex children learn to control voluntarily between ages 2 and 4

years. In adults, the urge to void is felt when the bladder fills with about 200 mL of urine. When the bladder fills with 350 to 400 mL of urine, pressure from the urine volume stimulates specialized nerve endings in the bladder wall, called stretch receptors, which in turn stimulate a reflex arc at the second to fourth sacral segments of the spinal cord. Finally, the bladder wall contracts, strengthening the urge to void (Fig. 9-2). Without conscious control, urine would enter the urethra, the external sphincter would relax, and voiding would occur. Voiding remains under voluntary control until bladder volume approaches 700 mL, when most people lose the ability to delay micturition.

Neural Voiding Mechanisms. Messages are sent along neural pathways between the cerebral cortex and the sacral segments of the spinal cord as the bladder fills with urine and during the act of voiding (see Fig. 9-2). If environmental conditions are not suitable for voiding, messages from the brain will inhibit the reflex arc and lead to voluntary contraction of the external bladder sphincter. If conditions are favorable, the brain will send a message encouraging the external sphincter to relax, and urine will be voided. Brain messages also direct the bladder to contract until all urine has been expelled from the bladder.

Neural Pathway Disruptions. Disease and injuries may cause lesions along the central neurogenic pathways involved in micturition (see Fig. 9-2). If the pathway from the frontal cortex to the pontine-mesencephalic reticular formation is disrupted, voluntary voiding may be affected. Brain tumors, organic brain syndrome, cerebrovascular accident, and head injuries can cause such disruptions. Consequently, the bladder may empty secondary to involuntary reflex contraction of the bladder wall and involuntary relaxation of the urethral sphincter, or voiding may occur at inappropriate times because of scrambled brain messages, a condition known as *upper motor neuron bladder* or *reflex bladder*.

Injury to the neural pathway from the pontine-mesencephalic reticular formation to the parasympathetic nucleus in the S2–S4 area of the spinal cord (reticulospinal tract) may affect micturition coordination. Normally, the bladder wall contracts as the external urethral sphincter relaxes. If these actions are not coordinated and the bladder involuntarily contracts, the flow may be partially obstructed by a contracted sphincter. Incontinence accompanied by urine retention in the bladder results.

The corticospinal tract houses the neural connections between the brain and the pudendal nucleus. Injury to this pathway may affect the ability to voluntarily interrupt the urinary stream.

Damage to the pelvic nerve, which leaves the spinal cord to innervate the bladder, may cause areflexia, or the inability of the bladder wall muscle to contract. Consequently, urine is retained in the bladder, a condition also referred to as *lower motor neuron bladder, hypotonic bladder,* or *atonic bladder.*

The hypogastric nerve and the pudendal nerve are needed to stimulate external sphincter contraction. If these nerves are damaged, stress incontinence and decreased sphincter tone may result.

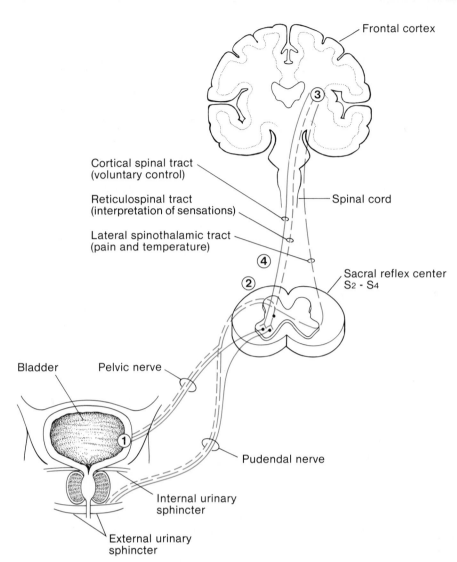

Figure 9–2. *Urine elimination: Neuromuscular mechanisms. (1) Bladder stretch receptors send messages to the brain signaling bladder fullness. (2) Spinal (sacral) reflex causes sphincter relaxation and detrussor contraction when bladder is full. (3) Voluntary controls inhibit the spinal reflex until the person is ready to void. (4) Motor impulses are sent to the detrussor and sphincters so that voiding occurs.*

THE HEALTH HISTORY AND INTERVIEW

The assessment of elimination begins by obtaining a history of the individual's bowel and urinary elimination patterns. Any perceptions of problems with excretory functions should also be considered and included in the health history. Factors that influence elimination patterns, such as activity, nutrition, pathology, medications and environmental factors, also should be noted. Provided the person is willing to discuss the intimate functions of bowel and urinary elimination, most of the health history may be obtained by interviewing the person. A straightforward and nonjudgmental approach will help minimize embarrassment and inhibitions.

Data included as part of the history pertaining to bowel elimination should help you make judgments about the following:

- Usual defecation pattern
- Self-care practices
- Factors influencing bowel elimination
- Altered bowel elimination patterns
- Responses to special situations, such as ostomies

Data included as part of the history pertaining to urinary elimination should help you make judgments about the following:

- Usual voiding pattern
- Self-care practices
- Factors influencing urinary elimination
- Altered urinary elimination patterns
- Response to special situations, such as urinary diversion

The interview guide shown in the accompanying display may be used to direct the collection of appropriate data.

If the person does not report any problems with elimination, and if you do not suspect problems based on the

Interview Guide Elimination

Bowel Elimination

Usual Pattern of Defecation

Number of bowel movements per day or per week _____
What time of day do you usually move your bowels? _____
Do you postpone defecation? _____
How would you define constipation/diarrhea? _____
Any recent change in bowel patterns? _____

Self-Care Practices

Do you do anything special to treat or prevent problems with defecation?
_____

Do you take any food to treat or prevent constipation/diarrhea? _____
_____

Do you use laxatives? _____ Suppositories? _____ Enemas? _____ Hemorrhoid remedies? _____

Factors that Influence Bowel Elimination

Any changes in usual routines/surroundings? _____
Current medical diagnosis _____
Previous hospitalizations/surgeries _____

Any of the following problems?	Yes/No		Yes/No
Ulcerative colitis	_____	Drug History	
Crohn's disease	_____	Laxatives	_____
Diverticuli	_____	Antidepressants	_____
Spastic colon	_____	Antihistamines	_____
Colon polyps	_____	Antiparkinsonians	_____
Hemorrhoids	_____	Tranquilizers	_____
Anal fissures, ulcers	_____	Narcotics	_____
Spinal injury	_____	Antibiotics	_____
Head injury	_____	Antacids	_____
Stroke	_____		
Multiple sclerosis	_____		

Symptoms of Altered Bowel Elimination

Do you have any problems with bowel movements? _____
Do you experience any of the following? _____ Rectal pain _____ Abdominal cramping _____ Straining with bowel movements
_____ Hard stools _____ Fewer than three stools per week _____ Blood in stools _____ Loose stools _____ Difficulty getting to
the bathroom in time _____ Stools that float in the toilet _____ Tenesmus _____ Flatulence

Urinary Elimination

Usual Pattern of Voiding

Approximate number of voidings per day _____ per night _____
Is this your typical pattern? If, no, why do you think there has been a change? _____
Approximate daily fluid intake _____
Daily caffeine intake _____
Are you taking diuretic medications? _____

Symptoms of Altered Urinary Elimination

Do you have any problems with voiding? _____
Do you experience any of the following? _____ Pain (in abdomen or pelvic area) _____ Frequent voiding _____ Difficulty starting
urine flow _____ Difficulty getting to the bathroom in time _____ Passing urine when you do not want to _____

Self-Care Practices

Do you do anything special to treat or prevent problems with voiding? _____
Knows Kegel's exercises? _____ Practices Kegel's exercises? _____
Any problems with ADLs? _____
UTI practices? _____ Increases fluid intake _____ Acidifies urine _____ Knows and practices appropriate perineal hygiene _____
Showers *vs.* bathing _____
Urinary hesitancy practices? _____ Uses trigger point stimulation _____ Uses Credé maneuver _____
Urinary incontinence management? _____ Restricts fluids _____ Follows regular, planned toilet schedule _____ Uses incontinence devices _____ Self-catheterization _____

(continued)

Interview Guide **Elimination (continued)**

Factors that Influence Urinary Elimination

Any changes in usual routines affecting urinary elimination? _____

Current medical diagnosis _____

Previous hospitalizations/surgeries _____

Number of pregnancies _____

Any of the following problems?	Yes/No		Yes/No
Enlarged prostate	_____	Drug History	_____
Female pelvic alterations	_____	Antidepressants	_____
Urinary tract infections	_____	Antihistamines	_____
Vaginal infections	_____	Antiparkinsonians	_____
Pelvic infections	_____	Belladonna alkaloids	_____
Venereal disease	_____	Phenothiazines	_____
Constipation	_____	Diuretics	_____
Spinal injury	_____		
Head injury	_____		
Stroke	_____		
Multiple sclerosis	_____		
Diabetes mellitus	_____		
Renal stones	_____		
Renal disease	_____		

person's history, then a screening interview may provide sufficient information about elimination functioning. A more comprehensive interview is indicated whenever a person reports elimination problems or is at high risk for altered elimination because of changes in habitual patterns, emotional stress, or immobility (see Interview Guide). Any person who suffers from bowel or bladder incontinence, which is a loss of voluntary control of bowel or urinary elimination, needs a comprehensive elimination assessment before bowel or bladder retraining is initiated.

Some people may be uncomfortable discussing elimination, others physically unable to answer questions. Patients with cerebral pathology, for example, may be unable to respond to interview questions but may still benefit from bowel or bladder retraining. In such cases, other available sources, such as patient records, family reports, and observations by other caregivers, may provide the necessary information.

The Interview: Bowel Elimination

USUAL DEFECATION PATTERN

Because bowel elimination patterns vary extensively among people, it is important to determine the normal pattern for each person. Basic questions to ask during the interview include the following:

On the average, how often do you move your bowels each day? What time of day do you usually move your bowels?

Because constipation and diarrhea are the most common types of altered bowel function, it helps to ask the person to define constipation or diarrhea in relation to his or her normal bowel habits. Infrequent defecation, such as two or three times a week, does not always indicate constipation, just as frequent defecation, such as three times a day, does not necessarily indicate diarrhea. For example, a bowel elimination pattern including defecation once every 3 days but without abdominal cramping, bloating, or difficulty passing stool can be considered normal for a given individual. For a person whose normal pattern includes a daily bowel movement, however, going without a bowel movement for 3 days may be abnormal. In addition to evaluating the normal frequency of defecation, ask about the usual appearance of the stool before making a diagnosis of Altered bowel elimination.

Any recent changes in bowel elimination, such as constipation or diarrhea, should be thoroughly assessed. Serious problems such as colon cancer may be associated with a persistent change in customary bowel function.

Asking the person about the usual time of day for bowel movements allows you to assess the regular pattern further. Many people move their bowels at the same time every day, such as after breakfast, in response to the gastrocolic reflex. Habitually ignoring this reflex may contribute to chronic constipation, because the defecation reflex becomes progressively weaker when ignored.

Bowel Elimination Pattern and Aging. Theoretically, physical aging does not alter bowel elimination, because the gastrointestinal tract does not deteriorate with age. In elderly persons, as in any age group, altered elimination is a symptom of another problem. Immobility and dietary changes may contribute to bowel problems in people of any age.

SELF-CARE PRACTICES

Self-care practices involving diet, fluid intake, exercise, and self-administration of over-the-counter preparations influence the bowel elimination pattern.

Diet and Fluid Intake. If the person reports infrequent, hard stools, it is essential to inquire about fluid intake. Adequate hydration is necessary to add weight, bulk, and softness to stools. Dehydration, either from inadequate intake or increased fluid losses, results in excessive water reabsorption from the intestinal chyme, usually resulting in hard feces and constipation. Drinking at least six 8-ounce glasses of fluids daily is recommended. Coffee, tea, and grapefruit juice are not included in the recommended amount because they act as diuretics and thus cause less fluid to be retained in the stool.

Also evaluate the ingestion of fiber. Two to four grams of fiber daily helps prevent constipation and subsequent hemorrhoid formation. Low-fiber diets have been associated with colon diseases, including diverticular disease, irritable bowel syndrome, appendicitis, and colon cancer. However, excessive fiber can contribute to or aggravate diarrhea. Dietary fiber can be increased by eating whole grain breads, cereals, raw fruits, and vegetables. For a more comprehensive diet assessment, a 24-hour dietary recall may be recommended (see Chap. 8)

Specific foods may alter bowel elimination. For example, prunes, which contain dihydroxyphenylisatin, may have a laxative effect on the bowel. Certain foods and spices can irritate the gastrointestinal tract and cause diarrhea in persons who lack the necessary enzymes for digesting those foods. In persons who have lactase deficiency, for example, milk ingestion may have adverse effects, including abdominal cramping, pain, and diarrhea.

Tube feedings may result in diarrhea, although such a complication can be prevented. In the enterally fed patient, diarrhea may result from formula contamination, lactose intolerance, hypertonic formulas, or administration of formula in the presence of low serum albumin levels.

Activity and Exercise. Bowel elimination is facilitated by good muscle tone in the abdominal and pelvic muscles, which are used during defecation to propel the stool. Good overall muscle tone also strengthens the muscles responsible for peristalsis. Immobility may cause muscle weakness, preventing mass peristalsis needed for defecation. Inquiring about exercise and activity may provide a clue to possible elimination problems.

Laxatives, Enemas, and Suppositories. Ask the person if he or she uses laxatives, enemas, or suppositories to promote a bowel movement. If the answer is "yes," determine how often this occurs and under what circumstances.

Using drugs, either prescribed or over-the-counter, to promote bowel elimination is a common and potentially harmful self-care practice, especially for elderly persons. In fact, 40% of Americans over age 60 have reported using laxatives on a weekly basis for constipation. If the person reports this practice, it is important to ask about the type and frequency of laxative use. The four classes of laxatives are lubricants, bulk-formers, saline cathartics, and stimulants. Often, stimulant laxatives may be associated with adverse effects. Stimulant laxatives act on nerve endings in the colon, increasing peristalsis, and if used over a long period, will disrupt the intrinsic innervation of the colon, which may contribute to constipation. Consequently, the person may become a chronic user of stimulant laxatives.

FACTORS INFLUENCING BOWEL ELIMINATION

Environmental Influences. Ask if there have been changes in the person's usual routines or surroundings that might influence bowel elimination. Recent changes in daily routine and surroundings can affect the bowel elimination pattern. Daily biologic rhythms may be affected by hospitalization, travel, or lack of time or privacy. Alterations may result in disrupted bowel elimination habits through either voluntary or involuntary suppression of the defecation reflex, possibly leading to a loss of this reflex. Unnatural positioning, such as having to use a bedpan in a supine position, may also inhibit bowel elimination.

Physiologic Influences. Review the person's past medical history for conditions that might influence bowel elimination.

Pathology. Neurologic deficits can adversely affect bowel elimination. For example, brain disease or injury may impair a patient's ability to communicate defecation needs to caregivers, resulting in fecal incontinence. Damage to the upper part of the spinal cord may affect the ability to control the defecation reflex. Because the reflex arc may still be intact, however, reflex bowel emptying may occur. Damage to the sacral segment of the spinal cord may result in a loss of reflex action. When external sphincters are relaxed, continual fecal incontinence may result.

If the bowel is obstructed by gastrointestinal disorders such as strictures, adhesions, hernias, volvulus, intussusception, polyps, neoplasms, or fecal impactions, bowel elimination may be affected. Diarrhea, constipation, or complete loss of bowel motility may occur, depending on the location and degree of the obstruction. Inflammatory gastrointestinal tract diseases such as Crohn's disease, ulcerative colitis, acute infections, and diverticulitis may cause diarrhea. Clues to such disorders are usually obtained when asking the client about the usual bowel pattern and whether any recent changes have been noted in bowel elimination.

Metabolic disorders such as hypothyroidism, hypocalcemia, and hypokalemia are associated with constipation. Chronic diarrhea may be observed with hyperthyroidism, diabetes mellitus, adrenal insufficiency, and hypercalcemia.

Medications. Review the person's medication history and identify drugs that might alter bowel elimination.

Anticholinergic drugs, such as tricyclic antidepressants, antidyskinetics used to treat Parkinson's disease, antihistamines found in many over-the-counter cough and cold remedies, and major tranquilizers may cause constipation

Table 9–1. Some Common Drugs With the Side-Effect of Constipation

	Generic Name	Brand Name
Antacids	Calcium carbonate	Tums
	Aluminum hydroxide	Amphojel
Analgesics	Morphine	
	Codeine	
	Oxycodone	Percodan
Anticonvulsants	Phenytoin	Dilantin
Antidepressants	Phenelzine	Nardil
	Amitriptyline	Elavil
Barbiturates	Phenobarbital	Nembutal
	Amobarbital	Amytal
	Secobarbital	Seconal
Belladonna alkaloids	Atropine	Donnagel
	Scopolamine	Hyposcine
Cytotoxic agents	Vincaleukoblastine	Vincristine
Diuretics	Furosemide	Lasix
Minerals	Ferrous sulfate	
Phenothiazines	Chlorpromazine	Thorazine
	Perphenazine	Trilafon
	Prochlorperazine	Compazine
	Thioridazine	Mellaril
	Trifluoperazine	Stelazine
Tranquilizers	Diazepam	Valium

(Table 9-1). These drugs decrease the smooth muscle tone of the colon, resulting in less frequent mass peristaltic movements. Opiate narcotics, such as codeine, morphine, and meperidine hydrochloride (Demerol), also decrease colonic motility.

Overuse of laxatives, including over-the-counter preparations, may irritate the bowel mucosa and lead to diarrhea or loss of muscle tone by disrupting the colon's intrinsic innervation, aggravating constipation.

Broad-spectrum antibiotics, including ampicillin, clindamycin, lincomycin, tetracycline, neomycin, and cephalexin (Keflex), may induce diarrhea by altering the bowel's normal bacterial flora. The magnesium-containing antacids, including magnesium hydroxide (Gelusil, Maalox), magaldrate (Riopan), and aluminum hydroxide (Amphojel), may also induce diarrhea.

Psychological Factors. As you interview the person, be attentive to any signs of psychological alterations. Feelings of boredom, uselessness, withdrawal, sadness, and depression are associated with a decrease in colonic motility that can result in constipation. Depressed people may not consume an adequate diet or exercise enough to promote bowel activity. Often stress increases sympathetic tone, which causes decreased colon activity. Occasionally, stress may be associated with diarrhea or a pattern of alternating diarrhea and constipation.

ALTERED BOWEL ELIMINATION PATTERNS

Ask the person if he or she is experiencing either constipation or diarrhea. If the answer is "yes," obtain a complete description of the altered pattern.

In addition to constipation and diarrhea, common symptoms of bowel elimination problems include pain, weakness, rectal fullness, bloating, and bleeding. The basic question to ask in eliciting this information is:

Do you have any problems or discomfort when you move your bowels?

Follow up with additional interview questions as indicated. Analyze any symptoms of altered bowel elimination by obtaining detailed descriptions from the client.

Pain. Pain in the lower abdominal quadrant may occur when the colon becomes distended with gas or fluid, causing the muscle layers to stretch. This results in colon contractions or spasms. The pain is usually crampy or colicky and may occur with either constipation or diarrhea.

Rectal pain is more localized to the perineum and is usually caused by stool being retained in the rectum. *Tenesmus* is rectal pain associated with the urge to defecate and a sensation of incomplete emptying after defecation. In addition to stool retention, other causes of tenesmus include rectal tumors and colonic inflammation. Hemorrhoids (varicosities of the veins draining the rectum and anus) may also be a source of rectal pain and itching, which increases during defecation.

Miscellaneous Symptoms. Urgency, weakness, and frequency are often reported when diarrhea occurs. Straining to defecate, rectal fullness, and bloating are associated with constipation. Changes in stool consistency or color may also be reported and must be thoroughly evaluated, as discussed elsewhere in this chapter (see section on examination of the stool).

SPECIAL SITUATIONS: OSTOMIES

Ileostomy. An ileostomy consists of a surgical diversion of the ileum through the outer wall of the abdomen. The stool excreted from an ileostomy is usually liquid or semiliquid because significant water reabsorption does not occur in the small intestine. The person may have limited control of bowel elimination and need to wear a collection bag or appliance to collect the semiformed or liquid stool. Stool volume is greatest following meals, when the bowel is most active. The person usually needs to empty the ileostomy appliance 4 or 5 times a day, with normal output being approximately 700 to 800 mL/day.

A special type of ileostomy, the continent ileostomy (Kock pouch), provides for greater, sometimes complete, bowel elimination control. A pouch that serves as a reservoir for stool is created from a small portion of small intestine, and the stool can be drained through a nipple valve that is surgically constructed at the abdominal surface.

Colostomy. A colostomy is created when the large intestine is diverted to the abdominal wall. Colostomies are most commonly created by altering the ascending or descending (sigmoid) colon. The stool that is evacuated from an *ascending colostomy* is liquid or semiformed because significant water absorption has not had time to occur. The person may have less control of bowel elimination than a sigmoid colostomy provides, and usually must wear an external drainage bag.

A person who has a *descending or sigmoid colostomy* usually eliminates formed stools at regular intervals and can control the bowel elimination pattern by dietary habits, so that continually wearing an appliance is unnecessary.

Evaluate ostomy characteristics and the resultant evacuation patterns by asking questions such as the following:

How many times a day do you need to empty the appliance (bag)? How much does this pattern vary from day to day? Describe the consistency of your stools. Is this typical? What types of foods/beverages cause problems for you? Can you tell me about it? What problems do you have in caring for your skin/stoma/appliance? How does your ostomy affect your feelings about yourself? work? family?

The Interview: Urinary Elimination

USUAL AND ALTERED VOIDING PATTERNS

Asking the person about his or her usual voiding pattern will establish individual baseline data for future comparison. A typical approach is to ask:

How many times a day do you void (go to the bathroom)? How many times do you void at night?

People are usually aware of changes in their voiding patterns and may wish to discuss symptoms at this point in the interview. Common problems include frequency, urgency, nocturia, enuresis, dysuria, hesitancy, and dribbling. If the client reports symptoms of altered bladder elimination, you should also ask whether he or she has observed changes in the urine, such as color and odor.

Frequency. If voiding occurs more often than usual, the person is experiencing *frequency,* often a normal response to increased fluid intake. Frequency that is not accompanied by painful voiding but is associated with large volumes of urine output may be a sign of diuresis, which occurs secondary to medication, alcohol, or caffeine ingestion, or poorly controlled diabetes mellitus. Follow up reports of frequency to determine probable cause; ask the client if he or she has made recent dietary changes such as ingesting more caffeine than usual.

Frequency may also be a sign of urinary tract infection, especially if voiding is painful, or it may occur secondary to stress or anxiety. If the person is unable to provide information about the voiding pattern, observe how often voiding occurs and compare it to an arbitrary norm of once every 3 to 6 hours.

Urgency. A sudden need to urinate, called *urgency,* may be associated with inflammation of the bladder or urinary tract. Urgency may contribute to incontinence if the person is unable to use bathroom facilities in time.

Nocturia. Ask about nocturnal or nighttime voiding. Excessive voiding during the night, called *nocturia,* may be secondary to congestive heart failure. Edema fluid that accumulates during the day more readily perfuses the kidneys when the person is resting, and results in greater urine production and excretion during the night. Furthermore, a person with congestive heart failure may have nocturia secondary to the effects of diuretic medications.

Enuresis. Bedwetting or *enuresis* involves involuntary voiding during sleep and can be normal in children under age 3 years. In older children, however, enuresis may represent a behavior pattern or may be associated with obstruction or infection of the lower urinary tract.

Dysuria. Pain associated with voiding, called *dysuria,* is symptomatic of numerous conditions, including urinary tract infection, urethral stricture, prostate disease, prolapsed uterus, and cancer of the cervix. Pain may also be felt over the bladder area in the case of bladder infections or overdistended bladders. Flank pain is associated with upper urinary tract infections and stones in the urinary tract. Analyze reports of pain in terms of location, character, duration, radiation, and aggravating and relieving factors.

Hesitancy. Difficulty starting the flow of urine, called *hesitancy,* may indicate a neurologic dysfunction or lower urinary tract obstruction. Medications such as antihistamines, which improve the tone of the bladder sphincter, may contribute to hesitancy.

Dribbling. Involuntary passage of urine, or *dribbling,* may indicate weak sphincter tone, hypotonic bladder, reduced bladder capacity, or sagging of the structures that support the bladder.

SELF-CARE PRACTICES

People with urinary problems usually have special concerns about how to manage such problems, including questions about changes in fluid intake and about activity and exercise. Assessing self-care practices helps evaluate urinary function, identify dangerous practices, and determine any learning needs.

Fluid Intake. Many people modify their fluid intake as a means of controlling bladder elimination. Restricting fluid intake in the evening, for example, will probably lessen the urge to void during sleep. Some people with incontinence may decrease overall fluid intake to control bladder elimination. However, such methods may aggravate the problem by concentrating the urine, which may irritate the bladder, cause infection, and increase the urge to void.

Activity and Exercise. Determine if the person practices special exercises to control bladder elimination. Bladder elimination is facilitated by good pelvic muscle tone, which is usually associated with strong bladder muscles. Bladder muscle contraction is important for starting and stopping urination. Pregnancy may weaken the muscles involved in micturition; weakening of the bladder sphincter may then result in stress incontinence. Pregnant women are often taught Kegel's exercises to tone bladder muscles.

Prevention of Urinary Tract Infections. When the history reveals a frequent occurrence of urinary tract infections, it is important to ask about the measures the person uses to prevent infections. For instance, ask the person:

What do you do to prevent (or manage) urinary tract infections?

Optimal self-care practices include the following:

- Increase fluid intake in order to induce frequent voiding, which helps dilute the urine and create a less favorable environment for bacterial growth.
- Acidify the urine by drinking cranberry juice, which also inhibits bacterial growth.
- Practice good hygiene (especially important for women), including voiding after intercourse, wiping the perineum from front to back after a bowel movement, and showering rather than bathing. All these practices prevent bacteria from entering the urethra.

Self-Treatment of Urinary Retention. If the person has a problem with urinary retention, ask how he or she manages this problem. For instance, ask the person:

What helps you start urination?

Optimal self-care practices include the following:

- Stimulate trigger points to initiate voiding. Different methods will work for different people, such as stroking the inner thighs, tapping the abdomen, pulling the pubic hair, massaging the sacrum, and manually stretching the anal sphincter.
- Use the Credé maneuver, which is manual expression of urine from the bladder by applying pressure over the suprapubic area, if the bladder cannot be emptied by trigger-point stimulation.

Urinary Incontinence. To evaluate self-care practices related to urinary incontinence, ask the following question:

What do you do to prevent (or manage) involuntary urination?

The person may report the following self-care practices:

- Restriction of fluid intake
- Planning a toilet schedule
- Wearing an incontinence pad or external catheter
- Using intermittent self-catheterization, for inefficient bladder emptying secondary to neurologic lesions
- Exercising the pelvic floor to strengthen it. For example, Kegel's exercises are carried out by consciously contracting the pelvic floor or levator ani muscles. These exercises are performed several times a day. Another exercise is to stop urinary flow voluntarily in midstream. Such exercises are helpful in treating stress incontinence.

FACTORS INFLUENCING URINARY ELIMINATION

Environmental Influences. Determine how surroundings influence the person's urinary elimination pattern. A person's surroundings at any one moment may affect the ability to urinate. A lack of toilet facilities or privacy, for example, may force a person to suppress the urge to urinate. Using a bedpan in a supine position may also inhibit voiding. Usually, men are more comfortable voiding in a standing position, whereas women prefer to void while seated.

The attitude of others can also influence urinary practices. For example, when caregivers such as physicians and nurses adopt an attitude that urinary incontinence is inevi-

table, more instances of incontinence occur. Fitting people with incontinence pads, such as Chux pads, also seems to promote incontinence. In institutions, incontinence in elderly persons may also be related to inability to reach toilet facilities in time.

Asking specific questions and observing behaviors are two major ways to evaluate environmental influences. The most direct approach for a hospitalized person is to ask how the urinary elimination pattern has changed since he or she entered the facility.

Psychological and Physiologic Influences. Psychological states and physiologic alterations may contribute to problems with bladder elimination. If bladder elimination patterns are abnormal, determine if any of these factors contribute:

- *Stress.* Observe the person for signs of stress and related psychological symptoms. Urinary frequency may be influenced by stress. Although the exact mechanism is unclear, some forms of urinary incontinence may have psychological factors as an etiology.
- *History of prolonged urinary catheterization.* Long-term use of urinary catheters may weaken the bladder's external sphincter muscle and the detrusor muscle, which is no longer stretched and exercised when the bladder is continually drained. Urinary incontinence following removal of an indwelling urinary catheter may be related to impaired bladder muscles.
- *Medications.* Medications that affect the autonomic nervous system may influence bladder elimination. Drugs that may cause urinary retention include antidepressants, antihistamines, antiparkinsonian drugs, belladonna alkaloids, and phenothiazines. Retention may be treated with drugs such as bethanechol chloride (Urecholine), which may be administered after abdominal surgery. Sedatives may cause people to sleep despite the urge to void and thus cause incontinence.
- *Pathology.* Urinary system infection may inflame mucosal tissues and prevent the bladder from expanding to normal capacity, causing urgency, frequency, or dysuria. Conditions that may obstruct the urinary tract and contribute to urine retention include fecal impactions, surgical swelling, masses, urinary calculi, and prostatic hypertrophy. Lesions of the central and autonomic nervous systems may also adversely affect bladder elimination.

SPECIAL SITUATIONS: URINARY DIVERSION

Urinary diversion refers to surgical alterations of the urinary system that cause urine to bypass the bladder. The most common types of urinary diversion are the ileal conduit, the ureterosigmoidostomy, cutaneous ureterostomy, and the nephrostomy (Fig. 9-3). Assessing urinary elimination patterns in persons with urinary diversion is essential to detect and treat any dysfunctional patterns and to identify learning needs.

Because ileal conduits, cutaneous ureterostomies, and nephrostomies result in continuous drainage of urine, the person must wear a collection device or appliance. If the diversion is a ureterosigmoidostomy, urine is excreted

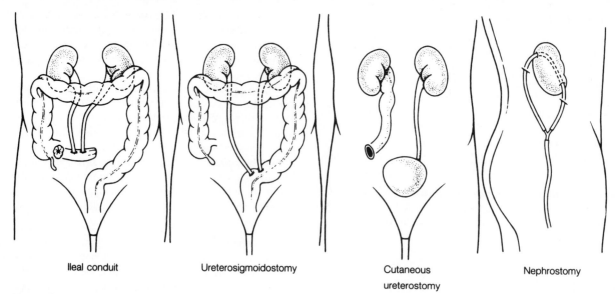

Figure 9–3. Methods of urinary diversion. (Brunner, L.S. & Suddarth, D.S. [Eds.] [1991]. *The Lippincott manual of nursing practice* (5th ed., p. 544). Philadelphia: J.B. Lippincott)

through the rectum. An optimal elimination pattern is to evacuate the urine from the rectum every 3 to 4 hours. During sleep, drainage is accomplished through an inserted tube or catheter. A person with a ureterosigmoidostomy often learns to distinguish voiding sensations from defecation sensations.

To assess urinary patterns in people with urinary diversions, ask questions such as the following:

How many times a day do you need to empty the appliance (bag)?
How much does this pattern vary from day to day?
What problems do you have in caring for your skin/stoma/appliance?
How has this procedure affected your feelings about yourself? work? family?

DIAGNOSTIC STUDIES

A complete evaluation of altered elimination patterns may include examination of specimens and special diagnostic procedures. The procedures for examining stool and urine specimens are discussed elsewhere in this chapter.

Additional diagnostic studies may be performed for persons with altered bowel elimination in order to diagnose pathologic conditions contributing to bowel changes. The most common diagnostic studies include the barium enema, proctosigmoidoscopy, and colonoscopy.

The functional status of structures involved in urinary elimination is further evaluated by selected urologic tests, including the intravenous pyelogram, cystometrogram, and electromyography; as advised by the physician. In addition, the bulbocavernous reflex may be tested. Results from these tests may be used to gain additional information about the status of the external urinary sphincter, bladder, ureters, and kidneys.

Barium Enema

A barium enema involves the instillation of barium, an x-ray contrast material, into the large intestine through the anus. X-rays are then taken of the colon and rectum to diagnose colorectal cancer, inflammatory bowel disease, polyps, and diverticula. Other diagnostic studies may be used to confirm a diagnosis of colorectal cancer, including colonoscopy and proctosigmoidoscopy.

Proctosigmoidoscopy and Colonoscopy

A proctosigmoidoscopy involves examination of the anal canal, rectum, and sigmoid colon through an endoscope inserted through the anus. Colonoscopy allows examination of the entire colon. The mucosa and structure of these areas can then be visualized. Tissue from suspicious lesions may also be biopsied with this instrument. Proctosigmoidoscopy is used to diagnose malignancy and inflammatory bowel disease and to locate the source of lower gastrointestinal bleeding.

Intravenous Pyelogram

The intravenous pyelogram (IVP) is a specialized radiograph used to study the renal pelvis, ureters, and bladder. Dye is injected into the urinary system to make the structures opaque and visible on radiographic media. Abnormal dye retention in the bladder usually indicates bladder neck obstruction. Stones or calculi that interfere with elimination can also be visualized. The IVP studies are also used to evaluate renal pathology that can effect urine production.

Cystometrogram

The cystometrogram provides information about bladder function. A two-way catheter is used to instill fluid into the bladder. The patient may feel the urge to void during fluid instillation. Reflex contractile voiding may also occur. This study measures bladder pressures and reflex activity, and indicates bladder contraction strength.

Electromyography

Electromyography helps determine muscular contraction strength of the external urinary sphincter in response to electrical stimulation. Pelvic floor muscles, which are important for urinary continence, can also be tested.

Bulbocavernous Reflex

A positive bulbocavernous reflex is associated with an intact voiding reflex, which is tested in the following manner: Place a gloved finger in the rectum, and squeeze the glans penis of the male or the clitoris of the woman. If the result is positive, the rectal sphincter will contract around your finger. The bulbocavernous reflex is not the same as the voiding reflex, but the innervation responsible for both reflexes originates at the same level in the spinal cord.

THE PHYSICAL EXAMINATION

Examination Focus

Physical examination techniques provide important information about elimination functions. The goals of the physical examination include determining bowel and bladder function, screening for functional and pathophysiologic causes of elimination problems, and identifying adverse effects of elimination problems. The data collected through physical examination, together with data obtained from the history, provide a basis for formulating nursing diagnoses or identifying problems that require interventions in collaboration with other care providers.

For example, a 70-year-old man who was staying at a long-term care facility while recovering from orthopedic injuries reported to the nurse that he had been dribbling urine for a week. This problem had caused him to stay in his room rather than engage in social activities. Physical examination revealed the following:

- *Abdominal examination:* Abdomen distended over symphysis pubis.
- *Genitourinary examination:* Urine stains on underclothing; strong urine odor. Inability to void volumes greater than 50 mL at a time. Urine residual 400 mL (determined by bladder catheterization that was advised by the physician).

Examination findings were consistent with the defining characteristics for the nursing diagnosis of Urinary reten-

tion. Additional physical examination data needed to be analyzed to determine the etiology of the diagnosis. The following physical examination findings helped identify the etiology:

- *Rectal and prostate examination:* Palpable hard, fecal mass; fills entire region of rectum that is palpable. Prostate: Smooth; not enlarged.
- *Neurologic examination:* Neurologic system intact.

Based on the findings, the nurse suspected that fecal impaction was obstructing the bladder neck and contributing to urine retention.

In order to evaluate elimination functions, a physical examination is conducted with emphasis on the following:

- General appearance
- Abdomen
- Anus and rectum
- Genitourinary structures
- Neurologic and musculoskeletal systems.

General Appearance

The general survey can provide cues about incontinence, self-care abilities, and fluid and electrolyte status.

Incontinence. Urine and stool have distinctive odors that are easily detected on the person's skin, clothing, or in the immediate environment. Such odors should be investigated further. Incontinence pads or appliances, such as external catheters, may be observed. Because incontinence may be an embarrassing and humiliating problem, the person may make great efforts to hide the problem. Strong perfumes or colognes might indicate an attempt to mask offensive odors.

Observations of sweating, restlessness, and abdominal discomfort, manifested verbally or by body position, may indicate bladder distension. People who have been incontinent or who have urinary retention should be monitored for these signs. Possibly, only one of these signs demonstrated consistently will signal a full bladder.

Self-Care Abilities. The ability to use one's hands and legs contributes to maintaining a normal elimination pattern. Obviously, hands and legs are needed to manipulate clothing and toilet facilities. Impairment involving the arms or legs should be noted during visual inspection.

The elimination pattern may also be affected by mental status. For example, a decrease in the level of consciousness or a confused state presents a risk for elimination problems. Severe depression and stress are also risk factors and may be revealed to some degree by the person's general appearance.

Fluid and Electrolyte Status. Severe fluid and electrolyte imbalances may be noted in conjunction with various elimination problems, but on general inspection the most obvious imbalance will probably be related to diarrhea.

Severe diarrhea, especially in very young or elderly persons, can deplete the body of sodium and water. Readily detectable signs include sunken cheeks, loss of skin turgor, and lethargy. Large potassium losses may also occur, resulting in apathy, lethargy, and weakness. These findings are manifested only as such conditions become extreme; therefore, prompt treatment and referral to a physician are indicated.

Associated Body System Alterations

Gastrointestinal System. Examine the abdomen to identify conditions associated with elimination problems. For example, a distended abdomen may indicate constipation or urinary retention. Bowel sounds usually increase with diarrhea and decrease with impaired peristalsis, a factor contributing to constipation. Decreased peristalsis may arise from hypoxic conditions and indicates a need to assess the cardiovascular and pulmonary systems (see Chap. 10). Techniques for abdominal examination are discussed in Chapter 8.

Examination of the anus and rectum may clarify the nature of bowel or urinary elimination problems. For example, the examination may reveal factors interfering with bowel elimination, such as hemorrhoids, or it may reveal factors interfering with urinary elimination, such as prostatic hypertrophy. A complete discussion of the anus and rectum examination is found elsewhere in this chapter (see "Physical Examination of the Anus and Rectum").

Genitourinary System. Genitourinary structures are examined to determine the functional status of structures involved in voiding urine. Alterations in these structures may contribute to urinary elimination problems. For example, a prolapsed uterus may contribute to urinary incontinence. For a complete discussion, refer to Chapter 15.

Neurologic and Musculoskeletal Systems. Examination of the neurologic and musculoskeletal systems is important when evaluating elimination because pathology in these systems may contribute to elimination problems. Sensory or motor deficits such as spinal cord injuries, cerebrovascular accidents, and neurologic disease, for example, can adversely affect both bowel and urinary elimination function.

Integumentary System. If a problem with incontinence exists, you should also examine the skin for signs of impaired integrity, which often results when the skin deteriorates because of contact with feces or urine.

BOWEL ELIMINATION

Anatomy and Physiology Overview

The primary structures one should consider when evaluating bowel elimination include the small and large intestine. The physiology of bowel elimination is discussed elsewhere in this chapter (see "Physiology of Bowel Elimination"). Physical examination techniques may be used to evaluate the status of these structures as well as some aspects of function. Peristaltic functions of the intestines are evaluated by auscultating bowel sounds (see Chap. 8, "Physical Examination of the Abdomen").

The terminal structures of the large intestine, beginning at the sigmoid colon, include the rectum, the anal canal,

and the anus (Fig. 9-4). The physical examination of these structures is commonly referred to as the rectal examination. The integument around the sacrum, gluteal cleft, and perineum (the external area between the vulva and anus or the scrotum and anus) should also be inspected during the rectal examination because of the proximity of these structures.

Anus. The skin of the anus, the outlet of the anal canal, is hairless and darker and moister than the skin surrounding the perineum, because the anus is a mucocutaneous junction. The mucous lining of the anal canal is usually not visible because the anus is held tightly closed by external and internal sphincter muscles. The mucous lining may be examined by exerting slight pressure on each side of the anus. Normally, the anus appears as intact skin without lesions.

Anal Canal. The anal canal is located between the anus and the rectum and is an epithelium-lined structure, 2.5 to 4 cm long. It is important to consider the angle of the anal canal when examining and inserting devices such as thermometers or rectal tubes: The anal canal lies along a line extending anteriorly from anus to umbilicus (see Fig. 9-4).

The internal and external sphincter muscles surround the anal canal and keep the terminal end closed except during defecation. The external sphincter consists of striated muscle under voluntary control and is innervated by the somatic nervous system. The nerve endings are very sensitive to painful stimuli, such as careless digital examination. The levator ani muscles of the pelvic floor augment the contraction of the external sphincter. The internal sphincter consists of smooth muscle controlled by the autonomic nervous system.

The external hemorrhoidal plexus, a vascular structure, is located in the tissue surrounding the anal canal. Vessel enlargement in the plexus is related to venous swelling or thrombosis, resulting in external hemorrhoids. Venous enlargement may occur secondary to increased hydrostatic pressure in capillary vessels, caused by various conditions, including portal hypertension, pregnancy, habitual straining during defecation, and prolonged standing. The proximity of external hemorrhoids to somatic nerve endings causes this condition to be potentially painful, especially during defecation.

Rectum. The rectum is a mucosa-lined structure 12 cm in length. The entire length of the rectum cannot be palpated by digital examination. The boundary between the anal canal and the rectum, called the anorectal junction or pectinate or dentate line, is not palpable. However, the diameter of the bowel lumen usually enlarges at this point and is palpable. The rectum extends posteriorly toward the sacrum, with the posterior wall of the rectum being oriented almost 90 degrees from the anal canal. Normally, the mucosa overlying the posterior wall is smooth. The zona hemorrhoidalis surrounds the anorectal junction and is slightly superior to it. In the underlying tissue, veins anastomose and form a ring around the anorectal junction. Congestion, dilation, and thrombosis of these vessels may result in internal hemorrhoids.

In men, the posterior surface of the prostate gland is palpable through the anterior rectal wall. The prostate consists of two lateral lobes divided by a slight indentation called

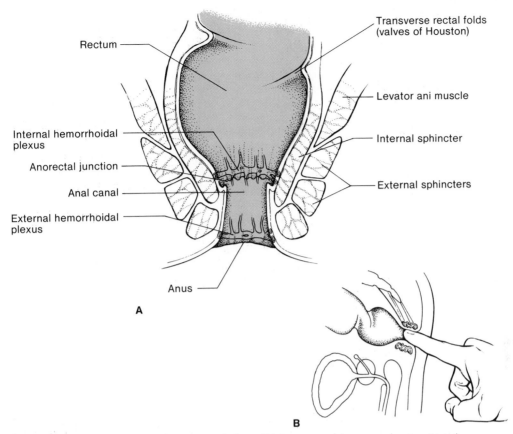

Rectum

Transverse rectal folds
(valves of Houston)

Levator ani muscle

Internal hemorrhoidal
plexus

Anorectal junction

Anal canal

External hemorrhoidal
plexus

Internal sphincter

External sphincters

Anus

A

B

Figure 9–4. (A) Gross anatomy of the anus and rectum. **(B)** Orientation of the anus and rectum. Note the angle of the anal canal and how the examining finger should be inserted.

the median sulcus. The entire gland weighs approximately 20 g and is 4 cm wide and 2.5 cm long. The prostate gland may become enlarged and compress the urethra, which may affect bladder elimination. The prostate gland is also susceptible to malignant growth and should be examined to screen for cancer.

The upper portion of the rectum is surrounded by several transverse folds of mucosa called the valves of Houston. These folds are palpable as ridges and are often mistaken for masses during the rectal examination. The valves of Houston may function to hold feces in the rectum when flatus is passed.

Physical Examination   *Anus and Rectum*

General Principles

The main techniques used in the anorectal examination are inspection and palpation. The areas examined include the peripheral and gluteal skin, the anal canal and rectum, and the prostate gland in men and the cervix and uterus in women. The presence and characteristics of any stool accumulations are noted.

To lessen the person's physical discomfort, your nails should be well-trimmed and no rings should be worn. Extreme pain during palpation is associated with fissures and hemorrhoids. *Do not force the examination if pain persists.* In such a case, consult a physician to determine if a lesion is present. A more extensive examination might require that the area be anesthetized. The physician may decide to inspect the anal canal and lower rectum with an anoscope, a speculum that allows epithelial and mucosal surfaces to be viewed.

Equipment

- Gloves (nonsterile examination type)
- Water-soluble lubricant (*e.g.,* KY Jelly, Lubrifax)

Minimizing Anxiety

For many people, the rectal examination is an uncomfortable and embarrassing procedure. A more comfortable atmosphere can be established by draping the person to lessen embarrassment and by offering simple explanations about the procedure and any sensations that may be elicited, such as the urge to defecate when the anal canal and distal rectum are palpated. Men should be warned that they may feel the urge to void when the prostate gland is palpated.

Hygienic Measures

Although you wear gloves during the examination, good handwashing is essential after the examination is completed. Take care not to contaminate the perineum with fecal material that may adhere to gloves. If the person has fecal impaction, liquid stool may ooze from the rectum during the digital examination. For people who are at risk for defecating during the examination, place a protective pad, such as Chux, beneath the buttocks. The person's skin should be cleaned after the examination, either by you or by the client.

Positioning

The person may assume any of several positions during the rectal examination. Selecting a position depends on examination purpose and the person's mobility.

The left lateral position (Sims's position) requires the person to lie on the left side with the upper leg flexed in a manner that brings the knee to the chest (Fig. 9-5). Masses (including fecal impactions) in the lower rectum can be easily palpated with the person in this position. The upper rectum may be difficult to palpate because this position will displace the upper rectum away from your finger. However, for a person who is confined to bed, this position is easiest to assume.

The knee-chest position (genupectoral position) requires the person to bend at the knees with the thighs upright and the head and shoulders resting on the examining table (Fig. 9-6). This position allows for optimal observation of the perineum and palpation of the prostate gland.

The standing position requires the person to stand at the end of the examining table and bend at the waist while supporting the upper body on the table (Fig. 9-7). Palpating the prostate gland is easier with the person in this position than in the knee–chest position.

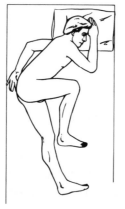

Figure 9–5. Left lateral (Sim's) position.

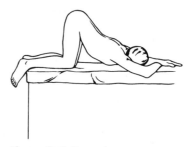

Figure 9–6. Knee–chest (genupectoral) position.

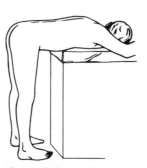

Figure 9–7. Standing position.

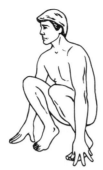

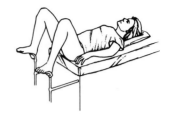

Figure 9–8. Squatting position.   **Figure 9–9.** Lithotomy (dorsosacral) position.

The squatting position requires the person to bend at the hips and knees, while leaning slightly forward and supporting the body weight with the hands and forearms (Fig. 9-8). Rectal prolapse (protrusion of the rectal mucosa through the anus) is most easily observed with the person in this position. It also allows you to palpate a more extensive area of the rectum and detect possible rectal–sigmoid lesions of the pelvic floor.

The lithotomy position (dorsosacral position) requires the person to lie on his or her back with the thighs flexed toward the abdomen and the legs pulled up on the thighs (Fig. 9-9). This position may also be achieved by placing the heels in stirrups attached to the table. This method is used for women undergoing pelvic and rectal examination, because the rectal examination is often conducted as part of the pelvic assessment in women. For men, however, the lithotomy position is not ideal because it does not provide the best position for palpating the prostate.

Examination and Documentation Focus

- *Perineal and gluteal skin:* Color and pigmentation, secretions or excretions, lesions
- *Anal canal and rectum:* Muscle tone, prostate gland or cervix and uterus, stool accumulation, tenderness, lesions, and masses

Examination Guidelines   *Anus and Rectum*

Procedure

Clinical Significance

1. INSPECT THE INTEGUMENT OF THE SACRUM, GLUTEAL FOLDS, AND PERINEUM.

   a. Position the person in the standing or left lateral position. If the lateral position is used, displace the buttocks with your nondominant hand. If the standing position is used, spread the buttocks apart with your hand. Use a small penlight to assess more easily the condition of the skin.

Deviations from Normal

A dimple or tuft of hair in this area may indicate a pilonidal cyst or sinus.

Pilonidal cyst (a cyst in the area of the sacrum or coccyx usually near the upper gluteal fold): This condition is congenital and forms when a small amount of epithelial tissue becomes trapped beneath the skin surface. Hair may grow from this tissue. The cyst is significant because it may trap debris, become infected, and lead to fistula formation.

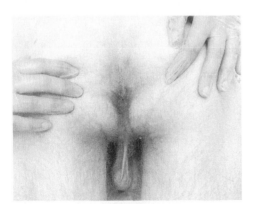

Inspection: Sacrum, gluteal folds, perineum

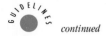

GUIDELINES *continued*

Anus and Rectum

Procedure

b. Inspect the perineum, noting any redness, excretions, or lesions including fissures, warts, hemorrhoids, and scars.

c. Inspect the perianal region and ask the person to perform a Valsalva manuever (bear down as though having a bowel movement). Then note any bulges, fissures, hemorrhoids, or polyps revealed by this manuever.

2. PALPATE THE ANAL CANAL AND RECTUM.

a. Relax the external anal sphincter. Use your nondominant hand to spread the buttocks. Your dominant hand should be gloved, with the index finger lubricated. Using the pad of the index finger of your dominant hand, exert slight, even pressure against the anus. This will relax the sphincter, and facilitate inserting your examining finger into the anal canal. Using the tip of the finger, rather than the pad, will cause greater pain and sphincter tightening.

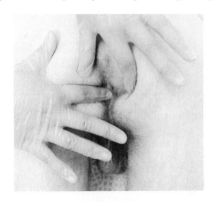

b. Palpate the anal canal. Insert your gloved examining finger into the anal canal, moving the finger in the direction of the umbilicus. Ask the person to tighten the external sphincter by squeezing around your finger so that you can assess muscle tone. To palpate, rotate your finger, which will expose the entire lumen of the anal canal. Stop the examination if the person experiences extreme pain.

Clinical Significance

Normal Findings

Perineal skin color matches the color of the surrounding skin. Skin immediately surrounding the anus may be darker (reddish brown), especially in children. The surface of the skin should be clear of fecal material. The anal area should be free of lesions or signs of skin irritation such as erythema or rashes.

Deviations from Normal

Excretions of fecal material may indicate poor hygiene practices. Other excreted substances, such as blood or mucus, should not be present. Possible lesions include protrusions, bluish discolorations, and fissures in the anal area. Skin tags (irregular flaccid skin sacs) may be noted around the anus if the client has a history of external hemorrhoids. Skin tags are usually benign and painless, forming as hemorrhoids expand through skin connective tissue and becoming flaccid when hemorrhoids resolve.

The digital examination may be painful if the external sphincter is not relaxed before the examining finger is inserted.

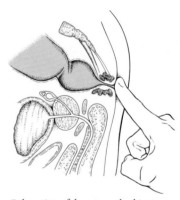

Relaxation of the external sphincter

Normal Findings

The external sphincter should remain closed until voluntary muscle contraction (as occurs during defecation) pulls it open. Good sphincter tone is present if the person can voluntarily contract the sphincter around the examiner's finger.

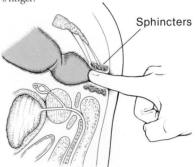

Sphincters

Palpation: Anal canal

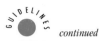

continued

Anus and Rectum

Procedure

c. Palpate the levator ani muscles. Advance your examining finger through the anal canal. At the anorectal junction, palpate the levator ani muscles on the lateral-posterior surfaces of the rectal wall.

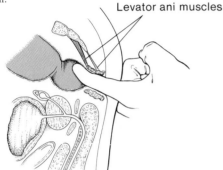

Levator ani muscles

Palpation: Levator ani muscles

d. Palpate the lateral and posterior rectal walls. Advance your examining finger and systematically palpate the right lateral wall, posterior wall, and left lateral wall of the rectum, noting any tenderness or masses. The posterior wall may be difficult to palpate because it extends furthest from the anal opening. Ask the person to bear down while you palpate the posterior wall, to expose any palpable masses higher in the rectum.

Clinical Significance

The levator ani muscles play an important role in bowel control. The muscles may be difficult to palpate, but should be smooth and firm.

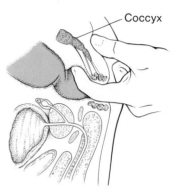

Coccyx

Palpation: Posterior rectal wall

Stool accumulation: Soft, formed stool may be palpable in the rectum; hard or putty-like stool may indicate fecal impaction.

Masses: Palpable masses are abnormal (see display "Anal and Rectal Masses"). Stool, tampons (felt through the anterior wall of the rectum), and the valves of Houston should not be mistaken for masses.

Anal and Rectal Masses

Note: Discovering a mass during the rectal examination warrants immediate referral to a physician. Further examination, including tissue biopsy, is often indicated to rule out a malignancy.

External Hemorrhoid

- May be visible at the anal opening unless thrombosed
- Small, shiny, bluish nodules
- May appear only when the person performs a Valsalva maneuver
- Tender to palpation

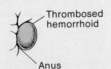

Thrombosed hemorrhoid

Anus

External hemorrhoid

Internal Hemorrhoid

- Located above the anorectal junction
- Not always palpable, unless thrombosed
- If palpable, should feel smooth and soft

Internal hemorrhoid

Rectal Prolapse

- Red mucosa protruding through the anus
- May appear only when the person performs a Valsalva maneuver

Rectal polyps

Rectal Tumor

- May be palpable anywhere along the anal canal or rectum
- Hard, nodular, irregular
- May or may not have a rolled edge
- Firmly embedded in surrounding tissue
- Nontender to palpation

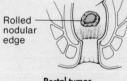

Rolled nodular edge

Rectal tumor

Rectal Polyps

- Small, rectal tumors
- Pedunculated polyps develop on a stalk and are freely moveable
- Sessile polyps lie close to rectal mucosa

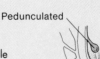

Pedunculated   Sessile

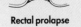

Rectal prolapse

continued   *Anus and Rectum*

Procedure

e. *In men:* Palpate the prostate and anterior rectal wall. Rotate the examining finger to palpate the anterior wall. Identify the lateral lobes and median sulcus of the prostate gland, noting size, tenderness, consistency (firm or boggy), and nodules.

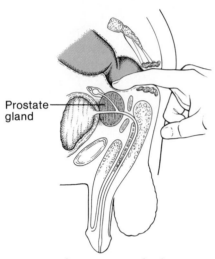

Palpation: Prostate gland

Clinical Significance

Normal Findings

The prostate is round, 4 cm wide and 2.5 cm long, with a palpable median sulcus or groove separating the two lobes. It should feel firm and be free of nodules and masses. When palpated, it should not cause tenderness, although it may cause an urge to urinate (see display, "Prostate Conditions").

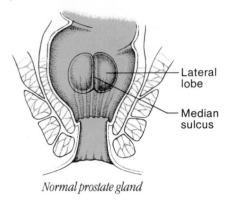

Normal prostate gland

Prostate Conditions

Benign Prostatic Hypertrophy

- Symmetric enlargement of the prostate
- Gland feels boggy
- Median sulcus may disappear
- Common after age 50
- May compress urethra and interfere with urination

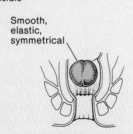

Smooth, elastic, symmetrical

Benign prostatic hypertrophy

Acute Prostatitis

- Prostate enlarged (may be asymmetrical)
- Tender to palpation

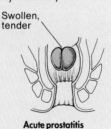

Swollen, tender

Acute prostatitis

Prostate Malignancy

- Palpable mass on prostate
- Hard, irregular, fixed
- May be painless on palpation
- May cause prostate to feel asymmetric

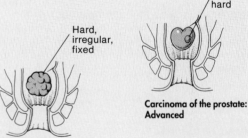

Hard, irregular, fixed

Irregular, hard

Carcinoma of the prostate: Single nodule

Carcinoma of the prostate: Advanced

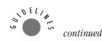

continued   **Anus and Rectum**

Procedure

   f. *In women:* Palpate the cervix. Examine the anterior rectal wall as part of the pelvic examination with the woman in the lithotomy position (this technique is described in greater detail in Chapter 15). Rotate the examining finger and palpate the anterior wall. Palpate the rounded tip of the cervix, noting any tenderness or nodules. Ask the woman to bear down in order to assess for uterine prolapse.

3. COMPLETE THE EXAMINATION.

   a. Slowly withdraw your examining finger from the rectum. Note the color of any stool adhering to the glove and check the stool for occult blood (see guaiac test, p. 208).

   b. Give the person tissue to clean the anus, or clean the perineum yourself as you finish the examination.

Clinical Significance

Cervix: A firm, round, smooth mass felt through the anterior wall; not tender on palpation.

Uterus: Difficult to palpate by rectal examination unless prolapsed.

Documenting Anus and Rectum Examination Findings

Example 1

Mr. H, aged 44, had an anorectal examination as part of his routine annual health assessment. The results were normal and recorded as follows:

> Perineal skin and anus clean and intact. Small amount of soft stool in rectum; no masses or tenderness. Prostate smooth, firm, nontender, and without masses; size 4 by 2 cm.

The same results may be summarized in a problem-oriented format:

  S: Reports no change in bowel elimination patterns; regular pattern—BM every AM after breakfast.
  O: Perineal skin and anus clean and intact. Small amount of soft stool in rectum; no masses or tenderness. Prostate smooth, firm, nontender, and without masses; size 4 by 2 cm.
  A: Normal anorectal examination results.
  P: Follow up with routine exams.
     Test stool for occult blood.
     Teach client significance of sudden change in bowel elimination pattern.

Example 2

Mr. G, aged 72, had an anorectal examination following reports of urinary hesitancy. The results were abnormal and recorded as follows:

> No masses, nodules, or stool palpable in rectum. Prostate enlarged and soft on palpation; unable to palpate median sulcus; no palpable prostate masses.

The same results may be summarized in a problem-oriented format:

  S: Reports "can't get my water going"; reports occasional constipation.
  O: No masses, nodules, or stool palpable in rectum. Prostate enlarged and soft on palpation; unable to palpate median sulcus; no palpable masses.
  A: Prostate enlarged—possibly related to benign prostatic hypertrophy.
  P: Refer to physician.

Example 3

Mrs. L, aged 55, had experienced intermittent constipation and noted bloody stools. The anorectal examination results were abnormal and the client was referred to her physician. The documentation was as follows:

> Firm, irregular, nonmobile mass palpated on posterior rectal wall 5 cm from anus; nontender to palpation; gross blood noted on examining glove.

Examination of the Stool

Feces form in the large intestine as water in the semiliquid chyme is absorbed across the intestinal wall. The final appearance of the stool varies among healthy people who have normal elimination function. In most instances, normal variations can be attributed to dietary differences.

The stool may be examined in the patient care setting or in the laboratory. In the clinical setting, the stool is examined to describe general characteristics and volume. General characteristics may indicate problems such as constipation or diarrhea. Bedside testing may also reveal the presence of occult blood in the stool.

The laboratory analysis of stool is more detailed and is directed at identifying and quantifying various substances such as fat, blood, organisms, and urobilinogen. Laboratory tests provide the following additional information about bowel and systemic problems:

- *Fecal fat* (normally <7 g/24 h). Documents malabsorption of fat (steatorrhea). The principal site of fat absorption is the small intestine.
- *Occult blood* (normally negative). Indicates hidden bleeding, especially in the bowel.
- *Ova and parasites* (normally negative). Microscopic examination of the stool may reveal parasitic ova, cysts, larvae, or trophozites. A positive test indicates infestation of the intestinal tract.
- *Stool culture* (usually reveals normal flora). Indicates the nature of pathogenic organisms.
- *Fecal urobilinogen* (normally (10–250 IU/100 g). Indicates hemolytic anemia (indicated by higher values) and biliary obstruction (indicated by lower values).

GENERAL PRINCIPLES

Stools should be evaluated by inspection, smell, and laboratory analysis.

Stool can be analyzed for occult blood by guaiac testing.

SPECIMEN COLLECTION

Stool collected for cultures must be delivered to the laboratory while still warm, usually within 30 minutes. Otherwise, stool may become overgrown with normal resident organisms that obscure abnormal organisms such as parasites. If the stool is being cultured for organisms such as bacteria, parasites, or viruses, three consecutive stool samples must be sent to the laboratory because organisms may not be passed with every stool. Stool collected for chemical analysis should be refrigerated if immediate delivery to the laboratory is not possible.

Stool specimens should be placed in a clean container and covered. Wax-lined containers should not be used for stools being analyzed for fat content because the wax can interfere with results. The container does not need to be filled unless the stool will undergo chemical analysis, in which case quantity is important. For example, fecal fat analysis involves determining the fat content of all stools excreted for a time period such as 24 hours.

BARIUM EFFECT

Barium is a radiopaque compound instilled into the lower bowel during certain x-ray studies. It is eventually excreted through the stool.

Barium in the stool will not interfere with most cultures, provided a relatively large stool sample is obtained. However, barium does interfere with cultures for parasites.

EXAMINATION AND DOCUMENTATION FOCUS

- Color
- Consistency and shape
- Volume
- Odor
- Composition

Examination Guidelines   *Stool*

Procedure

1. OBSERVE THE COLOR OF THE STOOL.

If food and drugs are ruled out as the reason for altered stool color, other causes should be investigated. Consultation with a physician may be indicated if any of the following colors are noted: black, maroon, gray, tan, clay, or yellow.

Clinical Significance

Normal Findings

Stool is light or dark brown as a result of the pigments stercobilin and urobilin, which are derived from the breakdown of bilirubin in the intestine. Certain foods and medications may alter normal color.

Dark brown to black: Indicates presence of iron pigments from large amounts of meat protein or iron-containing drugs.

Black: Indicates ingestion of licorice, anti-inflammatory drugs such as phenylbutazone and oxyphenbutazone, or bismuth compounds such as Pepto-Bismol.

Green: Indicates ingestion of spinach or senna laxatives. In children and infants, green stools indicate rapid transit of food through the bowel.

White or gray: Indicates ingestion of barium or drugs containing aluminum hydroxide, such as Amphojel.

Red: Indicates ingestion of beets or cocoa.

Deviations from Normal

Black or maroon: May indicate bleeding in the gastrointestinal tract. Blackened stool may also be tarry (melena).

Gray, tan, or clay: May indicate that bile, which contains bilirubin, is not being adequately produced or distributed, perhaps due to biliary tract obstruction.

GUIDELINES *continued*   ***Stool***

| Procedure | Clinical Significance |

Procedure

Clinical Significance

Yellow: May indicate excess fat in the stool, secondary to fat malabsorption syndromes.

2. NOTE THE CONSISTENCY AND SHAPE OF STOOL.

Normal Findings

Stools are usually soft because they are 75% water, and are tubular in shape like the rectum.

Deviations from Normal

Hard, nodular stools, which may be excreted as small, rocklike masses, may be the result of constipation or spastic colon. Fluid or mushy stools usually occur with diarrhea and may appear greasy because the fat content is high, perhaps secondary to fat malabsorption syndromes. Fat-infiltrated stools often float in the toilet because fat is light and buoyant. Stools that are narrow, flat, or ribbon-like, rather than tubular, may indicate rectal obstruction or spastic colitis. Such obstructions may be secondary to tumors, strictures, or hemorrhoids.

3. DETERMINE THE VOLUME OF STOOL EXCRETED WITH EACH BOWEL MOVEMENT AND IN A 24-HOUR PERIOD.

Normal Findings

A person who eats a healthy diet usually excretes an average stool volume of 100 to 200 gm/day. Not all people who ingest healthy diets defecate on a daily basis.

Deviations from Normal

Excessive volumes of watery stool may be noted with diarrhea. Low volumes are usually associated with constipation or prolonged fasting.

4. NOTE THE ODOR OF THE STOOL.

Normal Findings

Stool odor varies and is influenced by diet. Odors occur secondary to bacterial action in the colon. A sour odor may be noted in the stool of infants.

Deviations from Normal

Distinct changes in fecal odor are noted when stools contain excessive fat or blood. Cancers that invade the rectum or colon may cause a putrid or decaying odor.

5. NOTE THE COMPOSITION OF THE STOOL.

Normal Findings

Stool is normally composed of 75% water. The remaining dry matter consists of food residues, such as cellulose, fats, and proteins; bacteria (*E. coli*); inorganic salts; and residues from intestinal juices, such as pigments, and sloughed epithelial cells.

Deviations from Normal

Blood, mucus, parasites and foreign objects are not normal fecal constituents.

Bright red *blood* throughout the feces may indicate lower intestinal bleeding. Blood on the stool surface or on toilet paper may indicate rectal or anal canal bleeding, commonly caused by hemorrhoids and anal fissures. Occult blood is small quantities of blood in the stool that is not visible to the naked eye. Occult blood may be a sign of cancer or ulceration of the intestinal tract and requires further evaluation.

Mucus, although not always an abnormal finding, may be a sign of bowel inflammation. Mucus, diarrhea stools may be observed in ulcerative colitis, an inflammatory disease of the colon.

GUIDELINES *continued*   *Stool*

Procedure

6. IF INDICATED, TEST THE STOOL FOR OCCULT BLOOD (GUAIAC TEST).

   a. Properly prepare the patient.

   Diet Instructions: For testing conducted at home, instruct the person to alter diet 3 days before and during testing. Diet restrictions include all meat products, horseradish, and turnips. Before testing, the person should ingest high-residue foods such as raw vegetables, bran products, and nuts.

   Medication Instructions: Drugs may cause erroneous test results. If possible, anti-inflammatory preparations, steroids, or broad-spectrum antibiotics should not be taken before the stool is tested.

   Assess the patient's understanding of the procedures because this test must often be repeated several times at home.

   b. Assemble the necessary supplies. Presently, several commercial products are available. Stool is applied to specially prepared slides or filter paper and treated with a chemical solution that causes a color change.

   c. Apply a small stool specimen to slide or filter paper.

   d. Allow specimen to dry.

   e. Apply the required amount of developing solution to the slide or filter paper. Commercially prepared guaiac solution is commonly used.

   f. Wait the recommended time and read test results. The results should be read precisely 30 seconds after the solution is applied if commercially prepared guaiac slides are used.

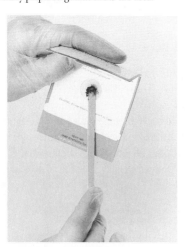

Stool application to guaiac slide

Clinical Significance

Parasites, including nematodes (roundworms) and tapeworms, may be visible on close examinaton of the stool. However, the ova and larvae of these organisms may be visible only with a microscope. Other microscopic organisms that may be excreted in the stool include protozoa and helminths.

Foreign objects, deliberately or accidentally ingested, may be found in the feces. This finding is most common in children.

This test is an important screening procedure for detecting gastrointestinal bleeding, which may indicate colon cancer or ulcer disease.

This test is based on detecting peroxidase activity in the hemoglobin molecule. Peroxidases in these foods can result in false positive results.

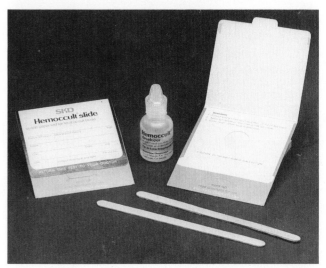

Commercial kit for testing stool for occult blood

Normal Findings

A negative result is indicated by no color change or a green color change, depending on the test.

Deviations from Normal

If occult blood is present, a blue ring will form around the stool specimen, indicating a positive result. A positive result should be followed by physician consultation. In addition, the test should be repeated several times to rule out a false-negative result or to detect intermittent bleeding.

Documenting Stool Examination Findings

Several descriptors may be used to document stool characteristics. The color, consistency and shape, and composition should be documented. The presence of occult blood revealed by guaiac testing is charted "guaiac positive." A sample documentation for a normal stool may be as follows: "Excreted soft, formed, brown stool on commode. Guaiac negative."

Descriptors for Documenting Stool Characteristics

	Normal Findings	Deviations from Normal
Color	Brown, tan, green-yellow	Black, maroon, bloody, white
Consistency and Shape	Soft, formed	Loose, liquid, hard, nodular, rocklike, stringy, greasy
Composition	No foreign particles	Blood, mucus, parasites, undigested food, guaiac positive

NDx

Nursing Diagnoses Related to Bowel Elimination Assessment

Constipation

The nursing diagnosis Constipation is defined as "the state in which the individual experiences or is at high risk of experiencing a delay in passage of food residue resulting in hard, dry stool" (Carpenito, 1989). Causes include change in life-style, immobility, and painful defecation.

The defining characteristics for constipation include decreased activity level; less frequent defecation than usual; hard, formed stools; palpable mass; a reported feeling of rectal pressure; a reported feeling of rectal fullness; and straining to defecate. Additional defining characteristics include abdominal pain; appetite impairment; back pain; headache; interference with daily living; and laxative use.

Constipation may be classified as Perceived constipation, or Colonic constipation. Perceived constipation occurs when the person makes a self-diagnosis of constipation and treats himself or herself with laxatives to assure a daily bowel movement. Colonic constipation refers to a bowel elimination pattern characterized by hard, dry stool.

Constipation Related to Change in Life-Style

History. Changes in a person's life-style may impair the response to the normal defecation reflex. Significant lifestyle changes include situations that cause or interfere with usual bowel elimination habits, such as travel or schedule changes and the use of laxatives or drugs that decrease colonic motility. Inactivity may also contribute to constipation. In addition, many disease processes can alter life-style

and bowel function. The person's chief complaint will often be infrequent stools rather than life-style changes. Consequently, you need to initiate a thorough nursing history.

The Physical Examination. The rectal examination may indicate a palpable fecal impaction. Abdominal distension may be noted, and may be accompanied by restlessness and an increase in flatulence.

Stool. The stool may be hard, dry, and formed. Stool size may vary.

Constipation Related to Immobility

History. A decrease in mobility is associated with decreased peristaltic activity and loss of muscle strength, both of which contribute to constipation. Hospitalization often limits mobility because of enforced bed rest and restricted activity resulting from the presence of tubes, intravenous lines, and other equipment used in therapy. The person may report infrequent, hard stools.

Physical Examination and Stool. See "Constipation Related to Change in Life-Style," above.

Constipation Related to Painful Defecation

History. Painful defecation may lead to a pattern of ignoring the defecation reflex. Patients frequently report hemorrhoids as the cause of this discomfort. Severe abdominal cramping may also make defecation painful. The patient may report infrequent stools, rectal itching, and straining during defecation.

Physical Examination. The anorectal examination may reveal conditions that cause painful defecation. Anal fissures or hemorrhoids may be visible or indicated by extreme pain when the anal canal is palpated. Further assess the rectum for other causes of painful defecation, such as prostatic enlargement, abscesses, and fecal impactions. The perineum may be excoriated.

Stool. The stool is often hard and dry. If lesions such as hemorrhoids are present, the stool may be streaked with bright red blood. The stool may be narrow if rectal masses or colonic dysfunction exists. Stools should be assessed for occult blood.

Diarrhea

The nursing diagnosis Diarrhea is defined as "the state in which the individual experiences or is at high risk of experiencing frequent passage of liquid stool or unformed stool" (Carpenito, 1989). "Untoward side effects" may be the cause of diarrhea and include factors such as infectious processes affecting the gastrointestinal tract, nutritional and malabsorption disorders, changes in life-style, drug side effects, and bowel surgery.

The defining characteristics for diarrhea include abdominal pain; cramping; increased frequency; increased frequency of bowel sounds; loose, liquid stools; and urgency.

History. Diarrhea results from hyperperistalsis of the small intestine or colon. Because diarrhea is a manifestation of over 100 clinical entities, determining the probable cause may be difficult. Investigate factors associated with infectious processes, obstructive neoplasms, ulcerative colitis, Crohn's disease, and malabsorption syndromes. The person may report frequent, loose, or watery stools, defecation usually more than three times per day, or pain and abdominal cramping with defecation. Loss of fluid and electrolytes accounts for complaints of weakness.

Physical Examination. Observable signs of dehydration include poor skin turgor, increased body temperature, hypotension, and weight loss. The rectal examination may reveal marked tenderness or a mass such as fecal impaction or tumor. Rectal examination with a proctoscope by a physician may reveal changes in the mucosal lining of the sigmoid colon that are characteristic of inflammatory diseases such as ulcerative colitis. Bowel sounds are usually hyperactive.

Stool. The stool may be liquid or mushy. Stool color, odor, and composition may indicate the probable cause.

Bowel Incontinence

The nursing diagnosis Incontinence is defined as "involuntary passage of stool." Etiologic factors include conditions that impair neuromuscular function of the colon, rectum, and anal sphincters. Cognitive and perceptual impairment may also be a contributing factor.

History. A person who is alert and oriented may not report fecal incontinence because of embarrassment. Therefore, you should ask questions during the interview to elicit this information, and to ascertain how frequently the incontinence occurs and to identify contributing factors such as neurological lesions or mental confusion. Question the person about factors relating to constipation, because fecal impaction is one of the most common causes of fecal incontinence.

Physical Examination. The rectal examination can provide information about muscle tone and sphincter strength. A fecal impaction may be palpated. A prolapsed anus or other rectal masses may contribute to incontinence. General muscle strength should also be assessed, although a weak and debilitated patient may not have the strength to contract anal sphincters. Skin excoriation may be noted around the anus and buttocks.

Stool. Stool consistency may range from formed to liquid. The appearance of the stool may help determine probable causes of incontinence.

Clinical Problems Related to Bowel Elimination Assessment

Inflammatory and Infectious Processes

Examining the anus, rectum, and stool may indicate inflammatory or infectious bowel or rectal disease, in which case the patient should be referred to a physician. Additional assessment, including stool analysis and culture, x-ray, and proctoscopic examination may be necessary. Understanding the signs and symptoms of certain pathologic conditions that affect bowel function will help you monitor the patient's response to the disease process and treatment.

Ulcerative Colitis. This inflammatory disease, of unknown etiology, affects the colon and rectum. Bloody, mucoid diarrhea with as many as 30 stools per day usually indicates ulcerative colitis. Defecation may be painful and is often accompanied by abdominal cramping and rectal tenesmus. The rectal mucosa usually become inflamed and may bleed easily. Signs of fluid and electrolyte depletion, including weight loss, fever, weakness, and fatigability, may also be present. This disease may involve a series of remissions and exacerbations.

Crohn's Disease. Also called regional enteritis, this inflammatory bowel disease easily can be confused with ulcerative colitis because it is also characterized by remissions, exacerbations, abdominal cramping, and diarrhea. Crohn's disease may affect the small or large intestine. The lesion it causes on the intestinal wall differs from the lesion caused by ulcerative colitis. In the early stages abdominal cramping occurs, usually aggravated by constipation and relieved by a bowel movement. In later stages, exacerbations are characterized by colicky pain in the right lower abdominal quadrant, fever, and abdominal tenderness. Diarrhea stools may occur. The disease invades the bowel mucosa, increasing the risk of fistula formation. Lesions of the anus, anal canal, and rectum are common.

Acute Gastroenteritis. This disease may also be characterized by diarrhea stools caused by pathogens that invade the intestinal tract. The pathogens may be viral, bacterial, or parasitic. Often the disease is self-limiting and will resolve spontaneously within 72 hours. Stool cultures may reveal the causative organism. The patient may appear ill; fever, signs of dehydration, and abdominal cramping often accompany attacks. Rectal examination results are usually normal, but diarrhea stools may cause skin excoriation.

Diverticulitis. This inflammatory process may occur when small pouches, called diverticula, form in the colon and are irritated by feces. The person's bowel elimination pattern may be characterized predominantly by constipation, occasionally alternating with diarrhea. Abdominal pain is usually relieved by a bowel movement. Stool testing will reveal occult blood in 20% of cases. Diverticula may bleed, resulting in massive gastrointestinal hemorrhage.

Malabsorption Syndromes

Malabsorption syndromes involve impaired absorption of fats, proteins, or carbohydrates across the intestinal wall. Malabsorption occurs to some extent with any condition causing rapid intestinal transit and diarrhea stools, as in Crohn's disease and acute gastroenteritis. Common malabsorption syndromes include celiac disease and nontropical sprue. People suffering from these diseases are unable to digest gluten and gliadin, proteins found mainly in wheat. Stools are high in fat content (steatorrhea), appear foamy, and may float. Diarrhea usually occurs as nonabsorbed substances pull excessive water into the bowel, causing distention and hyperperistalsis. The person may lose weight and become malnourished.

Hemorrhage

Gross or occult blood in stools is associated with gastrointestinal hemorrhage from diverse causes such as peptic ulcer disease, ulcerative colitis, diverticulosis, tumors, or hemorrhoids. Stools may become liquid if large amounts of blood enter the colon. Melena or black, tarry stools may be noted when bleeding originates in the small intestine. A maroon stool may indicate bleeding in the colon. Bright red blood within the stool or streaking the outside surface is associated with bleeding in the lower sigmoid colon, rectum, and anal canal.

Irritable Bowel Syndrome

Irritable bowel syndrome (IBS) or spastic colon is considered an elusive entity. Irritable bowel syndrome is characterized by recurrent abdominal pain and altered bowel elimination patterns. Although there appears to be intestinal motor dysfunction, no bowel pathology is found. Symptoms vary among people and in the same person from one time to another. Most people with this disorder have two or three of the six cardinal symptoms of IBS:

1. Relief of pain with defecation
2. Onset of pain associated with more frequent defecation
3. Onset of pain associated with looser stools
4. Distention of the abdomen
5. Rectal dissatisfaction (feeling of incomplete evacuation)
6. Passage of mucus with stools

Hyperplastic Growths

Colon and Rectum Cancer. The likelihood of developing colon, or rectum cancer increases between ages 40 and 60 years. If the condition is detected early, 90% of patients respond favorably to treatment. Often the earliest sign is a change in the bowel elimination pattern, either diarrhea or constipation. At later stages, rectal bleeding, abdominal

pain and distension, general malaise, and weight loss may be noted. Most rectosigmoid tumors are palpable during the rectal examination. The tumor is usually a hard, firmly embedded mass that may have an irregular border. Palpation of the mass rarely causes pain. The stool usually contains occult blood. Persons with a palpable rectal mass should be referred to a physician.

Prostate Cancer. Men over age 60 are at highest risk for prostate cancer. Initially, the patient may notice prostatic hyperplasia symptoms, including hesitancy and straining with urination, dribbling, and a decreased caliber of the urinary stream. Urine retention may occur as the enlarging prostate obstructs the bladder outlet. Rectal examination may reveal a hard, fixed, enlarged prostate gland. Nodular masses may be palpable.

URINARY ELIMINATION

Anatomy and Physiology Overview

The structures of the urinary tract include the kidneys, renal pelvis, ureters, bladder, urethra, and urinary meatus (Fig. 9-10). From the major calices of the kidney, urine drains into the renal pelvis and then into the ureter. The ureter from each kidney attaches to the bladder wall.

The urinary bladder is a hollow muscular organ that stores and expels urine. The size and shape of the bladder vary. When the bladder is empty, it is triangular-shaped and lies entirely within the pelvic structure. When the bladder is full, it is more spherical in shape and extends upward

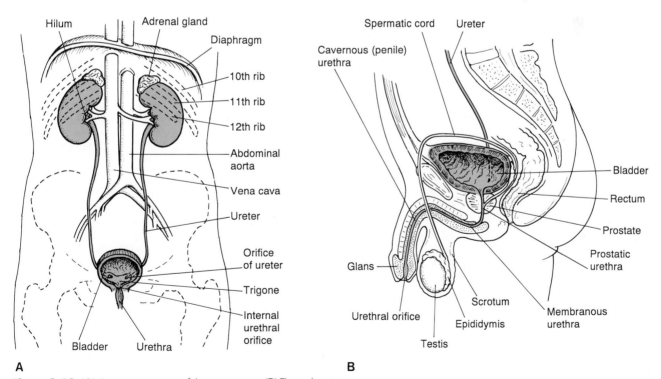

Figure 9-10. (A) Anatomic structures of the urinary tract. **(B)** The male urinary tract.

and anteriorly in the abdominal cavity. This causes the lower abdomen to appear distended.

The urethra extends from the urinary bladder to the urinary meatus. The male urethra traverses through the prostate gland and urinary alterations, such as retention, hesitancy, and narrow stream may be noted if the prostate gland is enlarged. The female urethra is relatively short compared to the male urethra. In women, good pelvic muscle tone is required to maintain voluntary control of the urethral sphincter.

The physiology of urinary elimination, including the role of the nervous system, is discussed elsewhere in this chapter (see "Physiology of Urinary Elimination").

Physical Examination   Urinary Structures

The kidney and ureters are generally not palpable, although a kidney may be palpated on very thin persons. Inflammation of the upper urinary tract is noted during the physical examination by using fist percussion over the lower back in the area over the kidney. This maneuver may be referred to as "eliciting costovertebral tenderness," because the percussion occurs on the lower back at the costovertebral angle (where the lower ribs meet the vertebral column). Tenderness and pain with this maneuver indicate inflammation.

An enlarged bladder is readily detected during the abdominal examination (see Chap. 8). Bladder enlargement may be detected by inspection, percussion, and palpation.

The examination of the urethra and related musculature is discussed in Chapter 15 (see "Examination Guidelines: Male Genitals" and "Examination Guidelines: Female Genitals and Pelvic Structures"). A pelvic examination is indicated in women with stress incontinence of urine to evaluate pelvic muscle tone.

Examination of Urine

Urine may be examined in the patient care setting or in the laboratory. At the bedside, urine should be evaluated by observing its appearance; noting its odor; and measuring volume, including voided volumes and residual volumes. Measuring urine volumes is especially relevant to assessing urinary elimination problems.

Analytic tests reveal information about specific gravity, pH, and urine composition. Test results are analyzed to identify problems. For example, an excessive white blood cell count may indicate infection; altered specific gravity may indicate dehydration or fluid overload; and polyuria may indicate endocrine or renal disorders. Urine may be cultured in the laboratory to determine the nature of infectious organisms.

General Principles Urine should be evaluated by inspection, smell, and laboratory analysis. Some analytic tests may be performed at the bedside using specific devices. For example, dipsticks may be used to determine urine constituents and pH. Dipsticks are specially treated plastic sticks that register important color changes when dipped into a fresh urine sample. The manufacturer's instructions are included on the container. Specific gravity is also tested in clinical settings.

Specimen Collection Urine specimens to be used in analytic tests or cultures should be clean-catch midstream specimens. Instruct the person to clean the area around the urinary meatus with soap and water, initiate and then stop the urinary stream, and resume urinating into the specimen collection container. Before he or she senses that the bladder is completely empty, the person should stop the stream again, remove the container, and finish voiding. If the urine will be cultured, it may be obtained by catheterization and placed in a sterile container. You must be extremely careful not to contaminate the inside of the sterile container by touching it.

The first morning specimen is most desirable for analysis because the urine is concentrated. To test for glucose, the second voided specimen should be used. However, urine glucose testing is being replaced by blood glucose monitoring, which is more accurate and easily performed with home testing devices. Urine may also be tested for occult blood and for the presence of protein.

Urine that will be sent to the laboratory should be refrigerated in order to slow bacterial growth or decomposition and should be analyzed within 1 hour.

Urine for analysis should never be collected from the bottom of a catheter bag because the urine will probably contain more sediment and be contaminated with bacteria, thereby distorting test results.

Examination and Documentation Focus

- Color
- Transparency
- Odor
- Volume
- Specific gravity
- pH
- Cells, casts, and crystals
- Electrolytes

Examination Guidelines   *Urine*

Procedure	Clinical Significance
1. OBSERVE THE COLOR OF THE URINE.	**Normal Findings**

Normal Findings

The normal color of urine ranges from pale to dark yellow because of the pigment urochrome. The variation in color reflects the urine concentration and the foods and drugs ingested. The normal color variations include pale yellow, colorless, bright yellow, yellow-orange, yellow-green, red, red-pink, and blue-green.

Pale yellow to colorless: Indicates urine is diluted because of increased fluid intake.

Bright yellow: May indicate ingestion of drugs such as acriflavine mepacrine, nitrofurantoin, and large doses of riboflavin.

Yellow-orange: Indicates ingestion of the drug phenazopyridine (Pyridium).

Yellow-green: Indicates ingestion of rhubarb.

Red: Indicates ingestion of beets or candies containing fuscin dye.

Red-pink: Indicates ingestion of phenolphthalein, a constituent of many over-the-counter laxatives.

Blue-green: Indicates ingestion of drugs containing the dye methylene blue.

Deviations from Normal

Colorless: Kidneys may not be concentrating the urine, as occurs in diabetes insipidus.

Yellow-orange: May indicate liver or gallbladder disease. Color changes are secondary to excess urobilin or bilirubin pigments.

Red, reddish brown, or brown-black: May indicate the presence of hemoglobin and be caused by trauma to urinary structures, reactions to blood transfusion, or lysis of red blood cells.

Brown to black: Indicates Addison's disease. The color change is due to urinary excretion of melanin.

Whitish cast: May represent bacteria or cell products of an inflammatory response (polymorphonuclear neutrophil leukocytes, or PMNs).

2. OBSERVE TRANSPARENCY OF URINE.

Normal Findings

Freshly voided urine is normally clear. Refrigerated urine or urine that is allowed to stand may become turbid as bacteria ferments. Urine contaminated with sperm or menstrual blood may appear cloudy.

GUIDELINES   *continued*   *Urine*

Procedure	Clinical Significance

Clinical Significance

Deviations from Normal

Cloudy urine (also called turbid urine) indicates the presence of abnormal cells or constituents such as excessive white blood cells (WBCs), calculi, pus, bacteria, or fats. In such cases, sediment may form at the bottom of the specimen container.

3. NOTE ODOR OF THE URINE.

Normal Findings

Urine is normally aromatic. Ingestion of multivitamins or vitamin B may cause a strong, sharp odor. Eating asparagus may give the urine a grasslike odor.

Deviations from Normal

An acetone odor indicates ketosis resulting from diabetic ketoacidosis and other starvation states. If the urine has an ammonia scent, the probable cause is infection, especially by *Proteus,* a bacterium capable of splitting urea into ammonia by-products. A smell of decay indicates infection and results from bacterial cell death. A musty odor is associated with phenylketonuria (PKU). A fecal odor indicates the existence of a rectal fistula.

4. MEASURE VOLUME OF URINE USING A CONTAINER CALIBRATED IN MILLILITERS.

Normal Findings

Normally 1200 to 1500 mL of urine is voided per day. Greater amounts may be voided if there is excessive fluid intake. Normally, the bladder can store 300 to 600 mL of urine before voiding becomes essential. Usually urine is not retained in the bladder after voiding.

a. Determine the residual volume, if indicated. Encourage the person to void and record the voided volume, then catheterize the bladder immediately and record the amount of urine obtained. This is the residual volume. Amounts greater than 50 mL indicate urine retention of high residual volume. Occasionally, a very high residual volume, such as 1000 to 3000 mL, may be obtained. In such a case, the bladder should be drained slowly by clamping the catheter after 800 to 1000 mL of urine are drained, then waiting, and releasing the clamp. Determining residual volumes by bladder catheterization may require a physician's prescription.

Deviations from Normal

Oliguria: In oliguria, less than 500 mL of urine is voided per day. The cause may be an elimination problem such as urine retention in the bladder or pathologic conditions related to urine production in the kidney. Determining residual urine volume (urine drained from the bladder by a catheter immediately after voiding) may help differentiate these oilguric states. Oliguria secondary to renal pathology usually does not result in significant residual volumes. On the other hand, if bladder function is impaired, which can occur when infection interferes with normal muscular contraction of the bladder muscles or when the bladder outlet is obstructed, then high residual volumes may be noted. Residual volumes exceeding 50 mL are generally considered abnormal. (See Measuring Urine Volumes.)

Polyuria: Polyuria refers to urine volumes of 2500 mL or greater per day, which may occur with diuretic therapy, endocrine dysfunction, or renal pathology. Cerebral pathology may undermine the influence of antidiuretic hormone (ADH), leading to increased urine production. The diuretic phase of renal failure may also be associated with large urine volumes.

b. Determine bladder capacity, if indicated.

Bladder capacity is the volume determined by adding the voided volume to the residual volume.

Deviations from Normal

A bladder capacity greater than 1000 mL may indicate urinary retention.

5. USING EITHER A HYDROMETER (URINOMETER) OR REFRACTOMETER, MEASURE THE URINE SPECIFIC GRAVITY.

Specific gravity is a measurement of urine density, a product of the volume of urine produced by the kidneys and the amount of particulate matter in the urine. In other words, specific gravity indicates whether urine is diluted or concentrated. Specific gravity correlates with urine osmolality.

GUIDELINES *continued*   *Urine*

Procedure

Hydrometer Procedure

a. OBTAIN A FRESH, WELL-MIXED URINE SAMPLE. When testing with the hydrometer, use enough urine to fill the container at least three fourths full.

b. PLACE THE URINE IN THE CONTAINER.

c. PLACE THE URINOMETER INTO THE CONTAINER OF URINE. Be certain that the urinometer floats freely without touching the sides of the container.

d. READ THE SCALE ON THE URINOMETER AT THE LEVEL OF THE MENISCUS. The value obtained is the urine specific gravity.

Refractometer Procedure

a. OBTAIN A FRESH, WELL-MIXED URINE SAMPLE. Use enough urine to cover the glass surface (usually only a few drops).

b. APPLY URINE TO THE REFRACTOMETER'S GLASS SURFACE. Use a dropper or syringe to transfer urine.

c. READ THE REFRACTOMETER SCALE. Place the cover of the instrument over the glass surface to which the urine has been applied. Point the instrument toward a light source. Look into the viewing end and read the scale at the demarcation line. The value obtained is the urine specific gravity.

Clinical Significance

Normal Findings

The normal adult range for specific gravity is 1.003 to 1.030, with the higher number representing more concentratred urine. The normal range for elderly people is between 1.016 and 1.022 because the ability to concentrate urine decreases with age.

Deviations from Normal

Urine specific gravity may be lowered with excessive urine production following increased fluid intake or ingestion of diuretic medications.

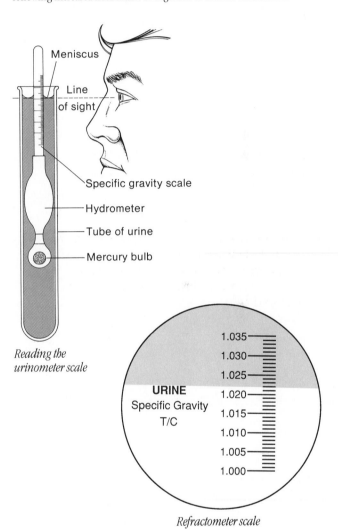

Reading the urinometer scale

Refractometer scale

Deviations from Normal

Increased urine specific gravity indicates decreased urine volume or an increased amount of particulate matter in the urine. The latter condition may be related to excessive glucose or protein, as in uncontrolled diabetes mellitus and nephrotic syndrome.

Decreased urine specific gravity occurs with diabetes insipidus, acute renal failure, water intoxicatin, and severe hypokalemia.

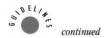

continued

Urine

Procedure

6. DETERMINE THE URINE pH USING A DIPSTICK.

7. EXAMINE THE URINE FOR CELLS, CASTS, AND CRYSTALS.

Cells, casts, and crystals are detected by microscopic urine examination but may be visible on gross inspection when large quantities are present.

Clinical Significance

Normal Findings

Urine is slightly acid with a normal pH of 5 to 7. A high intake of meat protein or foods such as cranberry juice may acidify the urine further. Urine that is tested early in the morning may be more acidic because a mild respiratory acidosis occurs during sleep, and the kidneys compensate by excreting more hydrogen ions. A more alkaline pH is noted in urine that is allowed to stand before it is tested. The bacterial action and the loss of carbon dioxide cause the urine to lose its acidity. Vegetarian diets may also cause alkaline urine.

Deviations from Normal

Increased alkalinity is noted with bacterial infections that are caused by organisms that split urea, such as *Proteus* and *Pseudomonas*. A more alkaline urine also occurs with respiratory alkalosis, because the kidneys attempt to compensate by excreting more bicarbonate ions, and with renal diseases such as chronic glomerulonephritis and renal tubular acidosis.

Increased acidity results from metabolic or respiratory acidosis because the kidneys excrete more hydrogen ions from the body, and from electrolyte disturbances such as hypokalemia and hypochloremia.

Normal Findings

Cells normally found in the urine include white blood cells (WBCs), red blood cells (RBCs), and epithelial cells from sloughing of dead cells in the urinary system. In normal urine, WBCs are more numerous than RBCs, with four or five WBCs and two or three RBCs per high power field. WBCs are more abundant in the urine of females.

Casts are molded elements formed by cellular or fibrous accumulations in urinary structures. Although casts are usually considered pathologic, an occasional hyaline cast may appear in normal urine. For example, hyaline casts may be observed in urine after strenuous exercise or diuretic therapy as well as in pathologic states such as inflammatory renal disease, but are usually considered normal if few in number and in the absence of other casts.

Crystals are normally formed in the urine and the type of crystal formed is pH dependent. In acid urine calcium oxalate, uric acid, and urate crystals may be present; in alkaline urine, phosphate and carbonate crystals may be noted. Although considered a normal finding, crystals indicate urinary calculi (stones).

Deviations from Normal

Cells: An increased amount of epithelial cells indicates renal tubule disease and associated cell necrosis. An increased amount of RBCs is associated with systemic bleeding disorders such as overcoagulation; renal disease and renal trauma, including trauma from Foley catheters; lower urinary tract pathology, including strictures, calculi, and bladder infections. An increased WBC count is found in most renal and urinary tract diseases. Bacteria are noted in urinary tract infections and in specimens contaminated by anal or vaginal excretions.

Abnormal casts are classified according to cell type and formation. Aside from the hyaline cast, the presence of casts in urine is abnormal and usually indicates renal pathology.

Crystals that contain cystine, tyrosine, or leucine are abnormal and may form large calculi that usually interfere with normal urinary elimination.

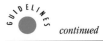

continued

Urine

Procedure

8. DETERMINE THE ELECTROLYTE COMPOSITION OF THE URINE USING A DIPSTICK.

Clinical Significance

Normal Findings

Normal urine should not contain glucose, ketones, or proteins.

Deviations from Normal

Glucose, ketones, and proteins in the urine are always abnormal. Proteinuria indicates kidney glomeruli damage. Glucosuria usually occurs secondary to hyperglycemic conditions such as diabetes mellitus (uncontrolled), and endocrine and liver disorders. Additionally, renal disease may prevent proper glucose reabsorption in the renal tubules and may cause glucose to spill into the urine. Ketones usually appear in the urine when the body breaks down fats for energy, as in starvation states, diabetes mellitus, vomiting and diarrhea, and conditions that increase the basal metabolic rate.

Documenting Urine Examination Findings

To document urine characteristics, note the color, transparency, odor, and volume. Dipstick results are charted + or − depending on whether a particular component is detected. Positive values are occasionally given a number to indicate magnitude, for example, "glucose, 4+."

Descriptors for Documenting Urine Characteristics

	Normal Findings	Deviations from Normal
Color	Straw, amber, yellow	Red, brown, orange, bloody
Transparency	Clear	Cloudy, sediment (specify color, *e.g.*, white, brown)
Odor	Aromatic	Ketosis, ammonia, fecal
Volume	1200–1500 mL/day	Anuria, oliguria, polyuria

NDx

Nursing Diagnoses Related to Urinary Elimination Assessment

Urinary Retention

The nursing diagnosis Urinary retention refers to the inability to empty the bladder, and may occur in the following conditions:

1. Hypotonic bladder (bladder muscle atrophy)
   a. Lesions affecting the motor roots of the S2–S4 spinal cord, such as occur with poliomyelitis, Guillain-Barré syndrome, trauma, tumor
   b. Lesions affecting the sensory roots of the S2–S4 spinal cord, such as occur in diabetes mellitus

2. Strong sphincter tone: Induced by drugs such as antihistamines and psychotropics
3. Urethral obstruction: Prostatic hypertrophy, surgical swelling, fecal impaction, vaginal and rectal packs

Assessment. When urine is retained in the bladder, the lower abdomen over the symphysis pubis may become distended. Urine output is significantly decreased or absent. Dribbling of urine or overflow incontinence may occur when the bladder fills to capacity. The person may experience a sensation of bladder fullness if the sensory fibers of the sacral spinal cord are intact, and may strain in an attempt to empty the bladder. Bladder capacity eventually increases, and residual urine volumes are usually high. Because of urine stasis in the bladder, the risk of infection increases. Urinalysis may indicate high concentrations of white blood cells and bacteria.

Total Incontinence

The nursing diagnosis Total incontinence, or uncontrolled incontinence, refers to an unpredictable or continuous urine loss. The following are contributing factors:

1. Loss of voluntary control mechanisms, such as occurs with cerebral pathology such as cerebrovascular accident (CVA), tumors, organic brain syndrome
2. Loss of neuronal control in pathways to the bladder, such as with severance or destruction of motor and sensory neurons below the voiding reflex arc (surgery, trauma)
3. Fistula formation

Assessment. Constant bladder flow may accompany total incontinence. The elimination pattern may also be characterized by urinary frequency, urgency, and nocturia. Incontinence is usually obvious unless a catheter or other appliance is used. Skin integrity is often impaired if urine comes in contact with the skin. Bladder capacity is usually decreased. Residual urine may not be observed.

Urge Incontinence

The nursing diagnosis Urge incontinence refers to urination that occurs immediately after a strong sensation to void. Urgency results from the following conditions:

1. Irritation of bladder stretch receptors, through infection, concentrated urine, neuropathies
2. Severe reduction of bladder capacity: May occur secondary to severe pelvic inflammatory disease or prolonged bladder drainage by an indwelling Foley catheter. The pressure of the uterus during pregnancy may also decrease bladder capacity.
3. Increased urine production, such as from diuretic therapy

Assessment. The bladder elimination pattern is usually characterized by urgency. Continence may be maintained if the person is able to reach toilet facilities quickly. If infection is the contributing factor, dysuria may accompany voiding. Urine analysis and culture may indicate bacterial growth.

Stress Incontinence

The nursing diagnosis Stress incontinence refers to the involuntary leakage of urine during momentary episodes of increased intra-abdominal pressure. The following are contributing factors:

1. Loss of the normal urethrovesical angle or muscular support structures, such as from multiple births, pregnancy, pelvic tumors, obesity
2. Weak sphincter tone due to childbirth, prolonged bladder catheterization

Assessment. Stress incontinence is more common in postmenopausal women and is associated with activities such as coughing, sneezing, lifting heavy objects, and climbing stairs. The amount of urine lost with each incontinent episode ranges from a few drops to large amounts. The pelvic examination may reveal cystocele or uterine prolapse.

Reflex Incontinence

The nursing diagnosis Reflex incontinence refers to incontinence related to a permanent neurologic lesion that causes voiding to be controlled by spinal cord reflex. It may occur in the following conditions:

1. When messages between the spinal cord reflex arc and brain are interrupted, such as in spinal cord injury, multiple sclerosis
2. When the spinal cord reflex is inappropriately inhibited or not inhibited, as in cerebral pathology, including CVA, tumors, organic brain syndrome.

Assessment. Predictable voiding patterns are usually noted. Voiding may be initiated by maneuvers that stimulate the reflex arc, including tapping the abdomen above the symphysis pubis, stroking the inner thigh, and pulling the penis or pubic hair. Residual urine volumes may be high.

Functional Incontinence

The nursing diagnosis Functional incontinence refers to the involuntary and unpredictable loss of urine. There is no warning sign such as urgency. This condition usually occurs because the client cannot reach bathroom facilities in time. People in unfamiliar environments and people with cognitive or motor deficits are at greatest risk.

Clinical Problems Related to Urinary Elimination Assessment

Many pathologic problems that contribute to urinary retention or incontinence are permanent alterations. In these cases, recognizing the pathology helps you make the correct nursing diagnosis and implement appropriate treatment. Recognizing potentially reversible pathologic conditions will help identify patients who must be referred to a physician.

Inflammatory and Infectious Processes

Acute lower urinary tract infection is usually characterized by dysuria, frequency, and urgency. Urine may be cloudy and voided in small volumes. Urinalysis may indicate bacteria and increased white and red blood cell concentrations. A urine culture helps to identify specific bacterial organisms.

Upper urinary tract infection is characterized by lethargy, fever, chills, headache, and occasionally vomiting. Abdominal pain and tenderness over the costovertebral angle may be noted. The urine usually contains bacteria as well as elevated white and red blood cell counts and increased amounts of protein. The serum white blood cell count is also usually elevated.

Prostatitis, inflammation of the prostate gland, may cause a lower urinary tract infection or may mimic this condition. Dysuria, frequency, and urethral discharge may be noted. The prostate examination may reveal an enlarged, boggy, and tender gland. Palpating the prostate may result in purulent urethral discharge. Pus cells and bacteria may be noted in the urine sample obtained after the prostate is palpated. Other symptoms include perineal pain and low back pain, which may be intensified with ejaculation or a bowel movement.

Urinary Stones

Urinary stones or calculi occur secondary to numerous conditions, including metabolic disease, urinary tract infection, and necrotic kidney disease. The signs and symptoms of urinary stones depend on where the stones are located in the urinary system. Kidney stones are often asymptomatic.

Stones that become trapped in the ureters usually produce intense, colicky pain in the lower back or abdomen that may radiate to the sides or legs. Back or abdominal muscle spasms may be noted. The person may experience mild shock. Urine may contain increased white blood cells and red blood cells and increased amounts of bacteria. Urine crystals may be present, providing information about stone type, such as uric acid or cystine.

Bladder stones irritate the bladder and may cause symptoms such as dysuria, urgency, and frequency. The stone may occlude the bladder neck, in which case the urinary stream may be interrupted. The bladder may become palpable as urine is retained. Urine may contain increased white and red blood cells, and increased amounts of bacteria.

Renal Failure

Acute renal failure occurs when normal kidney function suddenly ceases. The ensuing fluid and electrolyte imbalances may produce a life-threatening condition. Immediate

physician referral is crucial if you detect signs of acute renal failure during nursing assessment. The client may experience sudden oliguria. Urine examination reflects loss of kidney function. The urine may contain abnormal constituents such as protein and hemoglobin. Specific gravity is usually abnormally low (1.010–1.016). Systemic effects alter blood chemistry. For example, serum creatinine, blood urea nitrogen, potassium, and phosphate levels are usually increased. The person may experience anorexia, nausea and vomiting, hypertension, and fatigue.

ASSESSMENT PROFILE

Randy, aged 17, had mixed feelings about being discharged from the rehabilitation center. He had been hospitalized for several weeks after he had lost his footing and fallen 100 feet off the face of a cliff while hiking. The accident resulted in a complete transection of his spinal cord at the S2 level. His lower legs were permanently paralyzed, confining him to a wheelchair. Furthermore, Randy had lost control over bowel and bladder functions.

Randy had been incontinent of stool and unable to urinate voluntarily during the early phase of his recovery. Although he felt no pressure or urge to urinate, his bladder would fill with urine, which would dribble out without his knowledge. Eventually, Randy would become aware of the odor of urine.

The rehabilitation team taught Randy how to handle his elimination problems until he was able to control his bowel movements successfully and reduce accidents. However, he had less success with bladder control in that he retained urine in the bladder, resulting in overflow incontinence. The nurses taught Randy the Credé method, and Randy had prevented overflow incontinence by using this method up until 3 days before discharge, when he began to leak urine again. Consequently, his skin was beginning to break down from the irritating effects of the urine. The physician advised Randy's primary nurse to insert a catheter into the bladder to check for residual urine. A residual amount of 250 mL was found, and the urinalysis indicated signs of infection.

Although Randy was encouraged to continue using the Credé maneuver, intermittent bladder catheterizations revealed high residual amounts. The rehabilitation team suggested that Randy try intermittent self-catheterization to drain the bladder at regular intervals. Randy was upset about having to perform this procedure for the rest of his life. He felt ashamed and embarrassed, and he refused the team's efforts to teach him this new procedure.

Profile Analysis

Randy has a permanently altered elimination pattern as a result of irreversible damage to his spinal cord. While assessing the nature of the elimination problem and the response to related interventions is important, assessing additional responses that result from an altered elimination pattern is crucial.

Identifying the Assessment Focus

The nurses readily identified the necessary course for collecting data. People like Randy who have had spinal cord damage most often have urinary incontinence for one of the following reasons:

- Message transmission between the brain and the spinal cord reflex arc is interrupted, in which case voiding occurs after the bladder fills to a predictable point (Reflex incontinence).
- The bladder has become hypotonic, the detrusor muscle does not contract effectively, and urine dribbles constantly (Urinary retention).

Reflex incontinence is permanent but may become predictable as a result of bladder retraining. Data collection was aimed at detecting the problem of urinary retention. By performing a residual bladder catheterization and obtaining high volumes of residual urine, the nurses were able to confirm a problem with urinary retention.

Possible Nursing Diagnoses

Although the nurses were certain that Randy's altered bladder elimination problem was Urinary retention, they considered additional nursing diagnoses. For the person with a spinal cord injury, the altered elimination pattern presents a challenge to coping mechanisms and can effect the quality of life. Nursing diagnoses such as Ineffective coping and Self-concept alteration had to be considered because such human responses to altered elimination are common.

The nurses formulated additional nursing diagnoses and focused data collection on evaluating related cues:

Body image disturbance
High risk for infection
Impaired skin integrity
Urinary retention

Additional Data Gathering and Analysis

The nurses obtained additional data by assessing Randy's coping abilities and self-concept. The data indicated that Randy had an elimination problem that affected his self-esteem, and that his impending discharge was a stressor contributing to the disruption of previously acceptable bladder elimination patterns. Nursing interventions needed to be directed toward several different human responses in order to help Randy with the elimination problem. The nurses combined the pertinent data relating to Randy's elimination problem according to strengths and risk factors in the following manner:

Strengths

- Maintains control over bowel function.
- Has demonstrated ability to try alternative methods of bladder emptying and control.
- Performs self-care procedures sufficiently and is considered ready for discharge.

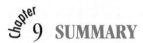

9 SUMMARY

Elimination pattern assessment should focus on:
- The person's concerns and behaviors related to waste elimination.
- Bowel and urinary elimination patterns.
- Factors influencing bowel and urinary elimination.
- Specimen characteristics of urine and stool.

Important principles to remember when assessing bowel and urinary elimination include the following:
- People may avoid discussing problems with elimination because of feelings of embarrassment or hopelessness. You should convey empathy and acceptance.
- Elimination patterns cannot be adequately described by merely quantifying stool and urine. Many factors influence elimination, and the relative impact of diet, activity, medications, life-style, and pathology should be evaluated.
- People are often concerned about bowel regularity, but wide variations exist in "normal" patterns.
- People who experience permanent alteration in bowel or bladder function have elimination patterns that can and should be described.
- Most people with bowel or bladder incontinence respond to bowel or bladder retraining, provided interventions are based on accurate assessment.
- Physical examination as a component of elimination assessment is aimed at determining bowel and bladder function in relation to elimination and identifying adverse effects of elimination problems. You should also examine body structures related to elimination to detect actual or potential pathology and make appropriate treatment referrals.

A number of information sources may be used to evaluate elimination patterns, including the following:

The interview, which focuses on:
- Usual voiding and defecation patterns
- Self-care practices related to bowel and urinary elimination
- Factors influencing bowel and urinary elimination
- Altered bowel and urinary elimination

Risks

- Suffers permanently altered bladder elimination pattern.
- Experiences significant stress related to effects of altered elimination pattern and impending discharge.
- Experiences threats to physical well-being: infection and impaired skin integrity.

Final Nursing Diagnoses

The ongoing assessment indicated cues supporting the originally formulated nursing diagnoses. These diagnoses were incorporated into Randy's care plan and appropriate interventions were planned.

Observations, which focus on:
- Self-care abilities
- General appearance
- Body system indicators of altered elimination
- Abdominal examination
- Anal and rectal examination

Specimen Evaluation
- Stool
- Urine

Evaluation of Diagnostic Test Results
- Barium enema
- Proctosigmoidoscopy
- Colonoscopy
- Intravenous pyelogram
- Cystometrogram
- Electromyography
- Bulbocavernous Reflex

Elimination assessment based on these principles and methods helps identify defining characteristics that might be present for the following nursing diagnoses:

Altered Bowel Elimination
Bowel incontinence
Colonic constipation
Perceived constipation
Diarrhea

Altered Patterns of Urinary Elimination
Altered urinary elimination
Functional incontinence
Reflex incontinence
Stress incontinence
Total incontinence
Urge incontinence
Urinary retention

Related nursing diagnoses may be identified, including
Body image disturbance
Risk for fluid volume deficit
Fluid volume deficit

RESEARCH *Hi*GHLIGHT

"What evidence is there that NANDA-approved diagnostic categories addressing elimination problems actually occur in clinical practice?"

One issue that has surfaced as nurses develop and refine nursing diagnoses is whether NANDA-approved nursing diagnoses have content validity, that is, whether the signs, symptoms, and etiological factors suggested by NANDA for each diagnosis actually exist in practice and apply to nursing clients. Discrepancies between a nursing diagnosis as defined by NANDA and the same nursing diagnosis as used by clinicians suggest that nurses are not clearly identifying and communicating their activities. Such discrepancies may arise because defining characteristics and etiologies, derived from the literature, do not reflect practice reality, or because the clinician lacks the expertise and experience to identify the signs and symptoms for a particular diagnosis. The following studies address content validity for diagnoses describing alterations in elimination.

In one study, not only did clients agree with the signs and symptoms for constipation previously identified by NANDA, but they suggested additional signs and symptoms. A study was designed to determine if three different age groups (older adults, middle-aged adults, and adolescents) described constipation in a manner similar to NANDA participants. The researchers also asked subjects about health practices related to constipation. Data were gathered from 300 subjects (100/group) using a tool designed for a previous study. Subjects were asked to describe the signs and symptoms of constipation, etiologies, and bowel elimination practices or behaviors. The subjects identified 22 signs and symptoms for constipation, including the 9 defining characteristics suggested by NANDA. Ten major factors contributing to constipation were reported:

Worried/upset	*Sweating*
Feeling down	*Antacid use*
Change in meal times	*Codeine use*
Missed meals	*Increased body temperature*
Usual foods not available	*Vomiting*

Reported bowel elimination practices, which varied among age groups, included use of laxative medications, alterations in diet, and exercise. Finally, the results indicated that older adults responded more to the defecation reflex than did adolescents. The researchers recommended that Sixth Conference NANDA participants refine the defining characteristics and etiological categories of constipation based on study results.[1]

In another study, nurses asked to identify signs and symptoms of urinary retention selected similar signs and symptoms when compared to each other and to a list derived from a literature review. Fifty-three staff

nurses responded to questionnaires designed to elicit their opinions about signs, symptoms, and causes of urinary retention. The subjects were asked to rate signs, symptoms, and causes from 1 to 5, on a Likert-type scale, to indicate how strongly each was related to urinary retention. A rating of 5 indicated the strongest relationship. A mean rank of 3 or greater was required before a sign or symptom was accepted as an indicator of urinary retention. Of the predetermined signs and symptoms, 74% were identified by staff nurses as indicators of urinary retention (see table). Staff nurses suggested additional indicators not listed on the original questionnaire, including residual urine volume of 150 ml or more, surgery, dysuria, and overflow incontinence. Nurses' acceptance of the proposed etiologies varied according to clinical specialty. Furthermore, nurses distinguished the concepts urinary retention and urinary incontinence. Based on the study results, the researchers suggested that NANDA participants refine the nursing diagnosis Altered patterns of urinary elimination to distinguish between retention and incontinence. This recommendation was followed and currently there are six distinct nursing diagnoses related to urinary elimination.[2]

Mean Rank of Signs and Symptoms Determined to Be Indicators of Urinary Retention

Mean Rank	Standard Deviation	Rank						
		0	1	2	3	4	5	
4.7*	0.50							Distension
3.6	1.42							Bladder percussion
3.2	1.28							Hesitancy
3.1	1.22							Decreased stream
4.4*	0.70							Small, frequent voidings
4.4*	0.94							No urine output
3.8	1.13							No filling sensation
3.0	1.44							Psychotropic agents
4.1*	0.87							Sensation of bladder fullness
3.9	0.96							Frequency
4.0*	1.00							Dribbling
3.3	1.11							Abdominal discomfort
3.1	1.03							Nocturia

*Critical signs and symptoms (indicators).
(Voith, A.M., Smith, D.A. [1985]. Validation of the nursing diagnosis of urinary retention. Nursing Clinics of North America, 20[4], 723–729)

(continued)

RESEARCH *Hi*GHLIGHT

"What evidence is there that NANDA-approved diagnostic categories
addressing elimination problems actually occur in clinical practice?"
(continued)

What significance do the studies have for health assessment?

Nurses formulate nursing diagnoses after systematically assessing for related signs, symptoms, and etiological factors. Studies such as these help nurses focus health assessment on relevant factors. Interestingly, McLane and McShane's study emphasizes *clients;* rather than *nurses'* perspective on health problems. For example, clients reported that the three most common etiological factors for constipation were being worried or upset, feeling down, and sweating. If nurses had been interviewed, the three most common etiologies would probably have been dietary alterations, immobility, and painful defecation. These differences indicate not only a need for additional research about etiologies but also the importance of assessing health from the client's perspective.

Can the studies' findings be applied to practice?

Nurses could use the additional defining characteristics and etiologies suggested by these studies to guide health assessment with minimal risk to clients. However, nurses should keep in mind that study recommendations, even if adopted by NANDA, are not conclusive. Acceptance by NANDA merely means that nursing diagnosis revisions should be further studied and tested. All such studies should be repeated before final judgments are made about accuracy and applicability of findings.

REFERENCES

1. McLane, A.M., & McShane, R.E. (1986). Empirical validation of defining characteristics of constipation: A study of bowel elimination practices of healthy adults. In Hurley, M.E. (Ed.). *Classification of nursing diagnoses: Proceedings of the sixth national conference.* St. Louis: C.V. Mosby.
2. Voith, A.M., & Smith, D.A. (1985). Validation of the nursing diagnosis of urinary retention. *Nursing Clinics of North America, 20*(4), 723-729.

Hopelessness
Ineffective coping
Risk for infection
Self-care deficit (specify type)
Self-concept alteration
Self-esteem disturbance
Altered sexuality patterns
Impaired skin integrity
High risk for impaired skin integrity

Additionally, you will develop skill at detecting and monitoring the following clinical problems:

1. Inflammatory and infectious processes of the anus and rectum
   a. Ulcerative colitis
   b. Crohn's disease
   c. Acute gastroenteritis
   d. Diverticulitis
2. Hyperplastic growths
   a. Colon and rectal cancer
   b. Prostate cancer
3. Malabsorption syndromes
4. Hemorrhage
5. Irritable bowel syndrome
6. Inflammatory and infectious processes of the urinary tract
   a. Upper urinary tract infection
   b. Lower urinary tract infection
7. Urinary stones
8. Renal failure

✳ CRITICAL THINKING

You are the contract nurse for an assisted living facility. Most of the residents are elderly, ambulatory, and able to feed, dress, and toilet themselves. During your weekly visit, you are asked to evaluate an 82-year-old female resident who has suddenly become incontinent of urine. She is ex-

Learning Exercises

1. Select and describe the approach you would use to determine the nature of this person's bladder elimination problem. Differentiate among the following: urinary retention, total incontinence, urge incontinence, stress incontinence, reflex incontinence, and functional incontinence.

tremely hard of hearing but otherwise healthy, with a medical history of congestive heart failure and hypertension. If this resident remains incontinent, she will require skilled nursing care. In order to intervene, you must first determine the nature of her incontinence.

2. Because of her hearing problem, you are unable to elicit a good history of this person's perception of her incontinence. Moreover, because she is not observed around the clock by care providers, you do not have data from other sources to help you understand her bladder elimination patterns. Given these limitations, plan and describe your strategy for ensuring a thorough and accurate assessment of this person.

3. Explain what you could learn about this person's problem from examining the physical surroundings.

BIBLIOGRAPHY

Abbott, D. (1992). Objective assessment ensures improved diagnosis: Principles and practice of urodynamics. *Professional Nurse, 7* (11), 740–742.

Barry, K. (1981). Neurogenic bladder incontinence: The consequences of mismanagement. *Rehabilitation Nursing, 6,* 12–13.

Berry, L. (1993). Incontinence and urinary problems. In D.L. Carnevali & M. Patrick (Eds.). *Nursing management for the elderly* (3rd ed.). Philadelphia: J.B. Lippincott.

Braunwald, E. et al. (Eds.). (1991). *Harrison's principles of internal medicine* (12th ed.). New York: McGraw-Hill.

Carpenito, L.J. (1993). *Handbook of nursing diagnosis* (5th ed.). Philadelphia: J.B. Lippincott.

Eastwood, H. (1983). Differential diagnosis of urinary incontinence in the elderly. *Geriatric Medicine Today, 2* (4), 19–28.

Fischbach, T. (1992). *Manual of laboratory and diagnostic tests* (4th ed.). Philadelphia: J.B. Lippincott.

Garrett, V.E. et al. (1989). Bladder emptying assessment in stroke patients. *Archives of Physical Medicine and Rehabilitation, 70* (1), 41–43.

Hahn, K. (1987). Think twice about diarrhea. *Nursing '87, 17* (9), 78–80.

Hahn K. (1988). Think twice about urinary incontinence. *Nursing '88, 18* (11), 65–67.

Holland, N.J., Wiesel-Levison, P., & Madonna, M.G. (1985). Rehabilitation research: Pathophysiology and management of neurogenic bladder in multiple sclerosis. *Rehabilitation Nursing, 10,* 31–33.

Mager-O'Connor, E. (1984). How to identify and remove fecal impactions. *Geriatric Nursing, 5,* 158–161.

McCormick, K. (1988). Urinary incontinence in the elderly. *Nursing Clinics of North America, 23* (1), 135–137.

McCormick, K., Newman, D.K., Colling, J., & Pearson, B.D. (1992). Urinary incontinence in adults. *American Journal of Nursing, 92* (10), 75–86.

McLane, A.M. (Ed.). (1987). *Classification of nursing diagnoses: Proceedings of the seventh conference.* St. Louis: C.V. Mosby.

McLane, A.M., & McShane, R.E. (1986). Empirical validation of defining characteristics of constipation: A study of bowel elimination practices of healthy adults. In M.E. Hurly (Ed.). *Classification of nursing diagnoses: Proceedings of the sixth national conference.* St. Louis: C.V. Mosby.

McLane, A.M., McShane, R.E., & Sliefert, M. (1984). Constipation: Conceptual categories of diagnositc indicators. In M.J. Kim, G.K. McFarland, & A.M. McLane (Eds.). *Classification of nursing diagnoses: Proceedings of the fifth national conference.* St. Louis: C.V. Mosby.

McShane, R., & McLane, A.M. (1988). Constipation: Impact of etiological factors. *Journal of Gerontological Nursing, 14* (4), 31–34, 46–47.

Novotny, R.W. (1984). Psychosocial implications of a neurogenic bladder. *Rehabilitation Nursing, 9,* 35–37.

Palmer, M.H. (1985). *Urinary incontinence.* Thorofare, NJ: Slack.

Palmer, M. (1988). Incontinence: The magnitude of the problem. *Nursing Clinics of North America, 23* (1), 139–157.

Ross, D. (1990). Constipation among hospitalized elders. *Orthopedic Nursing, 9* (3), 73–77.

Rottkamp, B.C. (1985). A holistic approach to identifying factors associated with an altered pattern of urinary elimination in stroke patients. *Journal of Neurosurgical Nursing, 17* (1), 37–44.

Smith, C. (1987). Investigating absent bowel sounds. *Nursing '87, 17* (11), 73, 76–77.

Tunink, P. (1988). Alteration in urinary elimination. *Journal of Gerontological Nursing, 14* (4), 25–30.

Voith, A.M. (1986). A conceptual framework for nursing diagnoses: Alterations in urinary elimination. *Rehabilitation Nursing, 11,* 18–21.

Voith, A.M., & Smith, D.A. (1985). Validation of the nursing diagnosis of urinary retention. *Nursing Clinics of North America, 20* (4), 723–729.

Weigel, J.W. (1988). Urinary incontinence. *Journal of Enterostomal Therapy, 15* (1), 24–29.

Wyman, J. (1988). Nursing assessment of the incontinent geriatric outpatient population. *Nursing Clinics of North America, 23* (1), 169–187.

10 Assessing Activity and Exercise

Examination Guidelines

Heart and Precordium

Arterial Pulses

Neck Veins

Nose and Sinuses

Lungs and Thorax

Bones, Joints, and Muscles

Assessment Terms

Activities of Daily Living
Metabolic Equivalents (METs)
Point of Maximal Impulse
Thrill
S_1
S_2
S_3
S_4
Opening Snap
Summation Gallop
Ejection Click
Friction Rub
Murmur
Physiologic Murmur
Pulse Deficit
Bruit
Allen Test

Jugular Venous Pressure
Hepatojugular Reflux
Tangential Lighting
Rhinitis
Crepitus
Fremitus
Adventitious Breath Sounds
Bronchophony
Whispered Pectoriloquy
Egophony
Claw Fingers
Opposition
Patella Ballottement
Bulge Sign
Drawer Sign
Homans' Sign

INTRODUCTORY OVERVIEW

Routine daily activities require energy expenditure and the ability to move freely in one's surroundings. Monitoring activity tolerance is aimed at identifying problems with activity and movement in susceptible individuals and identifying improvements in strength and endurance in people who exercise to improve their overall level of health. Cardiopulmonary and emotional responses to activity should be monitored in both health and illness states. Assessment of activity, activity tolerance, and exercise focuses on the person's usual daily activities, including exercise and leisure activities; ability to engage in activity; psy-

Jill Fuller and Jennifer Schaller-Ayers:
HEALTH ASSESSMENT: A NURSING APPROACH, Second Edition.
© 1990, 1994 by J. B. Lippincott Company.

chological and physiological responses to exercise; and risk factors that suggest reduced tolerance of activity.

Assessment Focus

Judgments about activity and exercise are based on data obtained by interviewing the person, reviewing results of laboratory and diagnostic tests, and examining major body systems whose physiologic functions are essential for activity and exercise. In addition, invasive monitoring instruments may be used to monitor physiologic functions.

The goals for assessing activity and exercise include the following:

- Obtaining a description of the person's typical activity pattern, including activities of daily living (ADLs)
- Determining if the activities are sufficient for meeting self-care needs
- Evaluating exercise habits and leisure activities in relation to promoting and maintaining health
- Identifying risk factors or conditions associated with activity intolerance
- Noting the person's physiologic, behavioral, and psychological responses to altered activity patterns.

The methods for collecting data applicable to these assessment goals are listed in the Assessment Focus.

Nursing Diagnoses

Assessment of activity and exercise patterns provides cues to the following nursing diagnoses:

Activity intolerance
Potential activity intolerance
Diversional activity deficit
Impaired home maintenance management
Fatigue
Bathing/hygiene self-care deficit
Dressing/grooming self-care deficit
Feeding self-care deficit
Toileting self-care deficit

The nurse should also evaluate major body systems, especially the cardiovascular system, pulmonary system, and musculoskeletal system, because the function of these systems is essential for activity and exercise. Examination of these systems may provide indicators for the following nursing diagnoses:

Ineffective airway clearance
Ineffective breathing pattern
Impaired gas exchange
Decreased cardiac output
Fluid volume excess
Altered (specify type) tissue perfusion (renal, cerebral, cardiopulmonary, gastrointestinal, peripheral)
Impaired physical mobility

KNOWLEDGE BASE FOR ASSESSMENT

Physiologic Responses to Activity and Exercise

Engaging in activity and exercise requires muscle contraction and a supply of energy. The most effective way to obtain energy is through the body's aerobic metabolic pathways, which require a constant oxygen supply. The physiologic response to activity and exercise is related to the body's attempt to meet oxygen requirements, which involves cardiovascular and respiratory responses. Musculoskeletal function is also an important determinant of activity capabilities.

OXYGEN DELIVERY

The supply of oxygen to muscle tissues depends on oxygen being diffused into the blood through the lungs and transported by hemoglobin molecules. Oxygen enters the body by diffusion across alveolar-capillary membranes in the lungs. Usually this process is not a factor in limiting physical activity unless there is underlying pulmonary dysfunction (such as excessive pulmonary secretions or edema that interferes with gas diffusion, altered lung ventilation, or obstructive pulmonary disease). In other words, for most people, getting oxygen into the body is not a problem affecting activity tolerance. Similarly, most people have adequate hemoglobin molecules to transport the oxygen.

Conversely, transporting oxygen to muscle tissue, which may occur at different efficiency levels, can be a factor that limits activity tolerance. The delivery of oxygen to muscle cells, where it enters metabolic, energy-producing pathways, depends on effective cardiac output and aerobic capacity.

CARDIAC OUTPUT

Cardiac output, the product of heart rate and stroke volume, is the amount of blood ejected from the left ventricle with each contraction. Resting cardiac outputs do not differ significantly among people; however, a person's maximally attainable cardiac output can be increased by regular exercise, thereby promoting activity tolerance. Exercise improves cardiac output by increasing stroke volume.

Assessing activity tolerance through the physical examination is based on understanding the physical signs of effective cardiac output. Normally, the heart rate increases as activity increases in order to raise the cardiac output and increase oxygen delivery to the tissues. The gradient for heart rate increase is greater in people who have had exercise training because they tend to have lower resting heart rates. Age-related norms have been established for exercise-induced maximal heart rates (Table 10-1). Exercise-induced maximal heart rates should be determined by taking the pulse 10 to 15 minutes after continuous aerobic

Assessment Focus **Activity and Exercise**

Assessment Goal	*Data Collection Methods*
1. Describe the person's typical activity pattern, including activities of daily living, leisure activities, and exercise habits.	*Interview* • Usual activities: What is the typical activity pattern? What modifications are needed for current activity abilities? • Exercise habits: Type, frequency, duration, intensity. *Initiate and Review Activity Record* • 3-day activity diary
2. Determine if current activity levels are sufficient for meeting self-care needs.	*Interview and Observe* • Ability to engage in self-care activities: Are there potential or actual self-care deficits?
3. Evaluate exercise habits and leisure activities in relation to promoting and maintaining health.	*Interview* • Exercise habits: Is the exercise pattern health-promoting? Does it promote cardiovascular adaptation? • Leisure activities: Is there time for leisure? Do leisure activities alleviate stress? *Physical Examination* • Exercise-induced maximal heart rate: Does this measurement compare favorably to recommended standards?
4. Identify risk factors or conditions associated with activity intolerance.	*Interview* • Distressing symptoms occurring with activity and exercise: Do symptoms suggest conditions known to influence activity tolerance? • Pertinent health history: Are there risk factors or pathologic conditions associated with activity intolerance? • Sleep and rest patterns (Chap. 12): Is activity tolerance compromised by sleep deprivation or fatigue? • Stress and coping patterns (Chap. 16): Are activity levels and exercise motivation adversely influenced by crisis, depression, or stress? *Physical Examination* • Measurement of vital signs: Are there alterations in vital signs suggesting Activity Intolerance? (*Example:* An adult respiratory rate of 36 breaths/min at rest) • Cardiovascular and pulmonary examination: Are physiological systems for meeting oxygen requirements during activity intact? • Musculoskeletal examination: Is mobility adequate or restricted? • Evaluation of other body systems (neurologic, gastrointestinal, and integumentary): Are there abnormalities that may contribute to problems with activity and exercise? *Review of Laboratory and Diagnostic Test Results* • Blood tests: What do test results suggest about cardiovascular, respiratory, and musculoskeletal functions? • Noninvasive and invasive cardiovascular tests, nuclear cardiac studies: What is the status of the cardiovascular system? • Arterial blood gas and pulmonary function studies: What is the status of the pulmonary system? • Muscle function studies: What is the status of the musculoskeletal system?
5. Identify physiologic, behavioral, and psychological responses to altered activity patterns.	*Interview* • Symptoms related to activity and exercise • Self-esteem (Chap. 13): Have altered activity patterns adversely affected self-esteem? *Physical Examination* • Vital signs, cardiovascular, respiratory, musculoskeletal, and integumentary systems: Are there abnormalities resulting from altered activity patterns?

Table 10–1. Age-Related Norms for Exercise-Induced Maximal Heart Rates*

Age	Maximal Heart Rate*	80% Maximal	60% Maximal
20	200	160	120
25	195	156	115
30	190	152	114
35	185	148	111
40	180	144	108
45	175	140	105
50	170	136	102
55	165	132	99
60	160	128	96
65	155	124	93

*Optimal physical fitness is associated with maximal heart rates 60% to 80% of age-related norms or 60% to 80% of the person's pretraining maximal heart rate. Pretraining maximal heart rate = 220 - age in years.

exercise, such as jogging or cycling. Optimal physical fitness is associated with maximum heart rates 60% to 80% of age-related norms or 60% to 80% of the person's pretraining maximal heart rate. A maximal heart rate that is lower than the norm indicates that cardiac output has been increased by stroke volume rather than heart rate, a positive adaptation to regular physical activity.

Using heart rate as an indicator of activity tolerance is most reliable when other aspects of cardiac function, such as contractility and left ventricular compliance, are normal. Failure of the heart rate to increase with activity or return to a resting level 5 minutes after the activity or exercise ends is considered abnormal. Also, a sustained high heart rate increases the heart's oxygen demands, which, if unmet, can tax the myocardium.

AEROBIC CAPACITY

Aerobic capacity refers to the maximal rate at which oxygen can be used, and may be measured during exercise testing by determining the peak oxygen consumption rate (VO_2 max), the maximum volume of oxygen the body extracts and uses from inspired air. A person's maximal oxygen consumption rate or aerobic capacity is a commonly used criterion for evaluating physical fitness. Genetic makeup largely determines aerobic capacity, but a number of other factors contribute and should be considered when you assess a person's activity tolerance.

Aerobic capacity can be increased by 20% in a person who engages in regular aerobic exercise. The following exercise pattern promotes aerobic capacity:

- *Type:* Continuous activity, such as running, cycling, stair climbing, swimming, or aerobic dancing
- *Frequency:* 3 to 5 days per week
- *Intensity:* 60% to 80% age-related maximum heart rate obtained and maintained during the exercise period

- *Duration:* 15 to 60 minutes, depending on intensity of the exercise

Diseases of the pulmonary, cardiovascular, or musculoskeletal systems may limit aerobic capacity. In such cases, oxygen debts may occur more readily and may be more difficult to compensate for, resulting in fatigue or, in extreme cases, cardiopulmonary compromise such as cardiac dysrhythmias, chest pain, or ineffective breathing patterns. However, people with such problems may improve aerobic capacity through individually prescribed activity and exercise programs. In addition, if a person's resting and maximum heart rates are lowered through exercise adaptation, myocardial oxygen consumption can be lowered, an accomplishment having significant implications for people with underlying cardiac disease.

Activity Assessment Using Metabolic Equivalents

Evaluating a person's activity and exercise capabilities in terms of maximum oxygen consumption rate may not always be practical because necessary data may not be available. In such cases, metabolic equivalents (METs) may be used to estimate oxygen costs for various activities. Table 10-2 presents METs for a variety of self-care, work, and leisure activities.

One MET is the average amount of oxygen a person consumes at rest, about 3.5 mL/kg of body weight/minute. When a person lies quietly at rest, the amount of oxygen consumed is 1 MET. A person who leads a sedentary life but who is not incapacitated by disease should be able to perform at least 10 METs of work with no adverse effects. Researchers continue to recommend activity levels in terms of METs for patients with disease limitations, such as acute myocardial infarction. The METs recommendations may be used to evaluate activity and exercise capabilities.

Metabolic equivalents are often used in prescribing exercise rather than in estimating activity capability. One of the problems with prescribing activity based on METs is that the guidelines fail to account for individual differences. For example, an obese person who sits up for the first time after surgery may consume a different amount of oxygen than would a thin person. Similarly, a person with high stress may use more oxygen during a particular activity than the MET guideline specifies.

THE HEALTH HISTORY

The assessment of activity and exercise functions begins by obtaining a history of the individual's patterns of activity, exercise, leisure, and self-care activities. Factors that interfere with usual or desired activities, such as disorders of the cardiovascular, respiratory, or musculoskeletal systems, and symptoms of these disorders should also be noted. Most, if not all, of the history may be obtained by interviewing the person. Additionally, records may be reviewed.

Table 10–2. Metabolic Equivalents (METs) Associated With Various Activities*

METs	Self-Care Activities	Work Activities	Leisure Activities
<3	Washing hands or face Shaving Brushing teeth Washing dishes Showering or bathing Driving	Sitting at desk Standing (store clerk)	Shuffleboard Fishing Billiards Archery Golf with cart Walking (<2 mph)
3–5	Carrying objects (15–30 lb) Cleaning windows Painting Mowing lawn with power mower	Stocking shelves Light carpentry Repairing cars Hanging paper	Social dancing Golf (without cart) Sailing Horsebackriding Tennis (doubles) Walking (3–4 mph)
5–7	Carrying objects (30–60 lb) Climbing stairs slowly Mowing lawn with push mower on level surface Gardening	Carpentry Shoveling dirt Using pneumatic tools	Badminton Light downhill snow skiing Light backpacking Skating Tennis (singles) Walking (4–5 mph)
7–9	Carrying objects (60–90 lb) Climbing stairs moderately fast Shoveling Sawing wood	Digging ditches Pick and shovel work	Canoeing Mountain hiking Fencing Jogging (5 mph) Rowing
>9	Carrying objects (>90 lb) Carrying loads upstairs Climbing stairs quickly Shoveling heavy snow	Heavy labor Lumberjack	Football Raquetball Cross-country skiing Basketball Bicycling (12 mph) Running (>6 mph) High-impact aerobics

*One MET equals the average amount of oxygen a person consumes at rest, about 3.5 mL/kg of body weight/minute. Actual energy requirements may vary depending on body size (e.g., obesity), physical condition, skill level, temperature and humidity, emotions, and intensity of the activity.

Data obtained by eliciting a history pertaining to activity and exercise functions should help you make judgments about the following:

- *Typical activities:* The usual activities the person engages in on a day-to-day basis. Is there a balance of required activities, leisure, and exercise? What is the capacity for self-care activities?
- *Physical fitness:* The individual's level of physical conditioning. Does the person have sufficient/optimal aerobic capacity, strength, or endurance?
- *Activity tolerance:* How well the person tolerates activity. Is there pain, discomfort, or dyspnea with activity?
- *Factors influencing activity tolerance:* Physiologic disorders, emotional problems, or environmental influences that interfere with the processes required for desired or essential activities

The Interview Guide shown in the accompanying display may be used to direct the collection of appropriate data.

During the interview, be especially attentive to the individual's beliefs and opinions. For example, note why the person may feel that certain activities are difficult, how he or she responds to activity problems, and whether he or she feels that efforts to solve problems have been effective.

Typical Activities

Ask the person to describe a typical day's activities, including exercise and leisure activities. Occasionally, it may be helpful if the person keeps an activity diary that may be evaluated after several days.

EXERCISE AND LEISURE ACTIVITIES

Be sure to ask the person about the quality and quantity of exercise and leisure activities. Many people who are able to independently carry out their daily activities may not be exercising or engaging in leisure activities. If such deficits are noted, continue to probe for possible causes, such as lack of time or motivation. For people who require long-term hospitalization or nursing home care, it is important to

Interview Guide **Activity and Exercise**

Typical Activities

Description of a typical day's activities:_____

_____

Usual leisure activities: _____

Amount of time spent performing leisure activities: _____

Do you have any problems managing your home? _____

Any problems with: _____ Eating or meal preparation? _____ Bathing? _____ Toileting? _____ Dressing or grooming? If so, describe (nurse assigns score): _____

Why do you think you have difficulty with these activities? _____

_____

Physical Fitness

Exercise Pattern

Type _____

Frequency _____

Intensity _____

Duration _____

Activity Tolerance

Describe any problems you experience with usual activities and exercise: _____

_____

Do you experience any of the following: _____ Chest pain _____ Arm pain _____ Leg pain _____ Joint, muscle or back pain

_____ Difficulty breathing (specify: dyspnea, air hunger, wheezing, orthopnea) _____ Cough _____ Numbness or tingling

_____ Lightheadedness _____ Fatigue or weakness _____ Palpitations

Factors Influencing Activity Tolerance

Current medical diagnosis: _____

Previous hospitalizations or surgeries: _____

Do you smoke? _____ If yes, estimated pack-years:* _____

Length of present hospitalization and amount of time out of bed per day (if applicable): _____

Any of the following problems?	Yes/No		Yes/No
Family history of heart disease	_____	Asthma	_____
Angina pectoris	_____	Pneumonia	_____
Myocardial infarction	_____	Musculoskeletal trauma	_____
Hypertension	_____	Arthritis	_____
Congestive heart failure	_____	Osteoporosis	_____
Rheumatic heart disease	_____	Weight-bearing problems	_____
Heart murmur	_____	Head trauma	_____
Heart/valve surgery	_____	Spinal cord injury	_____
Abnormal ECG findings	_____	Multiple sclerosis	_____
Stroke	_____	Myasthenia gravis	_____
Emphysema	_____	Sensory deficits	_____
Bronchitis	_____		

Pack-year = Packs per day × number of smoking years. Example: 2 packs per day × 10 smoking years = 20 pack-years.

---

evaluate what efforts have been made to involve the person in exercise and leisure activities. If such activities are lacking, try to identify the person's interests. This information is crucial when planning appropriate activities and interventions.

SELF-CARE ACTIVITIES

Self-care activities include feeding, dressing, toileting, and bathing. Using observation and interviewing, determine the degree of independence the person experiences in relation to these activities. If the person being interviewed demonstrates optimum independence and is managing a home or career, then you may not need to ask additional questions about self-care. However, it is important not to make assumptions without a sufficient data base. For example, a person with diabetes may appear to have no self-care deficits, but on further questioning may reveal that bathing is sometimes a problem because he or she has difficulty differentiating water temperatures. Because a diabetic person is at risk for neuropathy and impaired circulation, the nurse should consider how this might affect self-care abilities.

Ask specific questions about abilities to eat, bathe, go to the bathroom, dress independently, and maintain a home. If the person reports any problems, it may be helpful to ask him or her to perform certain activities to determine the specific nature of the problem. Determine whether or not the person uses assistive devices such as canes, walkers, or special tools to carry out activities.

Once a self-care deficit is identified, continue to investigate for a cause or contributing factors. The following factors influence a person's self-care abilities and should be considered during assessment:

- Age and developmental status
- Cultural values and beliefs
- Socioeconomic status
- Cognitive abilities and knowledge base
- Motivation
- Health status (including pathologic conditions)
- Health care environment (including imposed activity restrictions)

To assure consistency, you may use a standardized rating scale to communicate the degree of self-care abilities or deficits:

- *Level 0:* Is capable of performing all self-care activities independently. *Example:* A 25-year-old mother of a newborn infant cares for other children at home.
- *Level I:* Requires equipment or device in order to perform self-care activities independently. *Example:* A 68-year-old woman with residual right-sided weakness following a stroke uses special utensils to prepare meals and feed herself.
- *Level II:* Requires assistance or supervision from another person. *Example:* A 49-year-old man in CCU for treatment of myocardial infarction requires a nurse to assist him with a bed bath because his movement is restricted by IV and pulmonary artery lines and by prescribed activity restrictions.
- *Level III:* Requires assistance or supervision from another person and must use equipment or assistive device. *Example:* A 73-year-old woman with severe osteoarthritis must be transferred from wheelchair to raised toilet seat (device) by one person.
- *Level IV:* Is completely dependent on others for self-care and does not participate. *Example:* A comatose 18-year-old man with a closed head injury resulting from a motorcycle accident.

Physical Fitness

Ask the person to share his or her perceptions about physical fitness. For example, you may ask, "How do you feel about your physical fitness?" or "Tell me more about your exercise program." In addition, explore the person's perceptions about strength and endurance.

Once you have elicited data on the person's perceptions, ask specific questions to evaluate the quality of exercise. To determine if exercise activities are appropriate, you need data regarding the type of exercise, frequency, duration, and intensity:

- *Type:* Ask what type of exercise they engage in. For example, *endurance or aerobic exercise* (walking, running, cycling, swimming); *strengthening or anaerobic exercise* (weight lifting)
- *Frequency:* Ask how many times a week the person exercises.
- *Intensity:* Determine whether or not the person knows his or her pulse rate before, during, and after exercise. Ask about his or her perceptions about the intensity of the exercise.
- *Duration:* Ask how long each exercise session lasts.

Exercise patterns promote physical fitness if they meet the criteria for type, frequency, intensity, and duration discussed earlier in this chapter (see "Aerobic Capacity").

Activity Tolerance

Solicit information pertaining to the person's responses to activity and exercise. Use an open-ended approach (*e.g.,* "Tell me how you feel after walking two blocks" or "What types of problems have you experienced when you're active/exercising?"). Focus on reports of pain, discomfort, fatigue, dyspnea, or cough. The characteristics of these symptoms can often be a clue to underlying medical problems such as cardiovascular disease or pulmonary illness.

Cardiac Chest Pain. Cardiac chest pain occurs with angina, pericarditis, and aortic aneurysm. Angina occurs from an oxygen debt in the myocardium and may be precipitated by activity. The pain is often described as a squeezing, pressing, or tightening sensation; it is seldom described as sharp. The pain may also be precipitated by stress, hypoglycemia, or the ingestion of a heavy meal. Often, anginal pain radiates throughout the chest or to the arms or jaw, and may be difficult to pinpoint.

Pericarditis pain occurs when the membranes or pericardium around the heart become inflamed. Unlike episodic anginal pain, pericardial pain is persistent, sharp, and usually aggravated by deep breathing.

A dissecting aortic aneurysm usually causes a constant, intense, searing pain that may radiate to the back, anterior chest, or abdomen. It requires immediate medical attention.

Activity Tolerance Classification. For persons with cardiac disease, activity tolerance may be characterized by using the New York Heart Association's Functional and Therapeutic Classification System as follows:

- *Class I:* Person with heart disease who is asymptomatic. Ordinary physical activity does not cause undue fatigue, palpitation, dyspnea, or angina.
- *Class II:* Slight limitation of physical activity. The person has no distress at rest, but ordinary physical activity results in fatigue, dyspnea, or angina.
- *Class III:* Significant limitation of physical activity. The person has no distress at rest, but even low-intensity self-care activities cause fatigue, palpitation, dyspnea, or angina.
- *Class IV:* Symptoms at rest. The person may have angina or dyspnea even at rest, and any physical activity aggravates symptoms.

Pulmonary Chest Pain. Pulmonary chest pain is often called pleuritic chest pain because the pain is secondary to inflammation of the pleural surfaces lining the lungs and inner thoracic cage. Inflammation may be caused by infection, tumors, trauma, or pneumothorax. Breathing aggravates pleuritic pain, which is usually sharp or knife-like. To avoid or lessen the discomfort, the person may take shallow breaths and splint the chest (lean toward or put pressure on the affected side to minimize chest excursion). A person with pleuritic pain usually feels short of breath because of poor lung ventilation and gas exchange. Activity may be poorly tolerated because of the altered breathing pattern.

Claudication. Intermittent claudication is a sharp, cramping, squeezing pain that occurs in the legs in response to activity or exercise. The pain may result from ischemia, or oxygen deficit, and usually occurs in the presence of atherosclerosis in the major arteries supplying the leg. If the pain, which usually dissipates with rest, persists more than 10 minutes after rest, another cause may be indicated, such as arthritis. Intermittent claudication usually occurs in the calf muscles and is brought on by walking. The amount of walking that precipitates the pain indicates the severity of the arterial occlusion. Therefore, you should ask specific questions about the amount of walking that brings on the pain and the length of time the pain lasts.

Musculoskeletal Pain. Musculoskeletal pain is often associated with movement. It is important to determine if the pain is due to alterations in the joints (articular pain) or in the surrounding structures such as muscles, tendons, or bones (periarticular pain). If you suspect musculoskeletal pain, follow the special physical examination procedures described in Physical Examination of the Musculoskeletal System. Often, musculoskeletal pain is localized, as in the case of degenerative joint disease, which may produce pain in the knees, hips, neck, fingers, or back. If the pain can be reproduced by direct palpation, ischemia can be ruled out as the cause. Specific movements may also reproduce the pain. Articular pain may be associated with stiffness and swelling of the affected joint.

Fatigue and Weakness. Fatigue may be expressed as a lack of energy or "pep." You should explore whether it is caused by physiologic factors or by psychological factors such as depression or boredom. The duration of the fatigue is also an important factor. Fatigue that is relatively rapid and recent in onset and that cannot be associated with physical work may represent infection, a fluid balance disturbance, anemia, or a cardiac or peripheral circulatory compromise. In such cases, even minimal activity may cause fatigue. Chronic fatigue, especially if accompanied by symptoms of psychological distress, may be secondary to depression or anxiety. In this case, ask the person about events that occurred when fatigue first became a problem.

Weakness, often erroneously confused with fatigue, is a symptom associated with decreased muscular strength. Rarely of psychological origin, weakness may result from muscle or nerve dysfunction and requires more elaborate diagnostic testing.

Shortness of Breath. Shortness of breath, or dyspnea, may reflect cardiac, pulmonary, or psychogenic problems.

Hyperventilation, which occurs when an excessive accumulation of carbon dioxide is excreted, may occur during exercise or in other states of metabolic acidosis, and should not be confused with dyspnea.

You should ask whether the person has difficulty breathing when lying down (orthopnea), which may indicate severe congestive heart failure, asthma, pulmonary edema, chronic obstructive pulmonary disease (COPD), pneumothorax, or pneumonia. In persons with orthopnea, dyspnea can be relieved only in either a sitting or standing position.

Dyspnea during exertion may be related to impaired ventilation, which occurs with restrictive or obstructive pulmonary disease, diffusion defects, or ineffective breathing patterns. Dyspnea at rest usually occurs with severe cardiac disease rather than chronic pulmonary disorders. It is also associated, however, with acute pulmonary problems, such as asthma, pneumothorax, and pneumonia.

Cough. Coughing may indicate pulmonary or cardiac problems and should be evaluated further. If the cough is productive, evaluate the amount, consistency, and color of any expectorated material, and note the presence of blood.

Factors Influencing Activity Tolerance

A number of factors are associated with or known to contribute to activity problems. For example, a neuromuscular impairment may contribute to immobility, cardiovascular disorders may be associated with activity intolerance, and severe depression may explain a self-care deficit. The health history should include consideration of these factors, which are shown in the Interview Guide. Most of these factors are considered part of the person's past medical history (*i.e.,* previous illnesses, injuries, surgical procedures). Some practitioners choose to obtain a medical history during the opening moments of the assessment interview before proceeding to inquiries about specific health patterns (*e.g.,* activity and exercise). If this information was previously disclosed, it is not necessary to ask for it again. However, you should reevaluate this information in light of its significance to activity and exercise functions.

DIAGNOSTIC STUDIES

The major body systems that are considered during an evaluation of activity and exercise functions include the cardiovascular, respiratory, and musculoskeletal systems. In addition to physical examination of these systems, a number of diagnostic tests may be performed to evaluate structures and functions.

Common diagnostic studies to evaluate cardiovascular function include the following:

- Blood tests
- Noninvasive cardiovascular studies
- Nuclear medicine studies
- Invasive cardiovascular studies

Common diagnostic studies to evaluate respiratory function include the following:

- Arterial blood gas measurements
- Pulmonary function studies
- Oximetry

Common diagnostic studies to evaluate musculoskeletal function are as follows:

- Radiographic studies
- Arthroscopy
- Electromyography

Blood Tests for Cardiovascular Function

The complete blood count (CBC) should be evaluated with special attention to the hemoglobin (Hgb) and hematocrit (Hct) values. If these values are abnormally low, the person may be anemic, and cardiac output may increase to compensate.

A *lipid profile* measures serum cholesterol, triglyceride, and lipoprotein levels. Abnormalities may indicate a risk for coronary artery disease, generalized atherosclerosis, and lipid diseases.

Serum enzymes should be evaluated if acute myocardial infarction is suspected. Cell death in the myocardium results in release of specific enzymes: creatine phosphokinase (CPK), lactic dehydrogenase (LDH), serum glutamic-oxaloacetic transaminase (SGOT), and hydroxybutyric dehydrogenase (HBD).

Noninvasive Cardiovascular Studies

The posteroanterior (PA) chest radiograph should be evaluated to determine heart size and the orientation of the heart in the chest, and to identify any enlargement of individual chambers. Valvular and aortic calcifications can also be detected on PA chest films.

An *electrocardiogram* (ECG) graphically records electrical heart activity and provides information about cardiac rhythm disturbances, conduction defects, cellular death or injury patterns, and electrolyte status.

Holter monitoring is used to obtain a continuous ECG recording for an extended time period, usually 24 hours, in order to detect dysrhythmias. The person must wear the compact Holter monitor during usual activities.

The *exercise electrocardiography test* (*exercise tolerance test* or *stress test*) monitors the ECG as a person performs prescribed exercises such as climbing steps, riding a stationary bicycle, or walking on a treadmill. This test is used to diagnose angina or prescribe activities for people with cardiovascular deficits.

Echocardiograms involve placing a transducer, which acts as an ultrasound emitter and receiver, against the outer chest wall. The transducer is tilted at various angles in order to evaluate cardiac structures, especially the chambers and valves. This test evaluates cardiovascular function in people with valve disease, cardiomyopathies, congenital heart disease, coronary artery disease, aortic aneurysm, and left ventricular dysfunction.

Plethysmography detects deep vein thrombosis in the lower extremities. Pressure cuffs are applied to the leg, and the plethysmograph, a device that records a pressure waveform, is attached to the leg. Then cuffs are inflated to increase pressure in the vessels. If the pressure fails to return immediately to normal after the cuff is released, thrombosis should be suspected.

Nuclear Medicine Studies (Radioactive Isotope Evaluation)

In the *positron emission tomography (PET)* study, radioactive tracers are injected and then evaluated to determine the metabolic status of myocardial tissue. Positron-emitting compounds become tagged to metabolically active tissue and help to determine the location and exact size of a myocardial infarction, to distinguish reversible from irreversible myocardial injury, and to evaluate the effects of various treatments.

Thallium scanning helps to evaluate coronary artery disease after a radioactive tracer injection. Thallium accumulates in normal myocardium but not in areas that are not perfused. Ischemic areas show decreased radioactive activity or cold spots.

The *multiple-gated acquisition (MUGA) scan* counts radioisotopes as they pass through cardiac chambers. Injected technetium tags red blood cells. These data can be used to calculate the left ventricular ejection fraction or to provide information about ventricle wall motion.

In the *radioactive fibrinogen scanning test,* fibrinogen is incorporated into blood clots to detect deep vein thrombosis of the lower extremities. Twenty-four hours after the radioactive injection, the legs are scanned with a Geiger counter to detect excessive isotope uptake.

Invasive Cardiovascular Studies

Cardiac catheterization can be performed on either the right or left side of the heart. Pressures in the various cardiac chambers may be determined and blood samples may be obtained for blood gas analysis. This study may be used to evaluate left ventricular function, to measure cardiac output, and to confirm pathologic conditions.

Angiograms are radiographic studies of the heart chambers, arteries (arteriograms), coronary arteries (coronary arteriograms), or veins (venograms). Contrast medium is injected, and rapid-series x-ray films are obtained. Occlusive processes can then be readily identified.

Arterial Blood Gas Measurement

Arterial blood gases provide important information about the gas exchange that occurs in the lungs and the general effectiveness of respiratory function. The components of the arterial blood gas include the following:

- Partial pressure of oxygen (PO_2)
- Partial pressure of carbon dioxide (PCO_2)
- Bicarbonate level
- Percentage of oxygen saturation (SO_2)
- pH

Table 10–3. Normal Adult Arterial Blood Gas Values at Sea Level*

	Arterial	Mixed Venous
pH	7.40 (7.35–7.45)	7.36 (7.39–7.41)
PO_2	80–100 mm Hg	35–40 mm Hg
SaO_2	>95%	70%–75%
PCO_2	35–45 mm Hg	41–51 mm Hg
HCO_3^-	22–26 mEq/liter	22–26 mEq/liter
Base Excess	–2 to +2	–2 to +2

*PO_2 and SaO_2 values are lower at higher altitudes because oxygen tension is lower at higher altitudes.

The PO_2 indicates how much oxygen the lungs are delivering to the blood, and the PCO_2 provides information about how well the lungs eliminate carbon dioxide. The pH of the arterial blood indicates the acid–base level, or the hydrogen in concentration. The arterial blood gas measurements together indicate respiratory function. Abnormalities in blood gas levels may indicate a respiratory disorder or a metabolic problem. Table 10-3 presents normal values.

Pulmonary Function Studies

Pulmonary function tests (PFTs) are used to measure lung capacity and lung volumes. Normal ranges for the four distinct lung volumes and the lung capacities are summarized in Figure 10-1. Test results can help differentiate obstructive or restrictive pulmonary disease, determine if surgical anesthesia is risky, and monitor the patient's response to therapy.

Pulmonary function tests may be performed at the bedside by means of a spirometer, a device that measures volumes of air that move in and out of the lungs during ventilation. Another device, the inspiratory pressure manometer, may be used to measure various pressures generated during ventilation. Bedside PFT results are often combined with ventilatory pressure measurements to evaluate the patient's readiness to be weaned from mechanical ventilation. Such tests provide a means of evaluating the patient's ventilatory muscle strength and his or her ability to breathe spontaneously.

Oximetry

Noninvasive methods of monitoring oxygen and carbon dioxide levels in the blood are available. Oximetry measures the percent saturation of hemoglobin with oxygen. An indirect estimate of the PO_2 can be obtained based on the oxyhemoglobin dissociation curve. Oximetry involves the transmission of light impulses through tissue. Light absorption by the arterial blood in the tissue is proportional to the quantity of oxyhemoglobin in the blood. The oximeter converts these factors to a saturation reading. The oximeter is a clip-like device that may be attached to the earlobe or fingertips. Continuous readings can be monitored in order to evaluate the respiratory status of patients on ventilators or of persons undergoing pulmonary and cardiac stress testing. Oximetry is also useful for observing changes that occur with various respiratory treatments.

Radiographic Studies

The musculoskeletal system may be evaluated radiographically using a number of different modalities:

- *Diagnostic x-rays:* Used to diagnose fractures, degenerative conditions, impingement, or tumors
- *Magnetic resonance imaging (MRI):* Used to identify musculoskeletal trauma, tumors, and spinal conditions

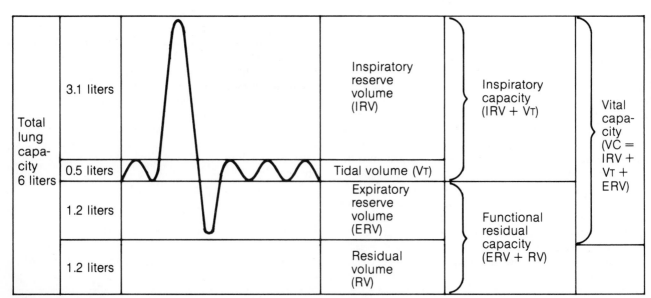

Figure 10–1. Lung volumes and capacities.

- *Computed tomography (CT scan):* Used to identify musculoskeletal trauma and other musculoskeletal disorders
- *Bone scintigraphy (bone scan):* Used primarily to identify metastatic processes in the bone
- *Myelography (myelogram).* Involves injection of radiopaque solution along spinal canal to identify abnormalities, including herniated discs or tumors.
- *Arthrography (arthrogram):* The radiographic study of joints after injection of a contrast material.

Arthroscopy

Arthroscopy is the direct examination of joint tissues through a special instrument called an arthroscope. Arthroscopy is considered a minor surgical procedure that requires anesthesia and invasive, sterile techniques. The joints most frequently examined using arthroscopy include the knee, shoulder, and elbow.

Electromyography

An electromyograph or electromyogram (EMG) is a graphic reading of nerve and muscle responses to electrical stimulation. The EMG indicates the status of nerves supplying muscles as well as muscle disorders (myopathies).

THE PHYSICAL EXAMINATION
Examination Focus

Examination techniques for activity and exercise focus on identifying any limitations to physical movement, the status of body systems essential for oxygenation, activity, and exercise, and physiologic responses to activity. In order to evaluate activity and exercise abilities and functions, a physical examination is conducted with emphasis on the following: general appearance; vital signs; and cardiovascular, respiratory, neurologic, and musculoskeletal systems.

General Appearance

During the general survey, note whether there are problems with movement by observing gait, posture, and obvious deformities such as missing limbs. Note the pattern of wear on the shoes, especially the heels, which could indicate abnormal walking movements. Prostheses such as walkers, canes, crutches, or artificial limbs should also be noted. Survey muscle mass and muscle tone, noting especially atrophied limbs.

Survey grooming. Appearance and general hygiene may reflect a person's ability to meet self-care needs. A neat and clean appearance indicates that the person is independent in activities of daily living or has compensated for any self-care deficits by using assistive devices or the help of another person.

Look for general signs of activity intolerance by observing facial expression and mental status. Be especially attentive to facial expressions of pain or anxiety associated with activity and movement. Determine whether activity interferes with level of consciousness, including states of alertness and orientation.

Note the general condition of the skin, especially color. Pallor and cyanosis reflect oxygenation problems and may be associated with activity intolerance.

Vital Signs

Evaluation of vital signs may help explain subjective reports of activity intolerance. For example, a person who reports feeling lightheaded after exertion may be noted to have an elevated pulse rate and hypotension. The vital signs also indicate tolerance or intolerance of activity. For example, an elevated pulse rate after activity should gradually return to resting levels. If it remains elevated, the person may not be tolerating activity.

Associated Body System Alterations

Cardiovascular, respiratory, neurologic, and/or musculoskeletal problems may predispose a person to problems with activity and exercise. An in-depth assessment of these systems is warranted when making overall judgments about activity and exercise. Examination of the cardiovascular, respiratory, and musculoskeletal systems is discussed elsewhere in this chapter.

The Neurologic System. Numerous neurologic dysfunctions, including sensory deficits such as impaired sight or hearing, contribute to activity and exercise problems. The nursing diagnoses that address self-care, mobility, and respiratory function may have neurologic etiologies. The neurologic system may be adversely affected by activity if cardiac output is not sufficient to maintain brain perfusion.

The Gastrointestinal System. Evaluating the function of the gastrointestinal system may reveal extensive cardiovascular pathology that interferes with activity and exercise. For example, severe right-sided congestive heart failure may lead to hepatic congestion and increased liver size. Abdominal vessel occlusion may also contribute to abdominal, ischemic pain during activity. The diminished oxygen supply to abdominal structures may be associated with nausea, vomiting, or constipation.

The Integumentary System. Both cardiovascular and pulmonary pathology, which interfere with activity and exercise, can cause changes in skin appearance. For example, circulatory problems may cause edema, loss of normal hair growth and distribution, or stasis ulcers. Chronic hypoxia may cause clubbing of the nails. Such integumentary changes should alert you that the person may be at increased risk for activity intolerance.

CARDIOVASCULAR SYSTEM

The cardiovascular system includes the following structures: the heart and blood vessels (arteries, veins, and capillaries). The autonomic nervous system plays a key role in influencing cardiovascular functions.

Anatomy and Physiology Overview

THE HEART AND GREAT VESSELS

The heart is a hollow, cone-shaped, muscular organ located beneath and to the left of the sternum. It is divided into a left and right side, each of which consists of an upper atrial chamber and a lower ventricular chamber. The chambers contract and relax in a syncopated rhythm that constitutes the beat of the heart. The atria are tilted slightly toward the back, whereas the ventricles extend to the left and toward the anterior chest wall.

The top of the heart is referred to as the *base,* whereas the conical bottom is called the *apex.* The apex is close enough to the chest wall to transmit a visible pulsation during ventricular contraction. The pulmonary artery, aorta and right ventricle face the anterior chest wall (Fig. 10-2). Heart size varies according to the size of the person. The size and shape of a person's clenched fist closely approximate the size and shape of his or her heart. The great vessels attached to the heart include the aorta, the pulmonary artery, the superior and inferior venae cavae, and the pulmonary veins (see Fig. 10-2).

BLOOD FLOW

Blood flows through the heart by way of a series of chambers and one-way valves (Fig. 10-3). The superior and inferior venae cavae return deoxygenated blood to the heart from peripheral veins. Blood enters the right atrium, which is a thin-walled, low-pressure filling chamber, passes through the tricuspid valve, and enters the right ventricle, which is a higher-pressure pumping chamber. Blood is then ejected from the right ventricle through the pulmonary valve and into the pulmonary artery, which carries blood to the lungs. Blood becomes oxygenated while flowing through the extensive capillary network of the lungs, before returning to the left atrium by way of the four pulmonary veins. The blood then passes through the mitral valve and finally enters the left ventricle, which is a thick-walled, high-pressure pumping chamber. Ventricular contraction

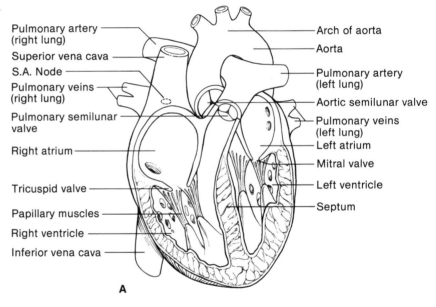

Figure 10–2. The heart and great vessels. (**A**) Anatomic representations usually show the atria on top of the ventricles. (**B**) This diagram represents actual orientation of heart structures in relation to the chest wall, showing the atria behind the ventricles, which project toward the anterior chest wall.

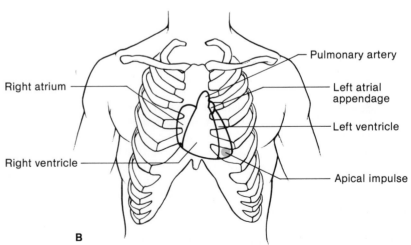

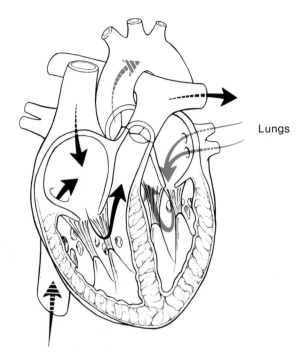

Figure 10–3. Blood flow through the heart.

Lungs

ejects the blood through the aortic valve into the aorta, which distributes blood throughout the body.

ALTERED BLOOD FLOW: MURMURS

Murmurs are abnormal heart sounds or vibrations. They may occur at any point in the cardiac cycle, and are caused by high rates of blood flow or turbulent blood flow over diseased valves.

Three main factors contribute to the intracardiac sounds called murmurs (see Fig. 10-4):

1. High flow rates through normal or abnormal valves
2. Forward flow of blood through a constricted or irregular valve or into a dilated vessel or chamber
3. Backward or regurgitant flow through an incompetent valve, septal defect, or patent ductus arteriosus

THE CONDUCTION SYSTEM

As electrical impulses cause heart muscle to depolarize, the heart's pumping chambers contract. This electrical impulse originates in the sinoatrial (SA) node near the right atrium and spreads through atrial conduction pathways to the atrioventricular (AV) node located at the interventricular septum (Fig. 10-5). This wave of atrial depolarization corresponds to the P wave on the ECG. The electrical impulse pauses at the AV node, allowing the ventricles to fill completely with blood before ventricular contraction. This phase of the cardiac cycle appears as the PR interval on the ECG. Next, the impulse travels rapidly through the bundle of His and down the left and right bundle branches to the terminal Purkinje fibers. The ECG configuration for this

phase is called the QRS complex. Repolarization of the ventricles corresponds to the T wave on the ECG.

ARTERIAL BLOOD VESSELS

The arteries are strong, compliant vessels that carry oxygenated blood away from the heart to peripheral tissues. The elastic properties of the arterial walls cause the arteries to stretch during systole and recoil during diastole. This results in a palpable arterial pulse and is the physiologic principle behind blood pressure measurement (see Chap. 6).

VENOUS BLOOD VESSELS

Veins are low-pressure vessels that carry deoxygenated blood to the heart. They have a larger capacity and thinner walls than arteries. Blood flow through the veins does not usually produce pulsations. However, pulsations may be noted in large central veins, such as the right internal jugular, and are caused by pressures generated in the right atrium during the cardiac cycle. Venous pulses have several distinct components, including the positive *a, c,* and *v*

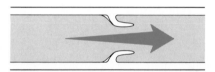

High flow

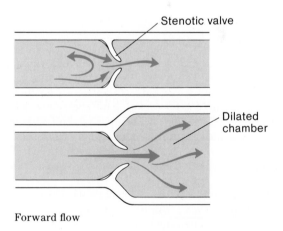

Stenotic valve

Dilated chamber

Forward flow

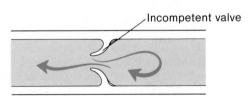

Incompetent valve

Backward flow

Figure 10–4. Origin of murmurs. (**Top**) High flow; (**middle**) forward flow through abnormal valves or chambers; (**bottom**) backward flow through abnormal valves or structures.

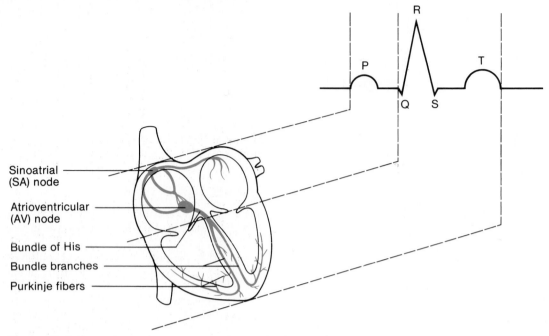

Figure 10–5. The cardiac conduction system in relation to the electrocardiogram.

Sinoatrial
(SA) node

Atrioventricular
(AV) node

Bundle of His

Bundle branches

Purkinje fibers

waves and negative descent waves, x and y (Fig. 10-6). Normally, only the a and c waves are readily detectable during the physical examination. The cardiac events generating these waves are discussed in the following section.

Veins distend when the intravascular volume increases; this may be noted in the great veins of the neck. See the section entitled Examination Guidelines: Neck Veins, later in this chapter.

THE CARDIAC CYCLE

The cardiac cycle includes all events between ventricular contractions (see Fig. 10-6). Understanding the cardiac cycle is important for assessing cardiovascular function because changes in blood flow during the cycle cause tension and vibration, which affect the heart valves and other structures. The sounds that are generated may be auscultated with the stethoscope. Electrocardiogram waveforms, pulsations in great veins, and arterial waveforms also correspond to events in the cardiac cycle.

Ventricular systole and diastole are the two major phases of the cardiac cycle. During heart auscultation, these phases can be distinguished by noting the heart sounds as "lub-dub": "Lub," or the first heart sound (S_1), signals the beginning of systole, and "dub," or the second heart sound (S_2), signals the beginning of diastole. When the heart rate is between 60 and 100 beats/minute, the cardiac cycle lasts approximately 0.86 seconds. Systole, the time between S_1 and S_2, is shorter than diastole. When heart rates are greater than 100 beats/minute, diastole shortens, and systole and diastole time periods become almost equal. The cardiac cycle can be traced from the beginning of diastole as follows:

1. Rapid Inflow. Blood flows into the atria from the venae cavae and pulmonary veins. This movement in-

creases the pressure in the atria over the pressure in the ventricles, which causes the AV valves to open and blood to flow rapidly into the ventricles.

Assessment Implications

- An abnormal heart sound, called the opening snap (OS), may occur during rapid inflow and is caused by the rapid opening motion of a diseased and stenotic mitral valve.
- The third heart sound, S_3, may be heard during rapid filling and results from sound vibrations generated when blood hits the ventricle walls. This heart sound is common in healthy young adults and children, and is called a physiologic S_3. In pathologic states, the vibrations may be generated by an increased volume load to the ventricles or by blood hitting a noncompliant ventricular wall. Third heart sounds are commonly noted with congestive heart failure.

2. Diastasis. During this phase, the inflow of blood from atria to ventricles continues, but at a much slower rate.

3. Atrial Systole. A wave of atrial depolarization spreads through the atria, initiating an atrial contraction, which forces the remaining 30% of blood into the ventricles, a process referred to as the "atrial kick."

Assessment Implications

- As pressure is transmitted to the venous system from atrial contraction, an a wave can be noted on the jugular venous pulsation (see Fig. 10-6).
- The P wave, PR interval, and beginning of the QRS complex can be noted on the ECG.
- An abnormal heart sound, called S_4, may be heard during atrial contraction. This sound is produced as blood

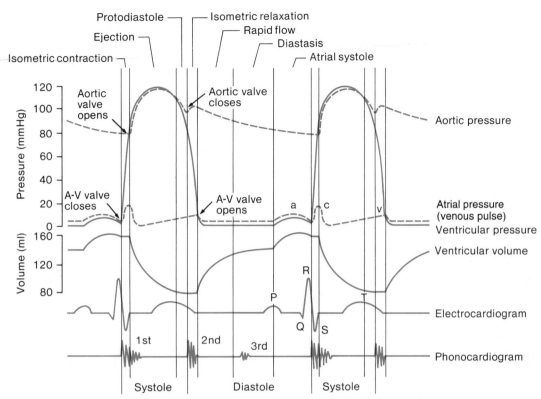

Figure 10–6. The cardiac cycle, showing changes in heart pressures and volumes, electrocardiogram, and phonocardiogram (graphic recording of heart sounds).

rapidly enters the ventricles because of increased blood volume or decreased ventricular wall compliance.

4. Isometric Contraction. Systole begins as pressure increases in the ventricle walls, forcing the AV valves to shut. The increasing pressures cause the downstream pulmonic and aortic valves to open. No blood enters or leaves the ventricles.

Assessment Implications

- The first heart sound, S_1, results from vibrations related to AV valve closure. Because two valves are actually closing, S_1 may be split into mitral and tricuspid components.
- When the valve closures transmit pressure to the venous system, a *c* wave is produced. The *c* wave is difficult to see when inspecting the jugular venous pulsations but may be noted if the pressure is recorded as a waveform.
- An abnormal heart sound, or ejection click, is produced when the tricuspid valves open, either when one of the valves is diseased or when ejection is rapid through a normal valve.

5. Protodiastolic Ejection. After the aortic valve opens, blood flows rapidly from the left ventricle. At the same time the right ventricle empties through the open pulmonic valve. When the blood flow ceases, the pressure in the ven-

tricles becomes lower than the pressure in the great arteries. Subsequently, blood flows back toward the ventricles, forcing the aortic and pulmonic valves to close.

Assessment Implications

- When the aortic and pulmonic valves close, a second heart sound, S_2, is produced. During inspiration, S_2 may be heard as a split sound as increased blood volume is returned to the right side of the heart, causing pulmonic closure to occur slightly later than aortic closure.
- The T wave can be observed on the ECG.
- If hemodynamic monitoring is being carried out, the dicrotic notch on the arterial waveform will correspond to aortic valve closure.
- A midsystolic click may be heard during the middle of protodiastolic ejection. This high-frequency, snapping noise is believed to be related to prolapsing or backward motion of the mitral valve leaflets during systole.

6. Isometric Relaxation. After the aortic valve closes, ventricle pressure falls, and the ventricles relax while maintaining a constant volume.

Assessment Implication

- Isometric relaxation corresponds with the *v* wave in the venous pulse, which results from the increased atrial pressure caused by venous return to the heart.

Physical Examination

Cardiovascular System

General Principles

Physical examination of the cardiovascular system involves the following:

- Precordial examination
- Arterial pulse examination
- Neck vein (venous pulse) examination

In addition, the skin is inspected during a cardiovascular examination to evaluate color changes, edema, and textures that might indicate cardiovascular disease (see Chap. 8). The liver may be evaluated in persons with congestive heart failure to evaluate the extent of pump failure.

Precordial examination focuses on the anterior chest wall and determining the status of underlying cardiovascular structures (the heart and great vessels). Precordial examination involves inspection, palpation, and auscultation. Percussion is rarely used because extracardiac factors such as the sternum and ribs interfere with heart evaluation. Occasionally, percussion may be used to evaluate the left ventricle border. However, a chest radiograph may provide more accurate information about the size of the heart.

During the precordial examination inspection and palpation usually precede auscultation. However, it may sometimes be helpful to perform the two simultaneously, especially when abnormal findings are noted. For example, if an abnormal pulsation is detected by inspection and palpation, it is helpful to auscultate while palpating the pulse or inspecting neck veins to learn where the pulsation falls in the cardiac cycle.

It is also important to note whether findings occur during early, middle, or late systole or diastole, as well as whether they occur intermittently or continuously. Also describe any variations with the breathing pattern.

Arterial pulses are generally assessed by palpating with the fingertips at points where an artery wall can be sufficiently compressed so that the artery's elastic recoil can be felt as pressure is transmitted from the aorta. Arterial pulses may also be detected by more sensitive equipment, such as Doppler ultrasound. Carotid and femoral arteries as well as the abdominal aorta should be auscultated with the bell and diaphragm of the stethoscope. Except for the carotids, pulses should be palpated bilaterally and simultaneously in order to make meaningful comparisons.

The neck veins are evaluated to determine the characteristics of the venous pulse in order to make judgments about the function of the right side of the heart. Jugular venous pulsations (JVP) and central venous pressure (CVP) can be determined by assessing the neck veins.

Jugular venous pulsations and CVP may be assessed by inspection as well as by invasive monitoring devices capable of producing a waveform or pressure scale reading. Inspection involves observing the column of venous blood in the internal jugular vein. Internal jugular vein pulsation can be distinguished from carotid artery pulsation by noting the difference in the type of stroke. The JVP is characterized by several low-amplitude and positive upstrokes as opposed to one brisk upstroke in the arterial pulse. To make this distinction, palpate the carotid artery on the opposite side while viewing the JVP. An alternative method is to ask the person to lie flat, which causes visible jugular vein distension. When the person sits up, the jugular vein distension will disappear because the vein will collapse. Pulsation from the internal jugular vein may also be identified by placing pressure on the neck just above and parallel to the clavicle. In about 20 seconds, the vein will fill, and the distension will become exaggerated.

Equipment

Stethoscope with bell and diaphragm
Ruler for measuring neck vein distention
Light source to provide tangential lighting
Doppler for detecting arterial pulses (optional)

Examining Room Preparation

To auscultate heart sounds accurately, the examination should take place in a quiet room. As with any procedure that requires the patient to be exposed, privacy as well as comfort should be maintained. The examination should be conducted with the person sitting or lying on a table or bed that will allow for various position changes.

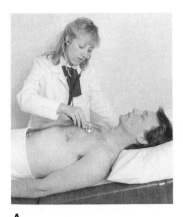 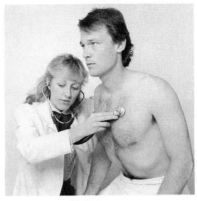 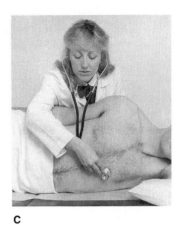

A   **B**   **C**

Figure 10–7. Precordial examination positions. (**A**) Supine position; (**B**) forward-sitting position; (**C**) left lateral decubitus position.

Exposure and Lighting	Tangential lighting, such as side lighting from a gooseneck lamp, is effective for casting shadows on the anterior chest or neck veins and thus making chest movements or venous pulsations more visible. The chest should be partially draped except during inspection when the entire precordium must be surveyed. Listening to heart sounds through clothing is unreliable and inadvisable.
Precordial Examination Positions	During the precordial examination, the examiner stands at the person's right side. If possible, the person's position is changed during the examination to bring underlying cardiac structures closer to the chest wall (Fig. 10-7).

The *supine position,* with the person's arms resting comfortably at the sides, will be adequate for most of the examination. The upper torso may be elevated to a 30-degree angle. The *forward-sitting position* will bring the base of the heart closer to the chest wall and is most effective for evaluating thrills and murmurs. The *left lateral decubitus position* will allow the apex of the heart to move closer to the chest wall and is best for detecting mitral valve murmurs.

Precordial Landmarks   Because the heart and great vessels are not visible, a system of precordial landmarks is used to guide the examination and provide locations for describing any sounds and pulsations observed during the examination. Heart sounds are created by valve movements and blood flow in the heart. Heart sounds are heard at the chest wall, but the area where you hear a sound may not be the area from which it originated. This is because blood flow transmits the sound away from its point of origin. Heart sounds originating with the valves are detected in the direction of blood flow at one of the following landmarks (Fig. 10-8):

The *aortic area,* located to the right of the sternum at the second intercostal space, represents the direction of blood flow from the aortic valve and the direction of sound transmission following closure of the aortic valve. Auscultatory findings related to the aortic valve may be heard at this point.

The *pulmonic area,* located to the left of the sternum at the second intercostal space, represents the pulmonic valve, which is located slightly lower than the second intercostal space. This landmark correlates with the outflow tract of the pulmonic valve.

The *tricuspid area,* located to the left of the sternum at the fifth intercostal space, represents the tricuspid valve, which is actually more superior and to the right of the sternum. The tricuspid area represents the outflow tract of the tricuspid valve and the direction of sound transmission following valve closure.

The *mitral or apical area,* located at the fifth left intercostal space just medial to the midclavicular line, represents a valve and a cardiac chamber. Blood flows from the mitral valve, which is superior and to the right, into the mitral or apical area. The apex of the left ventricle also lies beneath this area, and a pulsation may be palpated as the ventricle contracts.

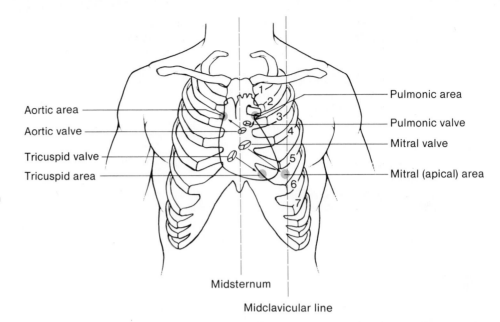

Figure 10–8. Heart sounds and precordial landmarks. Heart sounds are referred from valvular points of origin to the auscultatory or precordial landmarks. Sound travels in the direction of blood flow and may be heard at some distance from the valve.

Additional precordial landmarks may be useful during the examination (Fig. 10-9):

The *sternoclavicular area* overlies the sternum and its junctions with both clavicles, as well as portions of the left and right intercostal spaces. These structures can serve as a landmark for assessing the aortic arch and pulmonary artery, which are located to the left of the first intercostal space.

The *right ventricular area* overlies the heart's right ventricle, which faces the anterior chest and extends from the third intercostal space to the distal end of the sternum. The right lateral border of the right ventricular area overlies the right atrium. The left ventricle is located under the left lateral border.

Erb's point, the third left interspace, is included in the right ventricular area. Aortic and pulmonic valve sounds may be transmitted to this point.

The *epigastric area* represents the same anatomic region for both abdominal and cardiac examinations. Aortic or right ventricular pulsations may be detected in this area.

The *ectopic area* represents a landmark where abnormal precordial pulsations can be palpated in persons with left ventricular wall disorders secondary to angina or diffuse myocardial disease. Usually, such pulsations may be detected in the left midprecordium, just above the left ventricular apex. However, this location varies among people.

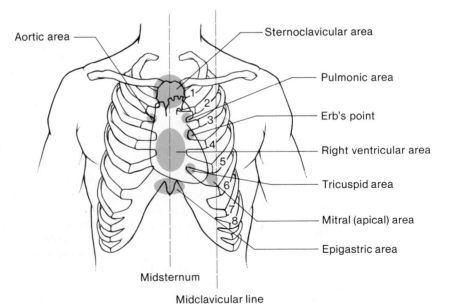

Figure 10–9. Additional precordial landmarks.

Examination and Documentation Focus (Precordium)	• *Inspection:* Pulsatile movements • *Palpation:* Pulsatile movements, vibrations • *Auscultation:* Heart rate and rhythm, heart sounds and murmurs
Examination and Documentation Focus (Arterial Pulses)	• Ease of palpation • Rate and rhythm of pulsation • Character of the arterial wall • Auscultatory findings • Contour and amplitude
Examination and Documentation Focus (Neck Veins)	• Pulse contour and amplitude • Distention • Height of venous pulsation

Examination Guidelines *Heart and Precordium*

Procedure

1. INSPECT THE PRECORDIUM.

   a. With the person supine, observe from the right side. (Viewing the person from the foot of the bed may also be helpful.) Note the precordial landmarks and visualize the position of the underlying structures.

   b. Observe each precordial area for abnormal heaves, thrusts, paradoxical movements, and pulsations. Also note the breathing pattern.

2. PALPATE THE MAJOR PRECORDIAL LANDMARKS.

   a. With the person supine, palpate each precordial area, aortic, pulmonic, Erb's point, tricuspid, mitral with the ball of the hand. Palpate pulsations with the fingertips. You may place the stethoscope lightly on the chest as you palpate, to time findings with the cardiac cycle.

Clinical Significance

Normal Findings

Apical pulse or PMI: Pulsation known as the apical pulse or point of maximal impulse (PMI) may be seen at the mitral area. This pulsation represents the outward thrust of the left ventricle during early systole and is caused by the heart wall recoiling as blood is ejected. A normal PMI is observed in the mitral area and should be no larger in diameter than 2 or 3 cm. However, during the later stages of pregnancy, this pulse may be noted above the fifth intercostal space because the diaphragm is displaced upward. The apical impulse may not be visible in all people, especially those who are obese or who have large breasts.

Deviations from Normal

Pulsations in the epigastric area may be noted in thin people. However, such a finding may be abnormal and should be further evaluated.

The ball of the hand is most sensitive to vibrations; fingertips are sensitive to pulsations.

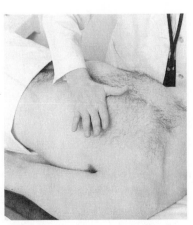

Precordial palpation with ball of hand

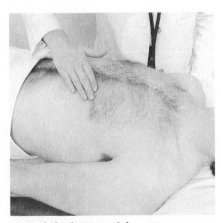

Precordial palpation with fingertips

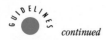 *continued*

Heart and Precordium

Procedure

  b. Note any pulsations, thrills, or rubs that must be further described in terms of location, amplitude, duration, and direction of impulse.

  c. You may palpate with the person in the forward-sitting position or left lateral decubitus position. However, changing to these positions at the end of the examination may be easier.

3. AUSCULTATE THE MAJOR PRECORDIAL LANDMARKS.

  a. With the person supine, systematically proceed from one landmark to the next in this sequence: aortic, pulmonic, Erb's point, tricuspid, mitral.

    Listen for several cardiac cycles at each landmark.

    Listen to each sound and try to block out all other sounds.

    Auscultate each area using the diaphragm and the bell of the stethoscope.

    At each landmark identify S_1 and S_2, normal splitting of S_1 and/or S_2, extra heart sounds and murmurs (see Display, "Abnormal Heart Sounds and Murmurs")

Clinical Significance

Normal Findings

Pulsatile movements: Normally, only pulsations over the mitral area corresponding to the PMI can be palpated.

Deviations from Normal

Vibrations: Palpable thrills, associated with murmurs, sound and feel like a purring cat and are not normal in any precordial area.

Heart rate: Normal resting heart rate is between 60 and 100 beats/minute but may be lower in people who are physically well-conditioned.

Rhythm: Usually rhythm will be regular, but it does vary in some persons, especially children and young adults. You may note an irregular rhythm that varies with respiration. During inspiration, venous return is greater and the heart rate may increase to compensate for the larger volume of blood. The rate will then decrease with expiration.

The diaphragm is used to detect higher-pitched sounds such as S_1, S_2, and aortic regurgitation murmurs. The bell is used to detect lower-pitched sounds such as S_3 and S_4.

Abnormal Heart Sounds

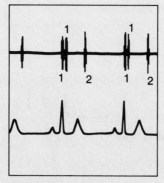

Widely split S_1

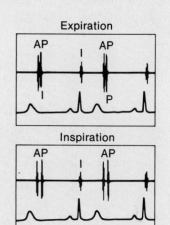

Expiration

Inspiration

S_2 splitting

Abnormal S_1 Splitting

Widely split first sound: S_1 may be abnormally split. Listen for a widely split S_1 with the diaphragm of the stethoscope.

This split may be secondary to electrical or mechanical causes, such as bundle-branch block and ventricular ectopy, that result in asynchronous ventricular contraction. A widely split first sound may be confused with other abnormal sounds, such as ejection clicks, that occur at this point in the cycle.

(continued)

Abnormal Heart Sounds *(continued)*

Abnormal S₂ Splitting

Second sound splitting: S₂ splitting during expiration is considered abnormal and may occur as either fixed splitting or splitting that is accentuated on inspiration. Use the diaphragm of the stethoscope at the base of the heart to detect this sound.

Splitting occurs because aortic and pulmonic valves close at least 0.03 seconds apart. Delayed pulmonic valve closure may be noted with right bundle-branch block or pulmonic stenosis.

Reserved second sound splitting (paradoxical split): Reversed or paradoxic S₂ splitting can be noted with expiration (unlike a normal or widely split second sound, which is detected on inspiration).

Paradoxical splitting occurs when the pulmonic valve closes first because of delays with left ventricular ejection related to left bundle-branch block or aortic stenosis.

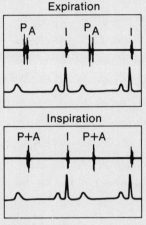

Expiration

Inspiration

Reversed S₂ splitting

Third Heard Sound (S₃)

The third heart sound, S₃, also called the ventricular gallop, is a low-frequency sound best heard using the bell of the stethoscope at either the apical area (for S₃ of left ventricular origin) or lower right ventricular area (for S₃ of right ventricular origin). The sound may be accentuated during inspiration (sounds like "Ken-tuc-ky").

S₃ is usually pathologic but may occur normally in young children or in people with high cardiac outputs. However, it is rarely normal in people over age 40 years. S₃ is associated with congestive heart failure and tricuspid or mitral valve insufficiency. This early diastolic sound represents rapid ventricular filling and is related to vibrations caused by blood forcefully hitting the ventricular wall.

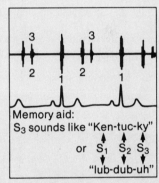

Memory aid:
S₃ sounds like "Ken-tuc-ky"
or S₁ S₂ S₃
"lub-dub-uh"

Third heart sound: S₃

Opening Snap (OS)

An opening snap (OS) is an abnormal early diastolic sound with a sharp quality, frequently mistaken for S₂ splitting or for an S₃. However, an OS will occur earlier than S₂ splitting or S₃. An OS will be detected at a higher pitch than S₃. This abnormal sound can be heard throughout the precordium and will not vary with respirations.

Opening snaps occur secondary to the opening of a stenotic or stiff mitral valve.

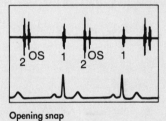

Opening snap

Fourth Heart Sound (S₄)

The fourth heart sound, S₄, also known as the atrial gallop, occurs near the end of diastole when the atria contract. Use the bell of the stethoscope to detect this low-frequency sound. Left ventricular S₄ sounds will be loudest at the apical area when the person assumes a supine or left lateral decubitus position. Right ventricular S₄ sounds will be loudest at the lower right ventricular area when the person assumes a supine position, and may increase in volume during inspiration (sounds like "Ten-nes-see").

S₄ occurs after atrial contraction and is caused by vibrations when blood flows rapidly into the ventricles. Vibrations result from the flow of a high blood volume or if the ventricle wall has low compliance. Associated conditions include coronary artery disease, hypertension, aortic and pulmonic stenosis, and acute myocardial infarction.

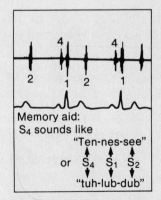

Memory aid:
S₄ sounds like
"Ten-nes-see"
or S₄ S₁ S₂
"tuh-lub-dub"

Fourth heart sound: S₄

(continued)

Abnormal Heart Sounds (continued)

Summation Gallop

When S_3 and S_4 occur simultaneously, the sound is called a *summation gallop*.

Summation gallops are associated with severe congestive heart failure.

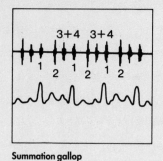

Summation gallop

Ejection Click

Heard just after the first heart sound, an *ejection click* is a high-frequency sound. This systolic sound can be heard widely throughout the precordium, unlike the more localized and lower-pitched S_4 sound.

Ejection clicks are produced by the opening of a diseased aortic or pulmonic valve or by rapid ejection through normal valves.

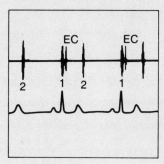

Ejection click

Midsystolic Click

The *midsystolic click* is a high-frequency, snapping sound that can be heard in middle or late systole. Listen for this sound over the mitral or apical area.

A midsystolic click is attributed to mitral valve leaflet prolapse during left ventricular ejection.

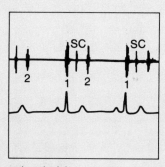

Midsystolic click

Pericardial Friction Rubs

This extracardiac sound is a high-pitched, scratchy sound that can be simulated in the following manner: grasp the stethoscope in the left hand with the diaphragm facing the palm. Rub the thumb of the right hand back and forth over the first and second finger metacarpal joints and listen to the simulated sound. Pericardial friction rubs are loudest at the left second, third, or fourth intercostal spaces and may be heard throughout the cardiac cycle, that is, throughout systole and diastole. There are three possible components of a pericardial friction rub: presystolic, systolic, and early diastolic. The rub is called *triphasic* if all three sounds are heard.

Pericardial friction rubs result from inflammation of the pericardial membrane.

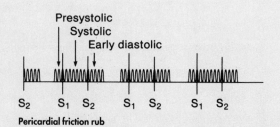

Pericardial friction rub

Murmurs

Criteria for Describing Murmurs

All murmurs should be evaluated in terms of timing, intensity, quality, location, radiation, ventilation, and the effect of position changes.

1. TIMING
   Does the murmur occur during systole or diastole? (Diastolic murmurs are usually pathological.) Describe the exact timing in relation to the cardiac cycle as follows:
   a. A pansytolic (holosystolic) murmur is continuous throughout systole.
   b. A midsystolic (ejection) murmur begins after S_1, peaks in midsystole, and ends before S_2.
   c. A protodiastolic murmur occurs early in diastole.
   d. A presystolic murmur occurs late in diastole.

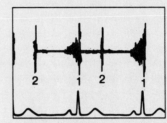

Pansystolic murmur

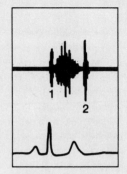

Midsystolic (ejection) murmur

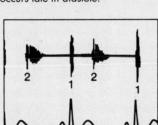

Protodiastolic murmur

Presystolic murmur

2. INTENSITY.
   How loud is the murmur? Use the following grading system to describe the murmur intensity:
   I—Barely audible
   II—Audible but quiet
   III—Clearly heard
   IV—Loud; may be associated with thrill
   V—Very loud; palpable thrill; may hear with stethoscope partially off chest
   VI—Very loud; palpable thrill; can hear without using stethoscope

3. QUALITY.
   What is the quality, pitch, and pattern of the murmur? Describe pitch using terms such as *high* or *low* and quality with terms such as *blowing*, *harsh*, or *musical*. *Pattern* refers to changes in murmur intensity.
   a. *Crescendo:* The murmur becomes progressively louder.
   b. *Decrescendo:* The murmur becomes progressively softer.
   c. *Crescendo-decresendo:* The murmur peaks in intensity.

4. LOCATION.
   Over which precordial landmark is the murmur loudest?

5. RADIATION.
   Is the sound of the murmur transmitted to other areas of the precordium? Murmurs usually radiate in the direction of blood flow.

6. VENTILATION AND POSITION.
   Is the murmur affected by inspiration, expiration, or position changes?

Murmurs are recorded as a fraction, with the grade as the numerator and "VI" (which indicates the grading scale used) as the denominator. Example: grade II/VI.

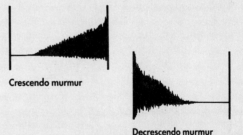

Crescendo murmur

Decrescendo murmur

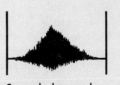

Crescendo-decrescendo murmur

Nursing Role

Your role in evaluating murmurs is to detect new murmurs and changes in existing murmurs. You should make appropriate referrals based on your assessment. Describe the murmur(s) in relation to the criteria described below. Although specific murmur diagnosis is often the cardiologist's responsibility, you should be able to recognize life-threatening murmurs, such as a mitral regurgitation murmur in the patient who has recently had a myocardial infarction. Such a murmur, often having a sudden onset, may indicate papillary muscle rupture. The ensuing left-sided heart failure is a frequent cause of death.

(continued)

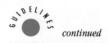 *continued*

Heart and Precordium

Murmurs (continued)

Common Murmurs

Physiologic Murmurs

- Nonpathologic murmurs also called physiologic or innocent murmurs
- Can only be detected during systole
- Normal during late pregnancy and in children
- Also associated with increased cardiac output states such as anemia or hyperthyroidism

Mitral Regurgitation

- Pansystolic (holostolic)
- Grade varies from I to V
- High-pitched, blowing murmur
- Heard at the apex with the person in the left lateral decubitus position
- May radiate to the back and left axilla
- Caused by backward blood flow through a "leaky" mitral valve
- Associated findings: S_3, diminished S_1, S_2 splitting

Aortic Stenosis

- Midsystolic ejection murmur
- Grade varies
- Harsh with a crescendo-decrescendo pattern
- Heard clearly at the aortic area with the person in the forward-sitting position
- May radiate to the neck and back
- Caused by blood flow over a narrowed aortic valve
- May be accompanied by a thrill in the aortic area
- Other associated findings: left ventricular lift, ejection click, and diminished aortic closing sound

Aortic Regurgitation

- Pandiastolic
- Difficult to hear—often graded I/VI
- Decrescendo, high-pitched, blowing
- Heard over the aortic area during exhalation (or holding breath) with the person in the forward-sitting position
- May radiate to the left sternal border
- Caused by backward blood flow from the aorta into the left ventricle
- S_3 and S_4 common; diastolic thrill may be palpable at the left sternal border

Mitral Sounds

- Usually middiastolic or presystolic
- Difficult to hear—less than grade III
- Low-pitched, rumbling quality
- Heard best at the apex with the person in the left lateral decubitus position
- Caused by blood flowing through a narrowed mitral valve during diastole
- Associated findings: Accentuated S_1, OS, diastolic thrill palpated at the apex

Procedure

4. IDENTIFY S_1 AND S_2.

   The first heart sound, S_1, may be heard as a single sound and will be loudest at the apex when the diaphragm of the stethoscope is used.

   The second heart sound, S_2, may be heard as a single sound and will be loudest at the base of the heart. Note intensity and any sound splitting.

Clinical Significance

S_1 represents the closing of the mitral and tricuspid valves.

S_2 represents the closing of the aortic and pulmonic valves.

Normal Findings

In a person with a normal heart rate and rhythm, the first and second heart sounds will be readily distinguished by the longer time interval between S_1 and S_2. Usually S_1 will be loudest at the mitral or apical area, and S_2 will be loudest at the pulmonic area. Also, S_1 may be heard almost simultaneously while palpating the upstroke of the carotid pulse.

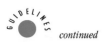

continued   ***Heart and Precordium***

Procedure

Clinical Significance

Noting such variations may help when identifying S_1 and S_2 in persons with rapid heart rates.

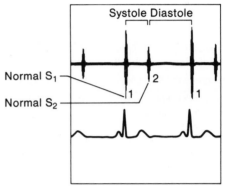

Normal heart sounds

5. IDENTIFY NORMAL SPLITTING OF THE FIRST AND SECOND HEART SOUNDS.

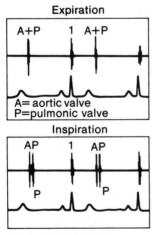

M_1 = mitral valve closure
T_1 = tricuspid valve closure

Split S_1: Normal variation

Split S_2: Normal variation

Because the left side of the heart normally contracts before the right side, two sounds are produced with S_1 (M_1 and T_1) and S_2 (A_2 and P_2). However, the time interval may be too short to differentiate these sounds.

Normal Findings

Split first sound: A split S_1 may be heard close to the tricuspid area or lower left sternal border (LLSB). There is no respiratory variation with a split S_1.

The two components of this sound, M_1 and T_1, are related to mitral and tricuspid valve closure, and occur 0.2 to 0.4 seconds apart.

Split second sound: Normal S_2 splitting, also called a physiological split, may be heard on inspiration. On expiration, S_2 is again heard as a single sound.

Inspiration increases blood return to the right side of the heart. At the same time, the pulmonary vasculature capacity increases, causing more blood to pool, thereby decreasing the amount of blood entering the left side of the heart. As a result, the left ventricle is emptied more rapidly than the right ventricle and aortic valve closure precedes pulmonic valve closure by about 0.04 seconds.

continued **Heart and Precordium**

Procedure

6. IDENTIFY EXTRA HEART SOUNDS AND MURMURS.
   a. Once S_1 and S_2 and any normal splitting patterns have been identified, concentrate on identifying any other extra sounds and murmurs that are timed in relation to the cardiac cycle and ventilatory pattern.
7. AUSCULTATE THE PRECORDIUM WITH THE PERSON ASSUMING DIFFERENT POSITIONS (optional).
   a. Auscultate with the person in the forward-sitting position.
   b. Auscultate with the person in the left-lateral decubitus position.

Clinical Significance

Extra heart sounds and murmurs may be abnormal (See Display, "Extra Heart Sounds and Murmurs").

Forward-sitting position brings the base of the heart closer to the chest wall.

Left-lateral decubitus position brings the apex of the heart closer to the chest wall.

Examination Guidelines   *Arterial Pulses*

Procedure

1. PALPATE THE CENTRAL AND PERIPHERAL ARTERIAL PULSES.
   a. Locate and palpate the following arterial pulses: carotid, brachial, femoral, popliteal, posterior tibialis, and dorsalis pedis.

   Carotid pulse: Locate the carotid pulse just medial to and below the angle of the jaw.

   Use light pressure.

Clinical Significance

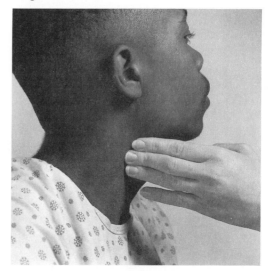

Palpation of the carotid pulse

Strong pressure stimulates the carotid sinus and may result in bradycardia, hypotension, or even cardiac arrest.

Avoid reduction in cerebral blood flow.

Never palpate both carotid arteries at the same time.

Arterial Pulses

Procedure

Clinical Significance

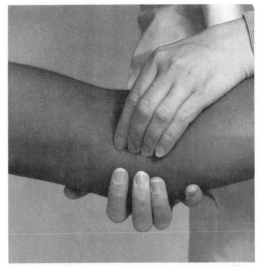

Palpation of the brachial pulse

Brachial pulse: Locate the brachial pulse just medial to the biceps tendon.

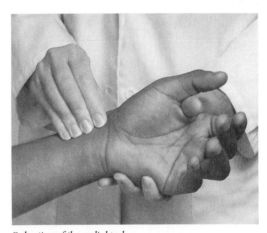

Palpation of the radial pulse

Radial pulse: Locate the radial pulse at the medial, inner wrist.

Femoral pulse: Locate the femoral pulse below the inguinal ligament.

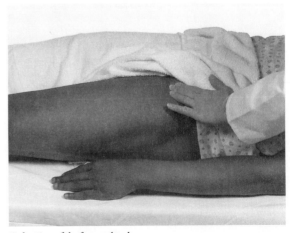

Palpation of the femoral pulse

Arterial Pulses

Procedure

Clinical Significance

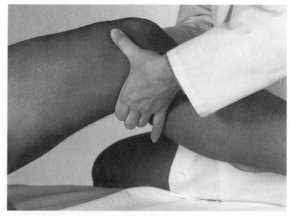

Palpation of the popliteal pulse

Popliteal pulse: Locate the popliteal pulse. Place the thumbs on the patella and the remaining fingers of both hands in the popliteal space. Hold the leg slightly flexed at the knee. Use firm pressure. The popliteal pulse is difficult to palpate.

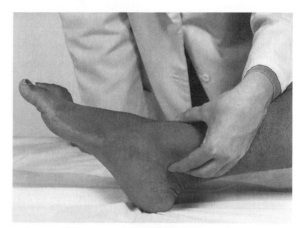

Palpation of the posterior tibial pulse

Posterior tibialis pulse: Locate the posterior tibialis pulse behind and slightly below the medial malleolus of the ankle.

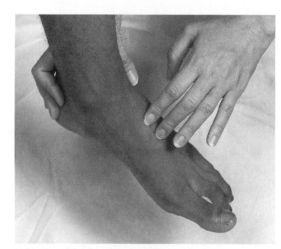

Palpation of the dorsalis pedis pulse

Dorsalis pedis pulse: Locate the dorsalis pedis pulse with the foot slightly dorsi-flexed on the top of the foot just lateral to the extensor tendon of the great toe.

b. Palpate, using the fingertips of the first and second fingers (or first, second, and third fingers).

Do not use your thumb. Because the thumb has a pulse, you may feel your pulse more readily than the patient's pulse.

c. Palpate left and right pulses individually as well as simultaneously. *Exception:* Never palpate both carotid pulses at the same time.

Simultaneous palpation of pulses on right and left sides helps you make comparisons. Findings should be identical. Asymmetric pulses suggest arterial occlusion.

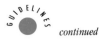

continued

Arterial Pulses

Procedure

d. Palpate each pulse to determine ease of palpation, rate and rhythm, character of the arterial wall, and contour and amplitude.

Ease of palpation: Note how easy or difficult it is to feel each pulse and how much pressure it takes to obliterate the pulse.

Rate and Rhythm: Observe the rate and rhythm of each pulse; compare with the apical (precordial) pulse.

Character of the arterial wall: Note how the arterial wall feels.

Contour and Amplitude: Note bounding of pulse, weakness, changes in upstroke and downstroke, and irregular patterns. Pulse contour and amplitude indicate volume and pressure relationships within the vessel and are difficult to assess by palpation. However, contour and amplitude may be assessed easily by examining pressure waveforms, obtained by intraarterial pressure monitoring.

Clinical Significance

Normal Findings

Arterial pulses should be easy to palpate and should not be easily obliterated by pressure from your fingers.

Deviations from Normal

Nonpalpable pulses: A pulse may be difficult to palpate in cases of atherosclerosis, which causes vessel stiffness and diminished artery wall elasticity. Nonpalpable pulses may also be related to cessation of blood flow and should be further evaluated with Doppler ultrasound.

Normal Findings

The pulse rate and rhythm should correlate with the rate and rhythm detected by precordial auscultation.

Deviations from Normal

Pulse deficit: A pulse deficit can be detected by simultaneously palpating a peripheral pulse and auscultating the precordial pulse. A pulse deficit exists if the peripheral pulse rate is slower than the precordial pulse rate. Pulse deficits indicate that myocardial contraction is not forceful enough to perfuse the extremities. This condition may be noted with cardiac dysrhythmias such as atrial fibrillation, atrial tachycardias, or premature ectopic depolarizations.

Normal Findings

The arterial wall will normally feel soft and pliable.

Deviations from Normal

The vessel wall may feel like a rope if atherosclerosis is present.

Normal Findings

Normal contour is characterized by a smooth upstroke. The dicrotic notch represents closure of the aortic valve.

Normal amplitude is represented by a pulse pressure (the difference between systolic and diastolic pressures) of approximatley 30 to 40 mmHg. This pulse is recorded "3+" on a 0 to 4 scale.

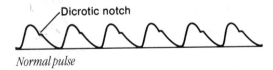

Normal pulse

Deviations from Normal

See Display, "Abnormal Pulse Patterns."

GUIDELINES *continued*   ***Arterial Pulses***

Abnormal Pulse Patterns

Pulsus Magnus

- Bounding pulse
- Increased pulse pressure
- Rapid upstroke and downstroke
- 4+ on a 0 to 4 scale
- Associated with atherosclerosis and hyperkinetic circulatory states as noted in hypertension, fear and anxiety, exercise, hyperthyroidism, anemia, patent ductus arteriosus, and aortic regurgitation

Pulsus Parvus

- Small weak pulse
- Decreased pulse pressure
- Delayed upstroke and prolonged downstroke
- 1+ on a 0 to 4 scale
- Associated with low cardiac output states such as cardiogenic shock, cardiac tamponade, and severe cases of aortic and mitral stenosis

Pulsus Alternans

- Heart rate is regular but the pulse alternates in size and intensity
- Difficult to assess by palpation; noted as the pulse is auscultated for blood pressure measurement
- Associated with a weakened myocardium and accompanying severe hypertension or left ventricular failure

Pulsus Paradoxus

- Exaggerated response to inspiration
- Normally, the pulse intensity or systolic pressure is lower during inspiration and is noted as a less than 10-mm Hg decrease in systolic blood pressure during inspiration
- A decrease of more than 10 mm Hg during inspiration indicates pulsus paradoxus
- Associated with severe heart failure, pericardial tamponade, severe lung disease, and constrictive pericarditis

Inspiration   Expiration   Inspiration

Pulsus Bisferiens ("Double-Beating" Pulse)

- Two pulses can be palpated during systole
- Associated with premature cardiac contractions, pericardial effusion, and constrictive pericarditis

Procedure

2. AUSCULTATE THE CAROTID AND FEMORAL ARTERIES.

   Auscultate for bruits, using the bell of the stethoscope.

3. PERFORM THE ALLEN TEST (optional).

Clinical Significance

The bell detects low-pitched sounds—bruits are low-pitched.

Normal Findings

Silent on auscultation

Deviations from Normal

Bruits: A bruit, the vascular equivalent of a murmur, can be heard as a blowing sound caused by restrictive blood flow through vessels. Bruits may be auscultated over the carotid and femoral arteries and the abdominal aorta, indicating occlusive arterial disease.

The Allen test is a method for determining the patency of the ulnar artery. The pulsation from the ulnar artery is difficult to palpate, yet in some clinical situations this artery must be assessed for patency. For example, when an intraarterial catheter is placed in the radial artery to monitor blood pressure, the ulnar artery must be patent to assure adequate collateral blood circulation to the hand.

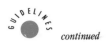

continued *Arterial Pulses*

Procedure

Occlude the radial artery with your fingers and ask the person to make a tight fist.

While you continue to hold pressure on the raidal artery, ask the person to open the fist and note whether the color returns to the hand.

Clinical Significance

This maneuver forces blood away from the hand and causes skin blanching.

Ulnar artery patency is indicated by color returning rapidly to the hand.

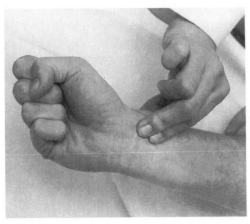

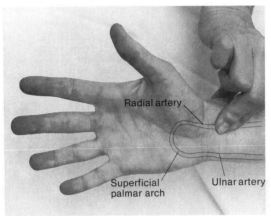

A

Allen test

B

Examination Guidelines   *Neck Veins*

Procedure

1. OBSERVE THE JUGULAR VENOUS PULSATION (JVP).

Observe the person from the right side.

Position the patient with the torso elevated 30 to 45 degrees and inspect the venous pulse. Turn the person's head slightly to the left.

Clinical Significance

The jugular veins are assessed by inspection because palpation obliterates the vein.

The right internal jugular vein is more visible than the left because of the proximity to the right heart.

The venous pulse is normally not visible with the person sitting fully upright. A flat position is undesirable because the vein is fully distended and pulsations are indistinguishable.

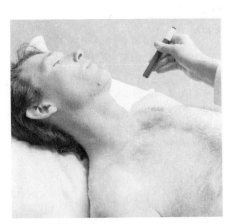

Neck vein inspection

GUIDELINES *continued*   **Neck Veins**

Procedure

Provide tangential lighting to the neck area.

Observe the jugular venous pulsation (JVP) for several cardiac cycles. Note distinct components of the venous pulse. Considerable skill is necessary to detect the distinct JVP components by inspection. However, such components are relatively easy to detect on a graphic waveform.

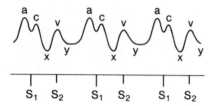

Jugular venous waveform in relation to S_1 and S_2

2. ESTIMATE CENTRAL VENOUS PRESSURE (CVP) BY MEASURING THE HEIGHT OF PULSATION IN THE INTERNAL JUGULAR VEIN.

   a. Choose a standard reference point from which to measure the height of pulsation in the internal jugular vein. The zero reference point, at the level of the right atrium, may be difficult to determine with accuracy. Therefore, use the sternal angle, which is approximately 5 cm above the right atrium, as the reference point.

   b. Measure the distance, in centimeters, from the sternal angle to the top of the distended jugular vein.

   c. Add 5 cm to the value obtained, for a rough estimate of central venous pressure.

3. CHECK FOR HEPATOJUGULAR REFLUX.

   With the person raised 30 to 60 degrees, compress the right upper quadrant for 30 to 60 seconds with your palm.

   The hepatojugular reflux is positive if the JVP level rises with this maneuver.

Clinical Significance

Tangential lighting accentuates shadows and makes any pulsations more visible.

Normal Findings

Normal JVP: Several pulse waves may be noted in the JVP that reflect pressure changes in the right side of the heart. Three positive waveforms include *a, c,* and *v*. The *c* wave, reflecting atrial systole, may be a distinct wave, or appear as a notch on the *a* wave, or be absent. The *c* wave is the largest positive waveform and may increase in amplitude during inspiration. The *c* waveform represents tricuspid valve closure. The *v* waveform represents right atrial filling.

The negative waveforms include *x* and *y*. The *x* descent occurs with ventricular systole as the height of the venous blood column declines. The *y* descent occurs when blood from the right atrium flows rapidly into the right ventricle.

Deviations from Normal

Abnormal JVP: Conditions that increase resistance to right ventricular filling, such as tricuspid stenosis, right ventricular failure, pulmonary hypertension, and pulmonary stenosis, may cause the *a* wave amplitude to increase (*cannon a waves*). Decreased amplitude *a* waves may be noted in clients with atrial fibrillation and ventricular pacemakers. Tricuspid regurgitation may increase *v* wave amplitude. Cardiac tamponade may cause an increase in both *a* and *v* waves.

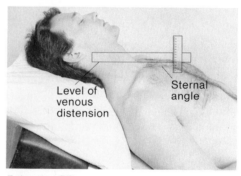

Estimating CVP

Normal central venous pressure is 3 to 5 cm above the sternal angle when the trunk is elevated 30 to 60 degrees.

CVP elevation may be attributed to right or left ventricular failure, pulmonary hypertension, pulmonary emboli, or cardiac tamponade.

Perform this maneuver if you suspect right ventricular failure.

The increased abdominal pressure increases venous return to the right side of the heart. If the right ventricle is impaired, pressure in the neck veins will increase.

Documenting Cardiovascular Examination Findings

Precordial Examination Findings

Example 1: Normal Heart and Precordium

Mr. L, aged 20, was examined at the college health center as a prerequisite for playing college basketball. The precordial examination findings were normal and were recorded as follows:

> No visible pulsations on anterior chest. PMI palpable at left 5th ICS; 2 cm in diameter. Heart auscultation: Regular rhythm, rate 68 beats/minute, S_1 and S_2 identified. No extra heart sounds, murmurs, or rubs.

The same findings may be summarized in a problem-oriented format:

S: Denies previous cardiovascular problems, including hypertension or rheumatic heart disease. No chest pain or dyspnea at rest or with activity.

O: No visible pulsations on anterior chest. PMI palpable at left 5th ICS; 2 cm in diameter. Heart auscultation: Regular rhythm, rate 68 beats/minute, S_1 and S_2 identified. No extra heart sounds, murmurs, or rubs.

A: No abnormalities detected on precordial examination.

P: Continue with routine follow-up examinations. Counsel about risk factors for cardiovascular disease; reinforce health benefits of present physical activities.

Example 2: Myocardial Infarction

Mr. H, aged 72, was a patient in the CCU following an acute anterior myocardial infarction 2 days ago. Heart sounds were auscultated several times a day. Examination findings were abnormal and were recorded as follows:

> Apical pulse regular, rate 80 beats/minute. S_4 heard at LSB, 5th ICS. No murmurs. Pericardial friction rub heard over left precordium, loudest at LSB, 5th ICS.

The same findings may be summarized in a problem-oriented format:

S: Reports occasional sharp anterior chest pain with deep inspiration. Reports pain has no pressure-like or squeezing quality.

O: Apical pulse regular, rate 80 beats/minute. S_4 heard at LSB, 5th ICS. No murmurs. Pericardial friction rub heard over left precordium, loudest at LSB, 5th ICS.

A: S_4 recorded on admission and not a new finding—probably indicates underlying heart disease. Pericardial rub is of new onset. Suspect post-MI pericarditis.

P: Inform physician about rub. Reinforce need to report chest pain and inform about probable cause of current pain. Continue cardiac auscultation q4h and as condition changes.

Documenting the Quality of the Arterial Pulse

To establish consistency, arterial pulses are graded using the following criteria:

0 = Absent
1+ = Diminished; thready; easily obliterated
2+ = Normal; not easily obliterated
3+ = Increased; full volume
4+ = Bounding; hyperkinetic

Example 1: Normal Findings

If all peripheral pulses are noted as normal, you may record your findings as follows:

> All peripheral pulses readily palpable and findings symmetric: 2+, regular rhythm, smooth contour, and brisk upstroke.

The results of examining normal carotid arteries may be recorded as follows:

> Carotid pulse regular rhythm, rate 72, 2+ (bilaterally) with brisk upstroke. No bruits.

Example 2: Cardiogenic Shock (Pulsus Parvus)

> All peripheral pulses diminished (1+). Delayed upstroke.

Neck Veins

Example 1: Normal Findings

The results of examining normal neck veins may be recorded as follows:

> JVP noted 2 cm above sternal angle with upper body elevated 45 degrees (CVP estimated at 7 cm). Distinct *a* waves observed. Hepatojugular reflex negative.

Example 2: Right Ventricular Failure

> Jugular veins distended in upright position. Hepatojugular reflex positive.

NDx

Nursing Diagnoses Related to Cardiovascular Assessment

Activity Intolerance

Activity intolerance is the inability to endure or tolerate an increase in activity. However, you should also consider the diagnosis potential for activity intolerance, to identify persons at high risk and prescribe appropriate activity restrictions for this problem. Causes of activity intolerance include cardiovascular and pulmonary disease and cardiovascular deconditioning, as well as noncardiovascular factors such as depression, chronic illness, and prolonged immobility. People may be screened for this problem by considering various aspects of a person's health history and physical examination.

If the patient has heart disease, the four levels of the New York Heart Association's Functional and Therapeutic Classification may be used to help predict the appropriate activity tolerance level (see p. 231). The patient's condition can be classified according to the severity of symptoms elicited during activity and exercise.

The most feasible way in the clinical setting to assess a person's activity capabilities is to monitor continuously his or her response to activity. Assess vital signs before, immediately after, and 3 minutes after monitored activities to determine the person's tolerance level. Note other physical changes as well as any symptoms the patient reports.

Vital Signs. Vital signs indicate an ability to tolerate activity and a normal or abnormal response to activity.

Normal

- *Resting level:* Pulse 60–100 beats/minute; blood pressure < 140/90; respirations < 20 breaths/minute
- *Immediately after activity:* Pulse rate and strength increased; systolic blood pressure increased; respiratory rate and depth increased
- *Three minutes after activity:* Pulse rate within 6 beats/minute of resting pulse

Abnormal

- *Resting level:* Pulse > 100 beats/minute; blood pressure > 140/90; respirations > 20 breaths/minute
- *Immediately after activity:* Pulse rate and strength decreased, irregular pulse; systolic blood pressure decreased or unchanged; excessive increase or decrease in respiratory rate
- *Three minutes after activity:* Pulse rate greater than 7 beats/minute over resting rate

Physical and Cognitive Changes. The following changes may also indicate poor activity tolerance: pallor, diaphoresis, cyanosis, incoordination, ECG changes, and confusion.

Symptoms. Activity intolerance may be associated with the following symptoms: fatigue, weakness, exertional pain, dyspnea, dizziness, and vertigo.

Decreased Cardiac Output

Decreased cardiac output occurs when the amount of blood pumped from the heart has decreased, adversely affecting peripheral tissue perfusion. The person should also be evaluated for conditions associated with a potential for decreased cardiac output, such as dehydration or dysrhythmias.

Symptoms. A number of reactions are associated with low cardiac output, including fatigue, weakness, dyspnea, syncope, vertigo, and coughing. Poor gastrointestinal tract perfusion may contribute to anorexia or nausea and result in constipation. Brain hypoxia usually results in dizziness and disorientation, and sometimes in loss of consciousness.

Physical Examination Findings. Decreased cardiac output may result in a lowered blood pressure, because the blood pressure is a product of cardiac output and peripheral resistance. Consequently, the sympathetic nervous system is stimulated, resulting in vasoconstriction, tachycardia, and decreased peripheral perfusion. You may note cool, diaphoretic, and possibly cyanotic skin. Urine output usually declines because kidney perfusion is compromised. Peripheral pulses may be difficult to palpate or may be diminished.

If cardiac output decreases because of poor left ventricular pump function, the blood in the left side of the heart will eventually back up to the lungs, right side of the heart, and venous system. You may note crackles on lung auscultation, an increase in CVP (jugular vein distention), a gallop rhythm, and peripheral edema.

Altered Tissue Perfusion

Inadequate tissue perfusion may be chronic or acute. Persons with chronic alteration in tissue perfusion should be evaluated by a physician for possible pharmacologic or surgical treatment. *Chronic alteration in tissue perfusion* is also considered a nursing diagnosis because nurses may treat associated functional deficits such as confusion, inability to ambulate safely, and impaired skin integrity. Acute alterations in tissue perfusion, such as acute arterial occlusion from a thrombus or embolus, are life-threatening clinical problems and not usually considered nursing diagnoses.

Chronic Altered Cerebral Tissue Perfusion

A chronic decrease in the brain's arterial perfusion is most often associated with circulatory system dysfunction, for example,

- Low cardiac output states such as congestive heart failure; cardiac dysrhythmias; Stokes–Adams syndrome
- Vessel occlusion related to cerebral vessel atherosclerosis (especially at bifurcations of the vertebrals and carotids); subclavian steal syndrome (decreased brain blood supply secondary to left subclavian or innominate artery occlusion)
- Other hypotensive states such as orthostatic (postural) hypotension; carotid sinus syndrome

History. Vertigo (dizziness) is a common symptom indicating inadequate brain perfusion. The person may report "blacking out," episodes of confusion, memory or vision loss, or other neurologic deficits. Ask whether symptoms are associated with position changes or with other activities. Sudden head movements may aggravate symptoms in persons with carotid sinus syndrome; sudden changes in body positions are associated with orthostatic hypotension. Often a history of prolonged immobility or bed rest contributes to orthostatic hypotension. Persons with subclavian steal syndrome may report that arm exercise precedes vertigo (or syncope).

Physical Examination Findings. Possible changes in function may be noted that are consistent with the person's history, such as restlessness, confusion, and altered mentation. Bruits may be auscultated over the vertebral or carotid arteries, indicating partial occlusion from atherosclerotic plaque. The absence of bruits, however, does not always indicate normal vessels. Orthostatic hypotension is indicated by the following blood pressure changes when the person moves from sitting to standing or lying to sitting: a decrease in systolic blood pressure of greater than 20 mm Hg and a decrease in diastolic blood pressure of greater than 10 mm Hg. To compensate, the pulse rate may increase. A blood pressure difference of more than 10 mm Hg in both arms may indicate brachiocephalic artery atherosclerosis.

Chronic Altered Cardiopulmonary Tissue Perfusion

Cardiopulmonary tissue perfusion may be decreased in disease states such as congestive heart failure, myocardial infarction, angina pectoris, and pulmonary edema. Poor heart and lung perfusion is associated with dysrhythmias, especially tachycardia, cardiac chest pain, dyspnea, and tachypnea.

Chronic Altered Gastrointestinal Tissue Perfusion

Blood shunting from the gastrointestinal system may occur with prolonged stress or shock. Inadequate perfusion of gastrointestinal organs may also be associated with severe congestive heart failure. Gastrointestinal motility may be adversely affected, and the person may report related symptoms such as constipation, nausea, and vomiting.

Chronic Altered Renal Tissue Perfusion

A decrease in renal tissue perfusion may occur when the blood supply to renal arteries or arterioles is decreased, as may occur with hypovolemia, congestive heart failure, shock, or thrombosis. The person may be oliguric, anuric, or edematous, and may display other signs that indicate renal failure, such as azotemia.

Chronic Altered Peripheral Tissue Perfusion Related to Interruption of Arterial Flow

Arterial flow interruption may affect tissue perfusion in upper or lower extremities. The history, symptoms, and physical examination findings vary, depending on the exact aterial lesion site. During assessment, you may note the following common features:

Claudication. Intermittent claudication, a cramping, squeezing pain that occurs in the affected extremity during activity, may be the symptom that causes the person to seek health care.

Atrophic Skin Changes. Atrophic skin changes may be noted over the affected extremities, including a decrease in subcutaneous fat and muscle mass; thin, tight, shiny skin; lack of hair growth; and slow-growing, ridged, thick nails. Such changes result from lack of oxygen. In people with unilateral vessel occlusion, atrophic skin changes easily can be noted by comparing one limb to the other.

Cool Skin Temperature. In patients with arterial occlusion, the skin may be cool or cold secondary to a decreased blood supply to the skin.

Skin Color Changes. Evaluate skin color by having the person raise the affected extremity and noting any color changes. Extremities with arterial occlusion are usually pale when elevated because gravity further reduces the blood supply. As the person lowers the limb, you may note dependent rubor (redness) as the capillaries refill. Cyanosis may occur in advanced stages as more oxygen is extracted from hemoglobin to compensate for the decreased blood flow. Prolonged skin blanching (>3 sec) after pressure is applied and then released at the nail bed indicates slow capillary refill.

Skin Lesions. Skin lesions associated with severe arterial insufficiency include ulceration and necrosis (gangrene). Such lesions are most often noted in areas of trauma such as shins, feet, and toes. Wound healing may be delayed.

Pulses Not Palpable. Pulses distal to the occlusion site may not be palpable.

Bruits. Bruits may be auscultated if vascular narrowing of major arteries causes turbulent blood flow. If you sus-

pect arterial occlusion, listen over all major arteries where pulses are being palpated.

Chronic Altered Peripheral Tissue Perfusion Related to Interruption of Venous Flow

Chronic venous insufficiency most often affects the lower extremities. This condition develops slowly and occurs because the venous valves become incompetent and fail to close completely. As a result, venous pressure increases, leading to the following physiologic changes: accumulation of edema fluid in surrounding tissues secondary to high hydrostatic pressures; rupture of small venules; atrophy of skin and tissue from inability of oxygen to diffuse into high-pressure areas; and eventual necrosis from ischemia. Such alterations contribute to the following assessment findings:

Pain. Pain may or may not be present and may be less severe than arterial occlusion pain. The person may experience a dull, aching pain in the lower extremities after standing for prolonged periods, which contributes to higher venous pressures. Itching is a common symptom, especially around the ankles.

Skin Changes. The skin may be edematous, but edema may be somewhat relieved by leg elevation. Atrophic changes may accompany the edema. The temperature and color of the skin may be normal in affected extremities. However, skin color may reflect possible cyanosis when the extremity is maintained in a dependent position. A brownish color, resulting from stasis pigmentation, may be noted over the lower extremities. This occurs as small vessels rupture and the red blood cell pigment hemosiderin, along with melanin, stains the tissues brown.

Painless ulcerations may form at the internal malleolus because the poorly perfused tissue is susceptible to injury. Healed ulcers may appear as thin scars that easily break down again with minor trauma. Skin ulcers are easily infected. The limb may also be eczematous. Gangrene usually does not develop.

Obscured Pulses. Although often obscured by tissue edema, pulses are usually palpable.

Clinical Problems Related to Cardiovascular Assessment

Cardiovascular examination may reveal many clinical problems such as heart murmurs, pericardial friction rubs, bruits, hypertension, and cardiac dysrhythmias. Some of these findings represent chronic conditions that you should monitor for changes. If you detect any abnormal findings, consult the physician.

Acute Arterial Occlusion

Acute arterial occlusion represents a medical–surgical emergency, requiring prompt assessment and diagnosis. Occlusion may occur secondary to embolism or thrombosis; the clinical signs depend on the site of occlusion. Although the signs are similar to those which occur with chronic alterations in tissue perfusion related to interruption of arterial flow, the onset is more sudden and irreversible. If the occlusion occurs in an extremity, the following signs may be noted: pain (sudden or gradual in onset), numbness, tingling, coldness, absence of pulses distal to the occlusion, pallor or mottling, superficial vein collapse, limb weakness, and parathesias. Eventually, skin blebs and gangrenous necrosis may occur. Pain may not be present in all cases. The most reliable assessment finding is the absence of a previously palpated (or auscultated) pulse.

You should regularly check the peripheral pulses of patients at high risk, such as those with mitral valve stenosis, atrial fibrillation, and transmural myocardial infarction.

RESPIRATORY SYSTEM
Anatomy and Physiology Overview

The pulmonary components of the respiratory system begin with the nose, mouth, and sinuses. Air is inhaled through the nose, where it is warmed and filtered before it enters the trachea and bronchial passages and passes into the lungs. The trachea is lined with mucus-producing cells that trap foreign material and with cilia (fine hair-like projections) that sweep mucus upward through the airway. Mucus is also moved upward by the cough reflex, which is especially strong at the bifurcation, or carina, where the trachea branches into the right and left mainstem bronchi. The right mainstem bronchus is shorter, wider, and more vertically aligned than the left mainstem bronchus. The bronchi divide into secondary branches that enter the lungs at the hilum. The bronchi gradually narrow into bronchioles and lead into alveoli in the lungs.

The lungs are spongy, elastic structures that occupy the thorax. The outer lung surface is covered by the visceral pleura, which is separated from the parietal pleura lining the chest wall by a layer of fluid (the intrapleural space). The area between the right and left lungs is referred to as the mediastinum. A normally functioning respiratory system relies on intact neurologic and muscular systems.

THE NOSE AND SINUSES

The nose and sinuses may be examined during the routine examination of the head or when a patient reports problems with these areas. Common problems associated with the nose include trauma, obstruction, and irritation or drainage secondary to colds and allergies. The primary symptom of sinus problems is pain that may result from inflammatory processes. Obstruction and dental disease are the most common causes of sinus inflammation.

The primary functions of the nose include olfaction and warming, moisturizing, and filtering inspired air. Olfaction is evaluated by testing the first cranial (olfactory) nerve (see Chap. 11).

Inspired air is warmed and humidified by passing through the three *turbinates* (Fig. 10-10). The turbinates consist of bony projections on the lateral walls of each nasal cavity. Only the middle and inferior turbinates are visible during physical examination. Turbinates are lined with ciliated epithelial cells, a large vascular supply, and mucus-secreting glands. The sinuses drain into the nose via small openings in the turbinates. When the turbinates are edematous, as might occur with a common cold, these openings may become obstructed. As a result, fluid may collect in the sinuses and provide a medium for bacterial growth. Pressure from fluid buildup contributes to the pain of acute sinusitis.

The four paranasal sinuses of the skull include the sphenoid, ethmoid, frontal, and maxillary sinuses (Fig. 10-11). Only the frontal and maxillary sinuses are accessible for physical examination. The sinuses normally are air filled and have no known function in humans; they are believed to be vestigial. The sinuses are lined with mucus-secreting cells and drain into the nose.

THORACIC LANDMARKS

The lungs are enclosed in the thorax and surrounded by the ribs. The sternum serves as the anterior thoracic border, whereas the thoracic spine borders the thorax posteriorly. The diaphragm forms the "floor" of the chest cavity and sits higher on the right side than on the left side. The right lung has three lobes and is larger than the left lung, which has two lobes. The lower lobe of the left lung curves slightly around and under the heart.

Chest landmarks for locating the underlying structures include the suprasternal notch at the top of the sternum between the clavicles; the sternal angle (angle of Louis), which is a palpable, slight outward projection of the sternum; 12 thoracic vertebrae; and 12 pairs of ribs (Fig. 10-12). The sternal angle is the starting point for counting ribs and intercostal spaces. The intercostal spaces have numbers that correspond to the overlying ribs. Identifying the ribs by palpation is usually easier along the midclavicular line, as opposed to the sternal border where proximal sternal cartilages may interfere. Only the cartilages of the first seven ribs attach directly to the sternum. The costal margin refers to the proximal rib surface that slopes down and away from the sternum. The costal angle is formed by costal margin intersections.

Imaginary lines are also useful for determining lung field location and include the midsternal line, midspinal line, left and right midclavicular lines (vertical lines from the midpoint of each clavicle), left and right anterior axillary lines, left and right posterior axillary lines, and left and right midaxillary lines that progress vertically from the left and right axillae apex (Fig.10-13).

Anteriorly, the lung apices extend approximately 1.5 inches above the clavicles. Posteriorly, the apices extend to the first thoracic vertebra. The inferior lung borders extend from the sixth rib, midclavicular line, to the eighth rib, midaxillary line. Posteriorly, the lower lung borders are located at the tenth thoracic vertebra (T10) on expiration and at T12 on deep inspiration.

The approximate location of the fissures that divide the lungs into lobes may be determined by noting the following landmarks. Posteriorly, the lungs divide into upper and lower lobes at an angle stretching from the spinous process

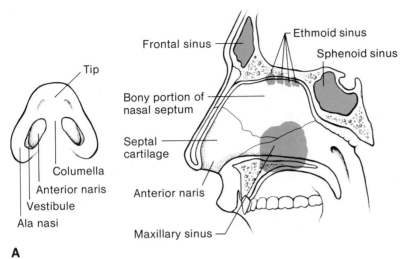

A

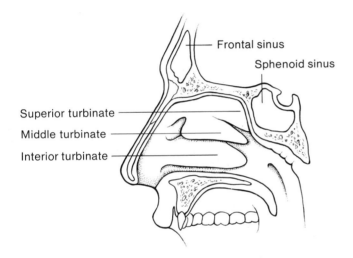

B

Figure 10–10. The nose and sinuses. (**A**) Cross-section of the nose. (**B**) Nasal turbinates.

Figure 10–11. The four paranasal sinuses of the skull.

Anterior

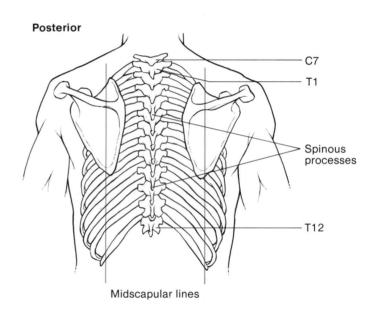

- Suprasternal notch
- First rib
- First intercostal space
- Angle of Louis
- Manubrium
- Xiphoid process
- Costal margin

Costal angle

Midclavicular lines

Figure 10–12. Landmarks of the anterior and posterior thorax.

Posterior

- C7
- T1
- Spinous processes
- T12

Midscapular lines

of T3 obliquely down and laterally. On the anterior surface, the lower lobes are divided from the upper lobes on the left, and from the upper and middle lobes on the right by bilateral imaginary lines extending medially and inferiorly from the fifth rib, midaxillary line, to the sixth rib, midclavicular line. On the right lateral chest surface, the right upper and right middle lobe division is located by a line drawn medially from the fifth rib, midaxillary line, to the fourth rib, midclavicular line.

VENTILATION MECHANICS

Inspiration and expiration occur as a result of pressure changes within the lungs. The inward pull of the lungs and the outward pull of the chest wall create a negative pressure that prevents the lungs from collapsing. During expi-

ration, when the lungs are at rest, lung pressure is equal to atmospheric pressure. During inspiration, the diaphragm contracts and moves downward. Then external intercostals pull the ribs up, and lung pressure becomes negative, allowing air to flow in. When the inspiratory muscles relax, lung pressure becomes positive, and air is expelled.

The diaphragm is the major muscle used during inspiration and is controlled by phrenic nerves from the third to the fifth cervical vertebrae. Accessory muscles, such as the trapezius muscles, scalenes, and sternocleoidmastoids, are used during extra inspiratory efforts; the abdominal muscles and internal intercostal muscles are used in extra expiratory efforts.

The compliance of the lungs and thorax also affects breathing and involves the ability of the lungs and thorax to expand and overcome their natural elastic recoil. Pressure is required to put a sufficient volume of air in the lungs

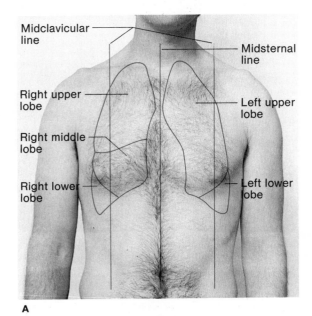

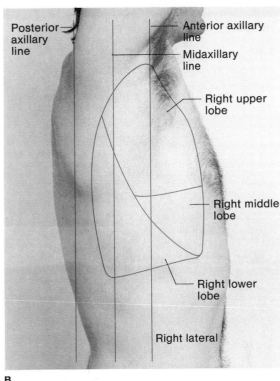

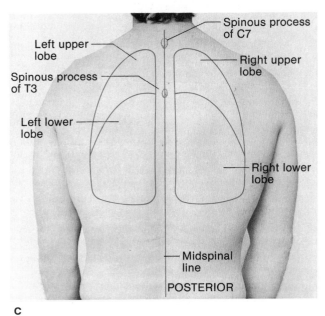

Figure 10–13. Reference lines for thoracic examination.

to overcome elastic recoil. Compliance is considered to be high or low depending on the pressure needed to expand the lungs. If the lung expands easily, for example, compliance is high, whereas if more pressure is needed to expand the lung, compliance is low, in which case the lung is called "stiff." Because of the surface tension in the fluid that lines the alveoli, these tiny air sacs tend to shrink. Surfactant, a phospholipid substance, is secreted by the alveoli to lower the surface tension. The decreased surface tension prevents alveolar collapse and reduces breathing efforts.

Respiratory muscle strength and compliance affect lung volumes, which vary with body size, age, and sex. The total lung capacity, or the amount of gas in the lungs after full inspiration, involves residual and tidal volumes and expir-

atory and inspiratory reserve volumes (see "Diagnostic Tests," Fig. 10-1).

- *Residual volume* is the amount of air remaining in the lungs after a maximal expiration.
- *Tidal volume* is the amount of gas inspired or expired during normal ventilation.
- *Expiratory reserve volume* is the amount of air that can be exhaled after a normal expiration.
- *Inspiratory reserve volume* is the amount of air that can be inspired above maximal inspiration.

The neurons of the respiratory center are located in the brain stem. The pons regulates the respiratory rhythm, and the medulla controls respiration rate and depth, which are affected by the carbon dioxide, hydrogen ion, and oxygen concentrations in the blood and body tissues.

In order for tissues to be oxygenated, the oxygen within the alveoli must be transported into the blood. Carbon dioxide and oxygen are exchanged across the alveolar–capillary membrane through the process of diffusion. The membrane has a large, thin surface area, approximately 1 μm thick, which allows gas to be diffused rapidly. Almost all of the oxygen in blood combines with hemoglobin in red blood cells. An adequate amount of hemoglobin is essential for tissue oxygenation. Carbon dioxide moves from the capillaries to the alveoli to be removed through respiration. While in the blood, carbon dioxide is transported in the form of bicarbonate.

Within the circulatory system, the right and left pulmonary arteries transport deoxygenated blood to the lungs from the right side of the heart and then branch into arterioles that lead into the alveolar–capillary network. The pulmonary veins transport oxygenated blood to the left side of the heart. The oxygenated blood is distributed throughout the body.

Physical Examination   *Respiratory System*

General Principles

The nose and sinuses are common sites for infection. Examine the nose and sinuses in persons with symptoms of upper respiratory infections, headaches, or breathing obstruction. The nose is inspected and palpated. The sinuses are inspected, using a light source for illumination, and palpated.

Inspection, palpation, percussion, and auscultation are used to assess the lungs and thorax. These techniques may be performed in the order cited, or they may be performed simultaneously, especially if abnormal findings are noted.

Equipment

Nasal speculum (optional)
Light source for transillumination of the sinuses
Stethoscope with diaphragm and bell

Positioning, Preparation, and Exposure

A quiet, warm room with adequate natural light is essential when examining the lungs and thorax. The person should assume a position that is comfortable and suitable and allows for easy examination of the anterior and posterior chest. If the person is short of breath, the head of the bed or examining table should be elevated. An equally comfortable position is to sit up and lean forward with arms supported on a table, especially if dyspnea is secondary to COPD. If such a position is impossible, the semi-Fowler's position can be used when the anterior chest is examined. This position allows the person to lean forward, supporting weight on the upper legs or on the side-rails (if confined to bed) while the posterior chest is examined. If the person's condition does not allow for any of these maneuvers, a side-lying position can be used to examine the posterior chest, and the supine position can be used to examine the anterior chest.

To reassure the person, explain the procedure as much as possible. Alleviating anxiety is important because apprehension could cause unnatural breathing. The person should undress to the waist; a woman should remove her bra. A loose-fitting examining gown may be used and a drape placed over the person to provide privacy.

Cues

Observing the person's general condition can provide important information about respiratory function. Alertness, level of consciousness, skin color, rate and depth of respirations, diaphoresis, nasal flaring, or breathing problems while speaking provide cues about respiratory function. Extreme agitation may indicate a low blood–oxygen level. During the general inspection, ask specific questions about the person's usual state of health and any signs of respiratory problems such as a cough, sputum production, fever, edema, fatigue, or shortness of breath. Also note any external sounds associated with breathing, such as wheezing, grunting, or grasping.

Examination and Documentation Focus (Nose)

- *Inspection:* Shape and configuration of external structures; position and integrity of nasal septum; color of the mucous membranes; color and swelling of the turbinates; discharge, lesions, masses, and foreign particles
- *Palpation:* Patency of the nares; displacement and tenderness along ridge and soft tissues

Examination and Documentation Focus (Sinuses)	• *Inspection:* Quality of transillumination • *Palpation:* Tenderness
Examination and Documentation Focus (Lungs and Thorax)	• *Inspection:* Trachea position, thoracic configuration and symmetry, ventilatory pattern, muscle movements, masses or lesions • *Palpation:* Symmetry of ventilatory movements, tactile fremitus, tenderness and masses, crepitus • *Percussion:* Percussion tones, diphragmatic excursion • *Auscultation:* Quality of breath sounds, voice transmission

Examination Guidelines   *Nose and Sinuses*

Procedure

1. INSPECT THE EXTERNAL NOSE.
   a. Note shape and configuration.

   b. Observe nares during ventilation.

   c. If nasal discharge is present, note the character (watery, purulent, mucoid), color, amount, and whether it is unilateral or bilateral.

2. EVALUATE NASAL PATENCY.
   Occlude the naris by placing your finger along one side of the nose. Ask the person to breathe in and out with the mouth closed. Repeat with the other naris.

3. INSPECT THE INTERNAL NOSE.
   a. Tip the person's head back and look through the nares to view the vestibule, septum, and inferior and middle turbinates. To enhance visualization of internal structures, place your thumb against the tip of the nose to move it. Hold a penlight in your other hand to illuminate the internal structures. A nasal speculum may facilitate inspection by dilating the outer naris, but such instruments are rarely recommended because they are invasive and may irritate tender tissue.

Clinical Significance

Normal Findings
The shape of the external nose varies greatly among people because of genetic differences and alterations secondary to trauma or cosmetic surgery.

Deviations from Normal
Deviations in the shape or configuration of the external nose generally are not significant unless indicative of recent trauma or associated with airway obstruction. Areas of recent swelling should be palpated for tenderness.

Deviations from Normal
Flaring of the nares indicates respiratory distress.

Deviations from Normal
Nasal discharge (rhinitis): Rhinitis has many causes, including the following:
1. Common cold—Clear, watery discharge of acute onset; associated findings include red, edematous nasal mucosa; purulent discharge may be noted after 3 to 5 days and represents secondary bacterial infection.
2. Allergies and hay fever—Clear, watery discharge that may be acute (hay fever) or chronic (allergic rhinitis); the nasal mucosa appears pale and edematous; allergic rhinitis may be accompanied by nasal polyps.
3. Cerebrospinal fluid rhinorrhea—Clear, watery discharge noted after facial trauma or basilar skull fractures; glucose-positive.
4. Sinusitis—Purulent discharge; usually unilateral following a cold; chronic sinusitis may result in unilateral or bilateral purulent discharge.
5. Foreign body—Unilateral purulent discharge.

Normal Findings
The nares should be patent. Normal nasal breathing should be quiet.

Deviations from Normal
Masses or foreign particles may interfere with airway patency.

Normal Findings and Deviations from Normal
Nasal septum: Deviation of the nasal septum is common. Severe deviation may interfere with patency. The septum should not be perforated.

Nares: The nares should be patent. Masses or foreign particles may interfere with airway patency.

Mucous membranes: The nasal mucosa is pink or dull red. A small amount of clear, watery discharge may be noted.

Turbinates: The turbinates should be nonedematous, without masses, and pink or dull red.

GUIDELINES *continued*   *Nose and Sinuses*

Procedure

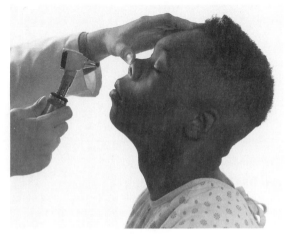

Inspecting the internal nose

   b. Note the color and condition of the nasal mucosa, the appearance of the turbinates, and the appearance of the nasal septum.

4. PALPATE THE SINUSES.

   a. Palpate the frontal sinuses. Press upwards from the eyebrows with your thumbs. Avoid pressing against the eye orbits.

   b. Palpate the maxillary sinuses with your thumbs or fingertips by pressing upward under the zygomatic processes (cheekbones).

Clinical Significance

Polyps: Polyps appear as small, penduncular masses and are associated with allergic rhinitis. Most polyps develop between the medial and inferior turbinates. Polyps may interfere with nasal patency and the sense of smell.

Epistaxsis (nasal bleeding): The nasal turbinates and mucosa have high vascularity. Therefore, epistaxis secondary to trauma or spontaneous rupture of blood vessels may be profuse. Epistaxsis may be associated with chronic sinusitis, nose picking, and cocaine abuse.

Deviations from Normal

Tenderness in response to palpation is associated with inflammation.

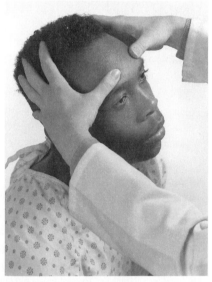

Palpating the frontal sinuses

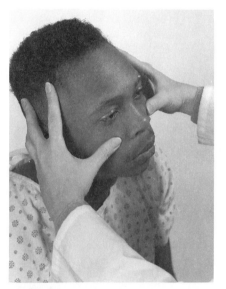

Palpating the maxillary sinuses

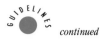

continued   **_Nose and Sinuses_**

Procedure

5. TRANSILLUMINATE THE SINUSES.

    If tenderness is elicited, transilluminate the sinuses to detect accumulation of fluid or masses.

    a. Transilluminate the frontal sinuses by pressing a bright light source (may use the otoscope light) firmly against the medial supraorbital rim. This procedure should be done in a completely darkened room.

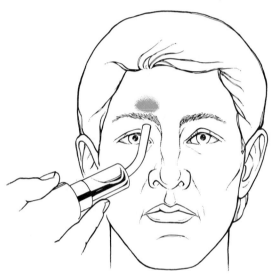

Transillumination of the frontal sinus

    b. Transilluminate the maxillary sinus by asking the person to tilt the head back and open the mouth. Press the light against the skin just below the medial aspect of the eye.

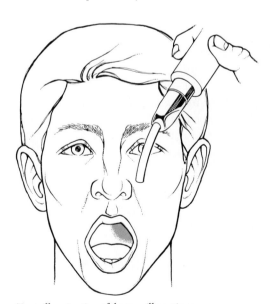

Transillumination of the maxillary sinus

Clinical Signficance

Normal Finding

A glow above the eye.

Deviation from Normal

No glow; may occur if the sinus is filled with fluid.

Normal Findings

A glow should be noted in the area of the hard palate.

Deviations from Normal

No glow.

Examination Guidelines   *Lungs and Thorax*

Procedure

1. INSPECT THE THORAX.

   a. Inspect the thorax with the person sitting upright and uncovered to the waist. Note the symmetry of the thorax, muscles used for ventilation, the ventilatory pattern, and skin condition. Proceed systematically, inspecting the anterior thorax and noting landmarks. Some landmarks are readily visible, particularly in a person with little body fat. Palpate to locate landmarks that you cannot see.

   b. Inspect the posterior thorax when you have completed all aspects of the anterior examination.

2. PALPATE THE THORAX.

   a. Use your fingertips to palpate the chest and intercostal spaces for tenderness, alignment, bulging, or retraction. As you palpate, note the amount of muscle mass over the chest wall. Palpate any masses or sinus tracts (rare, blind, tube-like structures opening onto the skin). Examine any reported tender areas last.

   b. To assess for crepitus, palpate with the fingertips, especially around any wound site or any tube that invades the chest, such as chest tubes or intravenous lines.

Clinical Significance

Normal Findings

Position of the trachea: The trachea should be located midline, without deviating to the left or right.

Thoracic configuration: In adults, the normal ratio of anteroposterior chest diameter to lateral chest diameter is approximately 1:2.

Chest movements: Each side of the chest should have equal upward and outward movement with inspiration. A downward movement of the diaphragm and an outward movement of the chest and abdomen should occur with each effective inspiration. The reverse should occur with expiration. Generally, women breathe with thoracic movement, whereas men and children usually breathe from the diaphragm (abdominally). In effective, normal breathing, accessory muscle use should not occur.

Deviations from Normal

Thoracic configuration: With aging, the dorsal curve of the thoracic spine may increase, resulting in an increased anteroposterior chest diameter. This "barrel chest" is a normal variant in older persons. An abnormal barrel chest may be noted in persons with COPD.

Impaired chest movements may occur with pain or abdominal distension. A paradoxical movement of the chest wall may be the result of fractured ribs.

Abnormal Ventilatory patterns: See Chapter 6, Display 6-1.

Masses and lesions: Masses or lesions in the neck or thorax are abnormal and require further investigation.

Normal Findings

The sternum, costal cartilages, ribs, intercostal spaces, and spine should not be tender on palpation. Muscles are palpable and should feel firm, smooth, and symmetrical.

Deviations from Normal

Palpable masses are abnormal.

Deviations from Normal

Crepitus, or crepitation, is a crackling sound produced when subcutaneous tissue containing air is palpated. Crepitus is an abnormal finding.

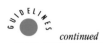

continued

Lungs and Thorax

Procedure

c. Evaluate tactile fremitus. Fremitus is vibration of the chest wall produced by vocalization. Ask the person to say "one, two, three" or "ninety-nine" while you palpate the thorax from left to right and then from right to left, using the heel or ulnar surface of your hand to detect vibrations. Usually, palpating with one hand works best to assess tactile fremitus, although both hands may be used to compare the left and right sides of the thorax. When evaluating the posterior chest, ask the person to fold the arms across the chest to move the scapulae partially out of the way.

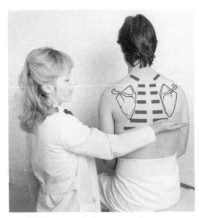

Evaluating tactile fremitus: Ulnar surface of hand

Clinical Significance

Always make comparisons between left and right sides.

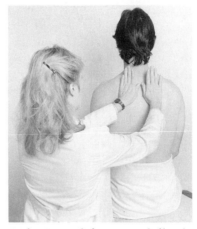

Evaluating tactile fremitus: Heel of hand

Normal Findings

Tactile fremitus: When the person speaks, tactile fremitus, a palpable vibration, should be felt on the chest wall. Fremitus is usually most noticeable where the trachea branches into the right and left mainstem bronchi in the upper chest near the sternal border. Fremitus is usually decreased or absent over the precordium.

Deviations from Normal

Increased tactile fremitus is associated with conditions favoring sound transmission in the chest, such as pneumonia with consolidation, atelectasis (with open bronchus), lung tumors, pulmonary infarction, and pulmonary fibrosis.

Decreased tactile fremitus is associated with conditions that interfere with sound transmission through the chest, such as pleural effusions, pleural thickening, pneumothorax with lung collapse, bronchial obstruction, tumors or masses in the pleural space, and emphysema.

3. EVALUATE THE CHEST EXPANSION

a. *Anterior approach:* To evaluate chest expansion anteriorly, place your hands over the anterolateral chest with thumbs extended along the costal margin, pointing to the xiphoid process. Ask the person to breathe deeply and note the movement of your hands.

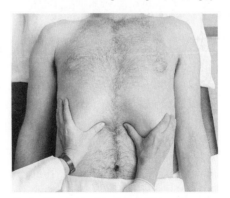

Evaluating chest expansion: Anterior approach

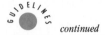
continued

Lungs and Thorax

Procedure

b. *Posterior approach:* To evaluate chest expansion posteriorly, place your hands on the posterolateral chest with your thumbs at the level of the tenth rib. Ask the person to breathe deeply and note the movement of your hands.

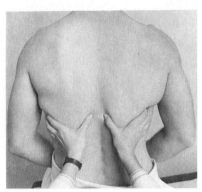

Evaluating chest expansion: Posterior approach

4. PERCUSS THE THORAX.

 a. Evaluate percussion tone over lung fields.

   Percuss the thorax from the apices to the bases, moving from the anterior surface to the lateral areas, and then to the posterior surface.

   Always compare findings between right and left sides of the thorax.

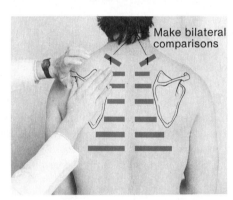

Make bilateral comparisons

Thoracic percussion

When evaluating the posterior chest, ask the person to fold the arms across the chest to move the scapulae partially out of the way.

 b. Percuss to determine diaphragmatic excursion. Locate the upper edge of the diaphragm by noting where the normal lung resonance changes to dullness when percussing the posterior thorax.

   Locate this point on the person's skin when the person is holding a deep breath and mark it. Then, locate this point on the person's skin following a deep exhalation and mark it. The difference between marks is the diaphragmatic excursion.

Clinical Significance

Normal Findings
Your thumbs should move an equal distance apart on each side as the person takes a deep breath.

Deviations from Normal
A lag in thoracic movement may indicate underlying lung or pleura disease.

Use percussion to determine boundaries of organs and to detect the relative amounts of air, fluid, and solid material within the underlying lung.

Normal Findings
Normal percussion tone: In adults, the lungs emit a resonant tone when percussed. Children's lungs are normally hyperresonant.

Deviations from Normal
Hyperresonance: A hyperresonant or tympanic note is produced when air accumulates in the lungs or pleural cavity. Examples: emphysema, pneumothorax.

Dullness: A dull or flat percussion tone is produced by vibrations from solid masses or fluid in the lungs. Examples: pneumonia, atelectasis, masses, pleural effusion, and hemothorax.

Normal Findings
The diaphragmatic excursion is the distance between the levels of dullness with deep inspiration and full expiration, and normally ranges from 3 to 6 cm. The diaphragm should be slightly higher on the right side.

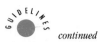

Lungs and Thorax

Procedure

5. AUSCULTATE THE LUNGS.

  a. Auscultate breath sounds.

When auscultating the lungs, mentally picture the lung segment located beneath the thoracic landmarks. To locate the lobes of the lungs, palpate thoracic landmarks. With the person in a lateral position, palpate the free-floating ribs or costal margins, and count four intercostal spaces upward to locate lower lung borders. Remember that when the person is supine, organs are displaced and lung expansion is altered.

Use the diaphragm of the stethoscope to auscultate the lungs. Ask the person to sit up, if possible, and to breathe slightly slower and deeper than normal, with the mouth open. Auscultate the anterior, posterior, and lateral lung fields. Listen to at least one full inspiration and expiration in each location that you auscultate.

Observe the client for dizziness and lightheadedness, which may indicate hyperventilation. If hyperventilation does occur, allow the client to rest.

Systematically listen to the chest, beginning with the apices and moving down to the bases in a zigzag, side-to-side manner. Compare one side with the other.

If the patient is unable to sit, auscultate the posterior and lateral lung fields while the person lies on first one side and then the other. Compare the findings from both sides.

Avoid misleading noises by placing the stethoscope firmly on uncovered skin. In addition, prevent the stethoscope or the person from moving during auscultation. To prevent extraneous sounds caused by the stethoscope moving over hair, dampen chest hair with a washcloth.

Clinical Significance

Auscultating the lungs helps to evaluate air flow as well as identify normal and abnormal breath sounds.

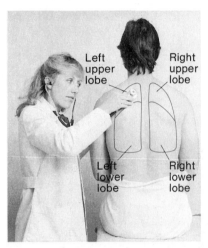

Lung auscultation

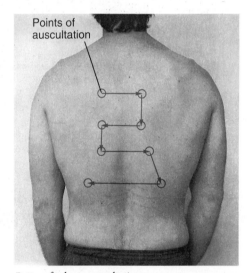

Pattern for lung auscultation

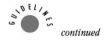
continued

Lungs and Thorax

Procedure

b. Note the quality of the breath sounds.

If you hear any abnormal breath sounds, note their location and where they occur in the ventilatory cycle. Ask the person to cough after the initial auscultation and note changes in adventitious sounds. If the person has complained of difficulty breathing, but you heard no abnormal sounds initially, check for adventitious sounds again after the person coughs.

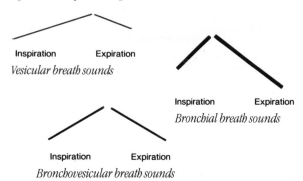

Clinical Significance

Normal Findings

Normal breath sounds: Normal breath sounds may vary according to the area auscultated. *Vesicular breath sounds* are low-pitched, soft, breezy sounds that can be heard over the lung fields of the anterior, posterior, and lateral chest. These sounds are usually longer and louder during inspiration than during expiration. *Bronchial breath sounds* are loud, high-pitched, and hollow and are a normal finding over the trachea. The inspiratory phase is shorter than the expiratory phase. *Bronchovesicular breath sounds* are found in the mainstem bronchi area and are heard anteriorly in the first and second intercostal spaces and between the scapulae posteriorly. The inspiratory and expiratory phases of bronchovesicular sounds are equal. They have a soft, breezy quality and are lower-pitched than bronchial sounds, but higher-pitched than vesicular sounds.

Deviations from Normal

See Display, "Abnormal (Adventitious) Breath Sounds."

Abnormal (Adventitious) Breath Sounds

Crackles

Crackles (formerly called rales) are soft, high-pitched, discontinuous popping sounds that occur during inspiration. The sounds are timed in relation to inspiration.

Crackles occur secondary to fluid in the airways or alveoli, or to opening of collapsed alveoli. Crackles in late inspiration are associated with restrictive pulmonary disease. Crackles in early inspiration are associated with obstructive pulmonary disease. *Fine crackles* in early inspiration are caused by small airway closure. *Coarse crackles* in early inspiration are associated with bronchitis or pneumonia.

Wheezes

Sonorous wheezes (formerly called rhonchi) are deep, low-pitched, rumbling sounds that are heard primarily during expiration and caused by air moving through narrowed tracheobronchial passages. Narrowing may be caused by secretions or tumor.

Sibilant wheezes (formerly called wheezes) are continuous, musical, high-pitched, whistle-like sounds that are heard during inspiration and expiration. They are caused by narrowed bronchioles and are associated with bronchospasm, asthma, and buildup of secretions.

Pleural Friction Rub

A *pleural friction rub* is a harsh crackling sound like two pieces of leather being rubbed together, and may be heard during inspiration alone or during both inspiration and expiration. This sound may disappear when the breath is held.

Pleural friction rubs are secondary to inflammation and loss of lubricating pleural fluid.

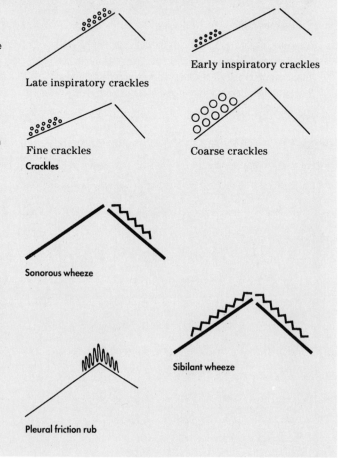

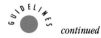 *continued*

Lungs and Thorax

Procedure

c. Auscultate for voice transmission.

Listening for voice transmission is an adjunctive technique used when abnormalities are found during inspection, palpation, percussion, or auscultation. Ask the person to say "one, two, three" or "ninety-nine," and auscultate the lung fields. To assess for egophony, ask the person to say "ee-ee-ee."

Clinical Significance

Normal Findings and Deviations from Normal

Normally, the sounds are muffled, but if the voice is transmitted loudly and clearly, lung tissue consolidation may be indicated. *Bronchophony* (loud, distinct voice transmission), *whispered pectoriloquy* (clear transmission of whispered sounds), and *egophony* (/e/ to /a/ change in sound) are normally heard over large airways (bronchi) and associated with abnormal conditions, including consolidation and pleural effusions.

Documenting Respiratory Examination Findings

Nose and Sinus Examination Findings

Example 1: Normal Nose and Sinus

Examination findings were normal and were recorded as follows:

> External bony structures of the nose without deformity. Nares both patent. Nasal septum midline. Nasal mucosa and turbinates pink, moist and without discharge or masses. Frontal and maxillary sinuses nontender.

Example 2: Upper Respiratory Infection

Examination findings were abnormal and were recorded as follows:

> Nares not patent, mouth breathing required. Copious, bilateral white discharge from nares. Nasal mucosa and turbinates swollen and bright red. Frontal sinuses nontender. Maxillary sinuses tender bilaterally. Unable to transilluminate maxillary sinuses.

Lung and Thorax Examination Findings

Example 1: Normal Thorax

Ms. S, aged 22, had a thorax examination as part of a routine annual health assessment. The examination results were normal and were recorded as follows:

> Trachea midline; AP to lateral chest diameter 1:2. Chest movements symmetric. Ventilation unlabored without accessory muscle use. RR 16 breaths/minute. No visible or palpable masses. Lungs sound clear to percussion and auscultation. Fremitus not evaluated.

These findings may be recorded in a problem-oriented record as follows:

S: Reports no cough, dyspnea, or chest discomfort; nonsmoker
O: Trachea midline; AP to lateral chest diameter 1:2. Chest movements symmetric. Ventilation unlabored without accessory muscle use. RR 16 breaths/minute. No visible or palpable masses. Lungs sound clear to percussion and auscultation. Fremitus not evaluated.
A: No abnormalities detected on thoracic exam
P: Routine follow-up examinations as indicated

Example 2: Suspected Pneumonia

Mr. J, aged 42, reports an acute onset of fever, chills, and a cough productive of red-brown sputum. Previously, he had a "cold" with a nonproductive cough. The physical examination findings for the thorax were abnormal and were recorded as follows.

> RR 20–24 breaths/minute; ventilation unlabored. Dullness percussed over right lower lobe; crackles heard over RLL; chest otherwise clear to A & P.

These findings may be recorded in a problem-oriented record as follows:

S: Reports fever and chills for last 24 hours. States he has a "cold" that started 3 days ago. In last 24 hours, developed cough productive of thick, red-brown sputum, "about a teaspoon" each time cough is productive.
O: Temp: 104°F. RR 20–24 breaths/minute; ventilation unlabored. Dullness percussed over RLL; crackles heard over RLL; chest otherwise clear to A & P.
A: Suspect pneumonia, possibly pneumococcal, on basis of sputum color and symptoms.
P: Refer to physician. Assist with ongoing diagnostic procedures: Obtain sputum sample for C & S; chest x-ray.

NDx

Nursing Diagnoses Related to Respiratory Assessment

Impaired Gas Exchange

Impaired gas exchange (IGE) involves an actual or potential decrease in the passage of gases (oxygen and carbon dioxide) between the alveoli in the lungs and the vascular system. Impaired gas exchange is characterized by a decreased PO_2, decreased hemoglobin saturation, or an increased PCO_2, as determined by arterial blood gas testing. Hypoxia, an inadequate tissue oxygen supply, and respiratory acidosis may accompany IGE.

History. Gas exchange across the aveolar–capillary membrane may be impaired under the following circumstances:

- Gas diffusion is blocked by secretions or fluid, such as those caused by mucus accumulation, inflammatory or infectious processes, or pulmonary edema.
- Loss of lung surface for gas diffusion, which occurs in cases of atelectasis, emphysema, tumor, and lobectomy
- Loss of lung elasticity and compliance, which occurs in cases of COPD and adult respiratory distress syndrome (ARDS)

In addition, extrapulmonary factors, such as pain, anxiety, and central nervous system depression, may affect pulmonary gas exchange.

To avoid inspiratory pain, which often occurs after chest or abdominal surgery, a patient may hypoventilate. As a result, secretions accumulate and atelectasis may occur. People with IGE may report feeling short of breath, fatigued, or disoriented.

Physical Examination Findings. Characteristic signs that indicate hypoxia, such as restlessness and dyspnea, may be noted with IGE. Initially, blood pressure, heart rate, and cardiac output may increase to compensate for the low PO_2. With increasing hypoxia, changes in mental status may occur, resulting in reduced responsiveness, drowsiness, and confusion as the pH drops and acidosis occurs. The respiratory rate increases initially, then becomes slow and shallow as the consciousness level decreases.

Hypoxia causes the skin to become diaphoretic and cooler as cardiac output decreases. Skin color and nail beds become dusky blue-gray to cyanotic (blue to purple). In people with dark skin, especially blacks, the mucous membranes in the mouth are a better indicator of tissue oxygenation. Observable signs that indicate dyspnea with IGE include an intolerance to lying flat. The person usually prefers to sit up with hands on the knees, or lean over a table. You will note an increased respiratory rate or increased respiratory effort with activity. Chronic IGE with carbon dioxide retention is associated with an increased anteroposterior chest diameter (barrel chest).

Ineffective Airway Clearance

The diagnosis of Ineffective airway clearance (IAC) is closely related to that of IGE because the former will eventually lead to the latter. Ineffective airway clearance occurs when partial or complete airway obstruction threatens to prevent air passing through the respiratory tract.

History. Ineffective airway clearance occurs in the same situations as IGE. Acute problems with airway clearance may be caused by improper positioning, edema of the upper airway structures, and mechanical obstruction such as choking.

Physical Examination Findings. Signs of ineffective airway clearance include a weak, ineffective cough; an abnormal respiratory rate, rhythm, or depth; dyspnea; wheezing; crackles; abnormal or decreased breath sounds; inability to remove secretions; and asymmetric chest expansion. A person with thick, sticky sputum, for example, may have difficulty removing the secretions because of an ineffective cough, resulting in increased breathing and changed respiratory rate or rhythm. Airway secretions may also produce

adventitious breath sounds. The factors mentioned under IAC could also contribute to IGE.

Ineffective Breathing Pattern

Ineffective breathing patterns occur from a loss of ventilatory function. Either hypoventilation or hyperventilation may accompany dyspnea. Hypoventilation decreases carbon dioxide exchange, which can cause respiratory acidosis. Hyperventilation increases carbon dioxide exchange, which can lead to respiratory alkalosis. Any chest pain that accompanies breathing difficulty will alter the breathing pattern. In turn, an ineffective breathing pattern may lead to IAC. Diagnosing Ineffective breathing pattern may be accomplished by observing any use of accessory muscles of respiration; shortness of breath, irregular respirations; hyperventilation; shallow, guarded, or rapid respirations; or difficulty breathing when not in an upright sitting or standing position.

Clinical Problems Related to Respiratory Assessment

Altered Elasticity and Compliance

Conditions that alter the lung's elasticity and compliance include COPD and ARDS. Chronic obstructive pulmonary diseases include asthma, chronic bronchitis, and emphysema. Wheezing, dyspnea, and a prolonged expiration phase are observable signs that indicate an asthmatic attack.

The patient with emphysema may appear as a "pink puffer," with a pink or flushed skin tone. The classic barrel chest is present, and the patient may be underweight and dyspneic. Emphysema involves decreased elastic recoil with increased lung compliance that causes air to be trapped in the alveoli.

Adult respiratory distress syndrome is diagnosed by chest radiograph and arterial blood gas analysis. Hypoxemia, which is refractory to oxygen therapy, indicates ARDS. Other signs include dyspnea, increased respiratory rate, tachycardia, and restlessness. A dry cough may be present. Rusty, frothy sputum that turns dark red may appear later in the disease process. Lung compliance is reduced in ARDS.

Inflammatory and Infectious Processes

Pneumonia is an inflammatory process, often having an infectious component. The patient may report chills, shortness of breath, pleuritic chest pain, fever, hemoptysis, and a cough that produces purulent sputum. Chest assessment may reveal crackles, wheezes, decreased breath sounds, and dullness on percussion. The diagnosis is confirmed through chest radiograph, blood cultures, sputum analysis, leukocyte counts, and arterial blood gas results.

Bronchitis may be acute or chronic. The person with chronic bronchitis is typically cyanotic and edematous, appearing as a "blue bloater." Dyspnea, wheezing, coarse crackles, and a chronic cough with sputum production are characteristics of chronic bronchitis.

Lung tuberculosis causes a cough that also produces purulent sputum, sometimes with traces of blood (hemoptysis). Fever and weight loss may also be noted. However, the patient may also be asymptomatic. The diagnosis is determined by chest x-ray findings, sputum culture, and a positive tuberculin test result.

A *lung abscess* may also cause fever and weight loss. Dyspnea, pleuritic chest pain, and a cough producing much bloody, purulent sputum may also occur.

Empyema (purulent material in a pleural space) may occur as a complication of respiratory infection, chest trauma, or surgery. Empyema produces shortness of breath, pleuritic chest pain, and fever.

Chest Trauma and Disease Alterations

Chest trauma or disease processes can cause anatomic and mechanical alterations in the lungs and thereby affect respiratory function. For example, blunt chest trauma may cause injuries, such as pneumothorax, tension pneumothorax, or flail chest. Penetrating trauma can cause a hemothorax (blood in the pleural space) or hemopneumothorax (blood and air in the pleural space).

Physical findings associated with a *pneumothorax* include limited respiratory excursion on the affected side and decreased or absent breath sounds. Crepitus may be present. Apprehension, dyspnea, and pleuritic chest pain may occur with a pneumothorax, which may be caused by a spontaneous or traumatic rupture of a lung bleb.

A *tension pneumothorax* may cause severe dyspnea and severe pleuritic chest pain. The trachea deviates toward the unaffected side, and the affected side reveals limited respiratory excursion and absent breath sounds. Cyanosis and shock may also be present.

A *flail chest* results from multiple rib fractures. The chest wall becomes unstable, resulting in inadequate respiratory exchange. Paradoxic chest wall movement may be noted. When the uninjured chest areas expand, the injured portion depresses. The injured area "flails out" during expiration. Only minimal air movement will be noted. The person will probably be dyspneic and cyanotic.

A *bronchial tumor* typically causes a cough. Dyspnea or chest pain may occur, with either pleuritic or dull discomfort. Other signs include tracheal deviation toward the normal side, absent breath sounds, and a dull or flat percussion note over the tumor area if the tumor is large. The person may be asymptomatic until the tumor has advanced into the pleura and chest wall or until distant metastases appear.

Pulmonary emboli are caused by venous thrombi fragments detaching and migrating to the lungs, or they may be caused by fat emboli associated with long-bone fractures. Pulmonary alterations vary with the size of the embolus. When an embolus occludes a pulmonary artery, alveoli are ventilated, but not perfused. Dyspnea is common. Tachypnea and tachycardia may also be present. Often the patient feels anxious and restless, but does not know why. If partial lung infarction occurs, pleuritic chest pain and hemoptysis may result. A massive pulmonary embolus usually causes sudden shock, cyanosis, respiratory distress and tachypnea, confusion, and anxiety. If the patient has a long-bone fracture or has had orthopedic surgery and then develops dyspnea, tachycardia, and a high fever, you should suspect a fat embolus. Petechiae usually appear over the thorax and upper extremities. Arterial blood gas analysis, chest radiograph, and ventilation–perfusion lung scan are commonly used to diagnose pulmonary emboli.

Pulmonary edema may occur gradually or suddenly. An initially dry cough usually progresses to a cough that produces pink, frothy sputum. Paroxysmal nocturnal dyspnea and orthopnea are present with gradual onset. Peripheral edema may be noted in the feet and ankles. Acute pulmonary edema causes dyspnea, tachypnea, and tachycardia. The patient's skin is cool, clammy, and cyanotic. Moreover, the person is usually apprehensive and must have the head elevated or sit up in order to breathe. Dry crackles may be heard first at the lung bases, progressing to wheezing, moist, bubbling adventitious sounds throughout the chest. Chest radiograph usually verifies pulmonary edema. Acute pulmonary edema is an emergency that requires immediate medical intervention.

Aspirating a solid object causes a cough, dyspnea, and wheezing. Respiratory distress, cyanosis, and the inability to speak indicate that an object is lodged in the airway. Aspirating materials such as water, gastric acid, or nasogastric tube feedings may cause an inflammatory reaction with decreased surfactant production and a resultant decreased lung compliance. Patients especially at risk for aspiration are those with a decreased level of consciousness and those without intact airway protective mechanisms.

Inhalation injuries result from smoke inhalation, thermal burns, or carbon monoxide poisoning. If the exposure is severe enough, mucous membrane edema and bronchospasms occur. Coughing, wheezing, dyspnea, and cyanosis are noted. Headache and depressed mentation may also be present, especially with carbon monoxide poisoning.

MUSCULOSKELETAL SYSTEM

Anatomy and Physiology Overview

The musculoskeletal system includes bones, muscles, and joints as well as supporting structures such as tendons, ligaments, cartilage, bursae, and fasciae. Bones provide support and levers for movement; joints act as fulcrums for the levers; and muscles provide the force to move bones around the joints.

BONES

The human skeleton is composed of 206 bones, 80 of which make up the axial skeleton, including the skull bones, vertebral column, sternum, and ribs. The 126 bones of the appendicular skeleton include the bones of the upper and lower extremities. Bones are further classified according to shape at maturity:

- *Flat bones* function mainly to protect the body, and include skull bones, ribs, sternum, scapulae, and pelvis. Flat bones cannot function as levers and therefore do not directly contribute to body movement.

- *Long bones* function as levers during movement and include the femur, tibia, fibula, phalanges, humerus, ulna, and radius.
- *Short bones* provide strength during movement and include the carpals and tarsals.
- *Irregular bones* include all other bones. The bones of the vertebrae are classified as irregular and have important functions for protection and mobility. Irregular bones of the face contribute to movements necessary for eating and facial expressions.

Bones and associated processes (enlargements or protrusions) often serve as landmarks during physical assessment.

Bone Processes

- *Crest:* A ridge or linear process, such as the iliac crest
- *Condyle:* A rounded process forming a joint surface, such as the knuckle
- *Head:* A rounded end of a bone separated from the main body of the bone by a constricted neck, such as the femoral head
- *Spine:* A pointed, slender process, such as the vertebral spines
- *Trochanter:* A large, rounded process for muscle attachment, such as below the head of the femur

- *Tubercle:* A small, rounded process, such as the tubercle on the clavicle, where the deltoid muscle attaches
- *Tuberosity:* A large, rounded process, but smaller than a trochanter, such as the ulnar tuberosity

Bone Formation. Bone formation is a complex, ongoing physiologic phenomenon. Ideally, an equilibrium exists between bone formation (deposition) and bone loss (resorption). Numerous factors may disrupt this equilibrium in persons with bone deformities or histories of spontaneous pathologic fractures, which are associated with high rates of bone resorption (Display 10-1). People on long-term bed rest are at higher risk for disproportionate bone loss because they do not perform activities that use long bones. Bone deformities are also attributed to hereditary disorders.

JOINTS

The joints, or articulations, are composed of tissues associated with the articulating bone surfaces. Body movements are impossible without joints, which are classified according to the degree of mobility:

- *Synarthroses* are immoveable joints, such as the fused suture lines noted on mature skulls.
- *Amphiarthroses* are joints with restricted movement, such as the pubic symphysis.

Display 10–1
Factors That Influence Bone Deposition and Resorption

Increased Bone Deposition
- Exercise, bone stress
- Growth hormone
- Fluoride*

Increased Bone Resorption
- Parathyroid hormone excess
- Vitamin D hormone[†]
- Adrenocortical steroid excess
- Calcium deficiency (dietary or malabsorption)
- Phosphorus deficiency (dietary, malabsorption, renal loss)
- Anabolic steroid deficiency (androgen, estrogen)
- Immobilization
- Acidosis
- Pregnancy and lactation
- Osteolytic neoplasms (including leukemia)
- Prostaglandins

Decreased Bone Deposition
- Immobilization, disuse, bed rest
- Growth hormone deficiency
- Adrenocortical steroid excess

Decreased Bone Resorption
- Calcium
- Phosphorus
- Parathyroid hormone deficiency
- Calcitonin
- Magnesium deficiency
- Anabolic steroids
- Alkalosis
- Mithramycin
- Diphosphates

*Excessive fluoride causes uncalcified osteoid deposition and produces osteomalacia.
[†] Osteolytic effect of parathyroid hormone requires vitamin D hormone.

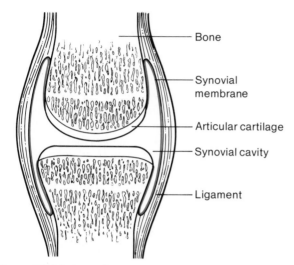

Figure 10–14. Synovial joint structure.

Bone

Synovial membrane

Articular cartilage

Synovial cavity

Ligament

• *Diarthroses,* or *synovial joints,* are freely moveable joints such as the shoulder, elbow, hip, and knee.

Physical examination should be focused on these joints.

Synovial Joints. In addition to the articulating bone surfaces, the joint is composed of a joint capsule, ligaments, muscle, and tendons (Fig. 10-14), and in some cases bursae or menisci. The *joint capsule* is a sac-like structure between bones bordered by the articular cartilage and surrounding ligaments. The outer layer of the joint capsule is fibrous; the inner, synovial layer secretes synovial fluid, which lubricates the joint and prevents friction during movement. *Ligaments, muscles,* and *tendons* provide joint stability. *Bursae,* pad-like structures that provide protection from friction, are located between moving surfaces such as bones, tendons, and ligaments. Bursae are associated with shoulder, elbow, hip, knee, and heel joints. *Menisci,* crescent-shaped pieces of cartilage, may be found between articulating surfaces of some joints, such as the knee and shoulder.

Synovial joints are classified according to the degree of movement:

• *Ball and socket joints* are most freely moveable and are created when the head of one bone fits into the concave surface of another bone; examples include the hip and shoulder.
• *Condyloid joints,* such as the wrist, move freely except for axial rotation. They are created by oval and elliptical bone surface articulation.
• *Hinge joints,* such as the elbow, interphalangeal joints, and knee, permit only forward and backward movements and are created by concave and convex bone articulation.
• *Pivot joints* permit bone rotation; examples include the atlas and axis joints of the head and the elbow.
• *Saddle joints,* such as the carpometacarpal joint of the thumb, are created when two bones with concave and convex surfaces articulate, joining in a reciprocal manner.
• *Gliding joints* permit sliding movements in all directions and occur when two bones with flat articulating

surfaces meet. The intervertebral joints and the carpal bones of the wrist are classified as gliding joints.

Intervertebral Joints. The moveable joints of the vertebral column do not have synovial fluid in the joint capsules between the articular surfaces as do other synovial joints. Intervertebral joints contain fibrocartilaginous discs with central, flexible cores (the nucleus pulposus) that function as shock absorbers between bones.

Joint Movements. Joints vary in the types of movement they can accommodate. During physical examination, joint movement or range of motion is evaluated for a particular joint:

• *Abduction:* Movement away from the midline of the body, such as raising an arm to the side or spreading fingers apart
• *Adduction:* Movement toward the midline of the body, such as lowering an arm
• *Flexion:* Bending at a joint, such as the hip, to create a lesser angle between two bones (sitting)
• *Extension:* Straightening a joint, such as the hip, to create an angle at or near 180 degrees between two bones (standing)
• *Hyperextension:* Extending a body part beyond anatomic position, such as tipping the head backward
• *Eversion:* Turning a body part outward, such as moving the foot at the ankle joint so that the sole faces outward
• *Inversion:* Turning a body part inward, such as moving the foot at the ankle joint so that the sole faces inward
• *Pronation:* Rotating the forearm so that the palm faces downward
• *Supination:* Rotating the forearm so that the palm faces upward
• *Rotation:* Turning a bone around an axis, such as moving the head from side to side
• *Circumduction:* Moving a limb to create a cone shape, with the joint forming the apex of the cone and the distal part of the limb tracing a complete circle
• *Protraction:* Moving a bone forward on a plane parallel to the ground, such as moving the lower jaw forward
• *Retraction:* Moving a bone backward on a plane parallel to the ground

Processes that may restrict normal joint movement include pain, muscle spasm, intervertebral disc herniation, fibrosis (contracture), and bony fixation.

Muscles. The skeletal or striated muscles provide force to move bones around the joints. They can be easily assessed during physical examination because the person can control contractions and relaxations. You should inspect and palpate skeletal muscles during the physical examination.

The microscopic fibers in a single muscle together form a large, central muscle body and are attached to bones either directly, by tendons (cord-like connective tissue), or by aponeuroses, which are broad, flat sheets of connective tissue. The distal end of the muscle is called the insertion and attaches to the bone being moved by the muscle's contraction. The proximal end of the muscle is the origin and attaches to the bone that is held stationary during movement.

Muscle Action. In response to neurologic stimulus, the muscle shortens in length, or contracts. As the muscle relaxes, it elongates. Movement is based on bone movements created by muscle contraction across a joint. Muscles are named in a manner that describes some feature associated with the muscle, such as the movement that is produced by the muscle, the orientation of the muscle fibers, the location of the muscle, the number of origins at the proximal end of the muscle, the shape of the muscle, or the point of attachment:

- *Muscles named for joint movement created by the muscle contraction:* Flexor hallucis brevis (flexes great toe); extensor carpi ulnaris (extends wrist); abductor digiti (abduct fingers); adductor magnus (adducts thigh); rotatores spinae (rotate vertebral column)
- *Muscles named for orientation of the muscle fibers:* Transverse thoracic (narrows the chest); oblique external abdominal (contracts abdomen)
- *Muscles named for their location:* Intercostals (draw ribs together)
- *Muscles named for the number of origins at the proximal end:* Biceps (flexes arm); triceps (extends forearm)
- *Muscles named for shape:* Trapezius (draws head back and to the side)

- *Muscles named for the point of attachment:* Sternocleidomastoid (rotates the head)

Signs of Muscle Dysfunction. Muscle dysfunction can result from a number of factors, including fluid and electrolyte depletion, overuse or disuse, malnutrition, and altered innervation. Clinical signs and symptoms that indicate muscle dysfunction include cramps, muscle strain, muscle atrophy, fasciculations, and tetany.

Cramps are caused by spasms of muscle fiber groups, often caused by dehydration and sodium or potassium depletion. *Muscle strain,* manifested by pain, stiffness, and swelling, usually results from excessive muscle use. Pain is often worse near the joint or associated ligaments. *Muscle atrophy* or wasting may result from loss of muscle innervation, malnutrition, or disuse. *Fasciculations* are twitches of muscle fibers and are noted as rapid movements of overlying skin. Twitches may occur spontaneously, indicating no muscle dysfunction, or may be associated with irritable muscle tissue. Degenerative nervous system disease is a common cause of fasciculation. *Tetany,* tonic muscle spasms, is most frequently noted in the extremities. Conditions causing hypocalcemia, such as parathyroid or vitamin D deficiencies, may cause tetany.

Physical Examination   *Musculoskeletal System*

General Principles

The musculoskeletal system varies significantly among different age groups (see Chaps. 19 and 20). In general, musculoskeletal assessment focuses on evaluating the extremities and the vertebral column. Evaluation of musculoskeletal function in relation to other body parts is integrated into the examination of other body systems. Part of the oral cavity assessment, for example, involves evaluating temporomandibular joint function; during the rectal or pelvic examination the muscles involved in bowel or bladder elimination are evaluated; and during pulmonary assessment the muscles involved in ventilation are examined. Muscles should be further evaluated to determine if movement is coordinated. Muscle assessment also involves evaluating neurologic function; this aspect of the physical examination is discussed in Chapter 11.

Assess the musculoskeletal system by inspection and palpation. Ask the person to report any pain, tenderness, or other sensations when musculoskeletal structures are palpated. Use special maneuvers, such as range of motion testing and muscle strength testing, to evaluate joints. Hold the palm of your hand over the person's joints during range of motion maneuvers to detect crepitation (grating) and deformities.

You should judge whether certain maneuvers or procedures are appropriate. In cases of suspected trauma, such as bone fractures, for example, range of motion maneuvers could cause considerable pain and aggravate the injury. In general, if light or deep palpation of a musculoskeletal structure causes pain, and the cause of the pain is uncertain, range of motion should not be evaluated until a cause for the pain can be determined. Similarly, if pain develops during range of motion testing, take special care to prevent further injury. In the case of injury to an extremity, you should examine the unaffected side first to determine the person's usual musculoskeletal function. Moving the neck and spine is strictly contraindicated if the person has had an accident that may have caused spinal injury.

Equipment

Metric tape measure
Goniometer (to measure joint angles)

Thorough Assessment Versus Screening Assessment

A thorough musculoskeletal examination is a lengthy procedure, involving evaluation of joint range of motion and skeletal muscle strength. A thorough examination may not be indicated for all persons or may not be tolerated because of fatigue or activity intolerance. If the person shows no overt signs of musculoskeletal dysfunction, then a screening examination may be sufficient. To determine whether a screening examination is appropriate, ask the person the following questions:

Do you have any pain or tenderness in an extremity or when you move? Does this pain affect your daily activities?
Do you have a history of injuries to any muscles, bones, or joints?

In addition, note any deformities apparent on general inspection, such as abnormal gait or stance and improper body alignment. In order to screen for musculoskeletal dysfunction, observe the manner in which the person walks, moves from a sitting to a standing position, shakes hands, and manipulates clothing. If such simple screening techniques indicate no musculoskeletal problems, the following components may be eliminated from the musculoskeletal examination: comprehensive testing of range of motion and muscle strength, and limb measurement.

Specific screening techniques, such as scoliosis screening in adolescents, may be used to detect musculoskeletal problems in certain high-risk groups.

Exposure

The person can remain gowned or draped during much of the musculoskeletal examination, especially when you assess distal parts of the extremities. Underwear can be worn when body alignment and spinal configurations are assessed.

Measurements and Comparisons

In a comprehensive examination, measurements and comparisons are useful in describing joint range of motion, muscle strength, and the length and circumference of the arms and legs.

Joint range of motion can be measured in degrees with a protractor device called the goniometer (Fig. 10-15). The zero reference arm of this device should be aligned with the neutral position of the joint. The person should move the joint through a specific range of motion and hold the final position while the other arm of the goniometer is moved to this position and the angle measured. This measurement may be compared to normal values. Record only values that deviate from normal by 10% to 20%. Differences in range of motion may be noted by comparing joint movement between left and right sides.

The length or circumference of the limbs may be measured with a cloth tape measure if there appear to be any inequalities between the right and left sides. Accurate measurements are necessary for different health care providers to make meaningful comparisons over a period of time. Serial measurements of limb circumference are most reliable when landmarks are specified or marks made on the person's skin with nontoxic markers to indicate tape measure placement. Measurement landmarks for the extremities may be designated as follows:

- *Entire arm:* Acromion process to the tip of the second finger
- *Upper arm:* Acromion process to olecranon process

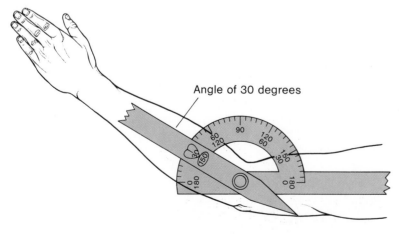

Angle of 30 degrees

Figure 10–15. The goniometer is used to measure degrees of joint motion. The zero point is placed at the extended anatomic position. This example shows 30 degrees of flexion at the elbow.

- *Forearm:* Olecranon process to ulnar styloid process
- *Entire leg:* Anterosuperior iliac spine to tibial malleolus
- *Upper leg:* Anterosuperior iliac spine to medial condyle of the knee
- *Lower leg:* Medial condyle of the knee to tibial malleolus

Musculoskeletal Pain

Although musculoskeletal pain is not considered normal, muscle pain, or *myalgia,* that results from overusing poorly conditioned muscles is usually benign. Crepitation (a grating sound) with joint movement is abnormal.

Musculoskeletal pain should be distinguished from visceral pain during the examination. Unlike visceral pain, musculoskeletal pain can usually be elicited by palpation, is aggravated by movement of associated structures, and usually does not have a characteristic pattern such as those observed with the pain of angina or pleurisy.

Examination and Documentation Focus

- Structural symmetry and alignment
- Ease and range of motion
- Muscle strength and tone
- Muscle mass
- Skin appearance over joints
- Deformities, pain, and crepitation

Evaluating Range of Motion

Every joint in the body has a normal range of motion, or maximum possible movement. Joint movements are described by range measured in degrees of a circle and by type of movement. When the range of movement is stated in degrees, the neutral joint position is 0 degrees. An example of range of motion description for a simple hinge joint, such as the knee, is "flexion, 130 degrees." Motion may be possible in several directions depending on joint type.

Differences in exercise levels, general health, and genetics account for normal differences among people. Generally, joint motion occurs with ease if the degree of movement is within 10% to 20% of the maximum possibility. Range of motion is normal if movement occurs without stiffness, pain, or crepitation. Joint movement past the normal maximum possibility may be abnormal, indicating ligament tears, abnormal connective tissues, or joint fracture.

Evaluating Muscle Strength and Tone

Muscle strength is graded on a 0 to 5 scale:

0—No detectable muscle contraction
1—Barely detectable contraction
2—Complete range of motion or active body part movement with gravity eliminated
3—Complete range of motion or active movement against gravity
4—Complete range of motion or active movement against gravity and some resistance
5—Complete range of motion or active movement against gravity and full resistance

Normal muscle strength is between 3 and 5 on this scale, and differs among people. Although the dominant side may be slightly stronger, muscle strength is usually equal bilaterally. In general, muscles that act as flexors and abductors are stronger than extensors and adductors.

Muscle tone can be detected during partial contraction of muscles, even at rest. Partial contraction is due to continual neural stimuli and keeps muscles ready for action. The muscles should appear firm or well developed. Twitching of muscle fibers in the relaxed state is not typical. An occasional, isolated twitch, however, is considered normal.

Examination Guidelines   *Bones, Joints, and Muscles*

Procedure

1. SURVEY GROSS MOTOR MOVEMENT AND POSTURE.

   Ask the person to walk across the room, or note the person's movements and stance when he or she enters the examining room. Note gross motor movements (gait, posture, or stance) and range of motion of joints used for walking.

   In addition to noting the style of gait, note the patterns of wear on the shoes, especially the heels, which could indicate unequal pressures or abnormal walking movements. Prostheses such as walkers, canes, crutches, or artificial limbs that may modify gait should also be noted.

Clinical Significance

Normal Findings

Normal gait is smooth and even and is usually accompanied by symmetrical arm swinging. In normal walking, the heel should gently strike the floor with the knee extended. Weight should then be smoothly transferred along the length of the foot toward the metatarsals. With the knee slightly flexed, the foot should lift off the floor. Walking movements should be coordinated.

Deviations from Normal

Abnormal gaits may be described as ataxic, hemiplegic, parkinsonian, scissors, spastic, steppage, or waddling. The different types of abnormal gait as well as the conditions associated with each are further described in the display, "Abnormal Gaits."

Abnormal Gaits

Ataxic Gait

The foot is raised high and strikes the ground suddenly with the entire sole. The person may stagger or fall to one side. Occurs with cerebellar disorders; alcohol or barbiturate toxicity.

Parkinsonian Gait (Festinating)

Body bends forward, rigid, with flexion of elbows, wrists, hips, and knees. Steps are short and shuffling with feet barely leaving the ground. May walk on toes as though pushed. Starts slowly and gradually accelerates. Sudden forward movement (propulsion) may continue until person can grasp some object for support. Occurs with Parkinson's disease and other basal ganglia defects.

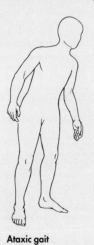

Ataxic gait

Hemiplegic gait

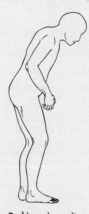

Parkinsonian gait

Scissors gait

Hemiplegic Gait

One leg is paralyzed. The paralyzed leg is abducted and swung around so that the foot comes forward and to the front, or the paralyzed leg may be dragged forward in a semicircle. Occurs with unilateral upper motor neuron disorder, as in stroke.

Scissors Gait

Legs cross at the thighs or knees with each step. Takes short steps. Very slow and awkward leg movements. Occurs with upper motor neuron disorders, as in stroke.

(continued)

GUIDELINES *continued*

Bones, Joints, and Muscles

Abnormal Gaits (continued)

Steppage Gait

Foot and toes lifted high with knees flexed. Foot brought to ground suddenly, heel first, with slapping noise. Person watches ground to know where to place foot. Occurs with peripheral neuritis, late stages of diabetes, alcoholism, and chronic arsenic poisoning.

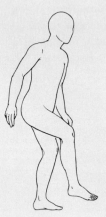

Steppage gait

Waddling Gait

Feet wide apart, and stride resembles that of a duck. Regular steps. Occurs with congenital hip displacement with lordosis, muscular dystrophy.

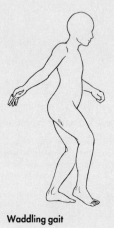

Waddling gait

Procedure

Note posture (stance). *Posture* or *stance* refers to the body position the person assumes when standing or sitting.

2. EVALUATE TRUNK MUSCULOSKELETAL STRUCTURES (vertebral column, paravertebral muscles, scapulae, pelvis).
   a. Ask the person to stand, facing you; note the alignment and symmetry of the spine, scapulae, and iliac crests. Observe the muscles for tone and note any visible spasms.

Clinical Significance

Good posture is characterized by proper alignment of body parts. Deviations from good posture, usually resulting from musculoskeletal or neurological pathology, may provide cues about the person's activity and exercise abilities.

Normal Findings

Normal alignment: Normal alignment is present if an imaginary line can be drawn through the ear lobe, shoulder, hip, femoral trochanter, center of the knee, and front of the ankle. The elbow, finger, ankle, and knee joints should be slightly flexed. Viewed from the front, the following structures should be at an even level: right and left shoulders; right and left iliac crests; right and left knees.

Symmetry: The bones and muscles on each side of the body are symmetric with respect to size, shape, and function. Surface features, such as trochanters, crests, and other bony prominences, should also be symmetric. Measured length and circumference of matching structures should also be equal. A 1-cm difference in length between left and right extremities is usually considered clinically insignificant.

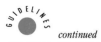 *continued*

Bones, Joints, and Muscles

Procedure

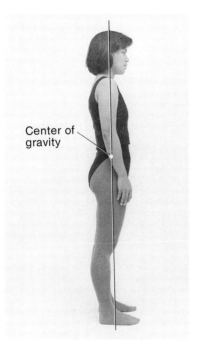

Normal musculoskeletal alignment: Side view

b. View the person from the side, and note spinal curvatures. Also note abnormalities, such as exaggerated curvatures or straightening of the lumbar curve of the spine.

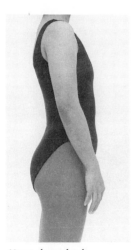

Normal vertebral column alignment

Clinical Significance

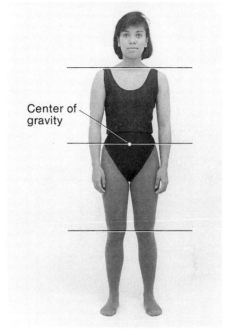

Normal musculoskeletal alignment: Front view

Normal Findings

Normal vertebral column alignment: Normally, when viewed from the side the vertebral column is characterized by concave curvature of the cervical spine, convex curvature of the thoracic spine, and concave curvature of the lumbar spine. The spine should be straight when viewed from behind the person. Exaggerated curvatures should be considered abnormal, even if oriented in a normal direction.

Deviations from Normal

Spinal deformities: Lordosis, abnormal concavity of the lumbar spine; *kyphosis,* abnormally increased rounding of the thoracic curve; *gibbus,* a projection along the vertebral column caused by a collapsed vertebra.

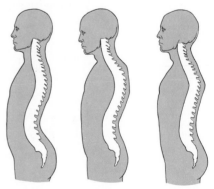

Spinal deformities: (left) *lordosis;* (center) *kyphosis;* (right) *gibbus*

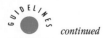

Bones, Joints, and Muscles

Procedure

c. Ask the person to bend forward at the waist. Stand behind the person and note the ease of mobility, the orientation of the supine and scapulae, and curvature of the spine.

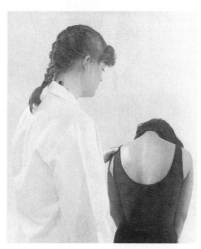

Spine inspection

d. With the person standing, sitting, or lying prone, palpate the vertebral column with the fingertips. Note any tenderness or bony deformities.

e. Lightly pound the length of the spine with the ulnar surface of your hand, and note any tenderness.

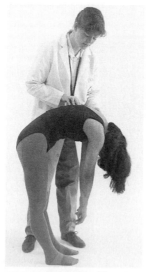

Fingertip palpation of the spine

Clinical Significance

Normal Findings

The entire spine should appear smooth and convex, and the vertebrae should remain midline.

Deviations from Normal

Scoliosis is lateral deviation of the thoracic spine best observed if the person bends at the waist from a standing position.

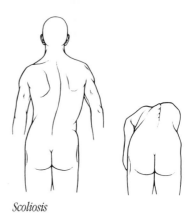

Scoliosis

Normal Findings

No tenderness elicited on palpation.

Deviations from Normal

Point tenderness (tenderness elicited on palpation); may indicate degenerative joint disease.

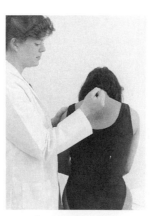

Fist palpation of the spine

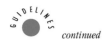

Bones, Joints, and Muscles

Procedure

3. TEST RANGE OF MOTION AND MUSCLE STRENGTH OF THE NECK.

  a. Check flexion and extension of the cervical spine by asking the person to touch the chin to the chest and then tip the head backward.

  b. To evaluate muscle strength, ask the person to repeat these movements while you press your hand against the person's forehead during flexion and against the occiput during extension.

  c. To evaluate cervical spine rotation, ask the person to turn the head toward the right and left shoulders while keeping the shoulders stationary.

  d. Then apply resistance to the temples and ask the person to repeat the movements, in order to assess muscle strength.

  e. Finally, to evaluate lateral bending of the cervical spine, ask the person to try and touch the ear to the shoulder while keeping the shoulders stationary.

  f. Then apply pressure to the person's right and left occiputs in order to evaluate muscle strength.

Clinical Significance

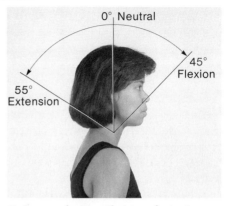

Neck range of motion: Flexion and extension

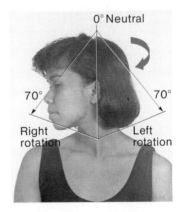

Neck range of motion: Rotation

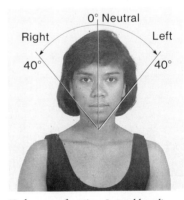

Neck range of motion: Lateral bending

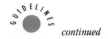 *continued*   ***Bones, Joints, and Muscles***

Procedure

4. TEST RANGE OF MOTION AND MUSCLE STRENGTH OF THE REMAINING SPINE.

   a. Ask the person to bend at the waist and evaluate forward flexion. Measure range of motion by determining the width of the angle between the neutral and flexed positions or by measuring the length between the fingertips and the floor. An alternative method involves measuring the change in length along the spine as the person bends forward. Place a tape measure from the spinous process of C7 to the spinous process of S1. Keep your hands on these landmarks, but allow the tape to slide through your fingers at S1 as the person leans forward.

   b. To evaluate spinal extension, ask the person to lean backward.

   c. Extensor muscle strength is best evaluated with the person in the prone position. Instruct the person to try to lift the head and shoulders while you apply resistance by placing your hand between the scapulae.

Clinical Significance

Normal Findings

Normally, the length should increase about 4 inches in adults. If length does not increase, you should suspect conditions that limit vertebral joint mobility, which cause the back to remain straight with forward flexion.

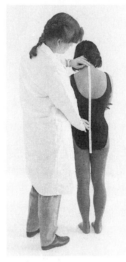

Evaluating spine range of motion: Upright

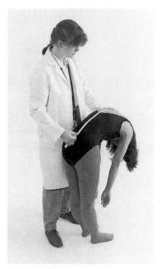

Evaluating spine range of motion: Bending over

   d. To evaluate lateral bending of the spine, ask the person to bend sideways as though to touch the hand to the side of the knee.

   e. Then evaluate spinal rotation as the person turns the head and the shoulders as one unit to the left and then the right while holding the pelvis stationary.

   f. Ask the person to repeat this maneuver while you place your hands against the right and left shoulders to evaluate muscle strength.

   g. *Special maneuvers.* Two special maneuvers, *Patrick's sign* and *Laseque's sign,* are indicated for persons with back pain. Because the person should be supine, you may postpone these maneuvers until you are ready to evaluate the lower extremities.

   Lasegue's sign is elicited by asking the person to raise one leg at a time off the examining table.

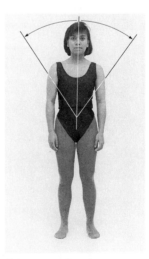

Spine range of motion: Lateral bending

Deviations from Normal

Positive Laseque's sign is indicated by pain in the back with this maneuver, and indicates back injury.

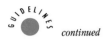

continued

Bones, Joints, and Muscles

Procedure

Patrick's sign is elicited by placing the heel of one foot on the opposite knee. Then, the hip of the flexed extremity is abducted.

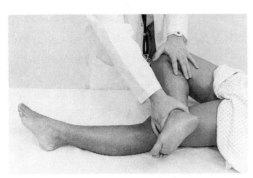

Assessing for Patrick's sign

5. EVALUATE SHOULDER MUSCULOSKELETAL STRUCTURES.

   a. With the person standing, sitting, or supine, inspect the shoulders from the front, and note right- and left-side symmetry. Inspect the skin over the clavicles for bulges or protrusions. Note the shoulder posture (erect, slumped, hunched).

   b. With your fingertips, palpate along the clavicles outward to the shoulders and note any discomfort or deformities. Visualize sternoclavicular and acromioclavicular joint locations as you move your fingers along the clavicles. Locate the greater tubercle of the humerus by palpating the shoulder as the person abducts and adducts at the shoulder, allowing you to differentiate between scapula and humerus at the glenohumeral joint. Ask the person to rotate the shoulder externally, and palpate just medial to the greater tubercle to locate the long head of the biceps. Palpate along this cord-like tendon, and note any tenderness. Finally, palpate the deltoid muscle.

Clinical Significance

Positive Patrick's sign is indicated by pain with this maneuver, and indicates sacroiliac joint disease.

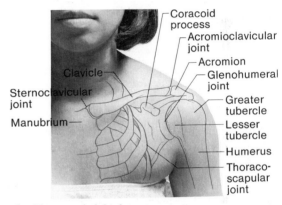

Shoulder musculoskeletal structures

Deviations from Normal

Skin bulges or protrusions are associated with clavicular fracture.

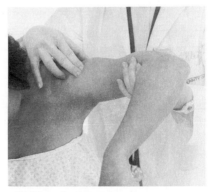

Shoulder palpation

Deviations from Normal

The deltoid muscle overlies the nonpalpable subdeltoid bursa; palpation may cause pain if *bursitis* is present.

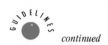 *continued*

Bones, Joints, and Muscles

Procedure

6. TEST RANGE OF MOTION AND MUSCLE STRENGTH OF THE SHOULDER.

   a. To evaluate flexion, ask the person to raise the arm anteriorly until pointing overhead.

   b. Apply resistance to the upper anterior arm just above the elbow. To test muscle strength, ask the person to repeat the shoulder flexion. Then apply pressure over the posterior surface of the upper arm just above the elbow to test muscle strength during shoulder extension.

   c. For abduction, ask the person to lift the arm laterally until the fingers point overhead.

   d. Apply resistance by placing your hand over the upper forearm just above the elbow.

   e. To test adduction, ask the person to bring the arm over the chest.

   f. Apply resistance over the medial aspect of the upper arm above the elbow to test muscle strength during adduction.

Clinical Significance

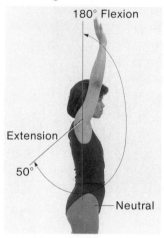

Shoulder range of motion: Flexion

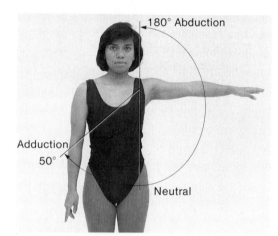

Shoulder range of motion: Abduction

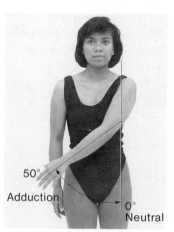

Shoulder range of motion: Adduction

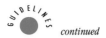

continued

Bones, Joints, and Muscles

Procedure

g. Finally, to evaluate external and internal shoulder joint rotation, ask the person to flex the elbow and raise the arm to shoulder level, holding the hand with the fingers extended and palm facing the floor. Note external rotations as the person rotates the forearm posteriorly, back and forth. Note internal rotation as the person rotates the forearm anteriorly so that the fingertips point to the floor.

7. EVALUATE ELBOW MUSCULOSKELETAL STRUCTURES.

Inspect and palpate the posterior elbow surface with your thumb and forefinger as the person bends the elbow at an angle of flexion just greater than 90 degrees while you support the forearm with your other hand. Note the medial and lateral condyles of the humerus and the olecranon process of the ulna. Note any bony deformities, and carefully compare opposite sides.

8. TEST RANGE OF MOTION AND MUSCLE STRENGTH OF THE ELBOW.

a. Instruct the person to hold the upper arm straight while bending at the elbow in a manner that allows the fingers to touch the shoulder. The opposite of this action is extension.

b. To test muscle strength, ask the person to repeat the maneuvers, and apply your hand to the medial surface and then to the dorsal surface of the wrist during both flexion and extension.

c. Finally, to test supination and pronation, ask the person to extend the forearm or rest the forearm on a flat surface with the palm facing down. Supination occurs when the person rotates the forearm so that the palm faces upward, and pronation occurs when the person rotates the forearm so that the palm faces downward.

d. To evaluate muscle strength during supination, apply resistance to the dorsal surface of the person's hand just distal to the wrist.

Clinical Significance

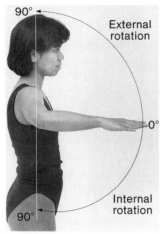

Shoulder range of motion: Rotation

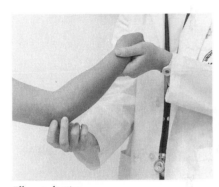

Elbow palpation

Deviations from Normal

The olecranon bursa lies between the condyles of the humerus and is not normally palpable but may be tender if inflamed. The ulnar nerve is palpable posteriorly between the olecranon process and medial epicondyle.

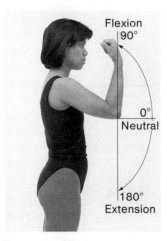

Elbow range of motion:
Flexion and extension

GU**IDELIN**ES *continued*   *Bones, Joints, and Muscles*

Procedure

    e. To evaluate muscle strength during pronation, apply resistance against the volar surface of the person's thumb.

    f. In addition to testing elbow range of motion and muscle strength, palpate the brachial pulse on the side opposite the olecranon process and check the bicep and tricep reflexes (see Chap. 11).

9. EVALUATE WRIST MUSCULOSKELETAL STRUCTURES.

    Grasp the person's wrist with both your hands so that both thumbs are over the dorsal wrist surface. Identify the bony processes of the radius (on the thumb side) and the ulna. Palpate the radiocarpal joint, a slight groove just distal to the radial process. With both thumbs, palpate remaining wrist bones.

10. TEST RANGE OF MOTION AND MUSCLE STRENGTH OF THE WRIST.

    a. To check flexion (palmarflexion) and extension (dorsiflexion), ask the person to bend the hand downward at the wrist and upward with fingers pointing up, respectively.

    b. To test muscle strength, place your hand against the volar surface of the person's hand during flexion and against the dorsal surface of the hand, over the carpals, during extension.

    c. To check radial wrist deviation, ask the person to hold the elbow aligned with the wrist and bend the wrist sideways toward the thumb side. Apply resistance by pressing against the person's thumb.

    d. Check ulnar deviation with the elbow and wrist in the same position, but instruct the person to bend the wrist sideways, away from the body.

    e. To test muscle strength, apply resistance along the person's little finger.

    f. In addition to evaluating the musculoskeletal structure of the wrist, palpate the radial pulse and check the supinator (brachioradialis) reflex (see Chap. 11).

Clinical Significance

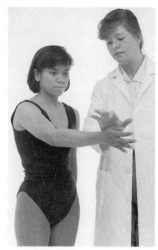

Evaluating muscle strength during elbow range of motion

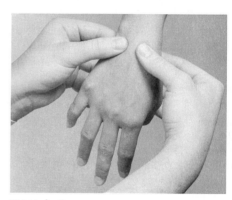

Wrist palpation

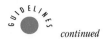

Bones, Joints, and Muscles

Procedure

11. EVALUATE HAND MUSCULOSKELETAL STRUCTURES.

    Focus hand assessment on the finger joints, which are susceptible to degenerative joint disease.

    With the person's fingers slightly flexed, use your thumb and forefinger to palpate the metacarpophalangeal joints, which feel like grooves just distal to the first knuckle. Then, palpate the interphalangeal joints.

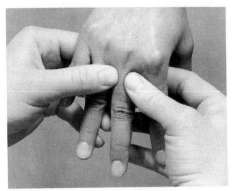

Metacarpophalangeal joint palpation

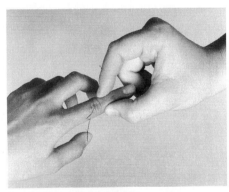

Interphalangeal joint palpation

12. EVALUATE RANGE OF MOTION AND MUSCLE STRENGTH OF THE FINGERS.

    a. To evaluate finger and thumb flexion and extension, ask the person to make a fist and then straighten the fingers.

    b. Test resistance to extension by placing your hand over the person's clenched fist before the hand is opened.

Clinical Significance

Deviations from Normal

Finger deformities include mallet finger (position of permanent flexion due to loss of extensor ability), boutonnière and swan-neck deformities (associated with rheumatoid arthritis), claw fingers (associated with injury to ulnar and medial nerves), and nodules (associated with osteoarthritis).

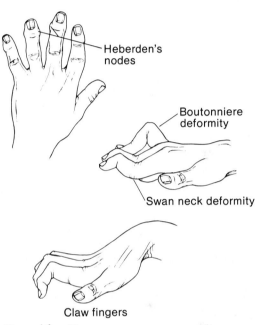

Finger deformities

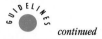
continued

Bones, Joints, and Muscles

Procedure

c. Test finger abduction as the person spreads the fingers apart and adduction as the person holds the fingers tightly together.

d. To test adductor strength, place your thumb against the person's index finger and your other fingers against the person's little finger.

e. To test thumb abduction and adduction, ask the person to move the thumb up and outward from the palm and then return the thumb to the neutral position.

f. *Special maneuvers.* If the person reports pain and burning in the hand, special examination maneuvers should be performed to rule out carpal tunnel syndrome.

Test for *Phalen's sign* by holding the wrist in flexion position.

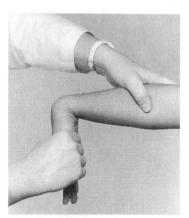

Testing for Phalen's sign

Test for *Tinel's sign* by tapping the palm of the hand (volar percussion).

Evaluate *opposition* by asking the person to touch the thumb to the fingertips of the same hand.

Clinical Significance

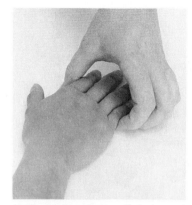

Evaluating muscle strength during finger range of motion

Deviations from Normal

Carpal tunnel syndrome results from pressure on the median nerve as it passes through the wrist. Signs include a positive Phalen's sign, a positive Tinel's sign, decreased sensation in the areas of the medial nerve distribution, atrophy of the thenar eminence, and weak opposition in the thumb of the affected hand.

Phalen's sign is positive if wrist burning is aggravated when the wrist is held in prolonged flexion, usually for 1 or 2 minutes.

Tinel's sign is positive if volar percussion produces tingling or shocklike pain.

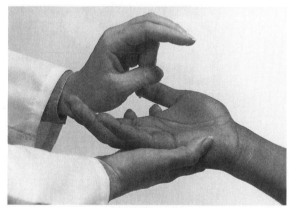

Tinel's sign

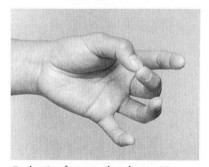

Evaluating finger-to-thumb opposition

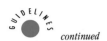 *continued*

Bones, Joints, and Muscles

Procedure

Clinical Significance

13. EVALUATE HOP MUSCULOSKELETAL STRUCTURES.

   Because the hip joint is essential for walking movements, evaluate gait and stance during the general inspection. The hip may be assessed with the person standing or supine. Range of motion maneuvers are the same for both positions. However, the person needs greater strength and balance to perform such maneuvers while standing.

   Palpate the hip joint and surrounding structures. Place your fingertips over the lateral aspect of the iliac crest with the palm of your hand over the lateral hip. The greater trochanter of the femur and the nonpalpable trochanteric bursa lie beneath the surface of your palm. Palpate around this process and note any joint tenderness or pain. Palpate the area surrounding the hip, thigh, and buttock muscles.

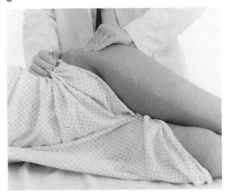

Hip palpation

14. EVALUATE RANGE OF MOTION AND MUSCLE STRENGTH OF THE HIP.

   a. To evaluate hip flexion, ask the person to lift the leg without bending at the knee.

   b. Check muscle strength by placing your hand over the anterior surface of the upper leg as the person repeats hip flexion.

   c. Note extension as the person returns the leg to the neutral position.

   d. Test extensor muscle strength by placing your hand over the posterior surface of the upper leg during hip extension.

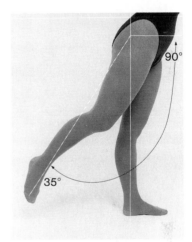

Hip range of motion: Flexion and extension

   e. To check abduction, ask the person to move the entire leg away from the body. Check adduction by having the person move the leg across the midline so that one leg lies over the other.

   f. Apply resistance over the lateral leg surface during abduction and the medial leg surface during adduction.

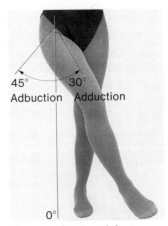

Hip range of motion: Abduction and adduction

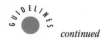
continued

Bones, Joints, and Muscles

Procedure

g. Finally, to evaluate external rotation, ask the person to turn the foot outward while holding the leg straight. To evaluate internal rotation, ask the person to turn the foot inward.

Clinical Significance

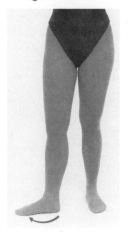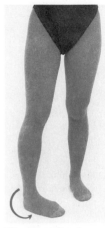

Hip range of motion:
External rotation

Hip range of motion:
Internal rotation

h. To test muscle strength, apply resistance against the lateral or medial aspects of the ankle.

i. *Special maneuvers.* The special maneuvers discussed with assessment of the trunk may be performed in conjunction with the hip examination because such assessments are based on hip range of motion maneuvers.

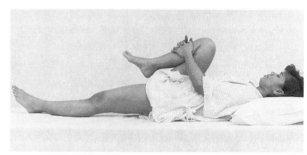

Thomas test

If you suspect a hip flexion contracture or note restricted range of motion, perform the *Thomas test.* Ask the person to assume a supine position and flex the knee, pulling it toward the chest.

15. EVALUATE KNEE MUSCULOSKELETAL STUCTURES.

The knee is most easily evaluated with the person seated, with the hips and knees flexed. However, the examination may be performed with the person supine. Apley's test should be performed with the person in a prone position (see p. 297).

Deviations from Normal

The Thomas test result is positive if the opposite leg flexes at the hip and knee with this maneuver. A positive result is abnormal and indicates a hip flexion contracture on that side.

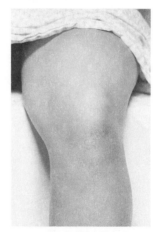

Knee musculoskeletal structure

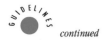 *continued*

Bones, Joints, and Muscles

Procedure

a. Inspect the front of the knee and note alignment, deformity, and the contour of the quadricep muscle and any atrophy of this muscle.

b. Focus palpation on the suprapatellar pouch, a sac-like structure separating the patella from surrounding structures.

To help make fluid more accessible to palpation, displace the pouch downward by placing one of your hands over the quadriceps at the top of the knee and exerting slight downward pressure.

Use your other hand to palpate along each side of the patella and over the tibiofemoral joint space. Palpate with the fingertips and stabilize the opposite side of the knee with the thumb of your examining hand. Displace the pouch upward by placing one of your hands over the lower part of the knee and applying slight pressure upward and inward. Palpate the area from the quadriceps to the patella with your fingertips. Note any tenderness, bogginess, edema, or thickening. If you suspect fluid, patella ballottement and evaluation for a bulge sign are indicated (see 16c).

c. In addition to evaluating the musculoskeletal structures of the knee, palpate the popliteal pulse, located at the back of the knee in the popliteal fossa, slightly lateral to the midline. Then check the patellar reflex (see Chap. 11).

Clinical Significance

Normal Findings

Normal contour, which may be lost with swelling, is indicated by hollows on each side of the patella.

Deviations from Normal

Fluid accumulation following injury or disease may be easily detected at the suprapatellar pouch.

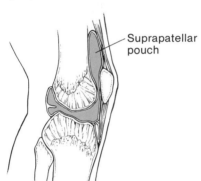

Suprapatellar pouch

Internal knee structure

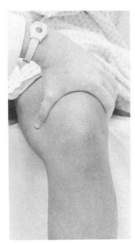

Displacing the suprapatellar pouch

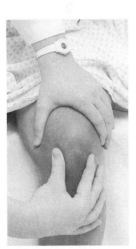

Palpating the suprapatellar pouch

16. EVALUATE RANGE OF MOTION AND MUSCLE STRENGTH OF THE KNEE.

a. To evaluate flexion, ask the person to stand and bend the knee, bringing the heel toward the buttocks. If the person is supine, the hip must also be flexed to perform this action. Note extension as the person returns the knee to the neutral position.

b. To test muscle strength of the knee during flexion, place your hand against the back of the ankle. During extension, move your hand to the front of the ankle.

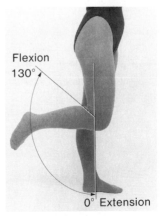

Flexion 130°

0° Extension

Knee range of motion: Flexion and extension

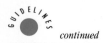
continued

Bones, Joints, and Muscles

Procedure

c. *Special maneuvers.* Two techniques may be used to check for fluid accumulation in the knee:

(1) To perform *patella ballottement,* place one of your hands over the quadriceps and apply downward pressure to distribute accumulated fluid in the suprapatellar pouch toward the patella. With the first and second fingers of your other hand, tap the patella against the femur and note the patella rebounding against your examining fingers.

Clinical Significance

Deviations from Normal

If the patella rebounds (ballots) against your fingers, fluid is present in the knee.

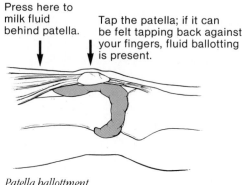

Patella ballottment

(2) To elicit a *bulge sign,* milk any suprapatellar fluid away from the medial half of the knee by using the ball of your hand to apply firm upward pressure along the medial side. Repeat this motion several times. Briskly tap the lateral side of the knee several times. Note the medial area where you just displaced fluid.

Deviations from Normal

A medial bulge with lateral tapping indicates fluid movement in the joint. In such a case, the bulge sign is positive.

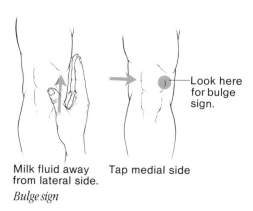

Milk fluid away from lateral side.

Tap medial side

Bulge sign

McMurray's test is used to detect meniscus injuries. With the person supine or seated, place one of your hands against the medial side of the knee to stabilize it. With your other hand, grasp the person's ankle and rotate the lower leg and foot inward while trying to extend the leg.

Deviations from Normal

The leg cannot be extended if a meniscus injury is present.

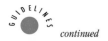

continued

Bones, Joints, and Muscles

Procedure

Apley's test also detects meniscus injuries and foreign or floating objects in the joint. The person should be prone with the knee flexed at 90 degrees. Grasp the person's foot and apply pressure. Then rotate the foot externally and internally.

Clinical Significance

Deviations from Normal

Knee locking or clicking and popping sounds indicate loose objects and injury.

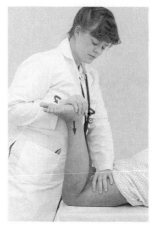

Apley's test

Knee stability is evaluated by attempting to move the knee in an abnormal manner. With the person supine, and the leg straight, grasp the thigh with one hand and the ankle with the other. Then, attempt to adduct and abduct the leg at the knee.

Exaluate the anterior and posterior cruciate ligaments by trying to elicit a *drawer sign*. With the person supine, flex the knee and grasp the lower leg firmly with both hands. Attempt to push the knee back and forth while stabilizing the person's foot by sitting on it.

Deviations from Normal

Movement with adduction indicates a tear of the medial collateral ligament, whereas movement with abduction indicates dysfunction of the lateral collateral ligament.

Deviations from Normal

Normally there is no movement. Forward movement indicates anterior cruciate tears, and backward movement indicates posterior cruciate tears.

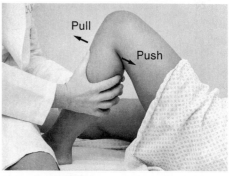

Testing knee stability

17. EVALUATE ANKLE MUSCULOSKELETAL STRUCTURES.

   a. With the person seated or supine, inspect the ankle and note any swelling or deformity. Compare the contour of the left and right ankles.

   b. To palpate, stabilize the ankle by cupping one of your hands behind the heel. Palpate with the fingers of your other hand.

   c. Palpate the posterior tibial pulse located slightly below the medial malleolus. Also test the Achilles reflex (see Chap. 11).

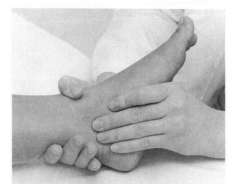

Ankle palpation

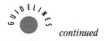

continued   ***Bones, Joints, and Muscles***

Procedure

18. EVALUATE RANGE OF MOTION AND MUSCLE STRENGTH OF THE ANKLE.

    a. To evaluate dorsiflexion, ask the person to bend the toes in the direction of the knee. Then, note range of motion as well as calf pain, which may indicate deep vein thrombosis in the lower leg (positive *Homans' sign*).

    b. Check resistance to dorsiflexion with your hand over the dorsal foot surface.

    c. To check plantar flexion, ask the person to point the toes.

    d. Evaluate resistance to plantar flexion by applying pressure over the ball of the foot.

    e. To check ankle inversion, ask the person to turn the sole of the foot inward at the ankle joint, and apply resistance to foot arches to check muscle strength.

    f. Check eversion as the person turns the soles of the feet outward at the ankle joint, and place your hands against the lateral aspect of the fifth metatarsal bones to check muscle strength.

Clinical Significance

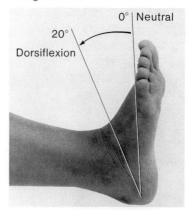

Ankle range of motion: Dorsiflexion

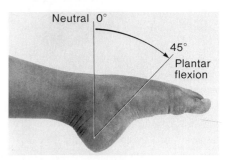

Ankle range of motion: Plantar flexion

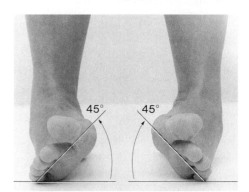

Ankle range of motion: Inversion

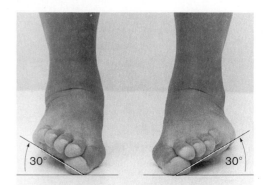

Ankle range of motion: Eversion

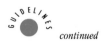 *continued*

Bones, Joints, and Muscles

Procedure	Clinical Significance

Procedure

19. EVALUATE FOOT MUSCULOSKELETAL STRUCTURES.

    a. Inspect the feet and note skin integrity, condition of the nails, and any deformities.

    b. Palpate the metatarsal bones and the metatarsal joints between the forefinger and thumb.

    c. The dorsalis pedis pulse is noted just lateral to the extensor tendon of the great toe.

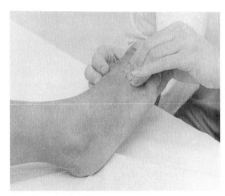

Metatarsal palpation

20. EVALUATE FOOT RANGE OF MOTION.

    a. Stabilize the foot by cupping one of your hands around the heel. Ask the person to turn the foot inward (adduction) and then outward (abduction).

    b. To evaluate the toes for flexion and extension, ask the person to bend and straighten the toes.

    c. To check abduction of the toes, ask the person to fan the toes apart; for adduction, return the toes to the neutral position.

Clinical Significance

Deviations from Normal

Foot deformities: Equinus and calcaneal deformities.

Toe deformities: Claw hammer toe.

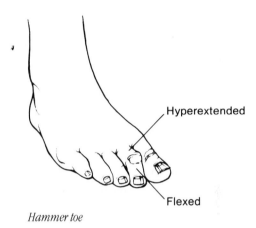

Hammer toe

Documenting Musculoskeletal Examination Findings

Documentation of musculoskeletal examination findings may reflect the overall status of the musculoskeletal system or may focus on specific body parts.

Example 1: Normal Musculoskeletal Function

Mr. W, aged 30, had a routine annual health assessment at the industrial clinic. The musculoskeletal screening examination findings were normal and were recorded as follows:

> Reports no previous musculoskeletal injuries or pain except for a sprained left ankle 3 years ago that healed without complications. Gait smooth and coordinated; extremities symmetric and posture upright. Range of motion required for general movement during examination intact; specific testing not done. Muscle strength 4 to 5; well-developed muscle mass. No visible musculoskeletal deformities.

These findings may be recorded in a problem-oriented format as follows:

S: Reports no musculoskeletal pain or movement limitations. Exercise program includes speed walking and using machine weights. Sprained left ankle 3 years ago that healed without sequelae.

O: Gait smooth and coordinated; extremities symmetric and posture upright. Range of motion required for general movement during examination intact; specific testing not done. Muscle strength 4 to 5; well-developed muscle mass. No visible musculoskeletal deformities.

A: No abnormalities detected by musculoskeletal screening exam.

P: Routine follow-up examinations as indicated. Evaluate exercise habits to see if he uses warm-up and cool-down periods to prevent muscle strain and injury.

Example 2: Ankle Injury

Mr. T, aged 38, reported to the emergency clinic with left ankle pain following a fall during a softball game. The lower extremity examination findings were abnormal and were recorded as follows:

Left ankle edematous and ecchymotic compared to right ankle. Guards left ankle by not bearing weight. ROM impaired because of pain but he is able to move ankle and toes. Left pedal pulse 3+.

These findings may be recorded in a problem-oriented format as follows:

S: "I twisted down on my ankle sliding into second base." Reports intense pain with weight bearing. Did not hear any snapping or cracking sounds when injured.

O: Left ankle edematous and ecchymotic compared to right. Guards left ankle by not bearing weight. ROM impaired because of pain but he is able to move ankle and toes. Left pedal pulse 3+.

A: Possible soft tissue injury to left ankle; need to rule out bone injury.

P: Immobilize left ankle; apply ice packs; notify physician; obtain x-ray if advised by physician.

NDx

Nursing Diagnoses Related to Musculoskeletal Assessment

Impaired Physical Mobility

Impaired physical mobility is a state in which the person experiences limitation in the ability to engage in independent physical movement.

History. The person may describe limitations in movement or activities. Listen for reports of pain, tenderness, or soreness with movement. Consider underlying pathology such as trauma, inflammatory diseases, or degenerative conditions. Determine what effect mobility problems are having on the person's capacity to carry out activities of daily living.

Physical Examination Findings. In general, a person with impaired physical mobility will exhibit the following: inability to move purposefully within the environment; limited range of motion; reluctance to attempt movement; decreased muscle strength. Impaired physical mobility caused by injury may be associated with the following physical examination findings: edema, bruising, or deformity at the injured area; guarding of injured part. When mobility is impaired because of inflammatory conditions of the musculoskeletal system, the following may be observed: edematous joints with enlargement and deformity; skin over affected areas that is warm and tender to palpation.

Clinical Problems Related to Musculoskeletal Assessment

Degenerative Joint Disease

Degenerative joint disease, also called osteoarthritis, is a disease manifested by degenerative changes in the articular cartilage, especially in the major weight-bearing joints (hip, knee, lower back) and hand joints.

History. Degenerative joint disease occurs more commonly in older people and is almost universal in people over age 75 years. Overuse of the joints has been indicated as contributing to the problem. Degenerative joint disease may be a long-term sequela to joint trauma. Symptoms of the disease vary with severity. Early in the disease, the person may report pain when the involved joint is subjected to stress. Later, the pain may be felt even at rest. The person may also report joint stiffness. The joints may be asymmetrically involved.

Physical Examination. The joints become limited in range of motion, and pain may be elicited with movement. Joint swelling or deformity may be present. There may be point tenderness over the affected joints. Occasionally, crepitations or crunching may be heard as the joint is moved.

Rheumatoid Arthritis

Rheumatoid arthritis is a systemic, autoimmune inflammatory disease of the body's connective tissue. Women are affected more often than men. The disease is most prevalent in the 30- to 50-year age group.

History. The person will typically complain of joint pain or stiffness upon arising in the morning. The joints are usually symmetrically involved. The joint pain may diminish throughout the day or it may stay the same. Painful episodes of the disease are cyclic. Remissions may be associated with decreased levels of activity. The small joints of the hands and the feet are usually the first joints to become affected.

Physical Examination. Examination of infected joints usually reveals signs of inflammation (swelling, warmth, redness). Passive motions and pressure elicit pain. Rheumatoid nodules may develop at or near the affected joint.

Bursitis

A bursa is a sac that is filled with a small amount of synovial fluid and located over a bony prominence (elbow, knee, greater trochanter of the femur). Bursae facilitate movement of overlying tendons and muscles. Inflammation of the bursa, through trauma or repeated use, is referred to as bursitis.

History and Physical Examination. The person usually can report a mechanism of injury for the affected joint, such as one involving repeated flexion and extension of the elbow. Movement of the affected joint results in pain and tenderness. Over the affected bursa, the area may be red, hot, and edematous with pain that may or may not radiate to surrounding areas.

Herniated Disc Syndrome

This is an acute problem that can occur in persons of any age, typically after age 30. The intervertebral disc of the spinal cord ruptures, compressing the nearby spinal nerves.

History and Physical Examination. The onset of symptoms is abrupt, and a snap may be felt in the back just prior to the onset of pain. There is low back pain that frequently radiates into the lower extremity. Numbness may be felt in the distribution of the sciatic nerve. The person appears in obvious distress and may have difficulty bearing weight on the leg in pain. The person is most comfortable sitting or lying flexed in the fetal position. The paravertebral muscles may be tender and in spasm. Straight leg raising in the supine position is painful. The person may be unable to lie supine with the affected leg straightened out.

ASSESSMENT PROFILE

● ●

Enrico Garcia, aged 26 years, was a patient in the coronary ICU with severe heart failure resulting from dilated cardiomyopathy. He had first experienced symptoms of heart dysfunction 4 years earlier after a viral illness. At that time, he was treated with digoxin, furosemide (Lasix), and warfarin sodium crystalline (Coumadin). Approximately 3 years later, hydrazine and captopril were added to the therapeutic regimen because of further deterioration. Five months before this hospital admission, Enrico had to leave his job because of increasing fatigue and dyspnea. While Enrico's condition was being evaluated to see if he should undergo a heart transplant, nursing efforts were directed toward maintaining cardiac function. Enrico's activities were restricted in order to prevent further cardiac decompensation. To evaluate the activity prescription, the nurses monitored Enrico's response to permitted activities. On bed rest he had no dyspnea; he felt well rested, with a pulse of 98 beats/minute, and his skin was warm and dry. While being transferred from bed to chair one day, however, Enrico became lightheaded and began to have trouble breathing. His pulse became weak and rapid at 160 beats/minute, and his skin was cool with cyanosis around the mouth. Enrico was returned to bed to rest. His symptoms persisted for 30 minutes.

For the patient with severe heart failure, even simple activities may further compromise physiologic function. Nurses monitor the patient's response to activity to prevent further deterioration, and in order to plan interventions that will improve activity tolerance by promoting rest, oxygenation, and cardiac function. Monitoring a patient's response to activity is complex and requires drawing conclusions more specific than statements such as "tolerated activity well" or "did not tolerate activity." Without more specific details about the person's response, planning appropriate interventions may be difficult.

Profile Analysis

Enrico experienced potentially life-threatening cardiorespiratory compromise in response to activity. In this case, the nurse should focus the assessment of activity tolerance so that timely interventions could be implemented.

Identifying the Assessment Focus

For a person with impaired cardiovascular or respiratory functions, the nurse should make a judgment about his or her capabilities before permitting activity. If the nurse believes that the person is at risk for activity intolerance, before permitting activity he or she should make a decision about what types of data to collect and about what signs of activity intolerance to consider valid and reliable.

Before moving him to the chair, Enrico's nurse noted that despite the severity of his illness, the patient's cardiovascular parameters were stable. Based on this assessment, Enrico was moved to the chair despite the risk of activity intolerance. Ongoing nursing evaluation of activity response focused on the following: watching the cardiac monitor for heart rate changes from baseline, resting levels, and cardiac dysrhythmias; noting signs of decreased cardiac output, such as changes in skin color, temperature, and moisture, all readily apparent by general observation; and evaluating blood pressure for cues to activity intolerance.

Formulating the Nursing Diagnosis

Evaluating Enrico's response to activity revealed several important cues. First, his heart rate increased, which in itself is not sufficient to identify activity intolerance because increased heart rate is a normal response to increased activity, contributing to the higher cardiac output needed to sustain activity. The nurse noted other cues, however, such as lightheadedness, weak pulse, and cool skin, indicating that cardiac output was not augmented. The nurse then made the appropriate decision to return Enrico to bed. Ongoing monitoring revealed that 30 minutes elapsed before Enrico's condition stabilized. Normally, heart rate should return to preactivity levels within 3 to 5 minutes.

Based on the nursing assessment, the nurse established the diagnosis of Activity intolerance. Enrico's activity prescription was modified to prevent further cardiovascular deterioration.

RESEARCH *Hi*GHLIGHT

Are adventitious breath sounds reliable indicators that tracheal suctioning is necessary?

Patients with artificial airways often require endotracheal suctioning to remove tracheobronchial secretions. Suctioning may irritate the mucosa, however, or place the patient at risk for hypoxia, which in turn can adversely affect cardiopulmonary status. Because of the risks involved, the nurse should use guidelines to help evaluate the patient's need for suctioning so that the procedure is performed only when indicated, rather than on a routine schedule such as every 1 or 2 hours. Suctioning routines that are based on a time schedule do not always result in aspiration of secretions. If no secretions are removed, the procedure may have been unnecessary.

One way to assess the patient's need for suctioning is to auscultate the lungs. Crackles over the large airways may indicate the presence of secretions.

Knipper designed a study to determine if auscultated crackles over the large airways correlated with the need for suctioning. Two suctioning protocols were compared to determine aspiration effectiveness. One protocol involved suctioning every 2 hours during a 4-hour period, and the other protocol involved suctioning only after lung crackles were auscultated. Patients with endotracheal or tracheostomy tubes were divided into two groups. One group was treated according to the timed-suctioning protocol and the other according to the auscultation protocol. In both groups, patients' lungs were auscultated every 30 minutes, and in both groups patients' suctioned secretions were measured.

Other studies have indicated that at least 0.5 mL of secretions must accumulate before crackles can be noted on auscultation. In this study, however, more than 0.5 mL of secretions were aspirated when crackles were noted. Suctioning when no crackles were present was associated with less than 0.5 mL of aspirate. Furthermore, when lung crackles were the basis for suctioning, some

patients were suctioned more frequently than every 2 hours, but in each case the aspirate was greater than 0.5 mL.

Based on this study, Knipper recommended that suctioning should be based on lung auscultation findings, because the presence of crackles was consistently associated with significant accumulation of secretions. Following this protocol could help ensure that patients are suctioned neither too infrequently nor too frequently, but rather, according to their clinical status.[1]

What significance does the study have for health assessment?

The study suggests that nurses should use chest assessment to make decisions in caring for patients with tracheal suctioning needs. Acting on assessment findings rather than according to an arbitrary schedule is more likely to benefit the patient while minimizing risk.

Can the study's findings be applied to practice?

Knipper summarized several limitations of the study, including the small sample size, which limits the possibility of generalizing the findings. Moreover, some patients with underlying pulmonary disease have abnormal lung sounds that may be difficult to differentiate from crackles associated with secretion buildup. Although it may not place patients at great risk to make suctioning decisions based on lung auscultation, the nurse should carefully monitor the patient's response to therapy based on this protocol and should make appropriate adjustments if needed.

REFERENCE

1. Knipper, J. (1984). Evaluation of adventitious sounds as an indicator of the need for tracheal suctioning. *Heart and Lung, 13*(3), 292.

Chapter 10 SUMMARY

Activity and exercise assessment should focus on evaluating the following:

- Usual daily activities, including exercise and leisure
- Ability to engage in activity
- Psychological and physiologic response to activity and exercise
- Potential for activity intolerance based on the presence of significant risk factors

Multiple data sources are used to evaluate activity and exercise patterns. The data base should consist of the following:

The Health History

- Typical activities
- Physical fitness
- Activity tolerance
- Factors contributing to activity problems

The Physical Examination Findings

- General appearance
- Vital signs
- Cardiovascular system
- Respiratory system
- Musculoskeletal system
- Neurologic system (see Chap. 11)

Assessment of activity and exercise patterns provides cues to the following nursing diagnoses:

Activity intolerance
Potential activity intolerance
Diversional activity deficit
Impaired home maintenance management
Fatigue
Bathing/hygiene self-care deficit
Dressing/grooming self-care deficit
Feeding self-care deficit
Toileting self-care deficit

Examination of the cardiovascular, respiratory, and musculoskeletal systems may provide indicators for the following nursing diagnoses:

Ineffective airway clearance
Ineffective breathing pattern
Impaired gas exchange
Decreased cardiac output

Fluid volume excess
Altered (specify type) tissue perfusion (renal, cerebral, cardiopulmonary, gastrointestinal, peripheral)
Impaired physical mobility

Additionally, the nurse develops skill at detecting and monitoring the following clinical problems:

Acute arterial occlusion
Heart failure
Ischemic heart syndromes
Altered lung elasticity and compliance
  COPD
  ARDS
Pulmonary infectious and inflammatory processes
  Pneumonia
  Bronchitis
  Abscesses
Anatomic or mechanical alterations of the thorax or lungs
  Chest trauma and sequelae: pneumothorax, tension pneumothorax, flail chest
  Chest or lung masses
  Pulmonary emboli
  Pulmonary edema
Degenerative joint disease
Rheumatoid arthritis
Bursitis
Herniated disc syndrome

✳ CRITICAL THINKING

A local business is sponsoring a "Wellness Program" and developing a screening program to evaluate wellness and physical fitness levels. The employees range in age from 18 years to 70 years. The sponsor is planning to complete each individual screening session within 20 minutes. Screening techniques commonly used by health clubs are being considered, including measurement of resting and exercise-induced heart rates, anthropometrics, flexibility, and blood pressure.

Learning Exercises

1. Determine and describe the types of information needed to make judgments about physical fitness.

2. If you were to add an additional screening option to this program, describe what it would be and specify your rationale for the addition.

3. Develop a plan for evaluating physical fitness for persons with physical disabilities who could not participate in some of the exercises included in a typical screening program.

4. Select and describe the aspects of the musculoskeletal, cardiovascular, and respiratory examinations you believe would be most useful when making judgments about physical fitness.

BIBLIOGRAPHY

Bennett, A.F., & Sauer, H.C. (1991). Special considerations in cardio-vascular assessment of the aged. *Nurse Practitioner Forum, 2* (1), 55–60.

Dougherty, C.M. (1985). The nursing diagnosis of decreased cardiac output. *Nursing Clinics of North America, 20* (4), 787–799.

Eakin, P. (1989). Assessment of activities of daily living: A critical review, part 1. *British Journal of Occupational Therapy, 52* (1), 11–15.

Erickson, B.A. (1986). Detecting abnormal heart sounds. *Nursing '86, 16* (1), 58–63.

Estok, P.J., & Rudy, E.B. (1986). Jogging: Cardiovascular benefits and risks. *Nurse Practitioner, 11* (5), 21–28.

Finesilver, C. (1992). Respiratory assessment. *RN, 55* (2), 22–30.

Forshee, T. (1986). Chest pain. *Nursing '86, 16* (5), 34–41.

Gehring, P.E. (1992). Vascular assessment. *RN, 55* (1), 40–48.

Gender, A.R. (1983). Development of a comprehensive nursing history and physical assessment program in a rehabilitation setting. *Rehabilitation Nursing, 8* (5), 17–21.

George, M. (1988). Neuromuscular respiratory failure: What the nurse knows may make a difference. *Journal of Neurosurgical Nursing, 20* (2), 110–117.

Gordon, M. (1976). Assessing activity tolerance. *American Journal of Nursing, 76,* 72–75.

Gordon, M. (1979). The concept of nursing diagnosis. *Nursing Clinics of North America, 14* (3), 487–496.

Guzzetta, C.E., & Dossey, B.M. (1983). Nursing diagnosis: Framework, process, and problems. *Heart and Lung, 12* (3), 281–291.

Herman, J.A. (1986). Nursing assessment and nursing diagnosis in patients with peripheral vascular disease. *Nursing Clinics of North America, 21* (2), 219–231.

Kim, M.J. (1984). Physiologic nursing diagnosis: Its role and place in nursing taxonomy. In M.J. Kim, G.K. McFarland, & A.M. McLane (Eds.). *Classification of nursing diagnoses: Proceedings of the fifth national conference.* St. Louis: C.V. Mosby.

Massey, J.A. (1986). Diagnostic testing for peripheral vascular disease. *Nursing Clinics of North America, 21* (2), 207–281.

Milde, F. (1988). Impaired physical mobility. *Journal of Gerontological Nursing, 14* (3), 20–24, 38–40.

Miller, P.G. (1985). Assessing C.V.P. *Nursing '85, 15* (9), 44–46.

Orem, D.E. (1991). *Nursing: Concepts of practice* (4th ed.). New York: McGraw-Hill.

Petty, T.L. (1986). ABCs of simpler pulmonary function assessment. *Nurse Practitioner, 11* (6), 50–60.

Rossi, L., & Leary, E. (1992). Evaluating the patient with coronary artery disease. *Nursing Clinics of North America, 27* (1), 171–188.

Rothenberg, M.H., & Graf, B.K. (1993). Evaluation of acute knee injuries. *Postgraduate Medicine, 93* (3), 75–82, 85–86, 149–151.

Staff. (1991). Assessing the lungs. *Nursing '91, 21* (11), 32C–32F.

Assessing Cognition and Perception

Examination Guidelines

Assessment Terms

Perception	Corneal Reflex
Cognition	Deep Tendon Reflex
Special Senses	Hyperreflexia
Visual Acuity	Reinforcement
Tonometry	Paresthesias
Extraocular Eye Movements	Mental Status
Consensual Reaction	Ophthalmic (Funduscopic) Examination
Accommodation	Otoscopic Examination
Convergence	Dermatome
Red Reflex	Romberg Test
Snellen Chart	Level of Consciousness
Jaeger Chart	Awareness
Audiogram	Confabulation
Whisper Test	Receptive Aphasia
Watch-Tick Test	Expressive Aphasia
Weber Test	Visual Analog Scale
Rinne Test	Facial Mask of Pain

INTRODUCTORY OVERVIEW

Perception is the process of acquiring information about the environment through the senses and interpreting sensory input in a meaningful way. *Cognition* is the act or process of knowing; it involves intellectual functions and associated operations such as memory, learning, motivation, reasoning and thinking, and following instructions. Perception and cognition are closely interrelated, and alterations in either process may affect the other one.

Communication, including communication through speech, involves sending and receiving messages. Alterations in cognitive and perceptual processes (such as those that result from lesions to the language areas of the cerebral cortex) or alterations of the special senses may interfere with communication. Communication is also an interpersonal

Jill Fuller and Jennifer Schaller-Ayers:
HEALTH ASSESSMENT: A NURSING APPROACH, Second Edition.
© 1990, 1994 by J. B. Lippincott Company.

process and may be influenced by the type of relationship one person has with another. Therefore, communication problems should be evaluated from the perspective of roles and relationships as well as cognition and perception.

Assessment Focus

Assessment of cognitive and perceptual functions focuses on the sensory organs and structures required for vision, hearing, taste, touch, smell, and position sense; cognitive functions, including learning style, language or communication capabilities, and thought processes; and sensory–perceptual experiences, such as pain, hallucinations, and altered thought processes.

Judgments about cognition and perception are based on data obtained through interviewing the person, reviewing diagnostic tests results, and examining the body systems and functions essential for sensation, perception, cognition, and communication. When a problem is identified, a person can be referred to a specialist for more thorough evaluation. For example, a person with a speech problem may be evaluated by a speech therapist, or a person with a hearing deficit may benefit from further testing by an audiologist.

The goals for assessing cognition and perception include the following:

- Determining the status of the special senses: sight, hearing, smell, touch, and taste
- Determining the status of the deep senses, including kinesthetic (position) and vestibular (balance) senses
- Noting the person's perceptions of self and surroundings
- Identifying persons at risk for injury because of sensory and perceptual alterations
- Recognizing signs and symptoms of sensory and perceptual alterations
- Noting the person's response to sensory and perceptual alterations
- Evaluating cognitive functions

The methods for obtaining data related to these assessment goals are listed in the Assessment Focus display.

Nursing Diagnoses

Assessment of sensory and perceptual functions, such as vision, hearing, taste, touch, and smell, may provide cues to the following nursing diagnoses:

Sensory–perceptual alterations (specify): Visual, auditory, kinesthetic, gustatory, tactile, olfactory
Unilateral neglect
Potential for injury

Assessment of pain perception may result in one of the following diagnoses:

Pain
Chronic pain

Evaluation of cognitive functions, including language and mental status, may provide cues to the following nursing diagnoses:

Impaired verbal communication
Knowledge deficit (specify)
Altered thought processes

KNOWLEDGE BASE FOR ASSESSMENT

Assessing sensory, perceptual, and cognitive functions requires an understanding of the structures and processes involved with vision, hearing, taste, smell, touch, pain perception, language, and thought. This includes an understanding of the sensory organs involved, the peripheral nervous system, and the central nervous system. Structural and functional aspects of these organs and systems are discussed throughout this chapter (see "Anatomy and Physiology" sections).

Dimensions of Cognition

Cognition refers to processes of thinking and learning. Thinking requires mental processes such as knowing and being aware. Learning encompasses both thinking and doing. Learning is used in connection with some aspect of behavior such as solving a problem or carrying out a skill. Assessment of cognition involves consideration of several parameters, including attention, thought processes, reality testing, orientation, language, memory, problem solving, and decision making.

Different levels of cognitive function can be identified. Variations in cognition function may be age-related (see Chap. 18). For example, babies may acquire knowledge through manipulation of the environment, whereas older children are capable of logical thinking. Cognitive ability may also vary according to a person's educational level, life experiences, and cultural experiences. Cognitive abilities may be temporarily or permanently impaired as a result of illness, stress, medications or abuse of substances such as alcohol or drugs. Therefore, when you conduct a cognitive assessment, you should consider factors that might be influential in the person's background and environment.

Dimensions of Perception

Perception, the process of interpreting reality and events, is a multidimensional phenomenon. Therefore, a broad knowledge base is necessary to guide the collection and interpretation of assessment data effectively. The following overview of the various dimensions of perception introduces concepts included in this knowledge base and suggests other areas of human function that should be considered during the assessment process.

Physiologic Dimension. The body houses mechanisms for receiving sensory stimuli from the environment, transmitting sensory impulses to the brain, discriminating the

Assessment Focus **Cognition and Perception**

Assessment Goal	Data Collection Methods
1. Considering the person's developmental stage, determine the status of the special senses.	*Interview* • Status of the special senses: Does the interview indicate actual or potential problems with the special senses? *Observation* • Performance of activities of daily living: Do sensory deficits (*e.g.,* impaired vision) influence the person's ability to perform activities of daily living? • Communication patterns: Do sensory deficits (*e.g.,* impaired hearing) influence the person's ability to communicate? • Mobility patterns: Do problems with the special senses influence the ability to move safely in the environment? *Physical Examination* • Cranial nerve examination: Are the cranial nerves involved with sight, hearing, smell, touch and taste intact? • Eyes and vision: Does examination of the eyes and vision testing indicate actual or potential sensory alterations? • Ears and hearing: Does examination of the ears and hearing indicate actual or potential sensory alterations? • Sensory examination: Are there actual or potential problems with the ability to perceive light touch, pain and temperature?
2. Determine the status of deep senses including kinesthetic (position) and vestibular (balance) sense.	*Observation* • Mobility patterns: Are there altered patterns of mobility indicating possible sensory-perceptual alterations? • Signs of injury: Altered deep sensory function place the person at greater risk for injury. Are there signs of physical injury? *Physical Examination* • Sensory examination: Is proprioception and balance intact?
3. Evaluate the person's perceptions of self and surroundings.	*Interview and Observe* • Body awareness: Are there cues indicating perceptual deficits such as one-sided neglect? • Visual-spatial awareness: Are there cues indicating problems with visual-spatial awareness? • Orientation and level of consciousness: Could alterations in mental status indicate perceptual problems? *Observation* • Responses to items evaluated by administering the Glasgow Coma Scale: The Glasgow Coma Scale provides data about the person's level of consciousness and ability to respond to sensory stimuli.
4. Identify risk factors for injury because of sensory-perceptual dysfunctions.	*Interview* • Any component of the interview may reveal this type of risk factor(s). *Observation* • The person's environment: Are there factors or conditions in the environment that might contribute to sensory overload or sensory deprivation?
5. Evaluate the person's responses to sensory or perceptual alterations.	*Observe and Test* • Abilities to communicate: Are comprehension and expressive abilities intact? *Interview and Observe* • Self-concept: Have sensory perceptual problems altered self-esteem?
6. Determine the status of cognitive functions.	*Observe and Test* The following tests of cognitive function are incorporated into mental status testing: • Recent/remote memory • Classification ability • Computation ability • Judgment • Ability to follow instructions

nature of the stimuli received, and formulating and performing reaction responses. Basic knowledge about ascending and descending neural pathways and brain functions is essential for understanding and assessing this aspect of perception. In this chapter, these physiologic concepts are discussed as they pertain to methods for assessing cognition and perception.

Cognitive Dimension. Nerve impulses reaching the brain activate various cortical association areas in brain tissue. A person's responses are shaped by his or her previous experiences, age, and intellectual abilities, with storage areas of the brain becoming activated and memory triggered by the nerve impulses. As past experiences are remembered, learned behaviors or conditioned responses to these stimuli are initiated, and meaning becomes associated with the sensory experience. Without memory and experience, or the cognitive processing of nerve impulses, a person would perceive many sensory stimuli as undifferentiated environmental events.

Personal or Cultural Dimension. An individual's personality and cultural background can influence perceptions. Usually, personal and cultural experiences enhance perceptual functions. For example, culture gives meaning to the words used when communicating with others. Personal experiences, family experiences, cultural norms, and the expectations of other persons serve as frames of reference to validate a person's perceptions. At times, owing to personal or cultural influences, an individual's perception of reality may not agree with society's standards. Such a person may be considered by others to be highly individualistic or unrealistic and unable to think clearly.

Behavioral Response Dimension. Everyone evaluates his or her own perceptions of reality. Reactions may be described positively as adaptive, goal-oriented, appropriate, or constructive, or negatively as inappropriate, nonadaptive, or destructive. Often negative reactions occur when incoming stimuli are perceived as unfamiliar, repetitious, boring, or meaningless.

THE HEALTH HISTORY

The assessment of cognition and perception begins by obtaining a history focused on the special senses, general neurologic indicators, and cognitive processes. The history is compiled on the basis of interviewing the patient or family members and reviewing records noting the past medical history and medication history. The interview also provides an opportunity to evaluate cerebral functions because you can observe the person's level of consciousness, orientation, thought processes, and communication patterns. Data included as part of the history should help you make judgments about the following:

- *Sensory functions.* Are there problems with the sensory modes such as vision, hearing, taste, touch, or smell? Is the person experiencing acute or chronic pain? How does the person perceive this pain, and how does it affect his or her daily functioning?
- *Neurologic dysfunctions.* Does the person report additional signs and symptoms of neurologic dysfunction

such as weakness, numbness, vertigo, dizziness, incoordination, or seizures?
- *Factors affecting cognition and perception:* Is the person taking medications that might influence cognition or perception? Are there other health problems that might adversely effect cognitive/perceptual functions?

The Interview Guide shown in the accompanying display may be used to direct data collection.

A screening interview may be sufficient if the person appears to have no sensory-perceptual alterations, as would be the case if the person were fully alert, communicated easily, ambulated readily, and displayed no signs of fatigue or irritability. A screening interview is based on questions about the status of the special senses, especially vision and hearing. The person is asked about participation in recommended screening programs for detection of visual or hearing problems and about any other problems with the special senses.

If the screening interview indicates potential or actual sensory–perceptual problems, or if the general survey indicates a problem (as might be evident if the person appears to have difficulty hearing or concentrating), then a more comprehensive and lengthy interview can be conducted. Problems with cognition, perception, and the special senses can pose barriers to the interview process. If, for example, thought processes are altered or communication abilities are impaired, questions may need to be rephrased in simpler words and ample time allowed for the person to respond. In such cases, the person should be encouraged to freely discuss important topics. It is especially important that the person with sensory deficits wear any necessary eyeglasses or hearing aids during the interview. Some people may feel threatened or be embarrassed by questions they think are designed to reveal sensory or mental incapacities. The interviewer should make an effort to be especially tactful and empathetic.

For persons experiencing altered thought processes, communication disorders, or other types of cerebral dysfunctions, the structured approach to interviewing suggested by the interview guide may not be useful. In these situations, an alternative approach to data collection may be applied (see "Cognitive Functions," p. 361).

Sensory Functions

To acquire data about the special senses, ask questions that focus on the functional status of the eyes and ears, the ability to taste, smell, and touch, and any problems the person identifies with the sensory organs. If sensory deficits are identified, the person should be interviewed about specific responses to the deficits. For example, the existence of problems with vision should lead the interviewer to ask about self-care abilities and the potential for injury; problems with hearing should prompt questions pertaining to the person's ability to communicate and interact with others; problems with position sense and tactile abilities should prompt questions about measures taken to prevent injury; and problems with taste and smell should initiate discussion of any effects on nutritional status.

Interview Guide **Cognition and Perception**

Special Senses

Eyes and Vision

Last eye examination _____

Last glaucoma testing? _____

Do you wear glasses/contact lenses? _____

Contact lens type and cleaning system _____

Any vision problems not corrected by eyeglasses? If yes, describe any measures taken for compensation _____

Have you experienced any of the following?

_____ blind spots	_____ itching
_____ cataracts	_____ loss of visual acuity
_____ diplopia	_____ pain
_____ discharge	_____ photophobia
_____ eye infections	_____ redness
_____ eyestrain	_____ visual blurring
_____ headaches	

If yes to any of the above symptoms/conditions, describe fully _____
_____

Ears and Hearing

Have you ever had an audiogram? _____

If yes, indication and results _____
_____

Hearing aid(s)? _____

Any problem with the hearing aid(s)? _____

Date of last hearing aid examination _____

Describe care of hearing aid _____

Any hearing problems not corrected by hearing aid? _____

If yes, describe any measures for compensation _____
_____

Describe hygiene/cleaning related to ears _____

Have you experienced any of the following? _____

_____ drainage

_____ ear infections

_____ ear ringing/buzzing/roaring

_____ pain/fullness

_____ pain with eating

_____ "swimmer's" ear

If yes to any of the above symptoms/conditions, describe fully _____
_____

Other Special Senses

Any problems with:

_____ ability to feel pain sensations

_____ ability to feel temperature changes

_____ smell

_____ taste

If yes to any of the above symptoms/conditions, describe fully _____
_____

Pain

Are you experiencing pain? _____

If yes, indicate location, quality, intensity, duration (acute or chronic), precipitating factors, interventions, and effectiveness _____
_____

How does pain affect your daily activities? _____
_____

(continued)

Interview Guide **Cognition and Perception (continued)**

Neurologic Dysfunctions

Any problems with weakness or numbness? _____
If yes, describe onset, duration, location, characteristics, and precipitating activities _____
_____

Any problems with headaches? _____
If yes, describe location, onset, duration, frequency, associated symptoms, any precipitating/aggravating/relieving factors _____
_____

Any problems with vertigo (sensation of rotary movements)? _____
If yes, describe onset, duration, frequency, associated symptoms, any precipitating/aggravating/relieving factors _____
_____

Any problems with dizziness? _____
If yes, describe the onset or any associated activities _____
Did you lose consciousness ("faint," "black out")? _____
Frequency, duration, associated symptoms, any precipitating/aggravating/relieving factors _____
Any problems with coordination? Balance? Gait? Falling? _____
If yes, describe fully _____
_____

Any history of seizures? _____
If yes, describe sequence of events, symptoms, precipitating factors, history of previous seizures, use of anticonvulsant medications _____
_____

Factors Affecting Cognition and Perception

Current medical diagnosis _____
Previous hospitalizations/surgeries _____

Do you have any of these conditions?	Yes/No	Drug History	Yes/No
Autoimmune disorders	_____	Alcohol	_____
Diabetes mellitus	_____	Antibiotics	_____
Ear disorders	_____	Anticonvulsants	_____
Endocrine disorders	_____	Antidepressants	_____
Eye disorders	_____	Antihypertensives	_____
Head injury	_____	Aspirin	_____
Heart disease	_____	Sedatives	_____
Hypertension	_____	Sympathomimetics	_____
Metabolic disorders	_____	Tranquilizers	_____
Neuralgias	_____		
Stroke	_____		

Eyes and Vision. When interviewing a person about the status of the eyes and vision, it is important to determine the person's adherence to a recommended schedule of eye and vision examinations. Determine the date of the last eye examination and refraction by an ophthalmologist. People over age 40 should be asked if they have undergone glaucoma screening, either by the air puff tonometry method or Schiotz tonometry, because it is recommended that this screening be performed annually for this age group. Inquire about use of eye medications or eyedrops, including over-the-counter preparations. If a person wears contact lenses, determine the type of lens used and the cleaning system.

Open-ended questions may be helpful when inquiring about a person's eyes and vision, such as:

How has your vision been lately?
In what ways have your eyes been bothering you?

Ask about vision changes such as blurring, diplopia (double vision), blind spots, loss of visual acuity, photophobia, pain, itching, burning, discharge, or redness. If any symptoms are noted or identified, ask specific questions about the onset of the symptoms and any aggravating or relieving factors.

People who wear eyeglasses may be in need of a change in their current prescription. This situation may be indicated by reports of eyestrain and headaches, usually frontal and occurring after prolonged visual activities. Bifrontal headaches in a person over age 40 years may be symptomatic of chronic glaucoma, and the person should be referred for tonometry.

If a person's visual deficits are not compensated for entirely by eyeglasses, inquire if this situation has affected daily activities. For example, a person who is required to wear an eye patch following surgery might be asked if this interferes with managing the home; a person who has loss of night vision would be asked if he or she is able to drive an automobile after dark.

Finally, inquire about pathologic conditions that affect the eyes and vision, such as cataracts, glaucoma, trauma, and infection. Also, ask the person if he or she has a history of hypertension, diabetes, or other disorders known to affect vision.

Ears and Hearing. During the interview, inquire about screening activities and health practices for care of the ears and hearing. Determine whether or not a person has had an audiogram; if the person answers that he or she has had one, determine the reason. Audiograms are sensitive tests of hearing acuity, and generally are administered if subjective hearing losses are noted through gross screening methods. Ask the person about ear cleaning practices. Attempts to remove earwax using cotton-tipped applicators are potentially harmful and may indicate a need for health teaching. Some persons who have recurrent otitis externa or swimmer's ear will rinse the ear canal with alcohol to remove water after swimming or bathing; this is not usually harmful. Finally, inquire about the use of hearing aids. If a hearing aid is used, ask the date of the last hearing-aid examination, and if the person experiences any related problems. Determine the person's method of caring for the hearing aid.

The interview provides an opportunity to inquire about specific hearing problems. However, a person with a hearing deficit may hesitate to disclose the problem, so be alert to other cues. Note whether the person speaks with a distorted voice tone, lipreads, pays special attention to the interviewer's gestures, listens with the head turned to one side, leans toward the interviewer, or displays a strained facial expression while listening to the interviewer speak.

During the interview, ask questions to elicit symptoms associated with disorders of the ear. Ask the person if he or she has experienced ear pain, ear pain when eating or talking, drainage from the ear, or a feeling of fullness in the ears. If such symptoms are present, ask additional questions about the onset and duration of the symptoms and about any exacerbating factors. If a person reports drainage from the ear, ask about color and odor.

Inner ear disorders may affect equilibrium and should be considered if a person reports loss of coordination while walking. Other symptoms of vestibular dysfunction include tinnitus and vertigo. Tinnitus is a buzzing, ringing, or roaring sensation in the ear. Vertigo is a sensation of rotary movement, indicated by sensations of "the room spinning."

Any history of diseases affecting the ear, such as frequent ear infections or systemic infectious diseases, viral illnesses, mumps, or meningitis, should be noted during the interview. Certain drugs are potentially ototoxic; therefore, a medication history should be obtained from a person who reports hearing problems. Drugs that are potentially ototoxic include antibiotics such as streptomycin, gentamycin, kanamycin, neomycin, vancomycin, and viomycin; diuret-

ics, especially ethacrynic acid and furosemide; antimalarial agents such as chloroquine and quinine; and aspirin.

Interview to determine if ear or hearing problems have affected the scope or quality of the person's usual activities. People with hearing losses may be most impaired. Although the client may not relate the effects of a hearing loss during the interview, family members may report that the person has become withdrawn and apathetic; paranoia also may be observed in the person who cannot hear adequately.

Taste and Smell. When the history reveals disorders of taste and smell, which often occur together, it is helpful to consider possible causes. Alterations in taste and smell may accompany systemic diseases such as cancer, liver disease, and kidney disease. However, elderly persons may experience diminished taste sensation as a normal age-related change. Olfactory disorders are also associated with upper respiratory tract problems. Taste and smell disorders may be indicated if the person reports using greater amounts of sugar and salt than in the past to enhance the flavor of food.

Touch. Assess tactile sensation during the interview by asking the person questions about temperature discrimination and abnormal skin sensation (*paresthesias*). People with peripheral neuropathies, such as those associated with diabetes mellitus, may lose the ability to discriminate temperature, which places them at risk for burns, especially from hot water. Ask if burns have occurred while bathing and whether precautions have been taken to prevent skin burns, such as testing bath water with a thermometer.

Paresthesias are abnormal skin sensations such as burning, tingling, or "crawling" that can be intense enough to cause considerable discomfort. People with peripheral nerve damage secondary to diabetes mellitus or demyelinating diseases such as multiple sclerosis are at greatest risk and may report these distressing sensations.

Trigeminal neuralgia, a disorder of cranial nerve V, may cause altered facial sensations, including severe pain, along one or more trigeminal nerve branches. Determine if the person has experienced such episodes of severe pain and if these episodes are triggered easily by touch or cold. Touch and temperature sensations from eating may precipitate an attack.

Pain. Because pain is a sensory capability of human beings, you should inquire about pain when eliciting a health history pertaining to cognitive and perceptual functions. If the person reports the presence of pain, and especially if the person feels that pain interferes with other functions, you should initiate a more thorough assessment of the pain experience. Methods used to assess pain are discussed elsewhere in this chapter (see "Examination Guidelines: Pain").

Neurologic Dysfunctions

During the interview, you should also screen for indicators of basic neurologic dysfunctions. Some of these indicators may be detected as you ask about the status of the special senses. For example, a person with visual disturbances may also report that headaches are experienced with blurred vision. In addition, you should ask whether or not there are problems such as weakness, numbness, headaches, vertigo, dizziness, incoordination, and seizures. These problems indicate problems with the nervous system that might contribute to cognitive and perceptual dysfunctions.

Factors Affecting Cognition and Perception

A number of physiologic alterations, in addition to alterations of the sensory organs, place a person at increased risk for cognitive and sensory–perceptual problems. Such conditions may be identified by taking a medical–surgical history during the interview or by obtaining this information from medical records. Physiologic alterations that increase a person's risk of experiencing sensory–perceptual problems include neurologic disorders such as a cerebrovascular accident, disruption of fluid and electrolyte balance, and hypoxic states. Additionally, immobility resulting from illness and injury may alter cognitive and perceptual functions, especially in the presence of sensory overload or sensory deprivation.

A person's medication history may also be pertinent in identifying factors that contribute to cognitive and perceptual problems. For example, tranquilizers, sedatives, and alcohol can alter levels of consciousness and thought processes. Certain antibiotics may be ototoxic. A drug history may indicate the use of drugs that affect sensory functions, either as a side effect or as a result of toxicity.

DIAGNOSTIC STUDIES

A complete assessment of cognitive and perceptual functions includes an evaluation of cognitive or mental status and the neurologic system. In addition to acquiring data by means of interviewing and physical examination, pertinent data may be obtained through diagnostic testing and procedures.

Standardized tools to evaluate or test cognitive function include the following:

- Mental Status Questionnaire (MSQ)
- FROMAGE Test
- Mini Mental Status Examination

Common diagnostic studies to evaluate neurologic function include the following:

- Blood tests
- Radiographic studies
- Electromyography
- Electroencephalography
- Evoked potentials

Cognitive Function Evaluation Tools

Standardized tests of cognitive function may be used in some clinical settings. These tests may provide a rapid way to gain information and may allow for easy follow-up comparisons when serial evaluations of cognitive function are desired. Standardized cognitive function tests should not be used for persons who are aphasic or for some other reason are unable to participate.

Be aware that some standardized tests are culturally biased or irrelevant. You should also consider that some tests lack performance norms for elderly clients, especially those clients who are over age 80. Standardized tests may need to be repeated several times before accurate diagnoses are made. A series of scores may be a better indicator of cognitive function than a single score.

Examples of standardized tests of cognitive function are presented below.

Mental Status Questionnaire (MSQ). The MSQ (Kahn and associates, 1960) is administered by asking the person 10 questions; errors are recorded to calculate a final score ranging from 0 to 10. Three levels of cognitive function are possible, with a higher score indicating greater dysfunction. The test has been criticized as inappropriate for persons, such as those in long-term health care facilities, who may view time or current events as less relevant to their lives than do persons living in their own homes.

FROMAGE Test. FROMAGE is an acronym for Function, Reasoning, Orientation, Memory, Arithmetic, Judgment, and Emotional State. Each category in the FROMAGE Test (Libow, 1977) consists of questions to ask the client or guidelines for the examiner's observations. Responses are scored, with higher scores indicating higher levels of dysfunction. This test has been criticized as being too subjective.

Mini Mental State Examination. In the Mini Mental State Examination (Folstein and coworkers, 1975), the person is asked questions focusing on orientation, memory, concentration, calculation, and language abilities. Test items are scored, and a maximum score of 30 indicates optimal function. Although the test takes only 5 to 10 minutes to administer, performance of the final portion requires that the person have reading and writing skills. For impaired persons, this portion may take longer or may be impossible to complete.

Blood Tests

Blood samples may be examined to aid in the diagnosis of a number of neurologic disorders. Usually the clinician uses his or her judgment regarding which blood tests are pertinent in confirming or ruling out a particular diagnosis. Blood tests may also be helpful in determining the cause of an unexplained loss of consciousness. For example, a person presenting to the emergency department in an unexplained coma may have blood samples evaluated for glucose, BUN, PCO_2, PO_2, pH, ammonia, sodium, potassium, chloride, calcium, and toxic substances (drugs, alcohol).

Radiographic Studies

The neurologic system may be evaluated radiographically using a number of different modalities:

- *Diagnostic x-rays:* Used to diagnose fractures, injury, or degenerative conditions causing neurologic dysfunction, pain, or motor and sensory impairment

- *Magnetic resonance imaging (MRI):* Used to identify neurologic trauma, malignancies, and cerebral or spinal cord infarction
- *Computed tomography (CT scan):* Used to identify cerebrovascular disturbances, brain lesions or malignancies, and other neurologic disorders
- *Cerebral angiography.* Involves the infusion of radiopaque material into the cerebral arterial system in order to evaluate the condition of the cerebral vessels
- *Positron emission tomography (PET):* Involves application of CT and radionuclide imaging to provide diagnostic information about cerebral functions and structures
- *Radionuclide scanning:* Involves the use of gamma scintillation counters and injection of radioisotopes to detect pathologic conditions of the brain and evaluate cerebral blood flow

Electromyography

An electromyograph or electromyogram (EMG) is a graphic reading of nerve and muscle responses to electrical stimulation. The EMG indicates the status of nerves supplying muscles as well as muscle disorders (myopathies).

Electroencephalography

An electroencephalogram (EEG) is a graphic recording of brain wave activity. It provides important diagnostic information about abnormal electrical activity in the brain and is used primarily in the diagnosis of epilepsy, brain death, and drug intoxication.

Evoked Potentials

Evoked potentials (EP) measure changes in brain wave activity in response to sensory stimulation. This test is used to evaluate visual and auditory problems, peripheral nerve disorders, and spinal cord injury.

THE PHYSICAL EXAMINATION

Examination Focus

The primary goals of the physical examination in relation to cognition and perception are to determine the status of the neurologic and motor pathways essential for perception and to evaluate sensory organs and related functions. Physical examination findings may be helpful as you consider etiologies for sensory–perceptual alterations. Additionally, the physical examination may reveal problems that are secondary to cognitive and perceptual dysfunctions. For example, you may detect signs of physical injury resulting from impairment of one or more of the special senses such as bruises on the legs of an elderly person from bumping into furniture because of poor vision. In order to evaluate cognitive and sensory–perceptual functions, a physical examination is conducted with emphasis on the following:

- General appearance and surroundings
- Eyes and vision
- Ears and hearing
- Cranial nerves
- Motor functions and reflexes
- Sensory and cerebellar functions
- Cognitive function
- Pain

The overall status of the neurologic system should be evaluated when making judgments about cognitive and perceptual functions. This includes an examination of the special senses, vision and hearing, as well as related structures, the eyes and ears. Additionally, examination of the neurologic system includes evaluation of the cranial nerves, motor functions and reflexes, and sensory and cerebellar functions.

An evaluation of cognitive function focuses on those processes controlled by the cerebral cortex. This includes level of consciousness, orientation, thought processes, and communication patterns.

Because pain is a human sensory capability, pain is evaluated in the context of cognitive and perceptual function. Pain can readily be assessed if the person discloses to you the nature of his or her personal pain experience, or you might detect evidence of pain by observing the person's nonverbal behaviors and body system responses.

General Appearance and Surroundings

A survey of the person's general appearance and surroundings may provide cues to sensory–perceptual problems or cognitive impairment.

For example, you may note that the person wears eyeglasses or hearing aids and deduce an impairment of the special senses of vision and hearing.

A person's facial expression may indicate some level of cognitive or perceptual dysfunction. For example, a flat affect may be a sign of apathy or depression, which in turn may be a sign or etiology for cognitive and perceptual dysfunctions. Patients suffering from chronic pain (a perceptual problem) may also develop a flat affect known as the "mask of chronic pain." Facial expression also indicates whether or not the person is attentive to various stimuli. You should note whether or not the person looks at demonstration activities, startles at loud, unexpected noises, or listens when you speak.

During general inspection, note condition of the person's skin and grooming, which may indicate level of functioning in relation to cognition and perception. For example, if the person has skin ulcers or burn scars, determine whether this is related to impaired tactile sensation, poor judgment, or other forms of sensory impairment. If grooming appears neglected on one side of the body, the person may have the perceptual dysfunction known as one-sided neglect.

As you survey general appearance you should also make observations of the person's surroundings and general environment. Environmental factors may contribute to sensory–perceptual problems, particularly sensory deprivation or sensory overload. You should also consider the status of other major body systems, especially if dysfunction might adversely affect cognitive and perceptual functions.

Make note of the quality of the sensory stimuli emanating from a person's surroundings, especially if the person is at high risk for sensory–perceptual alterations.

Sensory deprivation may occur as a result of decreased sensory input from the surroundings, or inability to extract meaning from the sensory input. An environment characterized by minimal, meaningless, or monotonous sensory input may contribute to this state, especially if the person has other impairments of the sensory system such as vision or hearing deficits. Environmental factors that may be associated with sensory deprivation include bed rest, lack of social interaction, darkness, or separation from familiar personal objects.

Sensory overload occurs when the person is bombarded with meaningless, confusing, or monotonous stimuli, such as frequently happens with patients in intensive care units. Equipment sounds, monitoring systems, continual interruptions, and constant lighting can contribute to sensory overload.

The environment should also be evaluated to identify factors that can be altered to contribute to optimal function for persons with cognitive or perceptual alterations. For persons with visual deficits, the surroundings are evaluated to determine if they are cluttered or have unnecessary barriers to safe ambulation. Be aware that people who have diminished hearing capability may prefer to increase the volume of television or radio above the normal level.

Associated Body System Alterations

Dysfunction of major body systems may adversely affect cognitive and perceptual functions. For example, if the cardiovascular and respiratory systems are impaired to the extent that oxygenation is affected, cognitive and perceptual problems may be observed. Orthostatic blood pressure alterations, carotid bruits (which may indicate that blood flow to the brain has been obstructed) or hypoventilation syndromes (which may cause CO_2 narcosis) can all contribute to cerebral dysfunction.

Similarly, hepatic or renal system disease can affect cognition and perception by altering the balance of essential electrolytes or chemical substrates required for brain metabolism. Significant changes in a person's mental status may be noted if these systems are impaired.

THE EYES AND VISION
Anatomy and Physiology Overview

Eye Structures and Functions. The eyes are set in fat-cushioned skull orbits. Openings in the six bones composing each orbit allow the passage of blood vessels and nerves. The major posterior opening, the optic foramen, permits passage of the ophthalmic artery and optic nerve (cranial nerve II), which are visualized during fundoscopic eye examination. Visual images are transmitted by the optic nerve to the occipital lobe of the cerebral cortex. Six extrinsic oculomotor muscles attach to the sclera near the ante-

rior portion of the eyeball and facilitate eye movement and rotation. Additionally, the extrinsic eye muscles help maintain a normal conjugate gaze, meaning that both eyes are midposition and oriented in the same direction in the resting state. During eye examination, testing the extraocular eye movements and eye position will enable you to assess the muscles and cranial nerves III, IV, and VI (oculomotor, trochlear, and abducens).

The visible, external eye structures, including ductal openings of the lacrimal sac, are shown in Figure 11-1. The lacrimal apparatus comprises the lacrimal gland, which produces tears to lubricate the eye; the puncta, located lateral to the inner canthus, which drain tears into the lacrimal canaliculus; and the lacrimal sac.

The conjunctiva is membranous tissue covering the inner eyelids (palpebral conjunctiva) and the sclera of the eyeball (bulbar conjunctiva). Except for its most anterior portion, the eyeball is surrounded by a tough, fibrous layer of sclera. The limbus marks the point at which the sclera merges with the cornea, a transparent structure that allows light to enter the eye to stimulate the retinal rods and cones. The sclera becomes discolored or jaundiced from certain systemic diseases such as liver disease.

The pigmented iris surrounds the pupil. The pupil changes size as the iris sphincter and dilator muscles and the ciliary muscle beneath the sclera are stimulated. These muscles, called the intrinsic eye muscles, are innervated by cranial nerve III (oculomotor) and nerve fibers from the ciliary ganglion. Pupil size is determined by the balance between sympathetic and parasympathetic discharge. Alterations in pupillary reflexes and size may indicate oculomotor nerve impairment. Pupillary responses may also be affected by seizure activity and certain drugs.

The anterior chamber, a fluid-filled space, is located between the cornea and pupil. Intraocular pressure (normally 20–25 mm Hg) is a function of fluid movement and drainage through the anterior and posterior chambers. If the canal of Schlemm becomes blocked, fluid backup and increased pressure may damage the retina and optic nerve. This condition, glaucoma, may develop slowly and insiduously as a person ages. Intraocular pressure measurements are used to screen for and monitor glaucoma before irreversible damage occurs.

The crystalline lens, which bends incoming light rays to project them to the retina, is not readily visible by inspection. If the lens develops opacities or cataracts, whitened areas may be visible through the pupil. Such changes are seen best through the ophthalmoscope, an instrument for viewing internal eye structures.

The most frequently examined parts of the inner eye include the retina and related structures. The retina, the eye's innermost layer, receives light rays from the lens. Light must pass through the nine retinal layers before reaching the cones (daylight vision receptors), or rods (dim-light vision receptors), which initiate a neural impulse ultimately perceived by the brain as a visual image.

Several retinal structures can be noted when viewing the optic fundus or the posterior eye wall through an ophthalmascope. The retina itself is transparent. The orange–red coloration seen through the ophthalmoscope results from the underlying, highly vascularized choroid layer. The

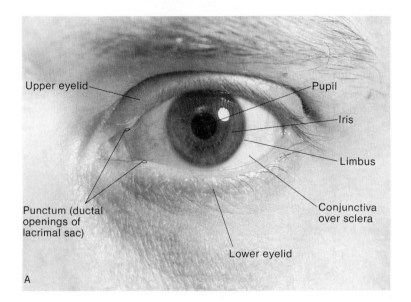

A

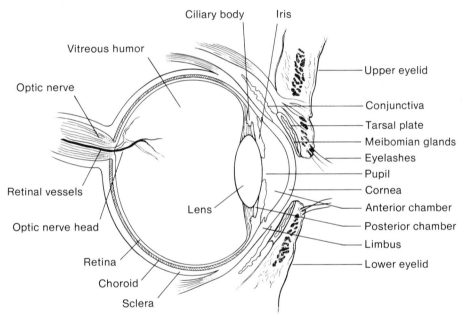

B

Figure 11–1. The eye. (**A**) Visible landmarks of the external eye. (**B**) Cross-section of the eye.

optic nerve leaves the retina through a site called the optic disc or the physiologic blind spot, thus named because it has no retinal neurosensory receptors. The optic disc is in the nasal quadrant of the fundus. The central depression in the disc is called the physiologic cup. Optic disc nerve tissues are continuous with brain nerve tissues. Consequently, brain swelling may be associated with visible disc swelling, a condition known as *papilledema*.

Also traveling through the optic disc are four sets of arterioles and veins, which bifurcate and extend toward the peripheral fundus. These retinal vessels are readily identifiable during examination. Systemic vascular changes, especially those resulting from hypertension and diabetes mellitus, may be detected by examining retinal vessels.

The retinal depression, or fovea centralis, is located adjacent to the optic disc in the temporal quadrant of the fun-

dus. The macula surrounds the fovea. The macula, the most darkly pigmented area of the retina, is highly concentrated with cones and represents the area of most highly resolved central and color vision.

Visual Perception. Light rays pass through the refractive eye structures (cornea, aqueous humor, lens, vitreous humor) to the retina. Accommodation occurs when the lens becomes thicker or thinner according to light rays transmitted from near or distant objects. Visual deficits known as refractive errors are common in many individuals. Myopia (nearsightedness) occurs when light rays converge before reaching the retina because the anteroposterior diameter of the eyeball is greater than normal. As a result, visual acuity for distant objects is diminished. Hypermetropia (farsightedness) occurs when the anteroposterior eyeball diameter is shorter than usual, which causes light rays to scatter beyond the retina. Accommodation processes compensate for this refraction error when the person is focusing on distant objects, but close images are blurred as compensation fails. Refractive errors are detected during examination by visual acuity tests.

Retinal neurosensory receptors receive the image refracted through the lens, initiating a photochemical reaction and a neural impulse that travels the visual pathways to the occipital cerebral cortex.

Nerve fibers from the retina enter the optic nerves, which pass through the optic foramen and meet just anterior to the pituitary gland at the optic chiasm. The medial fibers from each eye cross at the chiasm, and fibers from the lateral retina continue toward the brain uncrossed. The manner in which the fibers cross has great clinical and assessment significance. Characteristics of a particular visual deficit may be analyzed to determine what part of the visual pathway has been affected.

Physical Examination   *Eyes and Vision*

General Principles

The eyes should be examined using inspection and palpation. A special instrument, the ophthalmoscope, is used to inspect the interior ocular structures.

Visual acuity can be determined by special techniques that evaluate far vision, near vision, and peripheral vision. The equipment and procedures for testing visual acuity vary slightly, depending on characteristics of the person being tested. For example, when testing far or near vision in people who cannot read, appropriate substitutions are made for letter charts.

Equipment

- Penlight
- Cotton wisps and cotton-tipped applicators
- Ophthalmoscope
- Schiötz tonometer (optional; used to measure intraocular pressure)
- Snellen Chart for far-vision testing.
- Jaeger Chart for near-vision testing; newsprint and telephone directory print may be substituted for Jaeger chart
- Occlusive covers for individual eye testing (3 × 5 card, paper cup, or commercially available shields, which must be disinfected between uses)
- Ishihara plates (optional; used to test color vision)

Ophthalmoscope

Although several different brands of ophthalmoscope are available, all have similar features. The handle usually contains batteries for the light source, and can be unscrewed from the head and plugged into a wall socket for recharging. All models have a focus wheel to adjust the lens refraction. Initially, the focus is set on 0 diopters, meaning the lens neither converges nor diverges light rays. Depending both on your eyes and the client's, this setting should be adjusted to bring the fundus into sharpest focus. Then the focus wheel should be rotated toward positive numbers to bring near objects into focus. Some ophthalmoscopes have wheels for dialing different lens types. Generally, you will use the lens with the largest beam shining through clear glass. Slit-like beams and red glass are used during special examinations by the ophthalmologist. The ophthalmoscope is discussed further in Chapter 3.

Schiötz Tonometer

The Schiötz tonometer is an instrument that measures intraocular pressure. Nurses do not routinely use this instrument because more accurate methods for measuring intraocular pressure, such as applanation tonometry or air puff tonometry, are available through an ophthalmologist. The Schiötz tonometer footplate should be gently placed on the central cornea after first being zeroed on a test block (Fig. 11-2). A plunger will move along a scale to give a reading, which should be converted to mm Hg by consulting a chart. The instrument must be thoroughly disinfected after use.

Hygiene

Wash your hands before palpating the external eye structures. If signs of infection are present in one eye, be careful not to cross-contaminate the other eye. In such a case, wash your hands before examining each eye, and examine the infected eye last.

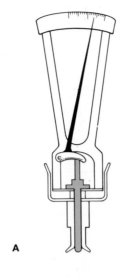

A

Figure 11–2. Schiotz tonometer. (**A**)The plunger (*blue*) measures the ease of indentation of the cornea. (**B**) Indentation of the anesthetized cornea by the plunger of the tonometer to measure ocular tension.

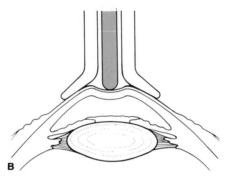

B

Pupil Dilation

The pupils must be slightly dilated for you to view the interior eye with the ophthalmoscope. Generally, this condition is achieved by darkening the room. Short-acting, mydriatic eyedrops can be used, but it is important for several reasons to first consult a physician. Mydriatics dilate the pupil by inducing temporary cycloplegia (paralysis of the ciliary muscle). Accommodation reflexes may also be lost, and acute glaucoma may be precipitated in a susceptible person. Additionally, iatrogenic pupil dilation may obscure the significant neurologic assessment parameter of pupil size and reactivity.

Examination and Documentation Focus

- *External eye:* Symmetry, shape, eyebrows, eyelids, eyelashes, skin integrity, infestations
- *Lacrimal apparatus:* Lacrimal sac and gland, puncta, tears
- *Conjunctiva:* Palpebral and bulbar
- *Sclera, cornea, and iris*
- *Pupil:* Color, size, pupillary reflexes, retinal light reflex
- *Retina:* Color and pigmentation, vessels, macula, optic disk
- *Eye movements:* Conjugate gaze, extraocular eye movements
- *Intraocular pressure*
- *Visual acuity:* Snellen test results, Jaeger test results, peripheral vision, gross vision

Examination Guidelines   *Eyes*

Procedure

1. INSPECT THE EXTERNAL EYE STRUCTURES.

   a. Stand facing the client (who should be sitting on the examining table). Inspect the client's eyebrows, lashes, and eyelids, and note eye shape and symmetry.

   b. Observe blinking, noting if there is complete closure of the lid. Note the eyeball position and any spontaneous eye movements.

2. INSPECT AND PALPATE THE LACRIMAL APPARATUS (optional).

   a. Look at the punctal openings just lateral to the inner canthus. Gently stretch the bottom eyelids with your thumb to better expose puncta and use a penlight to enhance visualization.

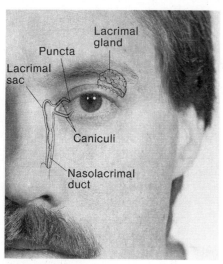

Lacrimal apparatus

Clinical Significance

Normal Findings

Eye shape and symmetry: Symmetry of the eyes and associated structures. Shape of the eyes varies from round to almond. In Asian persons, the skin fold over the inner canthus (the epicanthus) may cause eye shape to appear narrow. Eyes may appear rounded in some black persons because the eyeball protrudes slightly beyond the supraorbital ridge.

Eyebrows: Appearance may vary according to genetic background. No alopecia.

Eyelashes: Curve outward, away from the eye. No alopecia.

Eyelids: The upper lid does not cover the pupil when open, but may cover the upper portion of iris; eyelids should open and close completely without unilateral drooping or drag; spontaneous blinking should be observed every few seconds.

Deviations from Normal

See Display, "Structural Alterations and Disorders of the Eye."

Normal Findings

Puncta visible but without excessive discharge unless the person is crying or the area is momentarily irritated. Lacrimal sac and gland nonpalpable and nontender; eye surface moist.

Deviations from Normal

Excessive tearing

continued

Eyes

Procedure

b. If you suspect nasolacrimal duct blockage, indicated by excessive tearing, gently press over the duct with your index finger just inside the lower orbital rim. Note any discharge from the puncta. Proceed carefully because the area will be sensitive if inflamed. Repeat for the other eye.

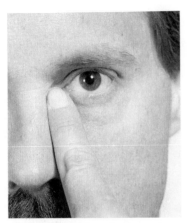

Lacrimal apparatus palpation

3. INSPECT THE LACRIMAL GLAND AND UPPER PALPEBRAL CONJUNCTIVA (optional).

a. Inspect the lacrimal gland by gently everting the upper lid. Ask the person to look downward with the eyes slightly open. Gently grasp the lid between your thumb and forefinger at the lid/eyelash junction. With your free hand, place a cotton-tipped applicator against the lower portion of the lid while pulling the eyelashes up to evert the lid. Be careful not to press the applicator against the eyeball.

b. Move the cotton-tip applicator away and hold the lid against the upper bony orbit to complete inspection. Note the small, visible portion of the lacrimal gland and at the same time, inspect the upper palpebral conjunctiva. Also note the appearance of exposed sclera.

c. Then, pull the lid lightly forward. The lid will resume normal position as you release and the person blinks.

d. Repeat this procedure on the other eye.

Clinical Significance

Deviations from Normal

Dacryoadenitis: Inflammation of the lacrimal gland. The upper, temporal eyelid may be swollen and red.

Dacrocystitis: Inflammation of the lacrimal sac. Associated with profuse tearing (epiphora), redness, swelling, and pain near the inner canthus. Dacrocystitis is associated with an obstructed nasal lacrimal duct, which may be congenital or acquired through trauma or infection.

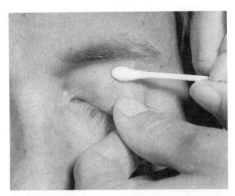

Eyelid eversion: Step a

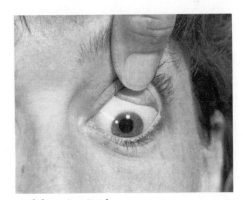

Eyelid eversion: Step b

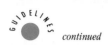 *continued*   *Eyes*

Procedure

4. CONTINUE INSPECTING THE INNER CONJUNCTIVA.

   Gently stretch the lower lid downward to see the lower palpebral conjunctiva. Note the appearance of the exposed sclera.

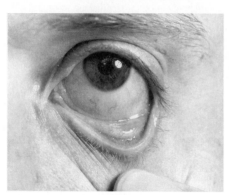

Lower palpebral conjunctiva inspection

5. INSPECT THE REMAINING VISIBLE OCULAR STRUCTURES.

   Continue to note the appearance of the sclera. Use a penlight to tangentially illuminate the lens and cornea. Inspect from several angles, noting surface features and opacities. Note and compare iris shape and color, and pupil shape and size.

6. EVALUATE EXTRAOCULAR EYE MOVEMENTS (EOMs).

   a. Instruct the person to follow your finger or pen with his or her eyes while keeping the head stationary. Move your finger or pen through the six cardinal fields of gaze, returning to the central starting point before pointing toward the next field. Remember that if you move too quickly, the person may have difficulty following.

Clinical Significance

Normal Findings

Palpebral conjunctiva: Pink, moist, and without lesions. Small vessels may be visible.

Sclera: White, pale yellow cast in some black persons.

Normal Findings

Appearance of bulbar conjunctiva: Transparent, allowing white sclera to show through. Small conjunctival blood vessels may be visible but normally are not dilated (bloodshot eyes).

Cornea: Smooth, clear, transparent; convex curvature.

Iris: Color varies: blue, brown, gray, green with markings. Shape is round.

Tests the function of cranial nerves III, IV, and VI.

Normal Findings

Extraocular movements: Voluntary movement of eyes through the six cardinal positions without nystagmus (involuntary cyclical movement of the eyeball). However, slight nystagmus when the eyes are at the far lateral position of gaze is within normal limits.

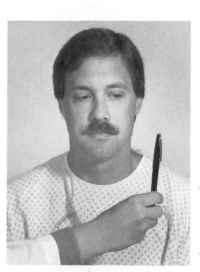

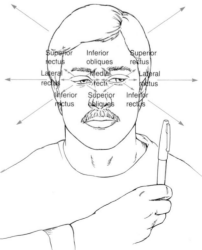

Assessing extraocular eye movements

nystagmus; wandering
strabismus

Eyes

Procedure

b. When the person looks toward the most distal point in the lateral and vertical fields, carefully note eyeball movements for normal conjugate movements and nystagmus.

7. TEST FOR STRABISMUS (cover-uncover test).

Ask the person to focus on your pen, which you should hold approximately one foot away, while you cover one of the person's eyes. Note any movement in the uncovered eye. As you remove the cover note any movement in the other eye.

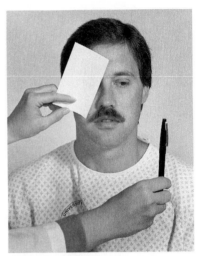

Strabismus testing

8. EVALUATE PUPILLARY REFLEXES.

a. *Pupillary light reflex.* Darken the room, or turn the person away from direct light sources. To obtain maximal pupil dilation, have the person focus on a distant object. Ask the person to cover one eye while you shine a light source from the side toward the pupil of the uncovered eye. Repeat testing with the other eye.

b. *Consensual reaction.* Shine the light source toward one eye from the side and observe both pupils. Both should constrict despite the fact that light is directed toward one eye. The constriction of the eye that is not receiving the direct light is the consensual response.

Clinical Significance

Normal Findings

Conjugate gaze: Eyes midposition when at resting position.

Normal Finding

The gaze remains on the pen during covering and uncovering, indicating good muscle strength the binocular vision.

Normal Findings

Appearance of pupils: Black, of equal size, round. Five percent of the population have slight inequality in pupil size (anisocoria), which is considered clinically insignificant.

Light reflex: Pupils constrict directly and consensually.

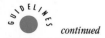 *continued*

Eyes

Procedure

c. *Accommodation and convergence.* Hold your index finger approximately 2 feet from the person's eyes. Ask the person to focus on your index finger as you move it toward his or her nose. The person should be able to watch your finger as it moves.

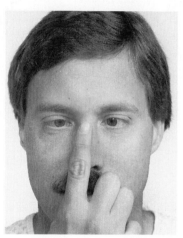

Testing accommodation and convergence

9. BEGIN THE OPHTHALMOSCOPIC EXAMINATION BY VISUALIZING THE RED REFLEX.

   a. In a darkened room, instruct the person to look at a distant point and keep his or her eyes focused there throughout the ophthalmoscopic examination.

   b. Grasp the ophthalmoscope with your right hand when you are examining the person's right eye. Check to see that the lens is set at 0, and turn on the light source.

   c. Position yourself at arm's length from the person; to assist your stability place your left thumb over the person's left eyebrow.

   d. From an angle about 15 degrees lateral to the person's line of vision, shine the ophthalmoscope toward the pupil of the right eye and look through the ophthalmoscope's viewing hole. Note the red reflex.

Clinical Significance

Normal findings

The pupils should constrict as you move the finger closer (accommodation) and the eyes should converge (cross). Accommodation is necessary for far-to-near focusing.

Normal Findings

The *red reflex* is the orange-red coloration of the fundus visible through the pupil.

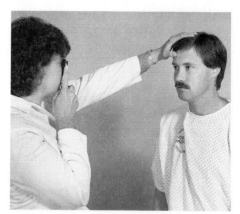

Ophthalmoscopic examination: Visualizing the red reflex

Deviations from Normal

Lens opacities (cataracts) may interfere with red reflex visualization. Cataracts appear as gray or white opacities, or may appear as black spots against the background of the red light reflex. Cataracts vary in size and configuration.

GUIDELINES

continued   ***Eyes***

Procedure

e. As you continue to look through the viewing hole and focus on the red reflex, move toward the person until your forehead touches your thumb on the person's forehead.

Clinical Significance

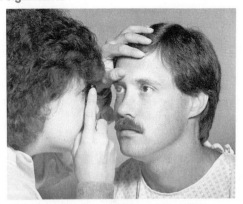
Ophthalmoscopic examination: Inspecting the anterior chamber, lens, and vitreous body

10. INSPECT THE ANTERIOR CHAMBER, LENS, AND VITREOUS BODY.

Inspect the anterior chamber and lens for transparency. Visualization may be made easier by rotating the lens toward positive numbers (+15 to +20), which are designed to focus objects closest to the ophthalmoscope.

Deviations from Normal

Hyphemia: The appearance of blood in the anterior chamber, which usually results from eye trauma. The red blood cells may settle and cause only the lower half of the anterior chamber to appear bloody.

Hypopyon: The accumulation of white blood cells in the anterior chamber, which causes a cloudy appearance in front of the iris. Secondary to inflammatory response accompanying corneal ulceration or iritis.

11. INSPECT THE OPTIC DISK.

a. Rotate the lens back to the 0 setting; then, focusing on a retinal structure such as a vessel or the disk, rotate the lens until you produce the sharpest focus.

The final setting will vary according to the specific characteristics of your eye structure and the client's eye structure. If the client is myopic, the eyeball will be longer and a negative setting will enable you to focus further back. Use the positive settings to visualize across the shorter eyeball distance that is associated with farsightedness.

b. If you do not see the optic disk, find a blood vessel and follow it in the direction in which the vessel thickens. This will lead you visually to the disk. Note that vessels have fewer bifurcations toward the disk.

c. Once the disk is visible, refocus if necessary to obtain the sharpest definition.

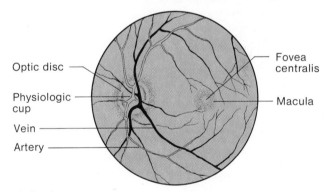
The fundus

Normal Findings

Optic disk: Round to oval with sharply defined borders; whitish or pink; 1.5 mm in diameter when magnified 15 times through ophthalmoscope. Physiological cup is slightly depressed and lighter in color than the remainder of the disk; cup occupies half of disk diameter.

Deviations from Normal

Papilledema: Swelling of the optic disk that occurs secondary to the venous stasis accompanying hypertension or increased intracranial pressure. Swelling obscures the disk margins and the physiological cup is no longer visible.

Glaucomatous cupping of the optic disk: Occurs when increased intraocular pressure is transmitted to the retina. The physiological cup enlarges, filling more than half the disk diameter.

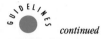

continued

Eyes

Procedure

12. INSPECT THE RETINAL VESSELS AND RETINA.

   a. Evaluate the retinal vessels that are distributed from the disk to the periphery. Four sets of arterioles and veins pass through the disk.

   b. Systematically inspect the retinal vessels by moving your line of vision through major retinal quadrants, using the person's pupil as an imaginary fulcrum.

Clinical Significance

Normal Findings

Arterioles: Progressively smaller diameter away from optic disk; bright red with narrow light reflex; 25% smaller than veins; no narrowing or nicking.

Veins: Progressively smaller diameter away from optic disk; dark red, no light reflex; occasionally pulsatile.

A-V ratio: Arteriole-to-vein ratio in relation to vessel diameter (A-V ratio) is 2:3 or 4:5.

Structural Alterations and Disorders of the Eye

Eye examination may reveal alterations or disorders of the external eye. Assessment includes determining if such alterations interfere with visual perception, comfort, or body image.

Exopthalmus

- The eyes appear to bulge with proptosis (downward eye displacement).
- Possible etiologies include cranial tumors and hyperthyroid disease.
- The condition may be detected by direct frontal inspection or by inspecting eye position while looking downward across the surface of the person's forehead.

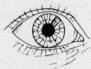

Exophthalmos

Enopthalmus

- A sunken eye appearance.
- May occur secondary to dehydration or following fracture of the orbital floor.

Ptosis

- Drooping of the upper eyelid.
- The most common causes include oculomotor nerve dysfunction (cranial nerve III) or sympathetic nerve dysfunction.
- May also be congenital.

Ptosis

Epicanthal folds

- Characteristic of certain races, such as Asian persons.
- Also noted in persons with Down's syndrome (trisomy 21).

Ectropion

- Marked eversion of the edge of the eyelid.
- The palpebral conjunctiva is exposed and susceptible to drying.
- If the punctum of the lower lid turns out, the eye no longer drains satisfactorily and excessive tearing occurs.
- Ectropion may occur following scar formation or secondary to muscle weakness.
- More often occurs in elderly persons.

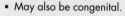

Ectropion

Entropion

- Inward turning of the eyelid.
- May be associated with *trichiasis,* or eyelash contact with the conjunctiva and cornea.
- Usually painful.
- Causes are the same as for ectropion.

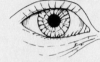

Entropion

Blepharitis

- Infection along the lid margins.
- Usually caused by *Staphylococcus aureus,* seborrhea, or a combination of both.
- The lid margins appear reddened and yellowish.
- Greasy scales may be noted.

Stye

- An infection occurs in the glands around the eyelash hair follicles.
- Associated with localized pain, swelling, and redness.
- A pustule usually forms on the eyelid margin.

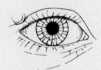

Stye

Chalazion

- Infection of the meibomian gland.
- Usually caused by *S. aureus.*
- Swelling and redness occur.
- No pustule formation.
- May be painless.

Chalazion

(continued)

Structural Alterations and Disorders of the Eye (continued)

Narrow Angle Glaucoma

- Associated with an anatomically shallow anterior chamber.
- Signs and symptoms include diffuse eye redness, pain, blurred vision, cornea clouding, moderate pupil dilation, and elevated intraocular pressure (40 mm Hg or more).

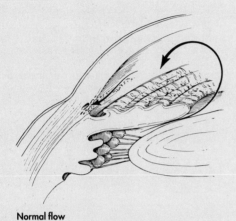

Normal flow

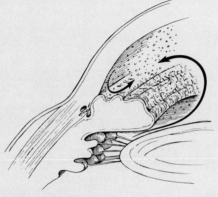

Narrow-angle glaucoma

Open Angle Glaucoma

- The size of the anterior chamber remains normal.
- The diagnosis is based on measuring intraocular pressure, which is usually elevated.

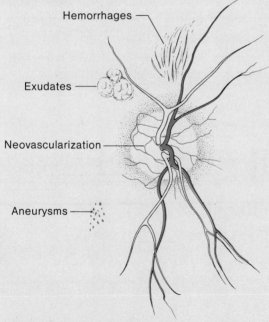

Hemorrhages

Exudates

Neovascularization

Aneurysms

Diabetic alterations of the fundus

Diabetic Alterations

Vascular changes associated with diabetes mellitus may contribute to fundoscopic changes, including:

- Round and flame-shaped retinal hemorrhages
- Venous dilation
- Microaneurysms
- Retinal detachment
- Neovascularization

Hypertensive Alterations

The retinal vessels and retinal background may be altered by hypertension. The Keith-Wagner (KW) classification system may be used to describe the severity and prognosis of the hypertension based on retinal changes. KW classifications, beginning with the least severe conditions are as follows:

- *KW1:* Minimal arteriolar narrowing and irregularity.
- *KW2:* Marked arteriolar narrowing and arteriovenous nicking (AV nicking). With AV nicking, the vein appears to stop abruptly on either side of the arteriole. This finding also indicates arteriosclerotic changes.
- *KW3:* Flame-shaped or round hemorrhages and fluffy "cotton wool" exudates noted on the retina. Cotton wool patches represent small infarcts.
- *KW4:* Any of the above signs plus papilledema.

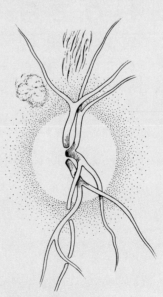

Hypertensive alterations

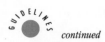 *continued*   *Eyes*

Procedure

c. Note any underlying retinal lesions as you inspect each quadrant. Also note the crossing points of arterioles and veins.

13. INSPECT THE MACULA

Ask the person to look directly into the ophthalmoscope light. Find the macula, which is temporal from the disk. The fovea, the center of the macula, should be approximately two optic disk diameters from the optic disk border. The macula may be difficult to see if the person's pupil is not sufficiently dilated.

14. ASSESS THE OTHER EYE.

To examine the person's left eye, hold the ophthalmoscope in your left hand. Place your right hand on the person's forehead and repeat the examination sequence.

Clinical Significance

Normal appearance of retina: The retina is transparent but the diffuse orange-red color of the choroid layer shows through; pigmentation may be darker in black persons. Spotty color alterations such as white patches may be abnormal.

Deviations from Normal

See Display, "Structural Alterations and Disorders of the Eye."

Normal appearance: Darker than the surrounding fundus; relatively avascular.

Examination Guidelines   *Testing Visual Acuity*

Procedure

1. TEST FAR VISION USING A SNELLEN CHART OR A COMPARABLE STANDARDIZED CHART.

Clinical Significance

The Snellen charts in the center and at right (*below*) may be more appropriate for testing illiterate adults and very young children.

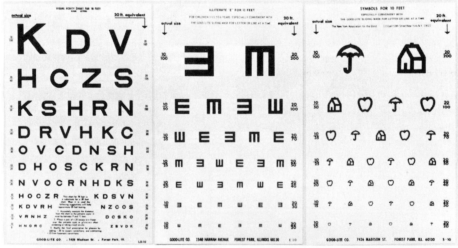

Snellen charts

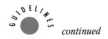

continued

Testing Visual Acuity

Procedure

a. The person should stand 20 feet from the chart in a well-lit area. The person may wear corrective lenses.

Ask the person to cover one eye with a shield while you test the other eye.

b. Ask the person to read the letters as you point to progressively smaller print. Note the last line that the person reads accurately.

c. Report vision acuity as a fraction, such as 20/20. The numerator indicates in feet the distance the person stood from the chart. The denominator indicates the distance at which the normal eye can read the line of letters. (This figure is printed next to each line of letters or figures on the chart.)

If the person wears glasses during testing, note that on the report. Record, for example, "20/30, corrected."

d. Repeat the testing procedure for the other eye.

2. TEST NEAR VISION USING A JAEGER CHART OR AN APPROPRIATE SUBSTITUTE.

a. Screen near vision acuity by asking the person to read from a Jaeger chart held 12 to 14 inches from the eyes.

b. If a Jaeger chart is not available, ask the person to read from a newspaper or a telephone directory.

3. TEST VISUAL FIELDS (PERIPHERAL VISION) BY CONFRONTATION.

a. Face the person being tested at a distance of 2 or 3 feet.

b. Ask the person to cover his or her left eye while you cover your right eye. Both you and the client should look at each other's uncovered eye.

c. Fully extend your left arm and bring your hand in along the main axes of the visual field (superior, inferior, temporal, and nasal). Move your finger as you do so, and instruct the person to indicate when the finger is first seen.

Clinical Significance

Reading glasses should not be worn because they distort far vision.

Covering the eye with the fingers is unreliable because of the possibility of looking through the fingers.

Normal Findings

Normal visual acuity: 20/20 vision (with or without corrective lenses).

Deviations from Normal

Nearsightedness: A larger denominator indicates impaired far vision. For example, if the person's vision is 20/100, this means that he or she needed to be as close as 20 feet to read what the person with normal vision would be able to read at 100 feet.

Normal Finding

Able to read Jaeger chart or newsprint at 12 to 14 inches.

Deviations from Normal

Farsightedness: Inability to focus on near objects due to impaired accommodation of the eye.

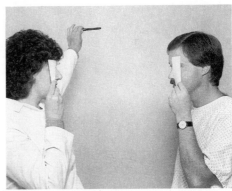

Peripheral vision testing

Normal Findings

Assuming your peripheral vision is normal, you and the client should see your finger at the same time.

Normal visual fields by confrontation:

- Temporal: extends 90 degrees from midline
- Upward: 50 degrees
- Nasalward: 60 degrees
- Downward: 70 degrees

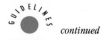

Testing Visual Acuity

Procedure

d. Repeat testing procedure on the other eye.

Clinical Significance

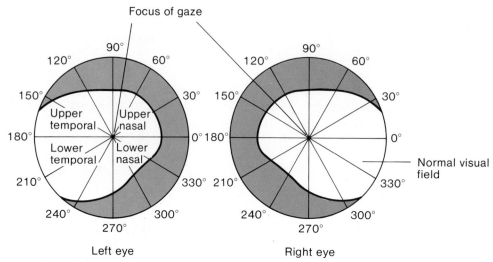

Normal visual fields by confrontation

4. TEST COLOR VISION.

Ask the person to view Ishihara plates or another color test.

Normal Finding

Able to discriminate and correctly identify different colors.

Documenting Eye Examination Findings and Visual Acuity

The results of a normal eye examination (not including visual acuity testing) may be recorded as follows:

> External eye structures symmetric, without lesions. Palpebral conjunctiva pink, moist; sclera white without injection. PERLA. Lens clear. EOMs intact and red reflex intact. Lacrimal apparatus nontender to palpation. Fundoscopic exam shows A-V ratio 2:3, round disc with sharp borders; no fundal lesions.

Examination findings are often recorded using abbreviations such as those shown in Display 11-1. Results of visual acuity testing may be recorded on appropriate forms or flowsheets or by using a method such as the one presented in Display 11-2.

NDx

Nursing Diagnoses Related to Eye and Vision Assessment

Sensory–Perceptual Alteration: Visual

A person's vision may be altered by numerous factors. Some alterations, such as myopia or hyperopia, are rela-

tively benign and do not significantly affect a person's sensory–perceptual abilities if corrective lenses are prescribed and used. Other alterations, such as those that occur with advancing age or secondary to pathology such as a stroke, may cause permanent changes in visual perception. Altered visual perception may contribute to loss of functional abilities such as the ability to drive, and may increase a person's risk for physical injury, social isolation, or disorientation.

Environmental or situational factors may also contribute to altered visual perception. For example, a person's position in bed, especially if the person is immobile, may be the sole factor determining his or her visual field. If, for prolonged periods of time, the person sees only the ceiling, bedrails, or partial views of care providers, sensory input may lose meaning, placing the person at greater risk for sensory deprivation or overload. This situation is especially likely to occur if the person cannot wear his or her corrective lenses. In addition, you should consider the visual overload that may result from excessive glare in a person's surroundings. Elderly people are especially at risk for visual alterations from glare.

Nursing diagnoses are usually formulated to describe the problems the person experiences as a result of visual alterations. For example, rather than the nursing diagnosis Sensory–perceptual alterations: visual, it might be more helpful to diagnose the person's responses such as Potential for injury or Self-care deficit.

Display 11–1
Eye Examination: Common Abbreviations

AV: Arteriovenous crossings in the retina
EOM: Extraocular eye movement
IOP: Intraocular pressure
J₃: Jaeger chart 3 print (print in phone book)
J₅: Jaeger chart 5 print (print in newspaper)
OD: Right eye (oculus dexter)
OS: Left eye (oculus sinister)
OU: Both eyes (oculus uterque)
PERLA: Pupils equal, react to light and accommodation
PERRLA: Pupils equal, round, react to light and accommodation

$\overline{cc}$: With correction (wearing glasses or contact lenses)
$\overline{sc}$: Without correction (without wearing glasses or contact lenses)
FC: Finger counting (indicates visual acuity—can client discern number of fingers held up by examiner?)
HM: Hand movement (indicates visual acuity—can client discern examiner's hand movements?)
LP: Light perception (indicates visual acuity—can client discern light from dark?)

Display 11–2
Documenting Visual Acuity

Documentation

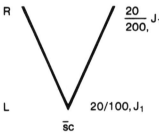
Example 1

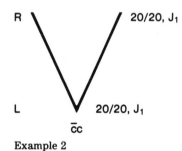
Example 2

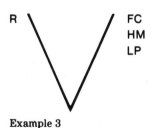
Example 3

Interpretation

Example 1: Snellen testing indicates 20/200 (right eye) and 20/100 (left eye) when tested without corrective lenses ($\overline{sc}$). Able to read Jaeger size 1 print (both eyes).

Example 2: Snellen testing indicates 20/20 (right eye) and 20/20 (left eye) when tested with corrective lenses ($\overline{cc}$). Able to read Jaeger size 1 print with both eyes.

Example 3: Able to see finger counting (FC), hand movement (HM), and has light perception (LP) with the right eye. No indication in this example if corrective lenses were used.

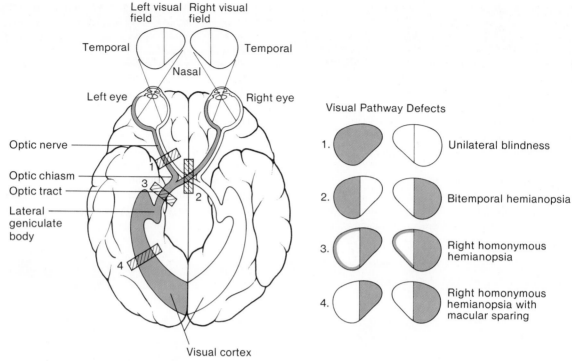

Figure 11–3. Visual pathways. Lesions at the numbered points correspond to the visual field defects shown on the right.

Clinical Problems Related to Eye and Vision Assessment

Visual Field Defects Caused by Alterations in Neural Pathways

The visual neural pathways may be pathologically altered by tumors, trauma, infectious diseases, and cerebrovascular accidents. Lesions along the visual neural pathways may result in partial or complete visual losses, depending on the location of the lesion (Fig. 11-3):

- *Unilateral blindness* may be caused by a lesion of one of the optic nerves.
- *Bitemporal hemianopsia* may be caused by lesions at the optic chiasm.
- *Left (or right) homonymous hemianopsia* may be caused by lesions at the right (or left) optic tract.

A person's perception of his or her surroundings will be affected by these changes. With bitemporal hemianopsia, for example, peripheral vision is impaired.

Visual Field Defects Caused by Alterations in Eye Structures

Many alterations in eye structures are associated with increasing age. The cornea may lose translucency, so that more light is required to produce an image on the retina; the sclera may lose opacity, permitting stray light rays to enter the eye and wash out visual images; "floaters," or black spots, may appear in the vitreous humor, distorting visual perception; pupils may dilate more slowly, requiring more time to adapt from light to darker environments. Such alterations may be permanent.

Pathologic alterations in eye structures may also affect visual perception. For example, black spots in the visual field may be an early sign of retinal detachment. As retinal detachment progresses, the person may describe a "black curtain" falling over the visual field. Blind spots or scotomas may occur in the visual field secondary to macular degeneration and glaucoma.

THE EARS AND HEARING

Anatomy and Physiology Overview

External Ear. The external ear includes the auricle and external auditory meatus (Fig. 11-4). The auricle, which is curved to receive sound waves, includes the helix, auricular tubercle, antihelix, antitragus, concha, tragus, and lobe. The external auditory meatus (or ear canal) is about 1 inch long and ends at the tympanic membrane, the border between the external and middle ear (Fig. 11-5). The ear canal is curved slightly, but may be straightened by gently pulling the auricle up and backward. Cerumen (ear wax) is secreted into the ear canal and may accumulate into a hardened brownish-black plug. The ear canal is supplied by many nerve endings and is extremely sensitive to touch, an important fact for you to remember during the examination.

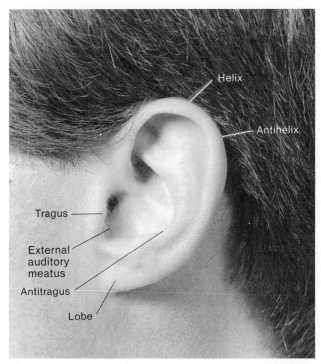

Figure 11–4. The external ear.

The tympanic membrane, or eardrum, is a fibrous, mobile tissue that forms the junction between the external and middle ear. Sound waves entering through the external ear cause the tympanic membrane to vibrate, which in turn transmits sound frequencies to the auditory ossicles of the middle ear.

Middle Ear. The middle ear is a bony cavity within the temporal bone that opens directly to the eustachian tube. The middle ear contains three ossicles or bones (the mal-

leus, incus, and stapes) and mastoid air cells. Except for the imprint of the malleus on the tympanic membrane, the structures of the middle ear are not visible during examination. Vibrations from the tympanic membrane are transmitted and amplified along the ossicles, which join the oval window of the inner ear. The mastoid air cells are air-filled spaces in the temporal bone that communicate with the middle-ear cavity and are lined with mucous membranes. These membranes can become inflamed by organisms transmitted from the upper respiratory tract through the eustachian tube, which connects the middle ear and the nasopharynx. When air enters the eustachian tube, air pressure on both sides of the tympanic membrane is equalized.

Inner Ear. The inner ear consists of the bony labyrinth, the semicircular canals, and the membranous labyrinth. The functions of the inner ear include hearing and equilibrium.

The bony labyrinth is the outer area of the inner ear and contains the vestible, cochlea, and semicircular canals. The membranous labyrinth, the inner area lining the bony labyrinth, contains the canals that transmit sound waves from the oval window. Semicircular canals maintain equilibrium; the utricle and saccule within the inner ear permit an individual to sense changes in gravity and linear acceleration. Auditory sensations are transmitted from the cochlea, which contains sensory cells, to the temporal lobe of the cerebral cortex by the cochlear division of cranial nerve VIII (acoustic). Position sensation is transmitted along the vestibular portion of the same cranial nerve.

Hearing Pathway. Sound waves must be conducted to the inner ear before sensory impulses are transmitted to the auditory areas of the cerebral cortex. This can be accomplished by means of air conduction or bone conduction; air conduction is more efficient. In air conduction, sound waves reach the external ear and travel the external canal to the tympanic membrane. The sound waves cause

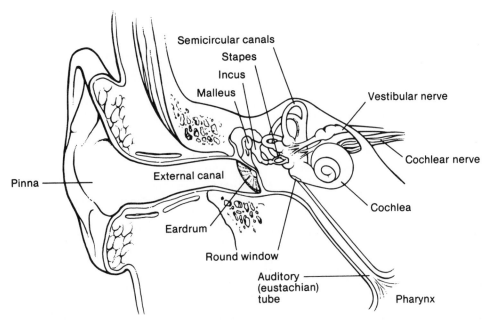

Figure 11–5. The middle and inner ear.

tympanic membrane vibration, which in turn vibrates the ossicles. The oval window vibrates, causing the inner ear fluid to move. This movement affects the basilar membrane of the organ of Corti, which is then activated. When bone conducts sound waves, the organ of Corti is activated, but bone sound waves must be more intense than those required for air conduction.

The neural component of hearing begins at the organ of Corti as the mechanical energy from sound waves is converted to an electrical or neural impulse. Nerve fibers in the cochlear branch of cranial nerve VIII are activated, carrying afferent impulses to the cerebral cortex. Many alternate afferent pathways carry auditory stimuli. Therefore, damage to a single neural pathway will not necessarily cause complete hearing loss.

Equilibrium. The functions of the inner ear are to maintain equilibrium and head position and to direct eye gaze. The three semicircular canals are oriented at right angles in three planes and have specialized cells capable of detecting movement in each plane. These sensations of movement are transmitted to the cerebellum, which rapidly initiates the skeletal muscle movements required to maintain balance and coordination.

Physical Examination   *Ears and Hearing*

General Principles

The ears should be evaluated by inspection and palpation. The otoscope is used to visualize internal ear structures. Equilibrium, a function of the inner ear, is evaluated as a component of the sensory examination (see pp. 356–360).

A person's hearing acuity may be evaluated during the physical examination by means of gross screening techniques such as observing the ability to hear the ticking of a watch and whispered voice sounds. Additionally, some tests enable you to evaluate the status of the conductive and sensorineural sound pathways. Additional inferences may be made about hearing by observing a person's responses to conversation and instructions. For example, note if the person must face you to comprehend verbal instructions; this could indicate that he or she is lip reading.

If you identify hearing deficits, refer the person for specialized audiometry testing.

Equipment

- Otoscope
- Watch (ticking)
- Tuning fork

Otoscope

The otoscope is used to illuminate and inspect the ear canal and tympanic membrane. Although different brands vary, most otoscopes have handles that contain batteries for the light source, a switch for turning on the light, a viewing window, and examining tips that can accommodate differently sized specula (disposable or nondisposable). Choose the largest speculum that can be inserted into the ear without causing pain. Reusable specula need to be thoroughly disinfected. Some otoscopes handles may be unscrewed from the head and plugged into a wall socket to recharge batteries.

A pneumatic otoscope is used to determine the mobility of the tympanic membrane. A rubber bulb is attached to the otoscope and the examiner squeezes it while visualizing the tympanic membrane. The squeezing action injects air, which normally causes the tympanic membrane to move in and out. Loss of tympanic membrane mobility is associated with middle-ear infection.

Tuning Forks

Tuning forks are used to test for conductive and sensorineural hearing losses. Differently sized tuning forks generate different sound frequencies. Usually, a tuning fork of 512 or 1024 Hz is used in examinations because the human ear can detect frequencies ranging from 300 to 3000 Hz. The frequency number is usually engraved on the instrument.

Activate the tuning fork by grasping its stem and striking the ends against your hand or other surface. Hold the instrument by the stem to avoid damping the vibration.

Cerumen Removal

Normally, cerumen dries and falls out of the ear. However, accumulation and impaction may occur if the ear canal is tortuous or extremely hairy. Attempts to remove cerumen with cotton-tipped applicators may be irritating and may push cerumen further

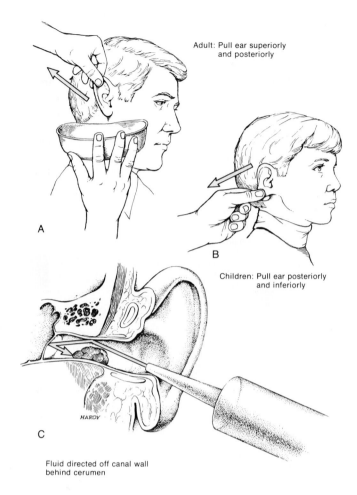

Adult: Pull ear superiorly and posteriorly

A

B

Children: Pull ear posteriorly and inferiorly

C

Fluid directed off canal wall behind cerumen

Figure 11–6. Ear irrigation. (**A**) The external auditory canal in the adult can best be exposed by pulling the earlobe upward and backward. (**B**) The same exposure can be achieved in the child by gently pulling the auricle of the ear downward and backward. (**C**) An enlarged diagram showing the direction of irrigating fluid against the side of the canal. *Note:* This is more effective in dislodging cerumen than if the flow of solution were directed straight into the canal. (Brunner, L.S., & Suddarth, D.S. [1991]. *The Lippincott manual of nursing practice* [5th ed.]. Philadelphia: J.B. Lippincott)

into the ear canal. Cerumen impaction is diagnosed on the basis of symptoms such as feelings of fullness in the ear, tinnitus, and reports of hearing loss (conductive). In such cases, the initial otoscopic inspection will reveal a large amount of hardened, dark-brown wax. Cerumen impaction interferes with the ability to hear and with visualization of the tympanic membrane, and may need to be removed by irrigation. However, irrigation is contraindicated if there is a history of eardrum perforation.

Before irrigating the ear, apply protective toweling to the shoulder and neck area. An irrigating syringe is filled with lukewarm water, because cold water may cause dizziness. The tip of the syringe is positioned just inside the ear canal and pointed toward the upper canal wall (Fig. 11-6). This position allows the irrigating fluid to accumulate behind the cerumen and eventually push it from the ear canal. The ear canal can be straightened by gently pulling upward and back on the auricle; irrigating fluid is injected repeatedly until the cerumen mass is dislodged. Discontinue irrigation if any pain or dizziness occurs. An emesis basin may be used to collect the irrigating fluid that will drain from the ear. If the cerumen is not dislodged by irrigation, an earwax-softening solution such as glycerin is applied for several days before the procedure is reattempted.

Examination and Documentation Focus

- *External ear:* Shape, size, position, skin integrity, response to palpation of the mastoid bone and tragus
- *External auditory meatus (ear canal):* Patency, discharge, inflammation, hair growth, cerumen
- *Tympanic membrane:* Color, surface characteristics, landmarks, light reflex, configuration
- *Hearing acuity:* Gross hearing, Weber test results, Rinne test results

Examination Guidelines   *Ears*

Procedure

1. INSPECT AND PALPATE THE EXTERNAL EAR.

   a. Inspect the external ear, noting skin integrity, shape, symmetry and ear position.

   b. Palpate the auricle between the thumb and forefinger, noting any tenderness or lesions.

   c. Palpate the mastoid process, which should be nontender. Tenderness is associated with middle ear inflammation.

   d. Press the tragus inward toward the ear canal to detect tenderness, which may indicate inner ear inflammation.

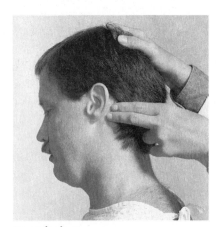

Mastoid palpation

Clinical Significance

Normal Finding

Left and right ears have equal size and shape. No skin lesions.

Ear position: The top of the ear should just touch or barely cross an imaginary line drawn from the outer canthus of the eye to the occiput.

Deviations from Normal

Lower-set ears may be associated with congenital kidney disorders or other chromosomal abnormalities.

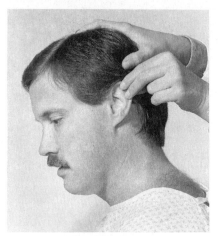

Auricle palpation

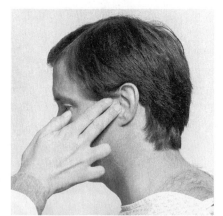

Tragus palpation

2. INSPECT THE EXTERNAL AUDITORY CANAL THROUGH THE VIEWING LENS OF THE OTOSCOPE.

   Note: If the person has symptoms of an ear infection (ear pain), inspect the unaffected ear first.

   a. Briefly explain the procedure. Ask the person to tip the head slightly toward the opposite shoulder (away from the side being examined).

   b. Choose the largest speculum the ear will comfortably accommodate and turn on the otoscope light.

Measures should be taken to avoid transferring infective material from one ear to the other on the speculum.

Aligns the ear canal with the examining instrument.

OPHTHALMOSCOPIC EXAMINATION

Normal Findings

RED REFLEX

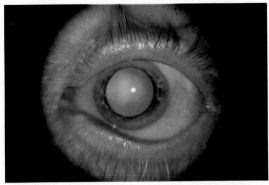

The red reflex is the orange-red coloration of the fundus that occurs when a small circle of light shines through the pupil. (Courtesy of Custom Medical Stock Photo, Inc. [Paula Ihnat])

ARCUS SENILIS

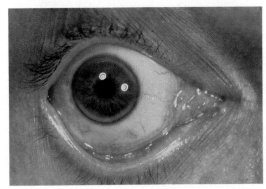

Arcus senilis is a grayish-white ring around the cornea that accompanies normal aging. In younger people it may be the result of hyperlipoproteinemia. (Courtesy of Custom Medical Stock Photo, Inc. [1993, National Medical Slide Bank])

Common Abnormalities

CATARACT

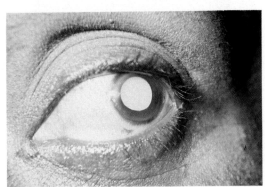

A cataract is a lens opacity that appears as a gray or white opaque coloration behind the pupil. The cataract will result in an absence of the red reflex. (Courtesy of Dr. William C. Byrne, OD, Optometric Eyecare Center, Fairless Hills, PA)

CHALAZION

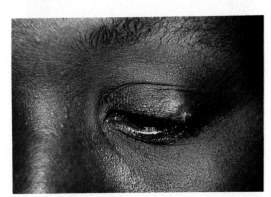

A chalazion is an eyelid mass that results from chronic inflammation of a meibomian gland. (Courtesy of Dr. William C. Byrne, OD, Optometric Eyecare Center, Fairless Hills, PA)

NORMAL FUNDUS: BLONDE

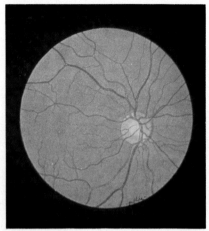

A lighter fundus is normal for a blonde. (Courtesy of American Optometric Association)

NORMAL FUNDUS: BRUNETTE

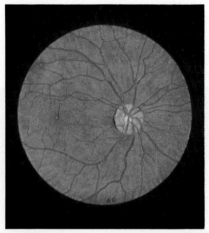

A darker fundus is typical for a brunette. (Courtesy of American Optometric Association)

NORMAL FUNDUS: DARK-SKINNED PERSON

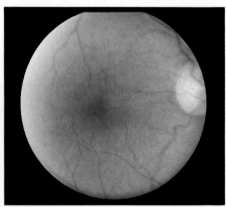

A much darker fundus is normal for a dark-skinned person. (Courtesy of Dr. William C. Byrne, OD, Optometric Eyecare Center, Fairless Hills, PA)

PAPILLEDEMA

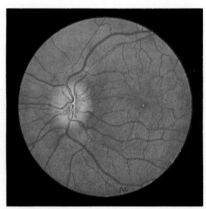

Papilledema is characterized by swelling of the optic disk that obscures the disk margins. The physiologic cup is no longer visible. This abnormality is caused by the venous stasis that occurs with increased intracranial pressure or hypertension. (Courtesy of American Optometric Association)

HYPERTENSIVE RETINOPATHY

Hypertensive changes result in hemorrhages and bursting blood vessels in the fundus. (Courtesy of American Optometric Association)

ARTERIOSCLEROTIC RETINOPATHY

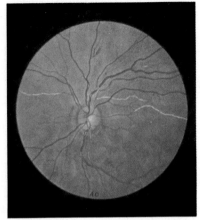

Arteriosclerosis can affect the fundal blood vessels, causing fatty deposits that appear as white streaks along the arteries. (Courtesy of American Optometric Association)

DIABETIC RETINOPATHY

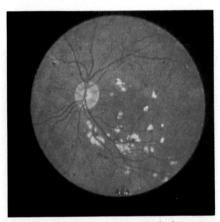

Diabetic changes result in characteristic waxy-looking retinal lesions, microaneurysms of the vessels, and hemorrhages. (Courtesy of American Optometric Association)

SOLAR RETINOPATHY

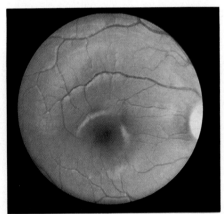

Solar retinopathy results from staring directly at the sun (as could happen when looking at an eclipse with the naked eye). (Courtesy of Dr. William C. Byrne, OD, Optometric Eyecare Center, Fairless Hills, PA)

GLAUCOMA

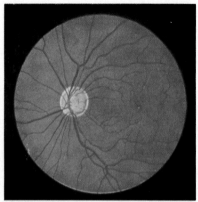

Glaucoma causes cupping of the optic disk when increased intraocular pressure is transmitted to the retina. The physiologic cup enlarges. (Courtesy of American Optometric Association)

DETACHED RETINA

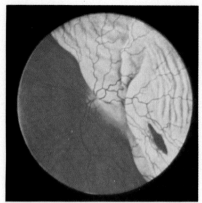

Retinal tears lead to cortical detachment as the vitreous fluid seeps through the bole to the subretinal space, pushing the retina away from the epithelium. (Courtesy of American Optometric Association)

OTOSCOPIC EXAMINATION

NORMAL TYMPANIC MEMBRANE

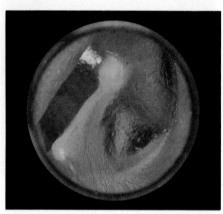

A normal tympanic membrane is pearly gray, with visible structures and light reflex. (Courtesy of Custom Medical Stock Photo, Inc. [1992, Childs])

RED, BULGING TYMPANIC MEMBRANE

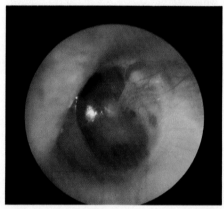

A bulging, red tympanic membrane obscures the typical landmarks, including the light reflex. It typically results from otitis media. (Courtesy of Custom Medical Stock Photo, Inc. [1991, Siu Biomed Comm])

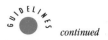 *continued*

Ears

Procedure

c. Grasp the otoscope with your dominant hand and hold it in one of two ways:

- For children and restless adults, place the hand that is holding the otoscope handle against the person's head to help stabilize the instrument.
- For cooperative persons, you may hold the handle so the instrument is in an upright position; stabilization efforts are unnecessary.

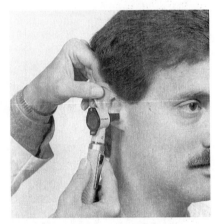

Otoscopic examination: Cooperative person

With your free hand, grasp the superior portion of the auricle and gently pull up, out, and back if the patient is an adult. The auricle is pulled downward in young children and infants.

d. Insert the otoscope and gently advance it to inspect the external auditory canal membranes through the lens.

3. INSPECT THE TYMPANIC MEMBRANE.

a. Next, move the otoscope to examine the tympanic membrane. If this membrane is not initially visible, pull the auricle up and back again to further straighten the ear canal. Do not force the speculum in too distal a direction.

Cerumen may be present in the canal, partially obstructing the tympanic membrane. Again, gently realign the canal by moving the auricle and try to view around cerumen particles.

Clinical Significance

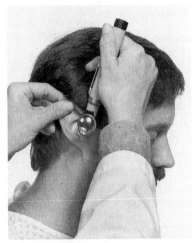

Otoscopic examination: Children, restless person

This maneuver should straighten the ear canal so that you can see the tympanic membrane.

Normal Findings

The adult ear canal is about 1 inch long. Skin is intact without redness or discharge. The canal is clear without obstructions. Hair growth is variable; hairs grow near outer third of the canal. Cerumen color and consistency vary depending on length of time since secretion. Fresh cerumen is light yellow, tan, or pink, and is soft. Old cerumen may be light to dark brown and is hard.

Quadrants of the tympanic membrane: Anterosuperior, posterosuperior, anteroinferior, and posteroinferior.

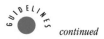
continued   ***Ears***

Procedure

b. Inspect the tympanic membrane and note major landmarks and color.

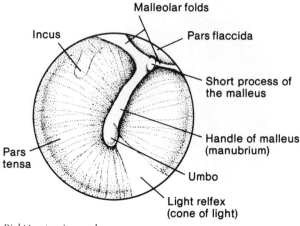

Malleolar folds

Incus

Pars flaccida

Short process of the malleus

Handle of malleus (manubrium)

Pars tensa

Umbo

Light relfex (cone of light)

Right tympanic membrane

c. Observe the movement of the tympanic membrane as the person performs a Valsalva maneuver (or when you inject air with the pneumatic otoscope).

d. Examine the other ear.

Clinical Significance

Normal Findings

Color: Pearly gray; shiny; diffuse white plaques over membrane are scar tissue from previous inflammations.

Surface: Continuous and intact; slightly transparent.

Landmarks: White light reflex (cone of light) projected over anteroinferior quadrant. Light reflex focused with well-defined borders (not diffuse). Following structures are visible: malleus (umbo and short process); pars tensa (taut portion of the tympanic membrane); annulus; pars flaccida (looser, superior fold of tympanic membrane); malleolar folds.

Configuration: Flat or concave (not bulging).

Deviations from Normal

Color: Redness; amber color

Surface: Perforated

Landmarks: No light reflex; inability to see landmarks

Configuration: Bulging or retracted.

Normal Findings

Movement of the tympanic membrane indicates a patent eustachian tube.

Examination Guidelines   *Hearing*

Procedure

1. VOICE/WHISPER TEST.

a. Stand slightly behind the person, close to the ear that you want to test. Ask the person to cover the other ear with his or her hand.

b. Whisper a few words, then ask the person to repeat what you said.

c. Repeat the test on the other ear.

Clinical Significance

A test of hearing acuity, especially ability to perceive high-frequency sound.

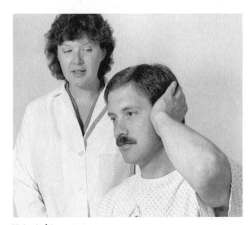

Voice/whisper test

Normal Finding

Ability to recognize the words of a whispered message from a 2-foot distance.

Hearing

Procedure

2. WATCH-TICK TEST.

   a. Stand behind the person. Instruct the person to cover the ear that is not being tested.

   b. Hold a ticking watch near the uncovered ear. Ask the person to say "yes" when he or she can hear the ticking and "no" when the ticking becomes inaudible. Move the watch until it is 2 feet from the ear.

   c. Repeat the test on the other ear.

3. WEBER TEST.

   a. Strike the tuning fork and place the stem firmly against the middle of the person's forehead or the top of the head at the midline.

   b. Ask the person where the sound is heard.

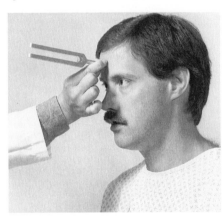

Weber test

4. RINNE TEST.

   a. Strike the tuning fork and place the stem firmly against the mastoid process.

Clinical Significance

A test of hearing acuity, especially the ability to perceive high-frequency sound.

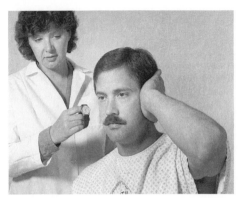

Watch-tick test

Note: Whispers and a watch's ticking are high-frequency sounds. These tests do not indicate a person's ability to perceive low-frequency sounds.

Tests perception of sound coming from the body's midline.

Normal Finding

No sound lateralization, meaning the sound of the tuning fork is heard equally in both ears.

Deviations from Normal

In unilateral conduction deafness, the sound is heard best in the affected ear; in sensorineural loss, the sound lateralizes to the unaffected ear. See Display, "Types of Hearing Losses."

Tests ability to perceive bone conduction versus air conduction of sound.

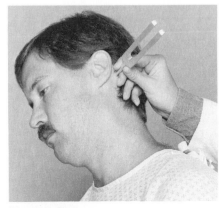

Rinne test: Step a

Types of Hearing Losses

Sensorineural Hearing Loss (Perceptive Deafness)

Associated Conditions

Conditions that disrupt *neural* hearing pathways: the cochlea, cranial nerve VIII, or the auditory portions of the cerebral cortex (bilateral lesions).

Causative Factors

- Congenital defects
- Maternal rubella
- Erythroblastosis fetalis
- Traumatic injury involving the inner ear or cranial nerve VIII
- Vascular disorders involving the inner ear
- Ototoxic drugs
- Bacterial and viral infections (meningitis, encephalitis, mumps, etc.)
- Meniere's disease
- Severe febrile illness
- Posterior fossa tumors
- Multiple sclerosis
- Presbycusis
- Prolonged or repeated exposure to loud sounds

Signs and Symptoms

- Delayed language and speech development (infants)
- Hearing loss that may be more severe in noisy environments
- May be associated with speaking loudly

Hearing Tests

- Whisper test and watch-tick test may indicate hearing loss
- Weber test usually shows sound lateralization to the good ear
- Rinne test should be positive (AC>BC)

Conductive Hearing Loss

Associated Conditions

Associated with external or middle ear problems that prevent normal sound transmission. Otoscopic examination is essential for detecting cerumen impaction, eardrum perforation, and otitis media.

Causative Factors

- Congenital ear malformations
- Traumatic eardrum perforation
- Trauma disrupting the ossicles
- Cerumen impaction
- Middle ear inflammation (otitis media)
- Otosclerosis

Signs and Symptoms

- Hearing loss that may be less noticeable in a noisy environment
- Normal tone of voice usually observed

Hearing Tests

- Whisper test and watch-tick test may indicate hearing loss.
- Weber test usually shows sound lateralization to the affected ear because this ear is less distracted by environmental noise and is therefore more perceptive to vibration.
- Rinne test should be negative (BC>AC) because vibrations passing through bone bypass the obstructive process.

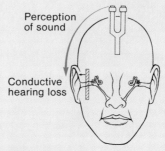

Weber test

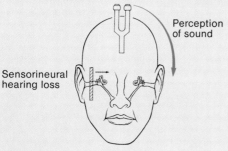

Weber test

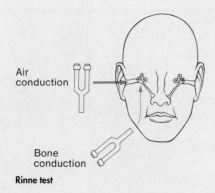

Rinne test

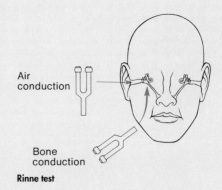

Rinne test

Mixed (Combined) Hearing Loss

Hearing losses may be secondary to ineffective conduction and sensory perception. Both air and bone sound conduction are impaired.

Procedure

b. Ask the person to report when the sound (or "buzzing") stops.

c. Then move the tuning fork, which will be vibrating weakly, near the external auditory meatus.

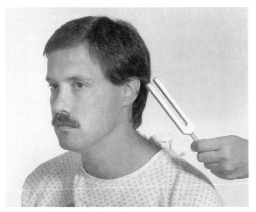

Rinne test: Step c

5. SCHWABACH'S TEST.

a. Strike the tuning fork and place it firmly against the person's mastoid process. Note the length of time before the person reports that the sound has stopped.

b. Then repeat the test, holding the tuning fork against your own mastoid process and note the length of bone conduction.

Clinical Significance

Normal Finding

The person should hear the sound of the tuning fork when it is placed in front of the ear. This indicates that air conduction of sound is greater than bone conduction (AC>BC; a normal result, called *Rinne positive*).

Deviations from Normal

Bone conduction of sound is greater than air conduction (BC>AC; an abnormal pattern, called *Rinne negative*). This is associated with a conductive hearing loss. See Display, "Types of Hearing Losses."

Compares the person's perception of bone conduction of sound with the examiner's. (The test assumes normal hearing abilities on your part.)

Deviations from Normal

Schwabach diminished: You hear the sound longer than the client, in which case the client may have a sensorineural hearing loss.

Schwabach prolonged: The client hears the sound longer, in which case he or she may have a conductive hearing loss.

Documenting Ear Examination Findings and Hearing

Example 1: Normal Ear

Kay, aged 10, had an ear examination as part of summer camp health assessment. The examination was normal and recorded as follows:

> External ear skin without lesions; tragus and auricle nontender to palpation. Canals have small amount of soft yellow cerumen; noninflamed. Both TMs pearly gray, shiny; Light reflex intact and landmarks discernable. Able to identify whispered voice, no sound lateralization, AC>BC.

The same examination may be summarized in a problem-oriented format:

S: Mother reports no history of ear infectons or hearing problems. Does not use cotton-tipped swabs or similar devices for ear cleaning.

O: External ear skin without lesions; tragus and auricle nontender to palpation. Canals have small amount of soft yellow cerumen; noninflamed. Both TMs pearly gray and shiny. Light reflex intact, and landmarks discernible. Able to identify whispered voice, no sound lateralization, AC>BC.

A: Ear exam and hearing acuity within normal limits.

P: Reinforce current routines and routine screening visits.

Example 2: Cerumen Impaction

Mr. T, aged 79, reported to the nurse that his left ear felt full and hearing acuity was diminished. The examination was abnormal and recorded as follows:

> Left ear canal impacted with dark-brown, hard cerumen. Unable to visualize TM. BC>AC on left side; AC>BC on right. Sound lateralization to the left side. Does not hear whispered sound on left, but can on right.

The same examination may be summarized in a problem-oriented format:

S: "I don't hear very well on this side [left], and my ear feels plugged."

O: Left ear canal impacted with dark brown, hard cerumen. Unable to visualize TM. BC>AC on left side; AC>BC on right. Sound lateralization to the left side.

Does not hear whispered sound on left, but can on right.

A: Tests of hearing acuity indicate conductive hearing loss, probably from cerumen impaction.

P: Consider cerumen removal if no contraindications.

Example 3: Ear Infection

Andrew, aged 8, had an URI for the last week and developed left ear pain 12 hours ago. The ear examination was abnormal and recorded as follows:

Right ear canal clear, TM pearly gray with discernable landmarks and light reflex. Left ear canal clear, TM erythematous and slightly convex. Unable to see light reflex or landmarks. Patient reports pain with left tragus palpation.

The same examination may be summarized in a problem-oriented format:

S: Mother reports history of URI for 1 week; began pulling left ear and having ear pain last evening.

O: Temp: 101° F (PO); P: 98; RR: 18. Right ear canal clear, TM pearly gray with discernable landmarks and light reflex. Left ear canal clear, TM erythematous and slightly convex. Unable to see light reflex or landmarks. Reports pain with tragus palpation.

A: Suspect acute otitis media (left side).

P: Consult with physician for treatment. Instruct mother re: antibiotic therapy; worsening of symptoms.

NDx
_____

Nursing Diagnoses Related to Ear and Hearing Assessment

Sensory-Perceptual Alteration: Hearing

A person's hearing may be altered by a number of factors, some of which are not amenable to nursing intervention. For example, sensory–perceptual alteration: Hearing related to the effects of aging, may not be a useful diagnostic label in planning nursing care. The nurse would have difficulty identifying realistic outcome criteria for this type of diagnosis. It might not be realistic to say that the person would achieve better hearing acuity as a result of nursing intervention. The nurse should determine the responses the person might have as a result of a hearing loss and specifically label the response, rather than the hearing deficit. For example, people with hearing deficits are at risk for Impaired communication or Social isolation.

Clinical Problems Related to Ear and Hearing Assessment

Otitis Externa (Swimmer's Ear)

Otitis externa is a painful inflammatory condition of the external ear caused by infective organisms, allergic reactions (such as contact dermatitis) or present as a variant of seborrheic dermatitis.

Risk Factors

• Prolonged moisture in the ear, most frequently caused by swimming
• Ear canal trauma, most often caused by cleaning or scratching

Signs and Symptoms

• Ear pain, especially near the external portion of the affected ear; pain may be aggravated by pushing on the tragus, or by chewing and talking
• Itching
• Scaling from the ear canal
• Conductive hearing losses may be noted if ear canal swelling is extensive and causes external canal blockage.
• Low-grade fever possible
• Proximal lymph node enlargement is possible, which may involve preauricular, postauricular, and upper cervical nodes.

Otoscopic Examination

• Inspecting the outer ear and external canal may reveal reddened and swollen skin surfaces.
• Serous exudate may be seen.
• The tympanic membrane should be normal unless otitis media is present.

Acute Otitis Media (Middle Ear Inflammation)

Acute otitis media occurs most commonly in infants and children as a sequela of upper respiratory tract infection.

Pathophysiology

Bacteria, especially beta-hemolytic streptococci, staphylococci, and pneumococci, as well as the *Haemophilus influenzae* virus, are easily transmitted to the middle ear along the eustachian tube.

Signs and Symptoms

• Ear pain (young children or infants may be irritable and pull or hold the affected ear)
• Feelings of fullness, pressure, or roaring in the ear
• Fever and chills are common.

Otoscopic Examination

• During the early stages, the only sign may be hyperemia of the blood vessels across the drum.
• Later, the drum may bulge outward as secretions collect in the middle ear.
• Bulging obscures the tympanic membrane landmarks, including the light reflex.
• The eardrum may be bright red.
• If the eardrum ruptures, purulent drainage may be noted in the canal.
• Eardrum perforation may be directly visible. It places the person at risk for developing chronic otitis media.

Serous Otitis Media

Serous otitis media may occur when sterile fluid accumulates in the middle ear. It may occur secondary to

• Eustachian tube blockage when pressure changes cause transudation of serous fluid
• Residual exudate accumulation from a bacterial otitis media

- A viral upper respiratory tract infection
- An allergic reaction, causing serous fluid exudation into the middle ear

Signs and Symptoms

- Usually little or no ear pain
- May have feelings of ear fullness or plugging
- Decreased hearing acuity possible and auditory function tests may indicate a conductive hearing loss
- Unnatural voice reverberation may be noted.

Otoscopic Examination

- The tympanic membrane may be retracted.
- Light reflex may be absent.
- Tympanic membrane color may be amber.
- A fluid demarcation line may be present.
- Air bubbles may be seen behind the tympanic membrane.

THE CRANIAL NERVES

Anatomy and Physiology Overview

Nuclei for the 12 paired cranial nerves originate in the brain, differentiating cranial nerves from spinal nerves, whose nuclei originate in the spinal cord. Cranial nerves are distributed mainly to the head and neck. Certain cranial nerves, like all spinal nerves, have both sensory and motor components. However, some cranial nerves have only sensory fibers and others have only motor axons.

Cranial nerve examination indicates the status of associated sensory or motor functions. Pertinent anatomic, physiologic, and functional features of the 12 cranial nerves are summarized in Table 11-1.

Table 11-1. Cranial Nerves

Number	Name	Structures Innervated by Efferent Components	Structures Innervated by Afferent Components	Functions
I	Olfactory	None	Olfactory mucous membrane	Nerve of smell
II	Optic	None	Retina of eye	Nerve of vision
III	Oculomotor	Superior, medial, inferior recti; inferior oblique; levator palpebrae superioris; ciliary; sphincter of iris	Superior, medial, inferior recti; inferior oblique; levator palpebrae superioris; ciliary; sphincter of iris	Motor and muscle sense to various muscles listed; accommodation to different distances; regulates the amount of light reaching retina; most important nerve in eye movements
IV	Trochlear	Superior oblique	Superior oblique	Motor and muscle sense to superior oblique; eye movements
V	Trigeminal	Muscles of mastication	Skin and mucous membranes in head; teeth; muscles of mastication	Nerve of pain, touch, heat, cold to skin and mucous membranes listed; same for teeth; movements of mastication and muscle sense
VI	Abducens	Lateral rectus	Lateral rectus	Motor and muscle sense to lateral rectus; eye movements
VII	Facial	Submaxillary and sublingual glands; muscles of face, scalp, and a few others	Same muscles; taste buds of anterior two thirds of tongue	Taste to anterior two thirds of tongue; secretory and vasodilator to two salivary glands; motor and muscle sense to facial and a few other muscles
VIII	Acoustic (cochlear and vestibular portions)	None	Cochlear organ of Corti; vestibular-semicircular canals, utricle, and saccule	Cochlear division is nerve of hearing; vestibular division is concerned with registering movement of the body through space and with the position of the head
IX	Glossopharyngeal	Superior pharyngeal constrictor; stylopharyngeus muscle; parotid gland	Taste buds of posterior one third of tongue; parts of pharynx; carotid sinus and body; stylopharyngeus muscle	Taste to posterior one third of tongue and adjacent regions; secretory and vasodilator to parotid gland; motor and muscle sense to stylopharyngeus; pain, touch, heat, and cold to pharynx; afferent in circulatory and respiratory reflexes
X	Vagus	Muscles of pharynx, larynx, esophagus, thoracic and abdominal viscera; coronary arteries; walls of bronchi; pancreas; gastric glands	Same muscles; skin of external ear; mucous membranes of larynx, trachea, esophagus; thoracic and abdominal viscera; arch of aorta; atria; great veins	Secretory to gastric glands and pancreas; inhibitory to heart; motor to alimentary tract; motor and muscle sense to muscles of larynx and pharynx; constrictor to coronaries; motor to muscle in walls of bronchi; important in respiratory, cardiac, and circulatory reflexes
XI	Accessory	Sternocleidomastoid and trapezius muscles; muscles of larynx	Sternocleidomastoid and trapezius muscles; muscles of larynx	Motor and muscle sense to muscles listed; shares certain functions of vagus
XII	Hypoglossal	Muscles of tongue	Muscles of tongue	Motor and muscle sense to muscles of tongue; important in speech, mastication, and deglutition

Physical Examination   *Cranial Nerves*

General Principles   Most cranial nerve functions involve the head and neck areas. Therefore, cranial nerve assessment should be performed in the early part of a head-to-toe examination sequence. Generally, cranial nerves should not be assessed alone but in conjunction with other major body areas or systems. For example, cranial nerves II, III, IV, and VI and the ophthalmic branch of cranial nerve V should be tested during eye and vision examination.

Equipment
- Small vials with familiar odors
- Snellen chart
- Ophthalmoscope
- Tongue blade
- Irrigation syringe (optional)
- Cotton-tipped applicator
- Safety pin

Examination and Documentation Focus
- Responses to external stimuli
- Motor functions
- Visual acuity
- Hearing acuity

Examination Guidelines   *Cranial Nerves*

Procedure

1. CRANIAL NERVE I (OLFACTORY).

   a. Ask the person to occlude one nostril at a time with the finger and to close the eyes.

   b. Present several familiar odors such as coffee, cloves, peppermint, or soap and ask the person to identify each. Avoid presenting irritating substances such as ammonia or vinegar. Remember that the ability to distinguish between odors is more important than the ability to make exact identifications.

2. CRANIAL NERVE II (OPTIC)

   a. Test cranial nerve II by testing visual acuity (see pp. 326–328).

   b. Examine the optic nerve, which ends in the retina, by using the ophthalmoscope (see pp. 322–323).

3. CRANIAL NERVES III (OCULOMOTOR), IV (TROCHLEAR), VI (ABDUCENS).

4. CRANIAL NERVE V (TRIGEMINAL).

   a. Test motor function of the trigeminal nerve. Place a tongue blade between the person's teeth on the right side and ask him or her to bite down. As the person bites, try to pull the tongue blade out. Repeat this procedure on the left side of the mouth.

   b. Alternatively, test motor function by asking the person to clench his or her teeth while you palpate the masseter and temporal muscles for firmness.

Clinical Significance

The olfactory nerve is not tested routinely.

Normal Findings
Identifies common smells with each nostril.

Deviations from Normal
Anosmia: Unilateral loss of smell. Associated with lesions to the olfactory nerve tract on the side being tested.

This nerve should be tested during eye and vision evaluations.

These nerves are tested by evaluating extraocular eye movements. The oculomotor nerve also innervates the intrinsic muscles that control pupillary constriction and accommodation. These functions are tested by evaluating pupillary light reflexes (see p. 321).

Normal Findings
Equal strength of bite bilaterally; no jaw deviation with teeth clenching.

Cranial Nerves

Procedure

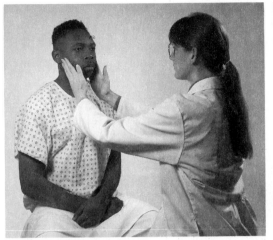

Trigeminal nerve: Testing motor function

c. Test sensory function.

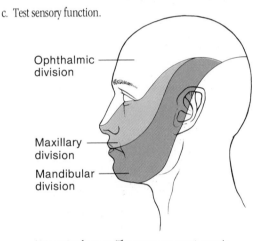

Ophthalmic
division

Maxillary
division

Mandibular
division

Trigeminal nerve: Three sensory components

d. Evaluate the sensory function of the ophthalmic division of the cranial nerve by testing the corneal reflex.

Hold the person's eye open and lightly touch the cornea with the tip of a cotton-tipped applicator that has been pulled into a thin strand. To ensure a reliable test, be careful to touch only the cornea and not the eyelashes or conjunctiva.

Clinical Significance

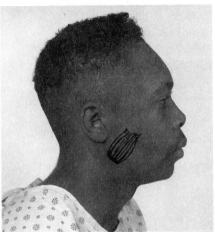

There are three major sensory components of the trigeminal nerve: ophthalmic, maxillary, and mandibular. All three sensory areas are tested.

This test also indicates the status of the motor division of the facial nerve.

Normal Findings
A strong, forceful blink.

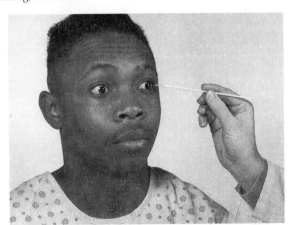

Testing the corneal reflex

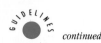
continued   ***Cranial Nerves***

Procedure	**Clinical Significance**

Procedure

e. Test all three sensory divisions of the trigeminal nerve by asking the person to keep the eyes closed while you alternately brush cotton across and lightly pinprick the facial areas innervated by the three sensory divisions. As you apply stimuli, ask the person to identify which sensation is being produced and the location to which it is applied.

5. CRANIAL NERVE VII (FACIAL)

   a. Test the motor division of the facial nerve by asking the person to perform voluntary facial movements such as frowning, smiling, wrinkling the forehead, puffing cheeks, and whistling.

   b. Test the strength of eyelid closure by asking the person to hold the eyes tightly closed. Then try to open the person's eyes.

   c. Test the sensory division of the facial nerve by evaluating the person's ability to discriminate tastes. Apply salt and sugar to both sides of the anterior tongue.

6. CRANIAL NERVE VIII (ACOUSTIC).

   a. Test the cochlear portion of cranial nerve VIII by evaluating hearing acuity (see pp. 336–339).

   b. Test the vestibular portion of cranial nerve VIII by performing the Romberg test (see p. 360).

   c. The vestibular portion of cranial nerve VIII may also be evaluated by performing the caloric test.

   With the person seated or with the head of bed elevated 30 degrees, inspect ear canal with otoscope to ascertain a patent canal and intact tympanic membrane. Irrigate the ear canal with ice-cold water. If client is conscious, use only a few drops.

7. CRANIAL NERVES IX (GLOSSOPHARYNGEAL) AND X (VAGUS).

   a. Test cranial nerve IX by touching the palatal arch with a tongue blade to elicit a gag reflex.

   b. Ask the person to open his or her mouth and say "ah."

   c. Cranial nerve X is also tested by evaluating speech quality. Ask the person to say, "kuh, kuh, kuh," "la, la, la," and "mi, mi, mi."

Clinical Significance

Normal Findings

Discriminates light touch and pinprick over skin innervated by the three divisions of the cranial nerve.

Normal Findings

Facial features are symmetric when performing voluntary movements. Symmetry also observed at the nasolabial folds.

Deviations from Normal

Bell's palsy: Lesion to the lower portion of the facial nerve resulting in ipsilateral paralysis.

Upper motor neuron lesions: Upper motor neuron lesions, such as stroke, may produce contralateral facial weakness, drooping, or paralysis.

Taste sensation is not tested routinely.

The caloric test is used to evaluate brainstem function in comatose persons. The test is rarely performed on conscious people because it may produce nausea.

Normal Findings (conscious person)

Nausea, horizontal nystagmus, vertigo toward unirrigated side, and "past-pointing" on irrigated side (person misjudges distance and points "past" the correct position when instructed to touch your fingertip with his or her fingertip).

These nerves are tested together because both have components that innervate the pharynx. Check them during the oral examination.

Normal Findings

The uvula remains midline and there is symmetric rising of the soft palate. This indicates normal function of cranial nerves IX and X.

Normal Findings

Speaks with clear voice.

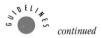

continued

Cranial Nerves

Procedure

8. CRANIAL NERVE XI (SPINAL ACCESSORY).

   a. Place your hands on the person's shoulders and ask him or her to shrug as you apply resistance.

   b. Inspect and palpate the sternocleidomastoid muscles, noting tone and symmetry.

   c. Ask the client to turn the head and touch chin to shoulder as you apply resistance. Test both sides.

9. CRANIAL NERVE XII (HYPOGLOSSAL).

   Ask the person to stick out the tongue. Note symmetry, atrophy, and involuntary movements.

Clinical Significance

Normal Findings

Raises shoulders against resistance.

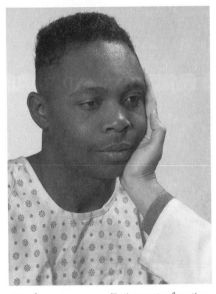

Spinal accessory nerve: Testing motor function

This nerve should be checked during the oral examination.

Normal Findings

Extends tongue along midline; no lateral deviation.

Documenting Cranial Nerve Examination Findings

If all 12 cranial nerve functions are normal, you may either specifically describe the normal response of each cranial nerve or make a broad statement indicating normal status of all 12 nerves. A specific description follows:

> *Cranial nerve VII (facial):* Symmetric facial features noted at rest and with performance of facial expressions.

The following is an example of a broad statement:

> Cranial nerves I–XII tested. All functions intact and appropriate responses noted.

Any abnormal findings should be described in detail. Record the type of stimuli applied or test performed and the response that was elicited.

NDx

Nursing Diagnoses Related to Cranial Nerve Assessment

For persons displaying abnormal responses to cranial nerve testing, the nurse should determine whether or not the nursing diagnosis Sensory–perceptual alterations is applicable. If a sensory–perceptual alteration is confirmed, you should then attempt to diagnose the response to any deficits. For example, if cranial nerve II (optic) is impaired and the person has a visual deficit, you might diagnose a response such as Potential for injury. Or, if cranial nerve IX (glossopharyngeal) is impaired and the person has lost his or her gag reflex, you might diagnose a response such as Potential for aspiration. Dysfunction of cranial nerve VII (facial) may alter the appearance of the face, and one side may be noted to sag or droop. In this case, you may diagnose the person's response as Body image disturbance.

Clinical Problems Related to Cranial Nerve Assessment

Cranial nerve dysfunctions can be associated with a number of disease entities. Impingement of cranial nerves secondary to trauma, tumors, or fluid accumulations may result in abnormal findings during the cranial nerve examination. Diagnosis and treatment are usually directed toward the underlying pathology.

MOTOR FUNCTIONS AND REFLEXES

Alterations in motor function are frequently observed in persons who are experiencing cognitive and perceptual problems originating with lesions to the cerebral cortex or spinal cord. Evaluating the motor system is an important part of a comprehensive neurologic assessment. Neurologic disorders may affect muscle bulk, tone, strength, involuntary reflexes, in addition to a person's ability to perform voluntary movements. Additional guidelines for musculoskeletal assessment are discussed in Chapter 10.

Anatomy and Physiology Overview

Voluntary movement is controlled by the motor cortex located in the frontal lobe of the cerebrum and the descending (motor) corticospinal tracts (Fig. 11-7). From the cerebral cortex, the descending tracts pass through the subcortical white matter and the internal capsule, an area between the thalamus and basal ganglia where motor nerve tracts converge before entering the brainstem. Because all motor fibers pass through the internal capsule, a stroke in this area will cause a greater loss of motor function than will occur with a cerebral hemisphere stroke.

Most corticospinal nerve fibers cross to decussate in the lower medulla and descend the spinal cord as the lateral corticospinal tract. A few fibers continue to descend uncrossed along ventral corticospinal tracts. Motor function is controlled predominantly by the crossed fibers, which accounts for clinical findings such as left-sided paralysis following right cerebral hemisphere damage. Before leaving the brain stem, the corticospinal tract fibers pass through a structure known as the *pyramid,* a compact bundle of nerve fibers in the medulla.

The descending fibers, known as the *upper motor neurons* (UMNs), form synapses with other efferent neurons, the *lower motor neurons* (LMNs), in the anterior horn of the spinal cord. The LMN directly innervates skeletal muscle and transmits the neural impulses essential for movement. Lower motor neurons, called the *final common pathway,* are influenced by one of two neural pathways: descending fibers originating in the brain; or afferent neurons of the reflex arc (neural pathways independent of the brain).

In addition to transmitting neural impulses for voluntary movement through the corticospinal tract, descending cor-

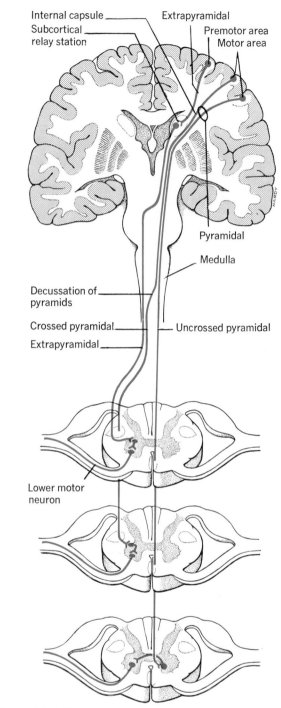

Figure 11–7. The motor cortex and motor tracts.

tical fibers transmit neural impulses that control muscle tone. For example, descending rubrospinal tract fibers facilitate flexor muscles and inhibit extensor muscles; pons and medulla descending reticulospinal tracts facilitate and inhibit stretch reflexes respectively.

Reflexes are involuntary motor movements or glandular secretions that are usually protective and adaptive in na-

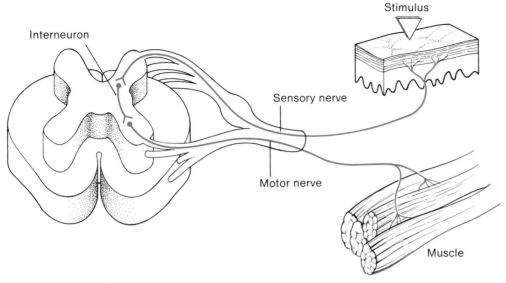

Figure 11-8. The reflex arc.

ture. The neural pathway involved in reflexes is the *reflex arc*. As noted in Figure 11-8, reflex arcs function independently of the brain. Reflex arcs may be monosynaptic (only two neurons and a synapse), or polysynaptic (more than two neurons). In either case, a sensory receptor in the skin or muscle is stimulated, and a neural impulse travels the afferent neuron to the spinal cord. An efferent neuron transmits the impuse back to an effector in the muscle or skin, which results in movement or glandular secretion. Were it not for inhibitory descending fibers from the brain, reflex activity would be more pronounced because the sensory receptors involved receive frequent stimulation.

Physical Examination

Motor System

General Principles

As a parameter for the assessment of neurologic function, motor system examination should focus on the following areas: degree of movement, strength and equality of movement, muscle tone, deep tendon reflexes, and superficial reflexes. This chapter section describes evaluation of deep tendon reflexes and superficial reflexes. Included in the deep tendon reflexes are the following: biceps, brachioradialis, triceps, patellar, and achilles. Superficial reflexes do not need to be assessed routinely but should be examined if neurologic or motor deficits are present.

Degrees of motor movement may indicate a person's level of consciousness; related assessment techniques are discussed in an earlier section of this chapter. Techniques for evaluating muscle strength and tone are discussed with musculoskeletal examination in Chapter 10. In addition, a person's gait, balance, and coordination may be tested to evaluate motor responses to proprioceptive sensory input in the cerebellum (see Sensory and Cerebellar Functions, p. 356).

Equipment

- Reflex hammer
- Tongue blade (optional)

Examination and Documentation Focus

Responses to applied stimuli, including the following:

- Type of movement
- Intensity
- Unexpected movements

Examination Guidelines   *Deep Tendon Reflexes*

Procedure

Note: Reflexes should be compared bilaterally.

Before You Begin

Practice using the reflex hammer. Deep tendon reflexes are tested by striking specific tendons with the reflex hammer. The hammer has a pointed end for small tendons and a blunt end for large tendons. Hold the instrument at the very end of its handle and allow the hammer to swing quickly and freely downward between the first and second fingers. Grasping the hammer too near its head will inhibit free movement.

Remember the principle of reinforcement. The person should be relaxed to elicit a deep tendon reflex successfully. If the reflex is diminished or absent, ask the person to use *reinforcement.* This method involves contracting muscles that are not being tested in order to relax the effector muscles that are being tested. For example, when testing the patellar reflex, reinforcement is accomplished by asking the person to lock the fingers and attempt to pull the hands apart.

Clinical Significance

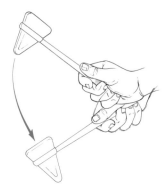

Using the reflex hammer

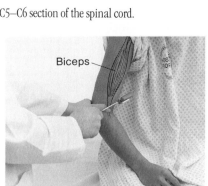

Reinforcement

1. TEST THE BICEPS REFLEX.

    a. Flex the person's arm slightly at the elbow and rest the forearm in your hand or on the person's leg.

    b. Place your thumb over the biceps tendon in the antecubital fossa.

Stimulates C5–C6 section of the spinal cord.

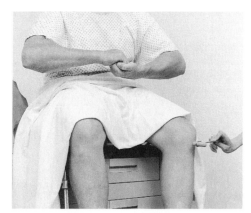

Biceps

Biceps reflex testing

    c. Strike your thumbnail with the pointed end of the hammer.

Normal Findings

Person's forearm flexes at the elbow.

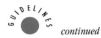

continued

Deep Tendon Reflexes

Procedure

2. TEST THE TRICEPS REFLEX.

   a. Flex the person's forearm at the elbow and hold the arm across the person's chest.

   b. Alternatively, allow the person's arm to hang loosely while you support it by placing your hand under the bicep.

Clinical Significance

Stimulates C6–C7 and C7–C8 sections of the spinal cord.

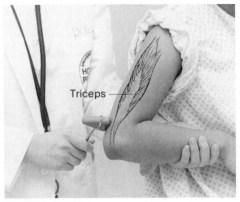

Triceps reflex testing

c. Strike the triceps tendon, located just above the olecranon process, with the blunt end of the hammer.

3. TEST THE BRACHIORADIALIS REFLEX.

   a. The person's forearm should be relaxed, palm facing down, and resting on the leg or supported by your hand.

Normal Findings

Forearm extends slightly at the elbow.

Stimulates C5–C6 section of the spinal cord.

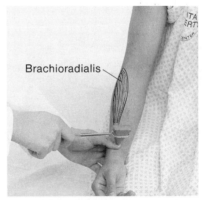

Brachioradialis reflex testing

b. Strike the brachioradialis tendon, located just above the styloid process of the radius.

4. TEST THE PATELLAR REFLEX.

   a. The person should be seated with the legs dangling or supine with the knees slightly flexed.

Normal Findings

Slight flexion of forearm at the elbow and forearm pronation.

Stimulates L2–L3 and L3–L4 sections of the spinal cord.

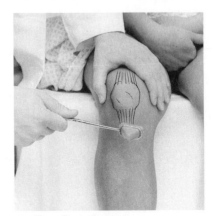

Patellar reflex testing

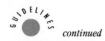

continued

Deep Tendon Reflexes

Procedure

   b. Strike the patellar tendon, located just below the knee-cap. Use the blunt end of the reflex hammer.

5. TEST THE ACHILLES REFLEX.

   a. Position the person in the same manner as you would for testing the patellar reflex.

Clinical Significance

Normal Findings

Leg extends at the knee.

Stimulates S1–S2 section of the spinal cord.

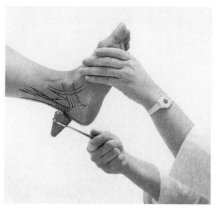

Achilles reflex testing

   b. Support the foot in a dorsiflexed position. Tap the Achilles tendon above the heel.

Normal Finding

Plantar flexion. This may be observed visually or felt by placing your hand against the sole of the foot as the reflex is tested.

Examination Guidelines   *Superficial Reflexes (Optional)*

Procedure

1. TEST THE UPPER/LOWER ABDOMINAL REFLEX.

   Lightly scratch or stroke the skin of the upper/lower abdominal quadrant with the handle of the reflex hammer or a tongue blade and note umbilical movement.

2. TEST THE CREMASTERIC REFLEX (MALES ONLY).

   Lightly scratch the inner, upper surface of the thigh and note testicular movement.

3. TEST THE PLANTAR REFLEX.

   a. Firmly stroke the outer border of the sole of the foot with the handle of the reflex hammer.

   b. Note the movement of the toes.

Clinical Significance

Upper abdominal: Stimulates T7–T8 and T8–T9 sections of the spinal cord.

Lower abdominal: Stimulates T11–T12 section of the spinal cord.

Normal response, upper abdominal: Umbilicus shifts upward toward point of stimulus.

Normal response, lower abdominal: Umbilicus shifts downward toward point of stimulus.

Stimulates T12–L1 and L1–L2 sections of the spinal cord.

Normal response: Testicle on the same side (ipsilateral) of stimulation rises.

Stimulates S1–S2 section of the spinal cord.

Normal response: Toes should flex (normal *adult* response); record the finding as Babinski negative.

Deviations from normal: If toes fan or extend, record the finding as Babinski positive, indicative in adults of cerebral dysfunction.

continued

Superficial Reflexes (Optional)

Procedure	Clinical Significance
4. IN PERSONS WITH NEUROLOGIC DEFICITS, TEST FOR THE PRIMITIVE REFLEXES—GRASP, SNOUT, GLABELLAR.	The primitive reflexes are indicators of cerebral pathology.
a. Test for the *grasp reflex.* Place your fingers in the palm of the person's hand.	*Abnormal reflex finding:* The person grasps your fingers but does not release the grasp when instructed.
b. Test for the *snout reflex.* Gently tap the side of the person's mouth.	*Abnormal reflex finding:* The person puckers the lips.
c. Test for the *glabellar reflex.* Gently tap the person on the forehead.	*Abnormal reflex finding:* The person blinks repeatedly after being tapped.

Documenting Reflex Examination Findings

The results of reflex testing may be documented by describing the type of movement noted when specific stimuli are applied to elicit a reflex. For example, you may describe a normal plantar reflex as follows:

> Toes flex following stroking sole of foot.

Deep tendon reflexes and plantar reflexes are more often described using a grading scale and diagram as shown in Display 11-3.

NDx

Nursing Diagnoses Related to Reflex Assessment

Persons displaying abnormal reflexes may have neurologic dysfunctions or electrolyte imbalances. Generally, these problems are not addressed by nursing diagnoses. However, the nurse should consider the types of responses (*e.g.,* anxiety) the person may be experiencing as a result of these problems. The response, rather than the neurologic deficit, becomes the focus when formulating nursing diagnoses related to reflex assessment.

Display 11–3
Documenting Reflexes

Grading Deep Tendon Reflexes

Deep tendon reflexes are graded on a scale of 0 to 4:

0   No response
1+ Diminished (hypoactive)
2+ Normal
3+ Increased (may be interpreted as normal)
4+ Hyperactive (hyperreflexia)

The deep tendon responses and plantar reflexes are commonly recorded on stick figures. The arrow points downward if the plantar response is normal and upward if the response is abnormal.

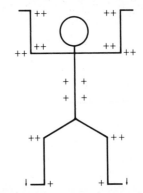

Recording deep tendon reflexes

Clinical Problems Related to Reflex Assessment

Reflex testing provides an indication of the status of the central nervous system in the conscious and unconscious person. Reflex responses may be helpful in distinguishing upper motor neuron and lower neuron pathology.

Damage to upper or lower motor neurons results in altered motor function; the examination findings and type of motor loss associated with each area differ (Table 11-2). Damage to upper motor neurons before decussation in the brain stem usually results in contralateral motor deficits, such as paralysis (hemiplegia) or weakness (hemiparesis). Upper motor neuron damage is also associated with hyperactive reflexes because inhibitory fibers are affected. Cerebral or brain stem dysfunction may result in complete loss of voluntary movements and abnormal reflex development or abnormal motor movements (see Table 11-2). Abnormal reflexes may include a positive Babinski reflex and grasp, snout, and glabellar reflexes. Although the exact mechanism is unclear, abnormal reflexes are believed to be primitive reflexes that are suppressed with nervous system maturation. Pathologic conditions may cause the primitive reflexes to reemerge.

Abnormal motor movements include decortication and decerebration. The clinical significance and assessment of these responses are discussed elsewhere in this chapter (see p. 365).

SENSORY AND CEREBELLAR FUNCTIONS

Anatomy and Physiology Overview

The sensory function tests that are presented in this section provide information about primary or cutaneous sensation and cortical integration of sensory impulses. The structures involved include peripheral spinal nerves, spinal cord sensory pathways, the thalamus, and sensory areas of the cerebral cortex. In addition, cerebellar processing of proprioceptive stimuli is discussed.

The two main types of sensations include exteroceptive, which is caused by stimuli outside the body such as pain, temperature, and touch, and proprioceptive, which is caused by inner body stimuli, such as position, kinesthetic, and vibration sense and touch responses.

Peripheral Nerves and Dermatomes. Specialized sensory cells in the skin, joints, muscles, and bones detect and then transmit sensory stimuli through peripheral nerve fiber networks. Eventually, fibers join peripheral nerve pathways that enter the posterior portion of the spinal cord as the posterior nerve root. This is the afferent or sensory division of the peripheral nervous system.

Table 11–2. Features of Upper and Lower Motor Neuron Disorders

Upper Motor Neuron
- Spastic paralysis
- Hyperactive reflexes
- Muscle weakness without atrophy
- Decorticate posturing (usually following brain hypoxia)
- Possibly frequent urination with reflex bladder emptying (reflex bladder)

Lower Motor Neuron
- Flaccid paralysis
- Muscle atrophy
- Muscle fasciculations
- Absence of reflex responses
- Possibly urinary retention with overflow incontinence (atonic bladder)

Each posterior nerve root is associated with a peripheral sensory network that supplies a strip of skin called a *dermatome* (Fig. 11-9). Although dermatomes appear to have distinct boundaries, some overlap between adjacent dermatomes may exist.

Sensory testing involves applying stimuli to the person's skin surface. Dermatomes should be used to describe specific spinal sensory nerves being tested in comprehensive and specialized examinations. If impaired cutaneous sensation is detected, the examiner should test other areas within the same dermatome. If the entire dermatome is involved but surrounding dermatomes are unaffected, the examiner should suspect a lesion of the posterior nerve root supplying the dermatome, such as posterior nerve root compression secondary to herniated nucleus pulposus. The client may experience pain, tingling, or numbness throughout the dermatome for the affected root.

Dermatomes may be used to explain other sensory phenomena such as referred pain syndromes. For example, clients with ischemic heart pain may feel pain in the jaw, shoulder, and upper extremity as well as the chest. As shown in Figure 11-10, such pain occurs because somatic sensory nerve fibers from the heart have central connections in common with afferent nerve fibers that correspond with arm, shoulder, and jaw dermatomes.

Spinal Cord Sensory Pathways. Sensory impulses enter the spinal cord through the posterior nerve root and travel toward the brain along major spinal cord sensory pathways, most of which cross the midline at some point before reaching the cerebral cortex. Clinically significant ascending sensory pathways include the following (Fig. 11-11):

- *The posterior columns (fasciculus gracilis and fasciculus cuneatus).* Sensory fibers enter the posterior horn of the spinal cord and ascend uncrossed to the medulla. In the medulla, the fibers cross and ascend through the midbrain to the cerebral cortex. Sensations conducted along these pathways include vibratory sense, kinesthesia and proprioception, two-point discrimination, and tactile localization.

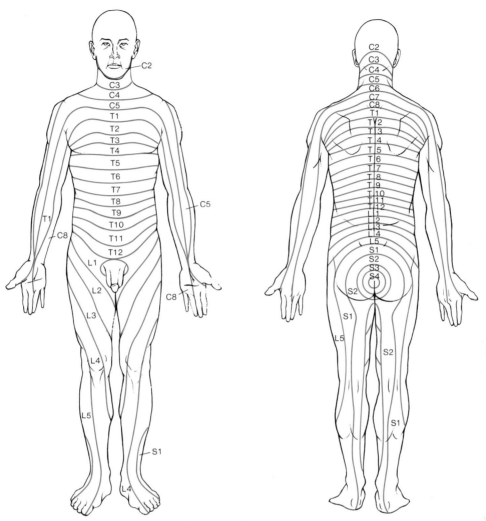

Figure 11–9. Dermatomes.

- *Lateral spinothalamic tract:* Sensory fibers enter the posterior horn and cross the midline at each segmental level of the cord before ascending toward the brain. Sensations conducted along this pathway include pain and temperature.
- *Anterior spinothalamic tract:* Fibers enter the posterior horn and cross the midline at each segmental level of the cord before ascending toward the brain along a route slightly anterior to the lateral spinothalamic tract. Sensations conducted along this pathway include light touch, pain, pressure, and temperature.
- *Posterior and anterior spinocerebellar tracts:* Fibers enter the posterior horn and ascend to the cerebellum, which senses proprioceptive stimuli influencing muscle tone and synergy. Cerebellar sensation impairment affects posture and coordination. Fibers of the ascending dorsal tract do not cross the ventral tract.

Contralateral and ipsilateral sensory deficits can be considered on the basis of sensory tract midline crossings and the location of the causative lesion. A spinothalamic tract lesion located above the crossing point within the spinal cord may cause contralateral sensory losses. For example, a cerebral infarct, causing damage to one side of the sensory cortex may cause the person to have sensory loss on the opposite side of the body. If the spinothalamic tract is damaged within the spinal cord at the crossing point, sensory losses may occur at the dermatome for the affected cord segment. A cord lesion that affects the posterior pathways below the crossing point in the medulla may cause ipsilateral loss of proprioceptive sensations. Because touch is both an exteroceptive and proprioceptive sensation and has alternate pathways to the brain, touch sensation may remain intact following spinothalamic tract lesions.

Thalamus. The thalamus, located in the lower inner portion of the brain, functions as a relay station for sensory and motor impulses traveling to and from the cerebral cortex and plays a role in consciousness and alertness. Incoming sensory stimuli are processed in the thalamus, but conscious interpretation of sensory stimuli, other than pain, does not occur at this level. The thalamus may facilitate cerebral interpretation of sensory stimuli by selectively masking or unmasking cerebral sensory receptive areas and

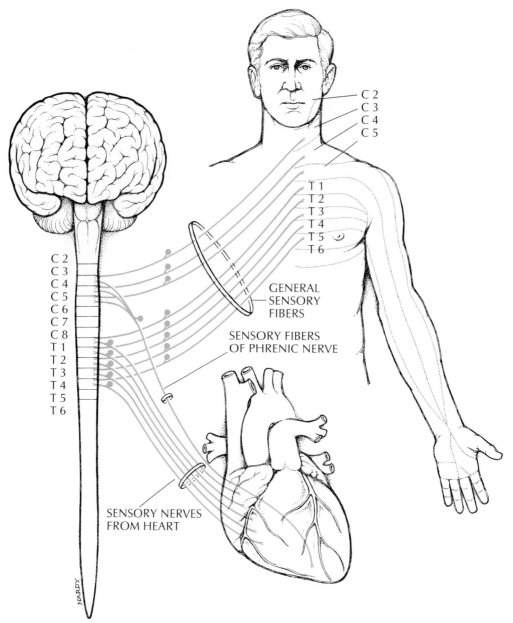

C 2
C 3
C 4
C 5

T 1
T 2
T 3
T 4
T 5
T 6

GENERAL
SENSORY
FIBERS

SENSORY FIBERS
OF PHRENIC NERVE

C 2
C 3
C 4
C 5
C 6
C 7
C 8
T 1
T 2
T 3
T 4
T 5
T 6

SENSORY NERVES
FROM HEART

Figure 11–10. Referred pain from the heart. (Capell, P.T., & Case, D.B. [1976]. *Ambulatory care manual for nurse practitioners.* Philadelphia: J.B. Lippincott)

delivering sensory input to the appropraite area of the cerebral cortex. Olfactory stimuli are the only sensory input that bypass the thalamus.

One type of sensory distortion known as "thalamic pain" may occur secondary to lesions of the posterior nuclei in the thalamus. The person experiencing such pain may not perceive single sensory stimuli such as light touch (pinpricks). However, repetitive or vigorous stimuli may cause considerable discomfort. Thalamic pain is usually more intensified when the offending stimuli occur in addition to unpleasant emotions.

Sensory Cerebral Cortex. The cerebral cortex, or gray matter at the outer surface of the cerebral hemispheres, is referred to as the sensorimotor cortex because both sensory and motor impulses are processed by cortex neurons.

Brodman divided the cerebral cortex into 47 different areas, correlating functional relations with anatomic locations (Fig. 11-12). Tactile sensations are perceived in the area over the parietal lobe or Brodman's areas 1, 2, and 3. Besides perceiving sensations, the gray matter makes distinctions between degrees of touch, temperature, vibration, and pain.

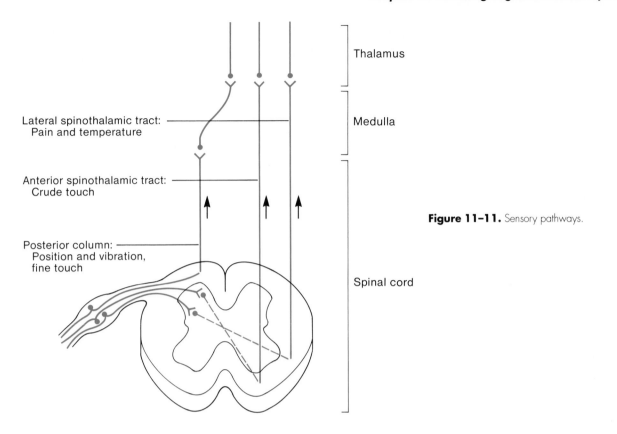

Lateral spinothalamic tract:
Pain and temperature

Anterior spinothalamic tract:
Crude touch

Posterior column:
Position and vibration,
fine touch

Thalamus

Medulla

Spinal cord

Figure 11–11. Sensory pathways.

Brodman's area 5, a somatic association area, formulates primary sensory stimuli such as tactile sensation into object images and then identifies such images. This process of knowing (or *gnosis*) involves comparing present sensory input with past experience. For example, somatic association areas must be activated when identifying a familiar object on the basis of touch.

Damage to any of these sensory areas may affect primary sensation or the person's abilities to recognize sensory stimuli (agnosisa). Sensory examination reveals associated deficits.

Cerebellum. Proprioceptive sensory impulses are sent to the cerebellum along the posterior and anterior spinocerebellar tracts. Cerebellar processing of such stimuli maintains coordination, posture, and balance. These cerebellar functions should be tested as part of the sensory examination.

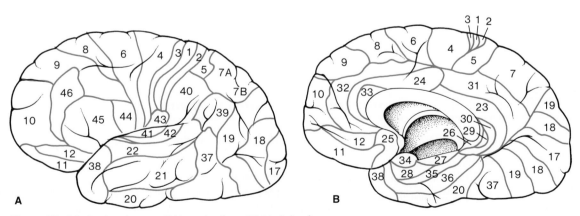

Figure 11–12. Brodman's areas. (**A**) Lateral surface. (**B**) Medial surface.

Physical Examination   *Sensory and Cerebellar Functions*

General Principles

Sensory testing involves applying stimuli to the person's skin surface and noting the person's ability to perceive and identify the stimulus. A complete sensory examination, involving sensation testing over the entire skin surface, is lengthy, and may tire the client and produce unreliable findings. Therefore, sensory testing should be conducted to assess major dermatomes, and conclusions about overall sensory function should be formed accordingly. For gross screening, test skin surfaces at the following areas: foot, lower leg, abdomen, hand, forearm, and face. If no sensory dysfunctions are suspected, fewer areas may be tested. Always compare the left and right sides of the body.

Persons requiring more extensive sensory testing include those who are experiencing rapidly increasing sensory loss, such as occurs with Guillain-Barré syndrome. In such cases, sequential dermatomes should be tested to determine the exact level of sensory deficits. More thorough assessment is also indicated for patients who report numbness, pain, or motor deficits and who have trophic skin changes such as hairless, thin, or shiny skin.

When testing sensation in a particular region, apply the stimulus in a distal-to-proximal manner, such as toes to foot to ankle. Sensation at the most distal site usually indicates that the corresponding spinal nerve tract is intact and precludes further testing within a dermatome. When a sensory deficit exists, you can pinpoint the exact level of dysfunction with distal-to-proximal testing.

Equipment

Sensory testing may be performed with the following stimuli:

- *Light touch:* Cotton wisps, soft brush, or fingertips
- *Pain:* Safety pin, needles (discard pin/needle after using), deep pressure applied by the examiner
- *Temperature:* Test tubes filled with hot and cold water
- *Vibration:* Tuning fork
- *Stereognosis:* Familiar objects, such as a key, comb, or pencil
- *Two-point discrimination:* Pins, needles, two-pronged caliper

Minimizing Cueing

Familiarize the person with each stimulus, such as cotton wisps, pinpricks, or the tuning fork, before the examination and then instruct the person to relax and close his or her eyes for the remainder of the examination. If visual cueing is allowed to occur, responses to tactile stimuli may be rendered invalid. Vary testing patterns and sequence so the person will not simply respond to a predictable pattern. Asking the person to identify a stimulus rather than asking whether or not the stimulus was felt can help eliminate suggestion. If a tuning fork is used to test vibration sense, eliminate audible vibratory noise by running the tap or turning on a radio.

Examination and Documentation Focus

- Ability to sense and discriminate light touch, pain, temperature, vibration
- Gnosis
- Proprioception and kinesthesia

Examination Guidelines   *Sensory and Cerebellar Functions*

Procedure	Clinical Significance
1. TEST LIGHT TOUCH SENSATION.	
a. Brush the person's skin with cotton, a soft brush, or your fingertips.	***Normal Findings***
b. Ask the person to identify the sensation and locate the stimuli (Where do you feel this?).	Identifies skin surface touched by the examiner. The ability to discriminate light touch may normally vary at different body areas. Symmetrical areas should have comparable responses.

Sensory and Cerebellar Functions

Procedure

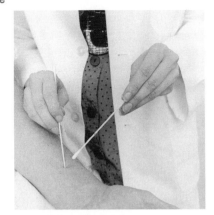

Testing light touch sensation

2. TEST SUPERFICIAL PAIN SENSATION AND THE ABILITY TO DISCRIMINATE SHARP AND DULL PAIN.

   a. Alternately apply a hypodermic needle point (sharp) and hub (dull) against the person's skin and ask the person to identify the stimulus.

   b. Use minimal pressure necessary to elicit a response, being careful not to pierce the skin.

   c. Pause several seconds between applying stimuli to allow the person to perceive each stimuli.

Clinical Significance

Hypodermic needles are preferred to sharp and dull ends of safety pins because sterile needles minimize potential for transmitting infection.

Normal Findings

Person can distinguish sharp and dull pain sensations.

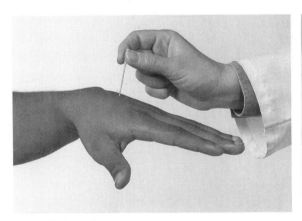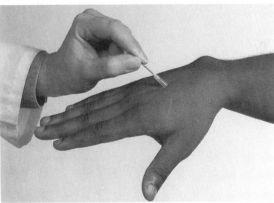

Testing pain sensation

3. TEST DEEP PAIN SENSATION.

   a. Grasp a tendon such as the Achilles or biceps between your thumb and forefinger and squeeze hard enough to elicit feelings of pressure or pain.

   b. If the patient is comatose, evaluate pain sensation by applying gradual pressure with a pen or reflex hammer handle over the finger or toe nail bed.

Intact sensory pathways will be indicated by facial grimace or decerebrate/decorticate posturing even when the patient is in a deep coma.

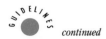
continued

Sensory and Cerebellar Functions

Procedure

4. TEST TEMPERATURE SENSATION (OPTIONAL)

   a. Test temperature sensation by alternately applying a test tube filled with warm water or cold water against the skin.

   b. Ask the person to identify whether the stimulus is warm or cold.

Clinical Significance

This test is unnecessary if pain sensation is within normal limits.

Normal Findings

Distinguishes warm and cold.

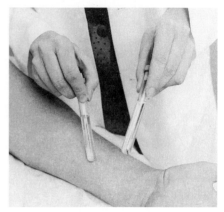

Testing temperature sensation

5. TEST VIBRATION SENSATION.

   a. Strike a tuning fork against your hand and apply the base to one of the person's bony prominences such as the clavicles, sternum, finger joints, wrists, ankles, or toes.

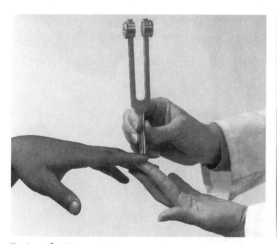

Testing vibration sensation

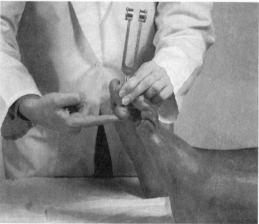

   b. Place your finger beneath the bony prominence if possible.

   c. Determine if the person senses the tuning fork vibration while it occurs as well as when the vibration stops. Tell the person to respond "buzzing" when the vibration is sensed and "no" when sensing pressure only.

This enables you to feel the vibration and evaluate the accuracy of the person's response.

Normal Findings

Identifies when vibration starts and stops.

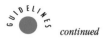

continued   *Sensory and Cerebellar Functions*

Procedure

6. TEST JOINT POSITION SENSE.

   a. Begin testing joint position sense of the most distal joints: the toes and fingers. Grasp a toe or finger on the sides and move it up or down.

   b. If the person does not sense joint position of toes and fingers, test more proximal joints.

Clinical Significance

Normal Findings

The person should be able to identify each move, no matter how slight, by the word *up* or *down* relative to the previous stationary position.

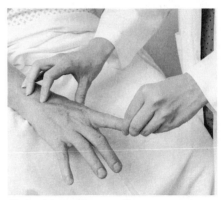

Testing joint position sensation

7. EVALUATE SENSORY ASSOCIATION.

   a. Evaluate *stereognosis.* Place a familiar object in the person's hand and ask the person to identify it by touch alone.

   b. Evaluate *topognosia.* Touch one of the person's fingers and ask the person to identify which one is being touched.

   c. Evaluate *graphognosia.* Trace a letter or number on the person's palm and ask the person to identify it.

Normal Findings

Gnosis: The ability to comprehend and recognize sensory stimuli.

The ability to identify familiar objects placed in either hand reflects the integrative functions of the parietal and occipital lobes.

Normal response: Client can identify which finger you are touching and whether it is on the left or right side of the body.

The ability to identify numbers indicates a functioning parietal node.

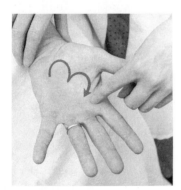

Testing graphognosis

8. CHECK TWO-POINT DISCRIMINATION.

   Press two needles or two points of a caliper against the person's skin. Ask the person the number of needles being felt.

Norman Findings

Person can sense whether one or two areas of skin are being touched.

Two points are discriminated at the following separations: fingertips, 2.8–5.0 mm; palms, 8–12 mm; dorsal surface of hand, 20–30 mm; chest and forearm, 40 mm; back, 40–70 mm; upper arms and thighs, 75 mm; shins, 30–40 mm.

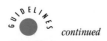 *continued*

Sensory and Cerebellar Functions

Procedure

9. EVALUATE CEREBELLAR FUNCTION.

   a. *Finger-to-nose-to-finger test:* Ask the person to touch the index finger to the nose while eyes are closed. Alternatively, ask the person to touch his or her fingertip to your fingertip.

   b. *Hand movements:* Ask the person to rapidly pronate and supinate the hands.

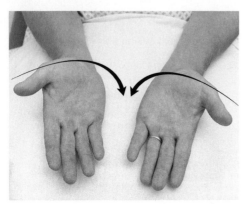

Testing cerebellar function

   c. *Romberg test:* Ask the person to stand with feet close together. First, while the person's eyes are open, note any swaying or difficulty in maintaining balance. Assist person with balance if necessary. Then ask the person to shut the eyes and note if the person moves.

   d. Evaluate gait (see Chap. 10, p. 281).

Clinical Significance

Normal Findings

Easily touches nose with finger when eyes are closed, and can touch fingertip.

Normal Findings

Diadochokinesia: The ability to perform rapid alternating movements.

Deviations from Normal

Adiadochokinesia: Inability to perform rapid alternating movements.

Normal Findings

Slight swaying is normal; if the person maintains balance, the Romberg test is negative.

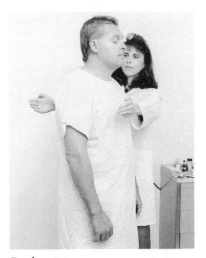

Romberg test

Documenting Sensory and Cerebellar Functions

If the examination indicates that sensory and cerebellar functions are normal, document your findings as follows:

> Able to sense and discriminate light touch, pain, temperature, and vibration at major dermatomes. Position sense and two-point discrimination intact. Able to sense joint positions with eyes closed. Can identify objects placed in hand and can identify figure traced on hand. Able to alternate hand movements rapidly. Romberg negative.

Abnormal findings should be described in detail, noting the dermatome(s) affected, the type of stimuli applied to elicit a response, and an exact description of the abnormal response. Descriptive terms used to describe abnormal sensory responses include the following:

- *Anesthesia:* Anesthesia is the absence of sensation and may occur secondary to stroke in varying degrees. A stroke in the thalamic area of the brain may result in complete, contralateral anesthesia. Complete anesthesia is less likely with cerebral hemisphere stroke because alternate sensory pathways remain unharmed. Complete spinal cord transection or pressure from spinal cord tumors may cause incomplete anesthesia. For example, pain and temperature sensation may be lost on one side of the body below the lesion.
- *Paresthesia:* Paresthesia refers to abnormal and unpleasant sensations such as burning, tingling, and crawling, which may occur as a result of contact with sensory stimuli or may occur spontaneously. Paresthesia results from incomplete peripheral nerve damage caused by tumors or diseases such as diabetes mellitus.
- *Hypesthesia (hypoesthesia):* Hypesthesia refers to abnormally decreased sensitivity in the skin and is usually caused by partial damage to peripheral nerves.
- *Hypalgesia:* Hypalgesia refers to a decreased pain sensation.
- *Analgesia:* Analgesia refers to an absence of pain sensation. The person may still feel pressure or touch.

NDx

Nursing Diagnoses Related to Sensory and Cerebellar Assessment

For persons displaying abnormal responses to sensory testing, the nurse should determine whether or not the nursing diagnosis Sensory–perceptual alterations (tactile) is applicable. If a tactile sensory–perceptual alteration is confirmed, you should then attempt to diagnose the person's response to any deficits. For example, persons with impaired tactile abilities may be at high risk for injury or tissue damage. Similarly, persons with cerebellar dysfunction may also be at risk for injury secondary to impaired balance or gait.

Clinical Problems Related to Sensory and Cerebellar Assessment

Abnormal findings in response to testing sensory and cerebellar functions indicate dysfunction of the central and/or peripheral nervous system. Additional diagnosis and treatment is directed toward the underlying pathology.

COGNITIVE FUNCTIONS
Anatomy and Physiology Overview

Cognitive functions, such as the ability to think, understand, communicate, and interact with the environment, are controlled by the cerebral cortex and require integrity of other neurologic structures such as the brain stem and sensory organs. Therefore, evaluation indicates the status of cognitive functions as well as related neurologic structures.

An evaluation of cognitive function focuses on appearance, behavior, orientation, speech patterns, memory, logic, and affect. A systematic assessment of cognitive function is based on observing the following: level of consciousness, awareness, thought processes, and communication abilities.

CEREBRAL CORTEX

The cerebral cortex is divided into four lobes: frontal, temporal, parietal, and occipital (Fig. 11-13). The cognitive functions discussed in this section primarily originate with the frontal lobe. The frontal lobe is divided into three functional areas: the prefrontal area, the motor area, and Broca's area. Psychic and cognitive functions, including personality, judgment, attention span, moral and ethical behaviors, drive, and depth of feeling, originate in the prefrontal area. Motor speech orignates in Broca's area. Speech functions are also controlled by Wernicke's area, located in the temporal lobe of the cerebral cortex.

SPEECH AND LANGUAGE

Speech and language functions are regulated by specific areas of the cerebral cortex. The left cerebral hemisphere is the dominant hemisphere for language function in over 90% of right-handed persons. Therefore, left hemisphere strokes are commonly associated with aphasia, whereas right hemisphere strokes are less likely to cause aphasia. In left-handed persons, the left hemisphere is dominant for language only 50% to 75% of the time.

Despite the concept of cerebral hemisphere dominance, it should be remembered that both hemispheres have some language function. The left hemisphere is responsible for propositional language such as word order, choice, and combinations to form phrases and sentences. The right

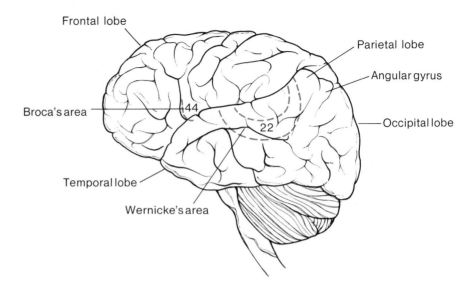

Figure 11-13. The cerebral cortex. Lateral view of the cerebral cortex showing speech areas.

hemisphere is responsible for affective language such as melody of speech, emotional tone, and intonation.

Wernicke's area (Brodmann's #22) is located in the temporal lobe of the dominant hemisphere and processes word symbols, which allows for understanding and interpretation. *Broca's area* (Brodmann's #44), located in the frontal lobe of the dominant hemisphere (see Fig. 11–13), func-

tions in the propositional language aspects and involves converting messages in the brain into words, phrases, and sentences in a manner consistent with grammatical rules. Another major speech and language area is located at the angular gyrus of the parietal lobe, which receives all incoming sensory stimuli and relates stimuli to language.

Physical Examination   *Cognitive Functions*

General Principles

Examination of cognitive functions focuses on the following: level of consciousness, awareness, thought processes, and communication abilities. Evaluation is conducted by means of observation or diagnostic testing (see "Diagnostic Studies," p. 312).

Level of consciousness refers to degree of wakefulness or arousability and is regulated by the reticular activating system (RAS) in the brain stem. In the strictest sense, consciousness is not the same as awareness. A person may be conscious but unaware of time or place. Level of consciousness is evaluated by observing a person's arousability, ability to speak and follow verbal commands, and motor abilities. Level of consciousness may be quantified in relation to the intensity of the sensory stimuli required to arouse a person.

Awareness refers to a person's ability to understand, think, feel emotions, and to appreciate sensory information about self and surroundings. At the highest levels of awareness, people are able to react purposefully to sensory input with both thoughts and actions. Awareness is evaluated by observing a person's level of orientation in relation to person, place, and time. Any perceptual deficits manifested by impaired awareness of self and surroundings are also noted.

Thought processes that are evaluated as part of the mental status evaluation include abstract thinking, problem solving, insight, memory, and judgment. These capacities are regulated by the frontal lobe of the cerebral cortex. Thought processes are evaluated by observing a person's ability to perform various cognitive tasks, such as interpreting statements, solving problems, memorizing, and making judgments. Several factors may influence a person's performance, such as the following:

- The amount of attention focused on the examiner
- The ability to understand the language or jargon used by the examiner
- Perceptual problems such as agnosia or aphasia
- Emotional withdrawal or depression

• The perception of certain questions or exercises as insulting, in which case a person may give the wrong responses out of anger, not as a result of impaired functioning

The influence of these and other factors should be considered throughout the evaluation process.

Communication processes include the person's speech patterns and ability to comprehend language. When speech and language problems are identified, a professional speech therapist may be consulted for specialized assessment and intervention. However, the nurse's assessment remains an important component of the clinical data base. Sudden changes in communicative abilities may indicate significant neurologic dysfunctions. Additionally, assessment helps you identify the specific nature of the communication problem. Accurate diagnosis facilitates optimal nurse–client communication between speech therapy interventions, or during more acute phases of illness when professional speech therapy is not a priority.

Because speech and language evaluation may be frustrating or embarrassing to the patient, assess communication processes only as often as necessary. Carefully record and communicate findings to avoid repeated assessments.

When your patient cannot communicate, ask family or friends about previous communication abilities and patterns and about vision and hearing abilities. Ask about reading and writing abilities because these areas will also be assessed. Assuming that a person has a cerebral disorder because he or she cannot read a passage in a book will be an erroneous conclusion if the person never learned to read.

Serial Evaluations

Serial evaluations of cognitive functions, especially level of consciousness, are recommended in patients with actual or potential alterations of cerebral structures and functions. This includes patients who are recovering from neurosurgical procedures and those with neurologic problems such as head injury, loss of consciousness, increased intracranial pressure, unexplained behavior or mood changes, seizures, and dizziness.

Serial evaluations of cognitive functions provide an index against which measurement can be made of the improvement or deterioration of a person's condition. Changes in the level of consciousness may be the earliest indication of significant changes in a person's condition.

Examination and Documentation Focus

• *Level of consciousness:* Response to sensory stimuli; degree of stimulation required to elicit a response
• *Awareness:* Orientation to person, place, time
• *Thought processes:* Abstract thinking, problem solving abilities, memory, judgment
• *Communication abilities:* Comprehension, writing, nonverbal communication

Examination Guidelines   *Level of Consciousness*

Procedure	Clinical Significance
1. DETERMINE THE INTENSITY OF STIMULI NECESSARY TO AROUSE THE PERSON.	
a. If the person is observed to be fully awake, no further testing is necessary.	
b. If the person appears asleep or unconscious, attempt arousal by applying progressively more intensive stimuli: calling the person by name, touching or gently shaking the person, applying painful stimuli.	Avoid unnecessary exposure to painful stimuli by first trying to arouse the person through verbal stimuli.
c. If it becomes necessary to subject the person to painful stimuli, the stimulus should be removed as soon as a response is noted. The following methods may be used: Apply pressure to the trapezius muscle by grasping the belly of the muscle between thumb and forefingers and squeezing. Apply pressure to the Achilles tendon by grasping the tendon between thumb and forefingers and squeezing.	Certain methods for applying painful stimuli should be avoided, such as vigorously rubbing the knuckles into the sternum ("sternal rub") and pinching the skin. Not only are these methods unnecessarily cruel, they also result in greater tissue damage and bruising.

continued

Level of Consciousness

Procedure

Apply pressure to the nail beds by squeezing the nail beds between your thumb and forefinger. Some examiners prefer to place a pen or pencil over the nail plate and squeeze the nail bed between the pen and forefinger.

Clinical Significance

Normal Findings

Fully Awake: Highest level of consciousness, characterized by the ability to respond to all types of sensory stimuli of minimal intensity. However, a person may be fully awake but still disoriented or forgetful.

Alert: Level of consciousness in which a person is fully awake and oriented as to person, place, time, and environment. Additionally, the person is capable of responding to verbal commands.

Deviations from Normal

Lethargic: Person appears drowsy or asleep most of the time but is capable of making spontaneous movements. It is possible to arouse the person, but gentle shaking of the person is usually required in addition to saying his or her name. Lethargic people tend to fall back to sleep easily and may become disoriented.

Obtunded: The person sleeps most of the time and makes few spontaneous body movements. More vigorous stimulation such as shouting or shaking is needed to arouse the person. The person is still capable of making verbal responses, but is less likely to respond appropriately to verbal commands.

Stuporous (Semicomatose): The person is unconscious most of the time and does not exhibit spontaneous motor activity. Strong, noxious stimuli such as pain are needed to elicit a motor response, which is usually a purposeful attempt to remove the stimuli. Verbal responses are limited or absent. A semicomatose person is rarely oriented or fully awake, even when the examiner is testing responses to sensory stimulation.

Comatose: The person cannot be aroused, even by applying painful stimuli. Some reflex responses to stimuli may be noted, such as the gag reflex. If no reflex responses occur, the person is in a deep coma.

A decline in the level of consciousness is associated with a progressive decline in the ability to purposefully respond to a stimulus.

2. DETERMINE MOTOR RESPONSES TO VERBAL OR PAINFUL STIMULI.

Ask the person to complete a simple task and note response. If the person does not respond to verbal stimuli, apply painful stimuli and observe the motor response.

Normal Findings

Ability to obey verbal commands: The person can move the extremities when asked or perform some other requested task such as squeezing and letting go of your fingers.

Deviations from Normal

Ability to localize or make purposeful movements: The person can withdraw from or attempt to locate and stop a painful stimulus. Any such attempt, whether successful or not, should be classified as purposeful movements.

Semipurposeful response: The person grimaces or briefly flexes the extremities in response to a painful stimulus, but makes no attempt to remove the stimulus.

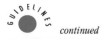

continued <u>*Level of Consciousness*</u>

Procedure

Clinical Significance

Flexor or decorticate posturing response: Flexion and adduction of the upper extremities with extension, internal rotation, and plantar flexion in the lower extremities. Decorticate posturing may occur in response to painful stimuli or may be spontaneous.

Decorticate posturing is associated with damage to the internal capsule of the brain or pyramidal tracts above the brainstem.

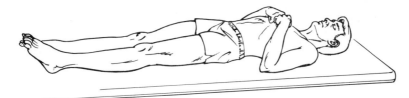

Flexor or decorticate posturing response

Extensor or decerebrate posturing: Rigid extension and adduction of one or both arms, and extension of the legs. Decerebrate posturing may occur in response to painful stimuli or may be spontaneous.

Decerebrate posturing is associated with little or no activity above the brainstem level and is a poorer prognostic sign than decorticate posturing.

Flaccid response: No motor response to painful stimuli and a weak or lax appearance of the extremities.

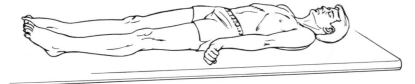

Extensor or decerebrate posturing

Examination Guidelines   *Awareness*

Procedure

1. DETERMINE ORIENTATION TO PERSON, PLACE, AND TIME.
   a. Note responses to the following questions to evaluate *temporal (time) orientation:*
      - What is the date (day, month, year)?
      - What day of the week is this?
      - What time of day is this (morning, afternoon, evening)?
      - What was the last meal that you ate (breakfast, lunch, dinner)?
      - What season is this?
      - What was the last holiday?

Clinical Significance

Deviations from Normal

When awareness is impaired, a person usually loses time orientation first, followed by place orientation and then person orientation. However, exceptions to this pattern may be noted.

People in unfamiliar environments, without time cues such as clocks, calenders, television, or newspapers, may lose track of time. The last four questions in this list may be a more appropriate means of evaluating such people.

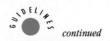

continued   ***Awareness***

Procedure	Clinical Significance

Procedure

    b. Note responses to the following questions to evaluate *locus (place) orientation:*

- Where are you now?
- What is the name of this building?
- What is the name of this city?
- What state is this?

    c. Note responses to the following questions to evaluate *person (personal) orientation:*

- What is your name?
- Who was just here to visit you?
- Who is this? (Indicate visitors or family members who are present).
- What do you do for a living?
- How old are you?
- Where do you live?
- What is your wife's (husband's) name?

2. EVALUATE FOR THE OCCURRENCE OF ONE-SIDED NEGLECT.

    a. Observe the person performing daily activities.

    b. Ask the person to read a page-width newspaper headline.

    c. Ask the person to draw a self-portrait or the face of a clock.

    d. Place several small, common objects on a table in front of the person. Ask the person to name the objects.

    e. Observe the person's pattern of ambulation.

Clinical Significance

Consider whether or not the person has been moved several times (*e.g.,* having been transferred through different hospital departments and nursing units). In such cases, the person may have difficulty naming the present or previous location.

Determine personal identity (name) and other personal data, including roles and life-style. Asking the person to name various health care providers may be an unreliable technique, especially if the patient has been in contact with many different people in one day, as occurs in acute care settings.

This type of evaluation is indicated for persons who appear to ignore sensory messages from the left side of the body.

Deviations from Normal

Ignoring one side when bathing, combing the hair, shaving, dressing, or eating is a sign of one-sided neglect.

A person with one-sided neglect may omit words from the left side of the page.

The left side of the drawing is incomplete or missing altogether with one-sided neglect.

One-sided neglect is associated with failure to name objects on the left side of the table.

Persons with one-sided neglect often bump into things on the affected side.

Examination Guidelines   *Thought Processes*

Procedure

1. EVALUATE ABSTRACT THINKING OR CLASSIFICATION.

    a. Test lower-level abilities for abstract thinking by asking the person to classify common objects according to use. For example, spread the following objects on a table: pen, pencil, comb, brush, hairpin, spoon, napkin, and salt shaker. Then ask the person which things go together. Demonstrate by picking up the pen and pencil and explaining that both objects are used for writing.

    Another test for lower-level abilities is asking the person to sort a deck of cards according to suit.

Clinical Significance

Abstract thinking is the ability to interpret concepts and ideas, and enables a person to understand unfamiliar situations. The ability to interpret proverbs, engage in creative conversation, and understand a joke as humorous all require a capacity for abstract thinking.

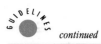 *continued*

Thought Processes

Procedure	Clinical Significance

Procedure

b. Test higher levels of abstract thinking by asking the person to interpret proverbs.

Example: Ask the person what is meant by the expression, "The early bird catches the worm."

c. Ask the person to describe similarities and differences between objects, such as a tree and a flower.

2. EVALUATE THE ABILITY TO SOLVE PROBLEMS AND CONCENTRATE.

a. *Problem solving:* Ask the person to perform an arithmetic calculation. For example, ask how many lemons can be purchased for $4 if lemons are priced at 5 for $1.

b. *Concentration:* Test concentration by asking the person to count backward from 100 by 7's (the serial 7's test). Alternatively, ask the person to count to 20 by odd numbers only.

3. EVALUATE MEMORY.

a. Test *immediate memory.* Ask the person to remember three numbers, such as 7, 0, and 4. Then, 1 or 2 minutes later, ask the person to recite the numbers.

If the person has difficulty with this task, offer a simpler test of immediate memory or retention. Give the person a set of instructions and observe the response. For example, ask the person to pick up a pencil with the right hand and place it in the left hand.

If the person cannot retain all the parts of this instruction, then simplify again, and ask the person just to pick up the pencil in the right hand.

b. Test *recent memory.* Ask the person what he or she had for breakfast or if anyone came to visit that day.

c. Test *distant memory.* Ask the person general questions about the remote past, such as year of birth, types of surgery he or she has had, or where he or she grew up. Verify the person's answers with a family member or the health record.

Ask general questions about the remote past that involve general knowledge. For example, ask the person to name the American president who was assassinated in the early 1960s, or what two countries America fought against in World War II.

Clinical Significance

Choose proverbs that are appropriate to the person's cultural background and educational level.

A response such as "birds eat early in the morning" is considered concrete, whereas the ability to think abstractly is demonstrated by a reply suggesting that people who pursue things in a timely or aggressive manner are more likely to be rewarded for their efforts.

Choose problems that are appropriate for the person's educational level.

Memory is the ability to store thoughts and learned experiences and retrieve previously learned information.

Tests of immediate memory or recall indicate whether or not a person can register information in the memory cortex. Ability to respond successfully to tests of immediate memory indicates that immediate recall is intact and that the person understands your message. This rules out other problems, such as receptive aphasia and apraxia, which might interfere with the person's ability to make appropriate responses.

Tests of recent memory indicate whether or not a person has the ability to recall new information a short time after it is presented.

Deviations from Normal
Recent memory loss is called *anterograde amnesia.* The person may register information (as manifested by repeating phrases) but forgets new information within minutes and does not remember recent events. Ultimately, the person becomes confused. Recent memory must be intact in order for the person to benefit from teaching efforts.

A person with recent memory loss, however, may have clear recall of temporally distant events.

Deviations from Normal
Retrograde amnesia is characterized by the ability to recall events only from the very distant past, such as childhood. In such cases, the person may live in reference to the distant past as though the recent past has not occurred.

Responses to general questions may be unreliable if the person regards the subject of the questions to be irrelevant to their concerns, or if the person's educational or cultural background is such that they would not have the information needed to answer correctly.

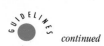

continued

Thought Processes

Procedure

d. Test for *confabulation*.

4. EVALUATE JUDGMENT.

   a. Observe the person and note if he or she makes appropriate use of surroundings. For example, check whether the patient knows how to call for assistance with the bedside call light, or whether the person's attire is appropriate for the current weather conditions.

   b. To assess judgment further, ask questions about hypothetical situations. For example, ask the person what he or she would do after noticing that smoke was coming from a trash can.

Clinical Significance

Deviations from Normal

Confabulation is the attempt to compensate for memory loss by using fictional information. In other words, the person may make up answers to questions and may even admit to this practice.

Judgment is the ability to comtemplate facts and ideas, and arrive at appropriate decisions or opinions.

Examination Guidelines   *Communication Abilities*

Procedure

1. EVALUATE COMPREHENSION.

   a. *Ability to hear:* Determine if there is any indication that the person is hearing impaired.

   b. *Ability to answer simple questions appropriately:* Determine if the person understands you by asking simple, open-ended questions such as the person's name, age, or address.

   c. *Ability to answer yes/no questions appropriately:* Continue with closed-ended questions, including some that are not reality-based, such as whether the person has a bird on his or her head.

   d. *Ability to follow simple directions:* Ask the person to respond to simple commands such as nodding the head or pointing to the door.

   e. *Ability to comprehend but unable to make a verbal reply:* Name an object and ask the person to point to it.

2. EVALUATE VERBAL EXPRESSIVE ABILITIES.

   a. *Ability to speak fluently:* Observe the person's speech for use of complete sentences or phrases. Note any slurring of words or facial drooping.

Clinical Significance

Deviations from Normal

Receptive aphasia (Wernicke's aphasia, sensory aphasia) is characterized by impaired comprehension abilities.

Receptive aphasias may occur in varying degrees. In the mildest case, the person may have difficulty naming only certain objects.

Deviations from Normal

An inability to follow commands is characteristic of *apraxia* as well as of receptive aphasia. Apraxia is the inability to perform certain motor movements even though paralysis, weakness, or loss of coordination are not evident.

The ability to comprehend in the absence of verbal abilities is evidenced in expressive aphasia.

Deviations from Normal

Expressive aphasia (Broca's, motor aphasia, nonfluent aphasia) is characterized by impaired speaking abilities. The speech may be nonfluent or telegraphic, or there may be a paucity of speech. The person may speak in a child-like manner, using only nouns and verbs, for example, "Me hurt," or "Get nurse." The person may struggle to form words, and may hesitate to produce sounds. *Telegraphic speech patterns* are characterized by short, choppy messages. There may be *preservation,* which is the tendency to repeat words or sounds; for example, "when, when, when."

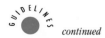
continued

Communication Abilities

Procedure	Clinical Significance

Procedure

b. *Repetition ability:* Observe the ease with which the person repeats words and phrases when instructed to do so. Note whether or not word substitutions occur with this task.

c. *Naming ability:* Point to specific objects, and ask the person to name them.

3. EVALUATE WRITTEN EXPRESSIVE ABILITIES.

a. *Simple writing tasks:* Ask the person to write his or her name and address.

b. *Complex writing tasks:* Ask the person to write a short paragraph. For example, ask the person to write about what he or she watched on television or what was served for lunch.

4. EVALUATE NONVERBAL COMMUNICATION ABILITIES.

a. Note the appropriate use of gestures.

b. Note the range of emotions shown in overall demeanor, facial expression, tone of voice.

c. Observe for *flat affect* (no signs of emotions).

d. Observe for *labile affect* (extreme fluctuations of moods or emotions).

Clinical Significance

Deviations from Normal

Repetition ability is poor with expressive aphasias because the person must struggle to form words.

Repetition ability is also poor with receptive aphasias because of *paraphasia errors,* for example, *pink* substituted for *sink,* and use of jargon.

Deviations from Normal

Naming ability may be impaired with both expressive and receptive aphasias.

Deviations from Normal

Writing abilities are poor with expressive aphasias. There is a paucity of written output that parallels speaking ability.

Deviations from Normal

Writing abilities are also poor with receptive aphasias, parallel with speaking ability. The person may be able to write, but the writing will lack meaning.

Documenting Cognitive Functions

Document cognitive functions with special attention to level of consciousness, awareness, thought processes, and communication. A concise description of a person with no alterations in cognitive functions might be as follows:

> Alert and oriented X 3. Thought processes intact. Comprehension and expressive abilities intact.

(*Note:* Oriented X 3 means oriented to three things: person, place, and time.)

For person's with altered levels of consciousness, describe your findings in detail in relation to the following assessment parameters: type of stimuli needed to arouse the person, behavior once aroused, verbal and motor responses. Consider the following example:

> Responds only after vigorous shaking and calling by name. Not oriented to person, time, or place when awake. Combative and does not follow verbal commands. Speech garbled—unable to discriminate words. Tries to remove painful stimuli.

Documentation of levels of consciousness, especially when serial evaluations are noted, may be facilitated by using a scoring tool such as the Glasgow Coma Scale (see Display 11-4).

NDx

Nursing Diagnoses Related to Cognitive Assessment

Altered Thought Processes

Altered thought processes refers to a state in which the individual experiences a disruption of cognitive functions such as conscious thought, reality orientation, problem solving, judgment, or comprehension. You should consider a number of factors before concluding that a person has altered thought processes.

First, you should realize that the diagnosis of Altered thought processes is based partly on your observations of the person's ability to make accurate statements about tem-

Display 11–4
Glasgow Coma Scale

Glasgow Coma Scale

The Glasgow Coma Scale is a standardized assessment tool that facilitates serial evaluations of level of consciousness in persons with actual or potential cerebral dysfunctions. It is a quick, objective, and replicable test of level of consciousness. Three level-of-consciousness parameters are evaluated: eye opening, best motor response, and verbal response. A score is given for each category and a total score determined, with the highest possible score being 15. Lower scores are associated with cerebral dysfunction. Some clinicians use this score to predict the prognosis of patients, although this method is not always reliable. Each category of the Glasgow Coma Scale may be scored as follows:

Eye Opening	Score	Best Motor Response	Score	Verbal Response	Score
Spontaneous	4	Obeys verbal commands	6	Oriented	5
To verbal stimuli	3	Localizes to pain	5	Confused conversation	4
To pain	2	Semipurposeful	4	Inappropriate words	3
No eye opening	1	Flexor response	3	Incomprehensible sounds	2
		Extensor response	2	Mute	1
		Flaccid	1	Intubated	0

Verbalization is not possible for an intubated patient, yet the patient may be fully awake and alert. When recording the Glasgow Coma Scale score of an intubated patient, write "T" next to the total score to indicate intubation (*example:* 9[T]).

poral events, his or her physical surroundings, and the people nearby. Use good judgment when interpreting a person's statements about person, place, and time. Some people may respond in a manner that you perceive as inappropriate, when in fact they are thinking clearly. For example, if you ask the person the day of the week, and he or she does not know, do not conclude that the person is disoriented (especially if the person is hospitalized) without further investigation. Concluding that he or she is disoriented might be as erroneous as concluding that a person who asks the date when writing a check is confused.

Second, you should realize that the nursing diagnosis Sensory–perceptual alteration has indicators similar to the diagnosis Altered thought processes. For example, both states may be characterized by disorientation, fear, and altered behavior patterns. Because intervention may differ depending on the diagnosis, you should take care to assure an accurate diagnosis.

If a person manifests perceptual distortions and such symptoms can be alleviated by helping the person correctly interpret sensory stimuli, the most likely diagnosis is Sensory–perceptual alteration. For example, the person who is exposed to unfamiliar sounds in an intensive care unit may develop auditory misperceptions such as mistaking the sound of aerosol oxygen devices for the sound of falling rain. If you can explain that this sound is not rain but is related to the equipment, and the person develops the in-

sight to interpret the unfamiliar auditory stimuli correctly, the nursing diagnosis would be Sensory–perceptual alteration. On the other hand, auditory hallucinations are auditory perceptions with no apparent basis in reality and usually represent altered thought processes. The person is not as likely to have such misperceptions corrected by explanations.

Alterations in thought processes may be characterized by both perceptual distortions and thought disturbances. However, Sensory–perceptual alteration is not characterized by thought disturbances. When choosing between the two diagnoses, you should carefully assess the nature of the person's thought processes and his or her response to your efforts to interpret stimuli.

Unilateral Neglect

A person may be oriented to person, place, and time but still have awareness deficits relative to self and surroundings. Unilateral neglect is an example of altered body and environmental awareness. This condition is associated with damage of the right cerebral hemisphere, particularly when left hemiplegia is present. The person ignores perceptions and sensations relating to or originating from the left side of the body, which has important self-care implications. In extreme cases, the person may eat food from only the right side of his or her dinner plate or may wash only the right

Table 11–3. Differential Diagnosis of Aphasias*

Type of Aphasia	General Speaking Ability	Repetition Ability	Naming Ability	Oral Reading	Auditory Comprehension	Reading Comprehension	Written Expression
Transcortical sensory (isolation aphasia)	Fluent; paraphasia; does not initiate speech on own; ecolalic	Good, despite poor comprehension	Poor	Poor	Poor	Poor	Poor (similar to Wernicke's)
Transcortical motor	Nonfluent; tries to prompt self with hands (like a conductor); does not initiate speech on own	Very good	Poor	Poor	Good	Fair to good	Poor (similar to Broca's)
Transcortical mixed	Nonfluent; ecolalic; does not speak unless spoken to	Relatively preserved in one setting; otherwise limited language skills	Poor	Poor	Poor	Poor	Poor
Anomic	Fluent; vague empty speech; circumlocution	Good	Poor	Good to poor	Fair to good	Good to poor	Good to poor
Broca's (motor, expressive, non-fluent aphasia)	Nonfluent; telegraphic; paucity of spoken output	Poor, struggles to speak	Poor	Poor	Good	Good to poor	Poor (parallels speaking ability) paucity of written output
Wernicke's	Fluent; disorganized; logorrhea (excessive spoken output); incorrect syntax (word order) and paraphesia	Poor due to paraphasia errors (e.g., *pink* for *sink*) and jargon usage	Poor	Poor	Poor	Poor	Poor (parallels speaking ability); excessive, meaningless writing
Conductive (fluent aphasia)	Fluent but with paraphesias; hesitations and repeated trials in approaching certain words	Poor in the context of good comprehension skills	Fair to poor	Poor due to paraphasic errors	Good	Good	Fair
Global (mixed)	Very poor; no output; nonfluent; may repeat one word or syllable	Very poor	Very poor	Very poor	Very poor	Very poor	Very poor

*Clinically, aphasia does not always fall into the discrete categories listed but may have elements of several types.
(Adapted from Pimental, P.A. [1986]. Alterations in communication: Biopsychosocial aspects of aphasia, dysarthria, and right hemisphere syndromes in the stroke patient. Nursing Clinics of North America, 21 [2], 325)

side of the body. Homonymous hemianopsia, a visual alteration characterized by blindness of the nasal half of one eye and the temporal half of the other eye, may accompany unilateral neglect.

Impaired Verbal Communication

Impaired verbal communication may be because of aphasia, which means a loss of language abilities. Many different types of aphasia have been identified, including Broca's, Wernicke's, conductive, global, transcortical sensory, transcortical motor, transcortical mixed, and anomic. It is helpful to know the type of aphasia a person has so that appropriate interventions can be planned. The diagnosis of a particular aphasia is complicated by the fact that many aphasias have overlapping features or do not fall into discrete diagnostic categories. The specific language symptomatology of the various aphasias is presented in Table 11-3.

Clinical Problems Related to Cognitive Assessment

Abnormal cognitive functions may indicate pathology of the central nervous system. Additional diagnosis and treatment is directed toward the underlying pathology.

PAIN
Anatomy and Physiology Overview

Sensory Component of Pain. Pain is initiated by conditions such as trauma, ischemia, hypoxia, or acidosis, which cause release of endogenous pain substances located in the vesicles or granules of peripheral nerve endings. The endogenous pain substances include substance P, somatostatin, kinins, prostaglandins, histamine, SRS-A, and thromboxanes. The release of these substances stimulates the nociceptors or pain receptors. The lowest-intensity stimulus that initiates the pain impulse transmission along efferent pathways is called the pain (nociceptive) threshold. The pain threshold is the same for all people.

Repeated stimulation of the nociceptors may result in sensitization to pain. Once sensitized, nociceptors continue to respond to painful stimuli, and eventually the pain may be perceived as more intense. Pain-relief efforts often involve minimizing continued endogenous pain substance release in order to prevent sensitization.

Pain sensations are transmitted to the brain primarily by the ascending lateral spinothalamic tracts, where two types of sensory nerve fibers are found. Myelinated *A-delta fibers* transmit sharp, highly localized types of pain that occur immediately with injury. Unmyelinated *C fibers* transmit pain sensations that are more diffuse and aching.

Pain fibers enter the spinal cord through the dorsal roots. The pain impulse then reaches a synapse in the substantia gelatinosa and crosses the cord by way of several short interneurons. Impulse transmission then proceeds along the lateral spinothalamic tract to the brain (Fig. 11-14).

When necessary, pain sensations may bypass the brain and pass through a reflex arc, causing an immediate motor response. For example, the action of quickly removing the hand after touching a hot stove occurs as a result of this mechanism.

Perceptual Component of Pain. Pain perception involves the thalamus and cortical association areas of the brain. Pain may be perceived in the thalamus, or the pain impulse may be projected along diffuse pathways to the cerebral cortex. The threshold for recognizing pain is physiologically the same for all individuals. However, several factors such as loss of consciousness and inhibition of pain

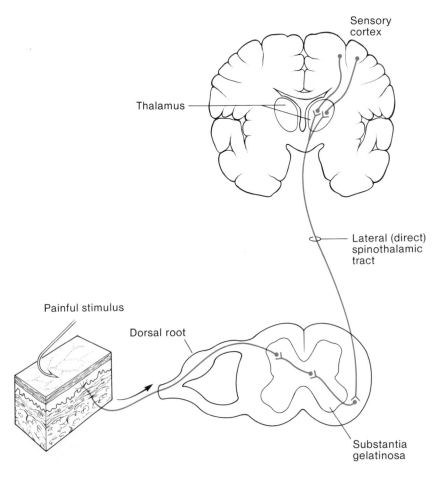

Figure 11-14. Sensory pathways and pain.

impulse transmission by endogenous opiates (endorphins) or exogenous opiates (morphine) may alter the perception of pain.

The pain experience, or a person's response to pain, is influenced by memories, personality, culture, and values. Pain tolerance, a learned and socially conditioned human response, is a cortical phenomena and varies among individual people.

Pain Responses. Pain responses, both psychological and physiologic, are initiated at the cortical level. Psychological responses to pain include fear, anxiety, depression, or anger. Neural impulses, conducted along descending pathways, initiate physiologic responses, including cardiovascular responses (increased heart rate and blood pressure), gastrointestinal responses (decreased gut motility and decreased saliva), and musculoskeletal responses (increased muscle tension). Pain responses are probably modulated by signals transmitted from the cerebral cortex.

Pain Theories

The *specificity theory,* first proposed by Max von Frey, holds that pain results from the stimulation of pain-specific fibers, and that when a particular pain fiber is stimulated, a predictable intensity of pain is produced. However, this theory does not account for individual differences in pain perception or the effect of emotions and cognitive processes.

The *pattern theory* proposes that pain results from the stimulation of nonspecific peripheral receptors. A pattern is coded at the peripheral site and then transmitted to the brain, resulting in pain perception. However, this theory does not account for peripheral nerve fiber specialization.

The *gate control theory of pain* (Melzack & Wall, 1965) proposes that the perception of pain is influenced by numerous physiologic and psychological variables. The status of the "gate," located in the dorsal horn in the substantia gelatinosa, affects the pain impulse. In other words, when the gate is open, pain impulses flow freely through the ascending pathways, thereby enhancing pain perception. When the gate is closed, the pain impulse is inhibited, diminishing pain perception. Gates may possibly be closed by factors that stimulate A-delta fibers, such as massage, cold, acupuncture, or transcutaneous electrical nerve stimulation. The gates are opened by C-fiber stimulation, which occurs secondary to tissue damage. Gate activity is also influenced by the cortical perception of pain. For example, distraction and guided imagery may close the gates, consequently altering pain perception.

Physical Examination · *Pain*

General Principles

A comprehensive assessment of pain requires an evaluation of the sensory, perceptual, and response aspects of pain. Nurses in particular should evaluate a person's perceptions and responses to pain because such human responses are most amenable to nursing interventions. Perceptions of pain are most reliably assessed when the person discloses to you the nature of his or her personal pain experience. You can gain additional information by observing the person's nonverbal behaviors and body system responses. However, not all people will readily reveal that they have pain or behave in classic pain-indicating ways. Careful interpretation of a person's behavioral or physiologic responses may be required. The pain experience is personal and subjective, and does not need to be validated by obtaining objective assessment data. This is consistent with McCaffery's (1979) definition of pain, "Pain is whatever the person says it is, existing whenever the person says it does."

Interviewing is a means of assessing the person's perceptions of pain. The initial interview should establish the presence of pain, pain characteristics, and what the pain means to the individual. If the person is reluctant to report pain, establishing the very presence of pain may be challenging. You need to distinguish between the pain experience and the individual's criteria for reporting pain.

You should also assess pain as a clinical symptom. In this sense, pain is a warning sign or the result of pathologic processes. Further evaluation is necessary for clinical diagnosis of the underlying problem.

Reluctance to Discuss the Pain Experience

A person who needs to be in control may attempt to become indifferent to pain and suffering. Such a person may be reluctant to discuss the pain experience openly, using stoicism as a coping technique. Additionally, the person may perceive pain as inevitable and may feel a loss of self-control when talking about pain or asking for pain relief. You should be careful not to judge these behaviors in relation to your personal values. Moreover, you should determine whether this represents an effective coping strategy. Even if the person does not openly discuss the pain experience, you may pro-

Display 11–5
The McGill-Melzack Pain Questionnaire

Descriptors fall into four major groups: sensory, 1 to 10; affective, 11 to 15; evaluative, 16; and miscellaneous, 17 to 20. The rank value for each descriptor is based on its position in the word set. The sum of the rank values is the pain rating index (PRI). The present pain intensity (PPI) is based on a scale of 0 to 5.

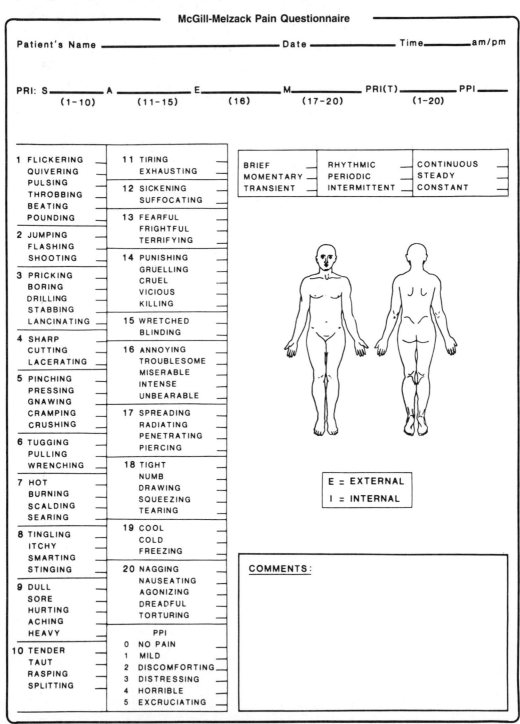

McGill-Melzack Pain Questionnaire

Patient's Name _____ Date _____ Time_____am/pm

PRI: S_____ A_____ E_____ M_____ PRI(T)_____ PPI____
    (1-10)   (11-15)   (16)   (17-20)   (1-20)

1 FLICKERING QUIVERING PULSING THROBBING BEATING POUNDING	**11** TIRING EXHAUSTING
	12 SICKENING SUFFOCATING
2 JUMPING FLASHING SHOOTING	**13** FEARFUL FRIGHTFUL TERRIFYING
3 PRICKING BORING DRILLING STABBING LANCINATING	**14** PUNISHING GRUELLING CRUEL VICIOUS KILLING
4 SHARP CUTTING LACERATING	**15** WRETCHED BLINDING
5 PINCHING PRESSING GNAWING CRAMPING CRUSHING	**16** ANNOYING TROUBLESOME MISERABLE INTENSE UNBEARABLE
6 TUGGING PULLING WRENCHING	**17** SPREADING RADIATING PENETRATING PIERCING
7 HOT BURNING SCALDING SEARING	**18** TIGHT NUMB DRAWING SQUEEZING TEARING
8 TINGLING ITCHY SMARTING STINGING	**19** COOL COLD FREEZING
9 DULL SORE HURTING ACHING HEAVY	**20** NAGGING NAUSEATING AGONIZING DREADFUL TORTURING
10 TENDER TAUT RASPING SPLITTING	PPI 0 NO PAIN 1 MILD 2 DISCOMFORTING 3 DISTRESSING 4 HORRIBLE 5 EXCRUCIATING

BRIEF RHYTHMIC CONTINUOUS
MOMENTARY PERIODIC STEADY
TRANSIENT INTERMITTENT CONSTANT

E = EXTERNAL
I = INTERNAL

COMMENTS:

ceed with the interview. It may be that the person is willing to discuss some characteristics of the pain despite reluctance to discuss its personal effects.

The following statements may be helpful when encouraging the person to discuss his or her pain:

Tell me about the pain you have experienced since the accident.

Most people have some pain following this type of surgery. I would guess this is also true for you, even though you don't show signs of pain.

Other people may be reluctant to discuss pain because they feel that silence is the most acceptable behavior. For these people, personal suffering may be increased by concealing pain. Be aware that your behavior or attitude may discourage an open discussion of pain. For example, patients who have been told that their pain cannot be entirely relieved and that they should stop asking for pain medication may think that you do not want to hear about their pain. The same message may be communicated if you close the door on the person who is crying with pain or if you delay in responding to the person's call light.

Barriers to Effective Pain Assessment

If you do not entirely understand pain expressions or pain-relief strategies, you may communicate to the patient that pain is inevitable and must be endured. In addition, if you believe that administering narcotics will lead to addiction, you may neglect evaluating the adequacy of prescribed narcotics. You should remember that the condition of people with acute pain may be effectively managed by consulting the physician and increasing drug dosage or frequency. In some cases, the most effective pain relief may occur with alternative strategies such as relaxation techniques, guided imagery, music, or distraction in addition to narcotics.

Pain-Assessment Tools

Ongoing assessment is essential to monitor pain-relief efforts and determine in what ways pain is affecting the patient. It may be helpful to make serial evaluations of pain with one of the pain-assessment tools developed for clinical use, such as the McGill-Melzack Pain Questionnaire (see Display 11-5). Pain-assessment tools may be used in their entirety and kept as a form in a patient's chart or can serve as reminders of what topics to discuss with the patient in less-structured interviews.

Examination and Documentation Focus

- Location, including point of origin and radiation
- Intensity
- Quality
- Onset and chronology
- Relieving factors
- Aggravating factors
- Effects of pain on other functions

Examination Guidelines   *Pain*

Procedure

1. LOCATION.

   a. Ask the person to point to the pain location or to mark the pain location on a figure drawing. Determine whether the pain radiates from its point of origin.

Clinical Significance

Pain location often provides clues about the cause of the pain or the type of pain being experienced. The following types of pain may be distinguished on the basis of location:

- *Somatic pain* originates in the trunk, extremities, skin, or bones. Somatic pain that is localized or that originates with cutaneous nerve fibers is called *epicritic pain* (*e.g.,* the pain that occurs after a first-degree burn). Deep somatic pain, which is not as localized, is called *protopathic pain* (*e.g.,* the pain that results from a sprained ankle). The patient may refer to somatic pain as external pain.

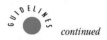

continued

Pain

Procedure

b. If you use a drawing to indicate the location of pain, separate pain sites can be labeled with letters or numbers. For example, headache pain may be #1 and abdominal pain may be #2. These numbers can then be used to categorize descriptive statements made by the person about pain.

c. Ask where the pain is most intense and whether the pain is perceived as internal or external.

2. INTENSITY.

a. Ask the person to rate the intensity of the pain being experienced. One of the simplest ways to rate pain is to ask the person to rate the pain on a scale of 1 to 10, with 10 representing the most intense pain ever experienced.

b. You may ask the person to rate pain and pain relief using visual analogue scales. Ask the person to mark an X on each scale representing present pain perception and pain relief. Serial comparisons of visual analogue scales help you evaluate the person's pain and pain interventions.

c. Alternatively, ask the person to describe the intensity of the pain.

Clinical Significance

- *Visceral pain* originates in the internal organs and is caused by factors such as ischemia, spasm, or acidosis. Visceral pain is often *referred pain* in that the pain radiates away from the pain origin, or the patient feels the pain at a location other than the origin. Unlike somatic pain, visceral pain cannot be sharply localized. The patient may refer to visceral pain as internal pain.

- *Phantom pain* is usually perceived to be in a missing extremity or body part. For example, the patient may feel right-lower-leg pain following an above-the-knee amputation. Nerve fiber alterations at amputation site probably contribute to this particular type of pain.

- *Causalgia* is an intense, burning pain following traumatic injury that involves the peripheral nerves of an extremity. The pain is severe in relation to the initiating trauma. Atrophic skin changes and bone demineralization may occur in advanced stages.

- *Neuralgia* refers to an intense, burning pain along the distribution of a peripheral nerve. The pain may occur after a nerve's "trigger zone" has been stimulated in the area of pain.

If a pain-rating scale is used, the same scale should be used in follow-up assessments in order to allow for meaningful comparisons.

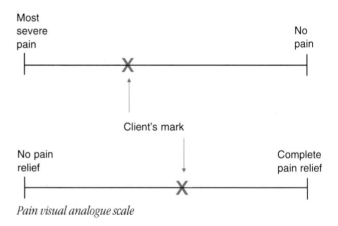

Pain visual analogue scale

Words such as none, mild, moderate, severe, or very severe may indicate intensity.

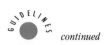 *continued*

Pain

Procedure	Clinical Significance
3. QUALITY.	
Ask the person to describe the quality of the pain.	Words such as pinching, pressing, gnawing, cramping, or crushing may describe pain quality.
Approaches such as "Describe what the pain feels like" are preferred over questions such as "Is the pain sharp?"	The use of open-ended questions will limit cueing or suggesting responses to the person. Limited information may be obtained by asking questions that only require a yes-or-no answer.
4. ONSET AND CHRONOLOGY.	
a. Ask about the time of onset and duration of pain.	Chronic pain may be perceived as having always been present. Acute pain may be associated with a more sudden onset.
b. Ask if the pain suddenly or gradually became more severe or if the pain is intermittent.	Pain that immediately reaches a maximum intensity may indicate tissue rupture. Ischemic pain gradually increases in intensity.
c. Ask whether or not the pattern of pain changes within a 24-hour period.	*Chronic pain* may follow diurnal rhythms. For example, because rheumatoid arthritis pain is aggravated by inactivity, the pain is usually more severe upon awakening. *Nocturnal epigastric pain* is associated with peptic ulcer disease.
	Colicky pain, which originates in hollow viscera, is a rhythmic, cramping pain.
6. RELIEVING FACTORS.	
Ask the person what, if anything, relieves the pain. Determine personal preferences in relation to pain relief strategies.	Pain relief may be obtained through the use of medications or by using alternative pain-management strategies such as guided imagery, massage, music, rest, or position changes.
7. AGGRAVATING FACTORS.	
Ask the person what makes the pain worse.	Some aggravating factors can be minimized. Consider the effects of sleep deprivation, anxiety, or environmental discomfort such as uncomfortable temperatures or noise.
Note the relationship between activity and pain.	Ischemic pain (angina, leg claudication) may be precipitated by activity.
8. EFFECTS.	
Ask questions such as the following:	Inquiring about the effects of pain helps the nurse identify problems with coping, relationships, and activities of daily living.
"What does this pain mean to you?"	
"Tell me how the pain has changed your lifestyle."	Concerns about addiction to narcotics, cost of medications, social interactions, and sexual activities are common in persons experiencing chronic pain.
"How has the pain influenced your everyday activities—eating, moving, sleeping?"	
"How has this pain influenced your relationships with others?"	
9. OTHER OBSERVATIONS.	
a. Note expressions of pain such as crying, withdrawal, moaning.	
b. Note physiologic signs of pain:	Pain may be present with or without physical signs.
Autonomic responses: Elevated blood pressure, heart rate, and ventilatory rate; cool, clammy skin; dilated pupils; nausea and vomiting.	
Musculoskeletal responses: Clenched fists, restlessness, guarding, muscle rigidity.	
c. Note facial expressions of pain: grimacing, "facial mask of pain."	*Facial mask of pain:* Flat or fixed facial expression; lusterless eyes; fatigued appearance. Associated with chronic pain.

Documenting Pain Assessment

The initial documentation of pain in the person's record should be thorough because all the qualities of the pain are considered in making a clinical diagnosis. Subsequent references may be more abbreviated provided the qualities of the pain remain the same. Documentation should include attention to the following: location, intensity, quality, onset and chronology, relieving factors, aggravating factors, and other effects. The pain experienced by a person suffering from angina might be described as follows:

> States pain is located in chest beneath sternum and radiates to left shoulder and arm. Pain is described as 8 on a 1 to 10 scale. Feels like pressure or a tight belt around the chest. First noticed pain at 0800 this morning while sitting at desk. Has never experienced this type of pain in the past. Pain was intermittent until 1 hour ago, when it became continuous. Nothing seems to make the pain better or worse. Finds it hard to breathe with the pain and noticed profuse perspiration since the onset of the pain.

NDx

Nursing Diagnoses Related to Pain Assessment

Acute Pain

Acute pain is considered self-limiting and purposeful in that it serves to alert a person to possible problems. Numerous factors initiate acute pain by causing tissue damage.

Pain History. The person may or may not verbalize pain perceptions. In the case of acute pain, verbal reports usually indicate that the pain had a sudden onset, and often a precipitating event can be identified (*e.g.,* "I felt the pain in my ankle right after I fell on the stairway."). The person may be able to describe the pain precisely and locate the site.

Observations. Autonomic responses that may be pronounced with acute pain include pallor, diaphoresis, and cardiovascular and respiratory alterations. Guarding is common. Depending on the nature of the pain, the person may decrease or increase the pace of activities or rub the affected part. The persons facial affect usually reflects anxiety or fear. Pain-relief strategies are usually effective for acute pain.

Chronic Pain

Chronic pain has a duration of greater than 6 months and may be a result of irreversible tissue damage. In this sense, chronic pain does not serve to warn the person of impending danger.

Pain History. The person may or may not verbalize pain perceptions. However, preoccupation with the pain experience is not uncommon. The pain may be reported as constant or intermittent and may be as intense as any acute pain experience. Rather than describing a specific onset of pain, the person may refer to the pain as being constant. The person may have greater difficulty localizing chronic pain and may describe it as an ache or soreness. Feelings of hopelessness, guilt, and frustration are common. Pain relief efforts may be unsuccessful.

Observations. With chronic pain, there is habituation to the autonomic nervous system reponses evoked by pain. Therefore, the person may no longer display acute physiologic signs of stress. The facial expression is frequently characterized by the facial mask of pain. The person may be irritable and angry or depressed.

ASSESSMENT PROFILE 1

● ●

David, aged 25, was recovering from a closed head injury received in a motorcycle accident. Recently, he was admitted to a rehabilitation nursing unit. The nurse caring for David noticed that when he was shaving or brushing his teeth, he would attend only to the right side of the body. He frequently appeared disoriented and would bump into things when ambulating.

Profile Analysis and Assessment Focus

Observation of David's self-care practices and orientation indicated a need for more thorough assessment and prompted the nurse to ask the following questions:

- What is the nature of the neurologic injury?
- How long has it been since the initial injury?

- How much functional improvement has there been since the injury?
- What is the current level of function in relation to feeding, grooming, and ambulation?
- If current functioning indicates regression, what factors may have influenced the client? Emotional upset? Stress of transfer? Less one-to-one nursing care? Unfamiliarity with caregivers?
- What is the patient's rehabilitation prognosis?

David demonstrated neglect of the left side of his body. The nurse observed that he did not shave the left side of his face or wash the left side of his body. The nature of his neurologic injury, which occurred 3 months ago, helped to explain his behavior. The right parietal lobe had been damaged, which is often associated with perceptual defects. The one-sided neglect had been noted since admission to the rehabilitation unit 1 week before and did not represent a recent change. Previous documentation of such behavior was not available. Disorientation may be associated with one-sided neglect. David had been fully oriented in the last few days, although fatigue and frustration appeared to contribute to transient disorientation.

The rehabilitation team felt that David's chance of recovering normal ability to perform daily living skills was excellent provided he received continuing therapy.

Possible Nursing Diagnosis

Based on the observed behaviors and history of the neurologic injury, the nursing diagnosis of Unilateral neglect was formulated.

Additional Data Gathering and Analysis

The nurse obtained additional data to be used in monitoring David's progress and planning interventions. David was asked to draw pictures of himself and common objects, such as a clock. In both cases, he initially drew only the right half of the image. However, three weeks later, he drew similar pictures with some attention to detail on the left side. One morning the nurse asked David to wash the neglected side of his body to see if he would respond to verbal cueing. Additionally, the nurse had David view himself in the mirror to see if he could identify areas neglected during hygienic care. Eventually, David showed increasing attention to the left side of his body and had fewer episodes of disoriented behavior.

ASSESSMENT PROFILE 2

Mrs. K, aged 75, was brought to the emergency department by her husband because she fell at home and lacerated her scalp. He reported that his wife has been "losing her memory" for the past 2 years and recently had left their home and had been brought back by the police. He reported that she neglected personal hygiene and had occasional fecal incontinence. Her husband stated that he was worried that she would injure herself further.

Profile Analysis and Assessment Focus

A more thorough evaluation should be made of Mrs. K's "memory lapses." A thorough health and medication history should be obtained to rule out any potentially reversible contributing factors. Mental status tests may be administered to evaluate judgment, memory, and other cognitive functions. The patient's emotional status and coping responses should also be evaluated. Additiona data should be obtained from both the patient and her husband. Finally, the husband's response to the patient's problems should be evaluated.

Possible Nursing Diagnosis

At this point, there are not enough data to make a nursing diagnosis relating to altered cognitive or perceptual functions. The immediate concern is with the patient's safety and emotional response to the emergency department admission. Appropriate diagnoses would include Potential for injury and Possible anxiety.

Chapter 11 Summary

The assessment of cognitive and perceptual functions is focused on the following:
- Sensory organs and structures required for vision, hearing, taste, touch, smell, and position sense
- Cognitive functions, including level of consciousness, awareness, communication abilities, and thought processes
- Sensory–perceptual experiences such as pain, hallucinations, and altered thought processes that may interfere with usual or desired activities.

Multiple information sources may be used to assess cognition and perception. The data base should consist of the following:

The Health History
- Information concerning the special senses
- Symptoms related to neurological dysfunction
- Pertinent physiological alterations and medications

The Physical Examination Findings
- General appearance
- Eyes and vision examination
- Ears and hearing examination
- Cranial nerve examination
- Motor function and reflex examination
- Sensory and cerebellar function examination
- Examination of cognitive functions
- Examination of pain

Reports from Diagnostic Studies
- Cognitive function (mental status) tests
- Blood tests
- Radiographic studies
- Electromyography
- Electroencephalography
- Evoked potentials

Assessment of cognition and perception provides cues to the following nursing diagnoses:

Impaired verbal communication
Dysreflexia
Knowledge deficit (specify)
Pain
Chronic pain
Sensory/perceptual alterations: Visual, auditory, kinesthetic, gustatory, tactile, or olfactory
Altered thought processes

Additionally, the nurse develops skill at detecting and monitoring clinical problems associated with the special sense organs. For example,

Eye/Vision Problems
- Structural alterations
- Infectious or inflammatory processes
- Anterior chamber pathology
- Fundi abnormalities

Ears/Hearing Problems
- Sensorineural and conductive hearing losses
- Infection or inflammation of the external or middle ear

✳ CRITICAL THINKING

The assessment of cognition and perception can be a complex and lengthy process. The assessment is complex because of the broad scope and specialized skill that is required. Also contributing to the complexity is the fact that the people who may be in greatest need of evaluation may be experiencing cognitive or perceptual deficits that interfere with optimal communication. A lengthy assessment is guaranteed if the clinician conducts a complete evaluation of the neurologic system.

Learning Exercises

1. You want to assess cognitive functions of a 32-year-old patient who has suffered a slight concussion. The patient speaks and comprehends Chinese only and you do not. Select and describe at least three options that might be implemented in this situation. Of these options, which is least likely to be helpful? Why? Which option is most likely to be helpful? Why?

2. Specify how you might use cranial nerve examination findings to plan nursing care.

3. Many nurses do not have time to routinely conduct a comprehensive examination of the neurologic system. Develop some criteria for determining the necessity of conducting an examination of deep tendon reflexes by an emergency room nurse.

4. You are unable to visualize the optic disk during an ophthalmoscopic examination. Identify several reasons why this might happen and recommend whether or not corrective actions will be helpful.

5. Determine and discuss the primary differences between assessing pain in a patient with a diagnosed condition versus an undiagnosed condition.

BIBLIOGRAPHY

Aradine, C., Beyer, J., & Tompkins, J. (1988). Children's pain perceptions before and after analgesia: A study of instrument construct validity and related issues. *Journal of Pediatric Nursing, 3* (1), 11–23.

Bashor, P.H. (1983). A nursing communciation assessment guide. *Rehabilitation Nursing, 8* (1), 20–21, 30.

Camp, L. (1988). A comparison of nurses' recorded assessment of pain with perceptions of pain as described by cancer patients. *Cancer Nursing, 11* (4), 237–243.

Carpenito, L.J. (1985). Altered thoughts or altered perceptions. *American Journal of Nursing, 85* (11), 1283.

Crosby, L., et al. (1989). Clinical neurologic assessment tool: Development and testing of an instrument to index neurologic status. *Heart and Lung, 18* (2), 121–129.

Folstein, M.F., Folstein, S., & McHugh, P.R. (1975). Mini-mental state: A practical method for grading the cognitive state of patients for the clinician. *Journal of Psychiatric Research, 12,* 189–198.

Hall, G. (1988). Alterations in thought processes. *Journal of Gerontological Nursing, 14* (3), 30–37, 38–40.

Hickey, J.V. (1992). *The clinical practice of neurological and neurosurgical nursing* (3rd ed.). Philadelphia: J.B. Lippincott.

Hoyt, K.S., & Sparger, G. (1984). Pain assessment by ED nurses. *Journal of Emergency Nursing, 10* (6), 306–311.

Huskisson, E.C. (1983). Visual analog scales. In R. Melzack (Ed.). *Pain measurement and assessment* (pp. 33–37). New York: Raven Press.

Jacques, A. (1992). Do you believe I'm in pain? Nurse's assessment of patient's pain. *Professional Nurse, 7* (4), 249–251.

Jess, L. (1988). Investigating impaired mental status: An assessment guide you can use. *Nursing '88, 18* (6), 42–50.

Kahn, R.L., et al. (1960). Brief objective measures for the determination of mental status in the aged. *American Journal of Psychiatry, 117,* 326–328.

Kane, R.A., & Kane, R.L. (1981). *Assessing the elderly: A practical guide to measurement.* Lexington, MA: Lexington Books.

Libow, L.S. (1981). A rapidly administered, easily remembered mental status evaluation: FROMAGE. In L.S. Libow & F.T. Sherman. *The core of geriatric medicine: A guide for students and practitioners* (pp. 85–91). St. Louis: C.V. Mosby.

Lower, J. (1992). Rapid neuroassessment. *American Journal of Nursing, 6* (92), 38–48.

McGuire, D.B. (1984). The measurement of clinical pain. *Nursing Research, 33* (3), 152–156.

Meinhart, N.T., & McCaffery, M. (1983). *Pain: A nursing approach to assessment and analysis.* Norwalk, CT: Appleton-Century-Crofts.

Melzack, R. (Ed.) (1983). *Pain measurement and assessment.* New York: Raven Press.

Melzack, R., & Wall, P. (1965). Pain mechanisms: A new theory. *Science, 150,* 971–979.

Melzack, R., & Wall, P. (1975). Psychophysiology of pain. In M. Weisenberg (Ed.). *Pain: Clinical and experimental prespectives* (pp. 8–23). St. Louis: C.V. Mosby.

Nikas, D.L. (1984). Neurologic assessment of altered states of consciouisness: Part III. *Focus on Critical Care, 11* (1), 54–58.

Perreault, J.A. (1985). Assessing for perceptual clarity: Closing the gap between theory and practice. *Rehabilitation Nursing, 10* (3), 28–32.

Pimental, P.A. (1986). Alterations in communication: Biopsychosocial aspects of aphasia, dysarthria, and right hemisphere syndromes in the stroke patient. *Nursing Clinics of North America, 21* (2), 321–337.

Richardson, K. (1983). Confusion: Recognition and remedy (Assessing communication, Part 5). *Geriatric Nursing, 4* (4), 237–238.

Savedra, M., Tesler, M., & Ward, J. (1988). How adolescents describe pain. *Journal of Adolescent Health Care, 9* (4), 315–320.

Shyder, M. (Ed.) (1983). *A guide to neurological and neurosurgical nursing.* New York: John Wiley & Sons.

Walker, J. (1992). Taking pains—pain assessment. *Nursing Times, 88* (29), 38–40.

Wyness, M.A. (1985). Perceptual dysfunction: Nursing assessment and management. *Journal of Neurosurgical Nursing, 17* (2), 105–110.

12 Assessing Sleep and Rest

Examination Guidelines

Bedside Sleep Pattern Observation

Assessment Terms

Sleep
Rest
REM Sleep
Non-REM Sleep
Sleep Cycle

Insomnia
Sleep Deprivation
Sleep (Bedtime) Ritual
Excessive Daytime Sleepiness
Polysomnographic Evaluation

INTRODUCTORY OVERVIEW

Sleep, rest, and relaxation satisfy basic human needs and have restorative powers. An inability to sleep or rest properly can rob a person of energy, vitality, and a sense of well-being.

Sleep disorders, ranging from occasional sleep deprivation to chronic insomnia, are common and may become more frequent as a person ages. Many people who experience disruption in their sleep patterns do not report the disruption to health care providers until their life-style is adversely affected by the problem.

Sleep and rest patterns should be assessed to identify actual or potential problems in satisfying basic sleep needs. Objectives of the evaluation include identifying the quantity and quality of sleep as seen from the individual's perspective; stimuli and circumstances that promote and inhibit sleep, rest, and relaxation; and psychological and physiologic factors indicating adequate sleep or sleep deprivation.

Assessing sleep and rest patterns is challenging because there are no simple tools to measure these behaviors. In addition, signs and symptoms associated with sleep deprivation, such as irritability or confusion, may also be associated with conditions unrelated to sleep.

Assessment Focus

Sleep patterns may be evaluated by (1) observing the person while he or she sleeps; (2) interviewing the person about his or her perceptions of sleep needs; and (3) reviewing, when possible or available, the results of a sleep laboratory evaluation (electroencephalograms, electrooculograms, and electromyograms). In addition, researchers have de-

Jill Fuller and Jennifer Schaller-Ayers:
HEALTH ASSESSMENT: A NURSING APPROACH, Second Edition.
© 1990, 1994 by J. B. Lippincott Company.

Assessment Focus Sleep and Rest

Assessment Goal	Data Collection Methods
1. Identify the person's perceptions about the quantity and quality of sleep and rest.	*Interview* • Usual sleep pattern • Altered sleep patterns
2. Identify factors perceived by the person to facilitate sleep and rest.	*Interview* • Sleep/bedtime rituals • Sleep environment • Sleep position
3. Considering environmental, physiologic, and psychological factors, identify possible causes of disrupted sleep.	*Interview* • All components of the sleep health history may be relevant *Observation* • Environmental stimuli: Are there environmental factors disrupting sleep? • Uninterrupted sleep time: Does the person have sufficient rest periods without interruption from health care providers? *Review of Medical Records* • Medical diagnoses: Do physiologic alterations interfere with sleep? • Medication history: Do medications interfere with sleep?
4. Identify signs and symptoms of sleep pattern disturbances.	*Interview* • All components of the sleep history may be relevant *Observation* • Person's appearance during designated sleep periods: Restless? Awake? • General observation including cognitive status, facial expression, speech pattern, movement, and posture: Are there signs of sleep deprivation? *Review Polysomnographic Data (if available)* • EEG, EMG, EOG, ECG, respiratory patterns: What are the characteristics of the sleep pattern disturbance?
5. Evaluate the effect of sleep pattern disturbances on physiologic, cognitive, and psychological functions.	*Interview* • Symptoms of sleep pattern disturbances *Observation* • Ability to carry out usual activities and functions

veloped formal questionnaires to collect data about sleep patterns.

The most basic information should be obtained through the interview and observations, with less emphasis on laboratory values and the physical examination. Evaluations conducted in a sleep laboratory may be costly and are not always possible or necessary. Nevertheless, such analyses can provide valuable information when the need arises. Specific sleep disorders such as sleep apnea, narcolepsy, insomnia, sleep-related seizures, sleepwalking, night terrors, gastroesophageal reflux, and nocturnal myoclonus may be thoroughly evaluated in the sleep laboratory.

The extent to which sleep and rest functions should be assessed is determined by the purpose of the assessment. The factors to be evaluated include the following:

• Factors that facilitate sleep and rest
• The quantity and quality of the person's sleep
• Possible causes of sleep disturbances
• Characteristics of any sleep disturbances
• Signs and symptoms of sleep deprivation
• Effects of sleep disturbances on other functions

The methods of collecting data for each of these areas are described in the Assessment Focus.

Nursing Diagnoses

Assessment of sleep and rest patterns provides cues to the following nursing diagnoses:

Fatigue
Sleep pattern disturbance

As you explore the factors contributing to sleep and rest problems, you may identify additional problems, especially the following:

Anxiety
Ineffective individual coping
Altered family processes
Fear
Pain
Dysfunctional grieving

Stress and other situational factors may have an adverse effect on sleep. An inability to cope with a pressing problem can lead to sleepless nights or periods of interrupted sleep. Physical pain, family arguments, fear or anxiety, and grief over the death of a loved one can all contribute to sleep pattern disturbances.

KNOWLEDGE BASE FOR ASSESSMENT

Sleep, a neural phenomenon, may be defined as a state of unconsciousness from which a person can be awakened by sensory or other stimuli. The fact that the person can be easily awakened distinguishes sleep from other unconscious states, such as coma or unconsciousness induced by general anesthesia. Although sleep produces a decrease in cortical vigilance, other essential physiologic and psychological functions continue during normal sleep.

Rest is a waking state characterized by feelings of physical and mental well-being that helps reduce damaging effects of psychophysiologic stress. Rest states vary greatly among people. For example, one person may find mild exercise restful, whereas another may not. Rest is promoted by such feelings as control, acceptance, and freedom from stress or physical discomfort. Because rest and sleep are interactive, people who cannot rest may have difficulty with their sleep patterns.

Sleep Neurophysiology

For adequate sleep to occur, certain neurologic structures in the brain must be intact, including the reticular activating system, the cerebral hemispheres, and the hypnogenic or sleep-producing areas located in the lower brain stem, anterior hypothalamus, and raphae and thalamic nuclei. These structures each influence physiologic functions in a particular way during wakefulness and in an opposing or antagonistic way during sleep. Additionally, neurotransmitters, including serotonin, norepinephrine, dopamine, and acetylcholine, influence sleep cycles. At present, the exact mechanisms that influence sleep and wakefulness are debated by scientists who continue to search for other biochemical influences and substances that may induce sleep.

Stages of Sleep

Sleep has been divided into several well-defined stages, beginning with the two major categories of rapid eye movement (REM) sleep, during which the eyes appear to move quickly under the eyelids, and non–rapid eye movement (non-REM) sleep. Non-REM sleep is further divided into four distinct stages (Table 12-1). Each non-REM and REM stage, as well as wakefulness, produce distinct brain wave patterns that can be traced by electroencephalogram (EEG) recordings (See "Diagnostic Studies-Sleep Laboratory Evaluation").

Sleep Cycles

During an average 8-hour sleep period, a person experiences four or five sleep cycles. An average cycle is 90 minutes long and is characterized by variable amounts of non-REM and REM sleep. This variance is determined by age and time relative to the overall sleep period (Fig. 12-1). Toward the latter part of the sleep cycle, REM, which may be 20 minutes in duration, dominates. Throughout the sleep cycle, the length of each sleep stage may be influenced by physical and mental states as well as medications.

The first sleep cycle follows the most orderly progression through the sleep stages. For example, stage I proceeds to stage II, followed by stage III, stage IV, and REM, which is always followed by non-REM. Thereafter, stage I may be absent, and the stages may occur in different orders. For example, stage IV may be followed by stage II and then REM sleep.

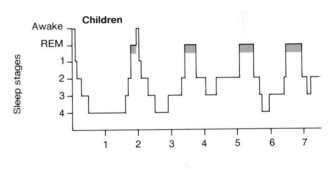

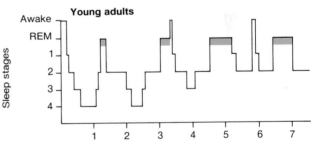

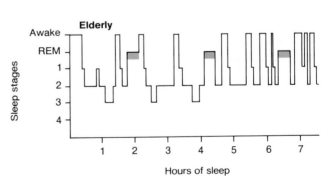

Figure 12-1. Typical sleep cycles. In children and young adults, stages 3 and 4 are reached early, with progressive lengthening of the first three REM periods and infrequent awakenings. Elderly adults show little or no stage 4 sleep, and awakenings are frequent. (After Kales, A., et al. [1968]. *Annals of Internal Medicine, 68,* 1078)

Table 12–1. Sleep Stages

Criterion	Wakefulness	Drowsiness	Non-REM Sleep				REM Sleep
			Stage I	*Stage II*	*Stage III*	*Stage IV*	
Electroencephalogram tracing	Rapid, irregular waves	Alpha rhythms	Uneven low voltage waves with frequencies of 2–7 cycles per second	Larger script with spindles and K complexes	Delta waves comprise 20%–25% of the tracing Occasional sleep spindles	Delta waves comprise more than 50% of the tracing	Wild oscillations; desynchronized beta waves similar to wakeful tracing
Subjective sensations	Alert, aware of environment	Serene, without deliberate thought, dream-like thoughts, floating images	None—if wakened may deny sleeping	None—if wakened may report vague dreams or reveries	None—dreams not reported by wakened subjects	None—dreams not reported by wakened subjects	None—wakened subjects usually report dreaming
Peripheral muscle tone	Moderate to high	Moderate	Moderate	Fair	Fair	Fair	Atony
Muscle activity	Voluntary, varying with basic activity/rest cycles	Diminished	Minimal to absent	Minimal to absent	Minimal to absent	Minimal to absent	Rapid conjugate eye movements
Duration	6 to 20 hours per day	Limited to a few minutes	Various	Various	Various	Various	5–20 min about every 90 min throughout sleep, each episode increasing in length as sleep progresses
Persistence		Very easily disrupted	Easily wakened	Not hard to waken	Hard to waken	Hard to waken and slow to arouse	Very hard to waken
Probable chemical mobilization in the brain	Catecholamine	Serotonin	Serotonin	Serotonin	Serotonin	Serotonin	Catecholamine
Physiologic signs	Normal waking patterns		Progressive slowing of the pulse and respirations and reduction of temperature and blood pressure from non-REM stages I through IV				Variable vital signs; irregular pulse and respirations; temperature is at its nadir; bursts of autonomic activity

(Spencer, R. [1993]. Clinical pharmacology and nursing management [4th ed.]. Philadelphia: J.B. Lippincott)

Sleep Functions

Although the exact functions of sleep remain speculative, certain theories have been proposed (Hartman, 1973; Oswald, 1976; Oswald, 1980). In general, sleep has an anabolic restorative function and facilitates "metabolic buildup." Experts also believe that sleep restores psychological functioning. Furthermore, sleep may be necessary for optimal functioning of the immune system.

Bone marrow and skin mitotic activity or cell division peaks soon after sleep begins. Hormones associated with growth and development are secreted in greater amounts during stages III and IV. Growth hormone secretion is interrupted if awakenings occur during the sleep period, because the pattern of growth hormone secretion is sleep-dependent and not a consequence of circadian rhythm. Strenuous exercise during the day has been associated with increased stage III and IV sleep periods, causing scientists to speculate that additional growth hormone secretion during these stages helps restore the body following physiologic stress (Oswald and associates, 1973).

Cerebral blood flow during REM sleep usually increases to levels above perfusion levels noted during wakefulness. This increased blood flow may be necessary to meet internal metabolic demands, which may be higher in children, who usually spend a proportionately greater time in REM sleep. During REM sleep, increased protein synthesis occurs, especially in the nervous system. Rapid eye movement sleep is associated with memory storage, memory consolidation, and learning.

People who are deprived of sleep usually have less ability to cope with psychological stressors; therefore, sleep probably functions to maintain well-being. Although early research indicated that REM deprivation was associated with psychiatric illness, later studies indicated that no long-term psychological effects were associated with REM sleep deprivation (Luce, 1965).

The knowledge that sleep has important functions raises questions that have clinical significance for nurses. For example, future research could focus on determining whether sleep disruption significantly alters existing pathologic processes, and if so, by what mechanisms.

Sleep Deprivation

According to scientists, a person is never 100% deprived of sleep because short episodes of "minisleep" will compensate for the sense of sleep loss. During such short sleep periods, which last only seconds, subjects in sleep deprivation studies were nonattentive and demonstrated EEG waveforms consistent with stage I, REM, or other sleep stages (Berger and Oswald, 1962).

Sleep deprivation results in impaired cognitive function and leads to mental fatigue, impaired memory, inability to concentrate, perception changes, and poor judgment. Personality changes include irritability, withdrawal, increased suspicion, confusion, disorientation, listlessness, and reduced emotional control. Neurologically, sleep deprivation is associated with mild nystagmus, hand tremors, ptosis, flat facial affect, and impaired speech patterns. Finally, sleep deprivation is associated with a lowered pain threshold and decreased production of catecholamine, corticosteroid, and hormones, which are essential for combatting stress.

Loss of REM sleep has been associated with specific effects, including hyperactivity, mood swings, agitation, and decreased impulse control.

Sleep deprivation alters subsequent sleep patterns, especially the type and length of the stages of sleep entered. When subjects in controlled studies were prevented from experiencing REM sleep and then were permitted to go back to sleep, they entered REM sleep within 4 to 10 minutes after falling asleep, rather than after the usual 90 minutes (Berger and Oswald, 1962). Furthermore, the amount of REM sleep obtained after REM deprivation may be 50% greater than baseline or normal amounts (REM rebound). Subjects who were deprived of stage IV sleep tended to gain additional stage IV sleep in subsequent sleep periods. If people who have been deprived of both REM and stage IV sleep make up stage IV sleep first, the problem of REM sleep deprivation may be aggravated.

Sleep and Rest Requirements

Although sleep requirements vary and change from infancy to old age, all people need periods of undisturbed sleep and rest during the 24-hour cycle, as outlined in Display 12-1. Sleep needs increase during periods of high metabolic need, such as following surgery or during starvation states. The right amount of sleep is the amount that results in optimal daytime function and minimal drowsiness.

Newborns sleep between 14 and 18 hours in a 24-hour period, and infants sleep 12 to 18 hours a day; for both,

---

Display 12–1
Sleep Requirements

Full-Term Infants

- 14–18 hr/day (newborns)
- 12–18 hr/day (infants)
- Average sleep periods are 3–4 hours
- Nighttime awakenings common
- 50% total sleep time (TST) is REM

1-Year-Olds

- 12 hr/night with AM and PM nap
- 30%–40% TST is REM
- Majority of TST is stages III and IV
- Sleep cycles 45–60 min long

2- to 5-Year-Olds

- 10–12 hr/night
- Progressive decrease in nap time
- Slight increase in REM sleep time
- Boys require more TST than girls
- Sleep cycles 45–60 minutes long

8- to 12-Year-Olds

- 8–10 hr/night
- 90-minute adult sleep cycle noted

12- to 14-Year-Olds

- 8–9 hr/night
- 20% TST is REM (growth spurts increase REM needs)

15-Year-Olds to Young Adults

- 6–9 hr/night
- 20%–25% TST is REM
- 50% TST is stage II

Older Adults

- 6–9 hr/night
- Progressive decrease in stage IV sleep
- Progressive nighttime awakenings
- Proportion of REM to non-REM sleep remains constant

50% of this sleep is REM. By the time a child reaches 1 year of age, REM sleep is reduced to 20% to 30%. Children spend most of their sleeping time in stages III and IV.

Young adults usually sleep 6 to 9 hours at a time, and spend 20% to 25% of their sleeping time in REM sleep. Fifty percent of their sleep time is spent in stage II, and the remaining time is spent in stages III and IV.

As people grow older, the amount of deep sleep they obtain decreases, and the total sleep period fragments. However, older adults need amounts of sleep similar to the amount younger adults need, ranging from 6 to 9 hours, depending on the individual. The proportion of REM sleep to the various stages of non-REM sleep remains constant from ages 20 to 60 years. The amount of time spent in stage IV usually declines rapidly, and by the time a person reaches age 50, it is reduced by 50%. Rapid eye movement sleep usually remains constant, but it is patterned more uniformly throughout the sleep cycle.

In elderly people, stage I time increases, but stages II and III remain unchanged. However, elderly women may spend more time in stage III sleep. Interestingly, 25% of 60-year-olds may experience little or no stage IV sleep. With this loss of restorative sleep, then, elderly people may exhibit signs and symptoms associated with sleep deprivation, including fatigue, headache, poor concentration, visual disturbances, forgetfulness, apathy, depression, coordination difficulties, and mood changes.

THE HEALTH HISTORY

The interview provides reliable data on the quality of sleep and rest, and alerts you to factors known to influence sleep and rest. Researchers have studied the correlation between what people report about their sleep patterns and what physiologic measures of their sleep pattern show, and they have found that, in most cases, the correlation is high. (See the Research Highlight at the end of this chapter.) For example, in people who report frequent periods of interrupted sleep, EEG changes often reflect this kind of sleep disturbance. Therefore, you should elicit information about a person's sleep patterns by asking appropriate questions during the interview. Understanding sleep neurophysiology as well as the variables that affect sleep is essential in formulating the appropriate interview questions.

The person's perceptions may reveal more about sleep quality than other methods of assessment. In other words, assessing sleep quality by observing the person sleep may not, in fact, be the most reliable approach. For example, you may report that the person slept all night based on observations that the patient remained supine in bed with eyes closed, yet the person may complain that he or she did not sleep during that time.

During the interview, you may choose to screen the person for sleep pattern disturbances by asking limited but relevant questions. If the person reports sleep–rest problems, you should conduct a more thorough interview (see accompanying display). In addition, you may ask the person to keep a log or diary of the number of hours slept each day for a period of a week or more. The following information should be recorded in a sleep log:

- Time the sleep period began (*i.e.,* when the person went to bed)
- Amount of time taken to fall asleep
- Number of awakenings during the sleep period and any perceived cause for waking up
- Time of final awakening

- Number of naps that were taken during the day and how long they lasted

Although obtaining the person's perspective about his or her sleep pattern is important, there are times when the person cannot respond to questions because of serious illness or impaired communication due to intubation or other treatment measures. Because such patients are frequently at great risk for sleep pattern disturbances, other sources of data should be consulted to obtain the necessary information. For example, information about medications and pathologic states that may affect sleep can be obtained from the patient's records. You can also interview the family about whether the patient has any bedtime habits that may promote sleep, such as saying prayers or drinking warm milk. Note any factors in the immediate environment that can disturb sleep, such as noises or light, and correct them if possible.

When the person can respond to questions about sleep patterns and sleep needs, the interview should explore the following points:

- Usual sleep pattern
- Altered sleep patterns
- Sleep or bedtime rituals
- Sleep environment
- Sleep position
- Factors that influence sleep
- Symptoms of sleep pattern disturbance

Usual Sleep Pattern

Sleep patterns vary greatly among people and may be attributed to differences in culture, family responsibilities, work schedules, and life-style. Cultural attitudes or personal differences can affect the amount of sleep obtained as well as the time period chosen for sleep. For example, a middle-aged, German–Russian farmer may work until midnight and rise at dawn, believing that work is more important than sleep. Such a person may sleep only 5 hours each night, yet feel well rested on awakening. Although this sleep pattern may be considered unusual, no real dysfunction may be indicated.

The interview questions should elicit specific information about the person's usual sleep pattern, including duration of sleep, usual time for falling asleep and for waking up, the number of awakenings, the causes for such awakenings, and whether naps are taken. It is also important to determine if sleep occurs other than at night. People who change work shifts often have difficulty sleeping or do not obtain enough sleep. How frequently the shifts change can also be a factor. A person who always works a night shift is less likely to suffer sleep disturbances than someone on a swing shift who probably does not have an opportunity to develop a typical sleep pattern. Other factors affect sleep, including family responsibilities such as caring for a newborn infant or a sick child or parent.

Determining whether the sleep pattern varies with respect to a particular day is also important. For example, many people sleep late on weekends and therefore disrupt

*Interview Guide*Sleep and Rest

Usual Sleep Patterns

How well do you sleep? _____

Usual sleep hours per 24 hour period? _____ Do you nap?
_____

Time of retiring _____ Time of arising _____

Is this your typical pattern? _____ If, no, what do you think
has caused a change? _____

Do you work rotating shifts or nighttime hours? _____ If yes,
what shifts do you work and how often do you rotate shifts?
_____

Describe sleep patterns in relation to shift work _____
_____

Do your weekend sleep patterns differ from weekday patterns?
How? _____

Altered Sleep Patterns

Do you have difficulty falling asleep? _____

What prevents sleep? _____

Number of nighttime awakenings _____

Cause of awakenings _____

Do you waken early and have difficulty falling asleep? _____

How do you make up for lost sleep? _____

Sleep/Bedtime Rituals

What is your usual routine before retiring? _____

(If sleeping in health care setting or any new setting) How has
your bedtime routine changed or been interfered with? _____
_____

Sleep Environment

Describe usual bedroom surroundings _____

Number/type of pillows _____

Number/ type of blankets _____

Usual noise levels _____

(If sleeping in health care setting or any new setting) What
things awaken you or prevent sleep in this setting? _____
_____

Sleep Position

In what position do you usually sleep? _____

What prevents you from sleeping in this position? _____

Psychophysiologic Influences

Current medical diagnosis _____

Previous hospitalizations/surgeries _____

Any of the following problems?	Yes/No
Enuresis	_____
Up to bathroom to void or defe-cate during sleep	_____
Use more than 1 pillow	_____
Wake with heartburn	_____
Leg jerking/muscle spasms	_____
Ulcers	_____
Cardiovascular problems	_____
Respiratory problems	_____
Rheumatoid arthritis	_____
Diabetes mellitus	_____
Migraine headaches	_____
Depression	_____
Thyroid disorders	_____
Renal problems	_____
Stress	_____
Drug History	
Caffeine (amount per day; inges-tion relative to sleep time)	_____
Alcohol	_____
Sleep aids	_____
Narcotics	_____
Barbiturates	_____
Antidepressants	_____
Amphetamines	_____

Sleep Pattern Disturbance Symptoms

Any of the following problems?	Yes/No
Excessive daytime sleepiness	_____
Nonrefreshing sleep	_____
Morning headache	_____
Snoring	_____
Difficulty initiating or maintaining sleep	_____
Nightly leg jerks	_____
Uncontrolled falling asleep	_____
Sudden awakening with a feeling of suffocation	_____
Nightmares	_____

their normal sleep time. You should also evaluate the quality of sleep by asking if the person obtains enough sleep and feels well rested on awakening.

Altered Sleep Patterns: Insomnia

Dissatisfaction with sleep quality may indicate a common sleep disorder known as insomnia. Insomnia is the inability to sleep, or the tendency to wake prematurely or too often. Insomnia does not always mean "no sleep"; many people who claim they are insomniacs sleep more than some people who have no complaints about sleep. If insomnia is a problem, ask additional questions to determine the type of insomnia.

Initial Insomnia. Normally, people need 5 to 15 minutes to fall asleep. A person with initial insomnia, the most common sleep disorder in young adults, often requires more than 30 minutes to fall asleep. Autonomic nervous system activity is higher during sleep in these people. Stress or anxiety may be a contributing factor, indicating a need to review the person's ability to cope with stress. Key interview questions are as follows:

Do you have difficulty falling asleep?

What do you think prevents sleep?

Intermittent Insomnia. In intermittent insomnia, electroencephalogram recordings may confirm that normal sleep patterns are characterized by several brief periods of awakening. However, the person may not perceive a sleep pattern disturbance or even be aware of awakening because sleep is easily resumed. In intermittent insomnia, the most common insomnia for all age groups, sleep is interrupted midcycle. The person is usually abruptly awakened by some stimulus, such as a baby crying, nightmares, the need to void, or pain. How quickly sleep is resumed depends on whether the person remains lying in bed or gets up to engage in some activity. Staying in bed is more likely to help the person fall back to sleep. Key interview questions are as follows:

Do you awaken frequently during the night/sleep period?
What do you think causes these awakenings?

Terminal Insomnia. Terminal insomnia, which becomes more common as people age, is characterized by early awakenings with an inability to return to sleep. Typically, the person may report final awakening as early as 3 or 4 AM. Terminal insomnia may be associated with daytime napping or retiring early. However, it may also be an important sign of depression, indicating a need to assess carefully the overall sleep pattern, coping abilities, and self-concept. A sleep log or diary may help identify naps and varied retiring times. Key interview questions are as follows:

Do you awaken early and find that you cannot go back to sleep?
Do you make up for lost sleep during the day by napping or retiring earlier?

General Causes of Insomnia. Insomnia may be chronic or transient and can develop from many causes. Stressful periods, pain, and environmental factors, such as extreme temperatures or shift work, may contribute to transient insomnia, as may drugs such as amphetamines or caffeine. Caffeine consumption is often the culprit because caffeine remains active in the blood stream for up to 12 hours after being ingested. Therefore, consuming caffeine with an evening meal may cause initial insomnia. Alerting people to this possibility can help to reveal the cause of their insomnia.

Sleep and Bedtime Rituals

Sleep or bedtime rituals include activities that a person engages in to prepare for sleep. Bedtime rituals may be brief, such as brushing one's teeth or washing one's face, or the rituals may be lengthy, such as reading, watching television, or eating. Illness and hospitalization can disrupt these procedures and make it difficult to fall asleep.

Asking the person to describe any pre-bedtime activities will help determine if sleep problems have occurred because routines have been disrupted or prevented. For example, you may say:

Tell me what you usually do an hour before going to bed.
How has your bedtime routine changed since coming here?

When a person is hospitalized, it helps to establish a bedtime routine to encourage rest and set the stage for sleep.

A routine may be as simple as changing the patient's gown and dimming the lights.

Sleep Environment

To assess sleep environment, ask the person to describe the usual bedroom surroundings, including type of bed and bed linens used, and the usual number of blankets and pillows. The pillow should support the head in alignment with the spinal column. If the person has cervical arthritis, a special cervical pillow may be needed, or rolled towels may need to be placed under the neck to maintain alignment during sleep.

Next, ask the person to describe room temperature and typical noise and lighting levels in the home environment during sleep. New noises, or sudden, obnoxious stimuli may inhibit or interrupt rest and sleep. For example, hospitalized patients are frequently subjected to unfamiliar sounds from equipment, staff, and other patients during the night. Their sleep is further disrupted when they are awakened periodically to have their vital signs measured or to be given medications. Unless or until they can adjust to these new routines, they will experience sleep disturbances.

Sleep Position

Some people prefer to sleep in a certain position, but may be unable to do so when they become ill or immobilized in some way. Some prefer to lie on their backs or stomachs or on their sides, or with legs curled or straight. Although such positions are rarely maintained throughout sleep, assuming them initially often facilitates falling asleep. Unnatural positions, such as the semi-Fowler's position, commonly used in acute care settings, may make it difficult for a person to fall asleep. If at all possible, you should help people assume their favored positions to promote sleep.

Factors Influencing Sleep

Psychological Influences. Ask the person if they perceive stress to be a factor disrupting their sleep pattern. Excessive demands at work or difficulty with personal relationships may contribute to sleep disturbances. See Chapter 16 for additional guidelines for assessing stress and coping.

Note whether there is a history of depression. Depression can disrupt sleep in different ways. Chronic depression is associated with a decrease in stage IV and REM sleep. On the other hand, acute depression, often experienced during grief, may be associated with delayed sleep onset, more rapid transition from one stage to another, more frequent awakenings, less deep sleep, and more REM activity but less total sleep time.

Physiologic Influences. Review the person's medical history for conditions that might disrupt sleep. Ask the person how sleep is affected by physical problems. For example, a duodenal ulcer may cause epigastric pain at night as a result of increased secretion of gastric acid that occurs throughout the sleep period, especially during REM sleep.

A person awakened by the pain may get up to eat or take antacids to relieve the discomfort. Nocturnal pain may also result from esophageal reflux, which may occur readily in the recumbent position. People with this problem may attempt to alleviate the discomfort by elevating the head of the bed or sleeping with additional pillows.

Angina is another kind of pain that may occur during REM sleep and may awaken the person. Increased activity of the sympathetic nervous system and variations in respiratory pattern can alter carbon dioxide and oxygen levels, and thereby contribute to REM-stage angina. Rapid eye movement sleep may also stimulate premature ventricular complexes (PVCs) in people with underlying cardiovascular disease. Congestive heart failure may be aggravated in a person lying in a recumbent position, which contributes to fluid accumulation in the lungs and leads to dyspnea. People with these cardiovascular problems may be afraid to go to sleep because they fear the pain.

Alterations in respiratory function are also associated with sleep pattern disturbances. Emphysema decreases ox-ygen saturation and increases carbon dioxide tension during sleep. The resultant alveolar hypoventilation may awaken the person or contribute to excessive somnolence (prolonged drowsiness). In children, asthma attacks may occur in the latter part of the sleep period, although not in stage IV. In adults, asthma attacks can occur in any sleep stage. Bronchial spasms frequently occur during REM sleep, and migraine headaches are known to originate during REM, as demonstrated on EEG tracings. Stage III and IV sleep time is decreased in persons with hypothyroidism and increased in persons with hyperthyroidism. Sleep disturbances also occur with chronic renal insufficiency, and with greater frequency before dialysis.

Medications. Review the person's medication history and identify drugs that might alter sleep patterns (see Display 12-2). Also, note the use of any drugs to induce sleep. Most sleep aids are physiologically effective for 2 to 3 weeks, after which time a placebo effect may occur. Many people with sleeping difficulties frequently change doctors as well as medications to facilitate sleep. You should care-

---

Display 12–2
Effects of Medication on Sleep

REM		*Stage IV*
Decrease REM Time		*Decrease Stage IV Time*
Ethchlorvynol (Placidyl) 500 mg	Morphine	Glutethimide (Doriden) 500 mg
Glutethimide (Doriden) 500 mg	Heroin	Pentobarbital sodium (Nembutal) 100 mg
Secobarbital sodium (Seconal) 100 mg	Alcohol	Diazepam (Valium) 10 mg
Pentobarbital sodium (Nembutal) 100 mg	Thiopental (Pentothal)	Reserpine 0.14 mg/kg
Methyprylon (Noludar) 300 mg	Nitrazepam (Mogadon)	Heptabarbital
Methaqualone (Quaalude) 300 mg	Dextroamphetamine	Chloral hydrate 1.5 gm
Diphenhydramine hydrochloride	Imipramine hydrochloride	Depression
(Benadryl) 50 mg	(Trofanil)	Hypothyroidism
Scopolamine 0.006 mg/kg	Amitriptyline (Elavil)	Dextroamphetamine and pentobarbital
Monoamine oxidase inhibitors (MAO)	Methadone hydrochloride	
	(Dolophine)	
	Meprobamate (Miltown) 1200	
	mg	
	Amobarbital	
	Heptabarbital (Medomin)	
Allow Normal REM Time	*Increase REM Time*	*Increase Stage IV Time*
Chloral hydrate 0.5 gm, 1 gm, 1.5 gm	Reserpine	Moderate to vigorous exercise carried
Flurazepam hydrochloride (Dalmane) 30 mg	LSD	out several hours before bedtime
Methaqualone (Quaalude) 150 mg		Antidepressants in the presence of
Chlordiazepoxide (Librium) 50 mg		depression
Diazepam (Valium) 10 mg		
Caffeine		

*These findings are for only the specific dosages listed.

(Fass, G. [1971]. Sleep, drugs, and dreams. *American Journal of Nursing, 71*[12],239)

fully assess medication types and dosages, and how long the person has been taking such medications.

Many sleep aids depress REM and stage III and IV sleep. When such drugs are discontinued, REM rebound and nightmares may occur. Medications such as diphenhydramine hydrochloride (Benadryl, a common over-the-counter sleep aid), barbiturates, and most antidepressants suppress REM activity. Hypnotics and barbiturates decrease the amount of REM sleep but may increase total sleep time. Antidepressants and amphetamines may abnormally decrease the amount of REM sleep. Many people withdrawing from these medications experience nightmares while "catching up" on REM sleep (REM rebound sleep).

Although few sleep medications allow normal sleep, some do not suppress REM sleep, including chloral hydrate, flurazepam hydrochloride (Dalmane), and methaqualone (Quaalude).

Caffeine and Alcohol. Caffeine may also cause sleep problems. A 24-hour food and fluid record may be needed to show the amount of caffeine ingested and the time it is consumed. Caffeine can have a stimulating effect up to 12 hours after ingestion.

Alcohol may contribute to insomnia, especially if consumed in large amounts. Initially, alcohol may have a sedative effect and induce sleep. However, the person may awaken within 3 or 4 hours, and REM sleep deprivation may occur. Linking alcohol ingestion with sleep pattern disturbances may be difficult because some people are reluctant to admit to alcohol ingestion and often believe that alcohol promotes sleep. Severe sleep pattern disruptions have been noted during alcohol withdrawal in alcoholics. During withdrawal, nightmares and physical activity, such as restlessness, may increase. Consequently, such people often fear sleep. Alcohol may be a contributing factor in the development of sleep apnea syndrome.

Symptoms of Sleep Pattern Disturbance

Although some 45 to 60 million Americans experience significant sleep problems, sleep deprivation problems may not be diagnosed because many people do not report sleep problems to health care providers. Because symptoms related to sleep disturbances are general, the person may not associate a particular set of symptoms such as mood alterations, cognitive impairment, and irritability with sleep disruption, and therefore may not mention such symptoms during the interview. However, the person may report symptoms such as fatigue on awakening or fatigue during the day, or difficulty falling asleep or staying asleep.

Symptoms most commonly associated with sleep pattern disturbances include the following:

- Excessive daytime sleepiness (EDS)
- Nonrefreshing sleep
- Morning headache
- Frequent nightly awakenings
- Nighttime leg jerks
- Difficulty falling asleep or staying asleep

You should ask additional questions based on the reported symptoms to determine possible causes. The following broad, open-ended statements or questions elicit the best results:

> Describe how you feel when you have not had a good night's sleep. How does lack of sleep affect you?

Ask the following three questions if the person complains of EDS:

> Have you had any unusual problems with your muscles? (Reports of cataplexy or weakness, especially weak knees during excitement, are associated with narcolepsy.)
> Do you snore? (If snoring is irregular, evaluate further for sleep apnea.)
> What medications have you used regularly in the past few months or years? (Chronic use of stimulants, hypnotics, and certain other drugs may lead to EDS.)

DIAGNOSTIC STUDIES

Sleep Laboratory Evaluation

Sleep laboratory evaluation involves the use of physiologic monitoring equipment to obtain data to characterize the person's sleep pattern and physiologic responses during sleep. An analysis of the data can reveal problems such as

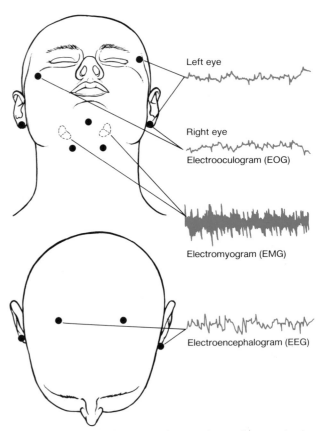

Figure 12–2. Sleep laboratory evaluation. Sleep is determined in the laboratory by measuring the electrical activity of the brain and muscles and the movement of the eyes, using techniques of electro-oculography, electromyography, and electroencephalography. Collectively, these measurements are called polysomnographic evaluation.

sleep apnea, narcolepsy, insomnia, myoclonus, paroxysmal contractions of the calf muscles that interrupt sleep, and other sleep disorders.

Before physiologic monitoring ensues, the person is interviewed to obtain information about the usual sleep pattern and factors influencing sleep, and a personality profile is constructed by administering questionnaires and psychological tests. In addition, the person may be asked to keep a sleep log or diary.

The basis of the laboratory assessment is a polysomnographic evaluation during one or more designated sleep periods. Polysomnographic evaluation includes the techniques of electro-oculography, electromyography, and electroencephalography (see Fig. 12-2). The electro-oculogram (EOG) records eye movements; the electromyogram (EMG) monitors muscle tone and activity; and the electroencephalogram (EEG) records brain wave activity. In addition, respiratory pattern, ECG findings, and arterial hemoglobin saturation may be monitored.

Electroencephalogram. The EEG provides a continuous recording of brain wave activity during the sleep period. Several electrodes are attached to the scalp, and a polygraph recording of the brain wave pattern is obtained on paper over a period of several hours. The recorded brain waves are then analyzed to determine the order and duration of the various stages of sleep. Sleep EEGs may be interpreted and described according to standard methods and nomenclature issued by the Association for the Psychophysiological Study of Sleep. Certain drugs as well as physical states may affect EEG patterns. For example, atropine may produce sleep-related EEG findings in a person who is awake.

Wakefulness is depicted on the EEG by random, low-voltage, rapid electrical activity, called beta and alpha waves (Fig. 12-3). Wakefulness is characterized by rapid eye movements and high muscle tone. People demonstrate waking behavior by being alert and aware of surrounding stimuli.

Stage I sleep represents the transition between wakefulness and sleep and may last only 5 minutes. Beginning with stage I, EEG patterns reflect activity progressively higher in voltage with lower-frequency waveforms until stages III and IV are reached. The EEG waveforms in stage I are called theta waves (see Fig. 12-3). The eyes will roll slowly from side to side, and heart and respiratory rates will usually decrease. Subjective feelings such as drifting or relaxation may be associated with this stage. A person may be easily awakened from stage I sleep by noise or other stimuli, and, if wakened, may deny having been asleep. Muscle tone is relatively high, and myoclonic jerks or sudden twitching in the face or extremities may be noted.

Stage II sleep, which lasts from 10 to 15 minutes, is a deeper sleep state. Greater effort is required to awaken a person in stage II sleep. The EEG pattern is characterized by delta waves, sleep spindles, and K complexes. Little or no eye movement may be recorded by EOG (see Fig. 12-3). Body processes, including metabolic rate and body temperature, continue to decrease during stage II.

Stage III sleep, a deeper, more restful sleep, is dominated by parasympathetic nervous system activity and lasts about 20 minutes. Delta waves, K complexes, and sleep spindles appear on the EEG (see Fig. 12-3). Because the brain wave tracing is slow and regular, stages III and IV are called slow-wave sleep (SWS). Parasympathetic activity accounts

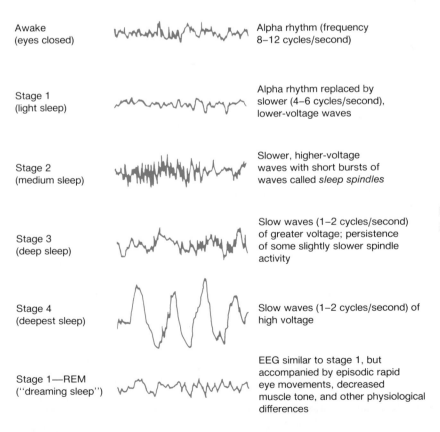

Awake (eyes closed)		Alpha rhythm (frequency 8–12 cycles/second)
Stage 1 (light sleep)		Alpha rhythm replaced by slower (4–6 cycles/second), lower-voltage waves
Stage 2 (medium sleep)		Slower, higher-voltage waves with short bursts of waves called *sleep spindles*
Stage 3 (deep sleep)		Slow waves (1–2 cycles/second) of greater voltage; persistence of some slightly slower spindle activity
Stage 4 (deepest sleep)		Slow waves (1–2 cycles/second) of high voltage
Stage 1—REM ("dreaming sleep")		EEG similar to stage 1, but accompanied by episodic rapid eye movements, decreased muscle tone, and other physiological differences

Figure 12-3. Sleep stages and associated polysomnographic recordings.

for decreased blood pressure and lowered heart and respiratory rates. In this stage, a person may be difficult to awaken.

Stage IV sleep, the deepest stage, is entered 15 to 30 minutes after a person initially falls asleep. The delta waves, noted during stage II, continue at an even slower rate (SWS) during stage IV. Muscle tone is relaxed, and the eyes remain still (see Fig. 12-3). Sleepwalking and bedwetting may occur in this stage. Respiratory and heart rates may be lowered 20% to 50% below waking levels, and the person may be difficult to awaken. Because restorative physiologic processes occur during this stage, including increased protein synthesis and increased secretion of growth hormone, sleep quality is judged by the amount of time spent in stage IV. People who report that they did not sleep, despite behavior demonstrating the contrary, may not have obtained sufficient stage IV sleep.

REM sleep is a relatively active sleep state that varies in duration and is dominated by sympathetic nervous system activity. Electroencephalogram waves reflect low-voltage and high-frequency electrical activity, similar to activity associated with wakefulness. At the same time, the muscles may appear relaxed, a sign indicating deep sleep (see Fig. 12-3). Because characteristics associated with wakefulness and deep sleep are present, REM sleep is also called *paradoxical* sleep. Episodic bursts of rapid eye movements, associated with vivid dreaming, are recorded by EOG, and such movements may be observed even though the person's eyes are closed. Sympathetic activity may contribute to increased blood pressure, increased heart and respiratory rates, and a subsequent increase in oxygen consumption, as well as to the great variability noted in each parameter. In addition, gastric secretion may increase, and steroid hormones are released. Penile erections may occur in males of all ages during this stage. The dreaming that occurs during REM sleep is qualitatively different from the dreaming that occurs during non-REM sleep, in that REM dreams are often bizarre or irrational, whereas non-REM dreams are usually more realistic and logical.

Electro-oculogram. The EOG records each eyeball position during sleep by measuring the potential difference between the cornea and retina. Small electrodes are placed at the orbital margins, and waveforms representing eye movement are traced on polygraph paper. Rapid eye movements are associated with REM sleep. Flat waveform lines usually are recorded during non-REM sleep. Frequent eye movements during REM sleep may indicate intense dreaming.

Electromyogram. An EMG is obtained by attaching small electrodes on the chin to record muscle tone. Face and neck muscles are usually hypotonic just before and during REM sleep. However, brief spikes of muscle activity may be noted, as a result of electrical discharge from the pons during REM sleep.

Miscellaneous Sleep Monitoring. The electrocardiogram (ECG) may be simultaneously monitored to detect sleep-induced cardiac dysrhythmias. Respirations may be electronically monitored and are useful in evaluating sleep apnea syndromes. All vital signs may vary between non-REM and REM sleep periods, which justifies using additional physiologic monitoring.

Sleep Questionnaires

Diagnostic evaluation may also include the administration of standardized tests. Sleep questionnaires measure and describe the characteristics of sleep from the patient's perspective. The person is asked to respond, usually in writing, to standardized questions about sleep quality and quantity, the number of awakenings, and the time needed to fall asleep. The information is similar to the information that may be obtained by interviewing. Questionnaires to evaluate sleep are often used in research studies as a means of collecting data quickly and in a consistent manner. Although such questionnaires may be used in the clinical setting, they have several disadvantages. Many acutely ill patients have difficulty completing a written questionnaire. Moveover, cognitive function may be impaired because of medications, procedures, sleep deprivation, and sensory overload or deprivation. Thus, the ability to complete a paper and pencil test is further compromised. Nevertheless, sleep questionnaires may be used with some patients or may serve as a basis for structuring interview questions. Table 12-2 summarizes features of sleep questionnaires that may be adapted for clinical practice.

Table 12–2. Sleep Questionnaires

Questionnaire	Description	Comments
Sleep pattern	11-item sleep and dream log. Measures presleep state of mind, sleep latency, awakenings, body movements, state of rest, sleep depth, and dream recall.	Easy to administer and score, even with acutely ill patients. Cannot be used for patients with impaired mental status.
Leeds sleep evaluation	10 questions grouped into 4 areas: ease of getting to sleep, perceived quality of sleep, ease of awakening from sleep, and quality of behavior after wakefulness.	Easy to administer, even with acutely ill patients. Has not been correlated with polysomnography.
St. Mary's Hospital	14-item questionnaire	Easy to administer and score. Cannot be used for patients with impaired mental status.
Richards Campbell	5-item instrument that uses a visual analogue scaling technique. Measures sleep depth, falling asleep, awakenings, returning to sleep, and quality of sleep.	Easy to administer and score. May be used in acute care settings. Correlated with polysomnography for 3 of 5 items.

NURSING OBSERVATIONS RELATED TO SLEEP AND REST

Examination Focus

During the physical examination, you may recognize signs of sleep deprivation and associated physical effects. In order to evaluate sleep and rest functions during the physical examination, special attention is directed toward the following:

- General appearance
- Cognitive functions

General Appearance and Cognitive Functions

During the general survey, note the person's facial appearance, speech patterns, gross motor movements and posture, and cognitive status.

Facial Appearance. A person who has been deprived of sleep may have a flat or expressionless facial affect because the facial muscles relax. Mild nystagmus (involuntary jerking movements of the eyeballs) and red conjunctivae may also be noted. Eyelid ptosis and dark circles beneath the eyes are common. The person may yawn frequently.

Speech Pattern. Sleep deprivation may contribute to thick or slurred speech, mispronunciations, and incorrect word usage.

Gross Motor Movements and Posture. Restlessness is associated with sleep disturbances and may be expressed by frequent changes in posture or position. Slight hand tremors may be noted along with possible impaired coordination, which, when combined with slurred speech, may give the appearance of drug or alcohol intoxication.

Cognitive Functions. Sleep deprivation is generally associated with progressive disorientation and decline in cognitive functions. The person may appear listless and lethargic rather than alert and aware. Attention span may be short. Other possible signs include irritability, apathy, and impaired judgment. Prolonged sleep deprivation can lead to visual hallucinations and psychotic behavior, especially paranoia (feelings of persecution).

Associated Body System Alterations

Sleep and rest dysfunctions will manifest primarily in two body systems: the neurologic system and the musculoskeletal system. Neurologic and musculoskeletal manifestations of sleep and rest dysfunctions have already been described and include cognitive changes, restlessness, irritability, flat affect, nystagmus, hand tremors, and incoordination.

Nursing Observations — *Sleep Pattern*

General Principles

The sleep pattern is evaluated primarily on the basis of the person's perceptions of sleep that are elicited during the assessment interview. Additional data may be obtained by actually observing the person and his or her surroundings during sleep.
In the in-patient health care setting, nurses have the opportunity to observe people at sleep and at rest. Often, nurses make judgments about the quality of the person's sleep based on intermittent observations. This method is valid provided the nurse makes every attempt to elicit and compare what the patient's perceptions of sleep quality were during the same observation periods.

Examination and Documentation Focus

- Environmental factors influencing sleep
- Body movements
- Uninterrupted sleep time
- Sleep behaviors

Examination Guidelines — *Bedside Sleep Pattern Observation*

Procedure

1. SURVEY THE SLEEPING PERSON'S ENVIRONMENT.

Note environmental stimuli that may promote or inhibit sleep.

Clinical Significance

Sleep Promoters
- Quiet
- Dark or subdued lighting
- Comfortable mattress and pillows
- Room temperature (personal preference varies)
- Presence of usual sleeping partner

GUIDELINES *continued*   *Bedside Sleep Pattern Observation*

Procedure	Clinical Significance
	Sleep Inhibitors
	• Noise (including voices)
	• Light
	• Irregular or soft mattress
	• Uncomfortable pillows
	• Extreme room temperatures
	• Roommates (especially if requiring treatments or confused)
	• Hospital routines (laboratory tests; vital sign measurement; medication administration)
2. OBSERVE BODY MOVEMENTS.	
Note the person's body movements during rest or sleep periods.	**Normal Findings**
	Expect to see periodic body movements during sleep. Position may be changed 20 to 60 times during an 8-hour sleep period.
	Deviations from Normal
If there is very little body movement observed, ask the person about sleep quality.	Absent or minimal position changes may indicate poor-quality sleep.
3. DETERMINE THE QUANTITY OF UNINTERRUPTED SLEEP TIME.	
Note the amount of uninterrupted sleep time the person experiences. Uninterrupted sleep time includes periods of time in which no one enters the patient's room or immediate surroundings.	People need at least 90 minutes to complete one full sleep cycle including REM sleep. In hospitals, some people are disturbed on an hourly basis and therefore are at high risk for sleep deprivation.
4. OBSERVE SLEEP BEHAVIORS.	
Note general appearance.	A person who is sleeping will usually lie immobile with eyes closed. Always validate by comparing your observations with the person's reports of sleep.
	Normal Findings
Note specific sleep-related behaviors.	Snoring, sleep talking
	Deviations from Normal
	Snoring associated with sleep apnea syndrome; sleep-walking; night terrors; enuresis; teeth grinding; apnea (see "Clinical Problems Related to Sleep and Rest").

Documenting Sleep Evaluation Findings

Sleep–rest assessment may be documented in the nursing progress notes or as a component of a problem-oriented record.

Example 1: Normal Sleep Pattern

Ms. G, aged 32 years, was interviewed about sleep and rest patterns as part of a routine health assessment at the community health clinic. Characteristics of her sleep and rest habits were recorded as follows:

Reports 6 or 7 hours of sleep between 2300 and 0600. Awakens once during night to care for infant but readily falls back to sleep. Awakens feeling refreshed; feels energetic during daytime activities; rarely naps. Presleep routine includes mending or needlepoint while watching television with husband, brushing teeth, checking baby, and letting cat outside.

These findings may be recorded in a problem-oriented record as follows:

S: 6 or 7 hours of sleep per night between 2300 and 0600, with one nighttime awakening to care for infant. Readily falls back to sleep. Rarely naps, feels energetic during day and wakens refreshed. "I feel I get enough sleep."

O: Alert and attentive throughout 20-minute assessment interview. Facial affect animated; eyes bright, clear conjunctivae.

A: Functional sleep–rest pattern; able to maintain desired life-style.

P: Follow-up with routine health screening in 1 year. Reinforce importance of regular daily cycling (regular retirement/wakeup times) in maintaining optimal sleep pattern.

Example 2: Sleep Apnea

Mr. S, aged 49 years, was observed overnight in the CCU following hospital admission for chest pain. The nurse observed irregular snoring and periods of apnea. When asked about sleep in the morning, Mr. S. reported long-standing fatigue. This and other data were summarized:

Noted to have apneic periods during sleep lasting 5 to 10 seconds. Irregular, loud snoring. Reports "wife always bothered by snoring"; excessive daytime sleepiness; and occasional morning headaches.

These findings may be recorded in a problem-oriented record as follows:

S: "I'm always tired; I must not sleep very well, although my wife says I snore all night long."
O: Obese male; high-risk age group for sleep apnea; apneic periods during sleep (5–10 sec). Snores irregularly.
A: Sleep dysfunction—possibly sleep apnea.
P: Discuss referral to sleep laboratory for additional evaluation when discharged from hospital. Consider aggravation of cardiovascular problems related to sleep apnea and increase nighttime surveillance while in CCU.

Example 3: Sleep Pattern Disturbance

Ms. P, aged 29, was evaluated at the student health center. Her primary reason for seeking health care was fatigue. She reported: "I'm always tired during the day, but especially on Mondays." Sleep data were recorded as follows:

Reports 6 hours of sleep on a good night and less than 4 hours of sleep on Friday and Saturday nights. Cites dating and school obligations as interfering with sleep; once asleep, has no difficulty staying asleep "unless I drank too much and then I'm up early, still feeling very tired." Denies use of sleep-inducing medications or caffeine. Reports occasional use of street amphetamines to "give me energy." General appearance: dark circles under eyes; frequent yawning; body slumped; short attention span during interview.

These findings may be recorded in a problem-oriented record as follows:

S: "I'm always tired during the day, especially on Mondays." Usual sleep pattern: "6 hours, uninterrupted, on a good night," and 4 hours on Friday and Saturday nights. Studies and social activities interfere most with sleep time. Occasional alcohol use causes early awakenings. "I take some speed if I get too tired and need some energy."
O: Dark circles under eyes; frequent yawning; body slumped; short attention span during interview.
A: Sleep pattern disturbance—possibly related to ineffective life-style management.
P: Discuss usual sleep requirements for age; explore alternative life-style patterns that will allow more time for sleep; discuss relationships between amphetamines/alcohol and sleep.

NDx

Nursing Diagnoses Related to Sleep and Rest

Sleep Pattern Disturbance

Sleep pattern disturbance can be defined as disrupted sleep that causes discomfort or interferes with a person's desired life-style. The indicators of this diagnosis include difficulty falling asleep; waking earlier or later than desired; experiencing interrupted sleep; not feeling well rested; and demonstrating behavioral or cognitive changes such as irritability, restlessness, disorientation, and lethargy. Possible physical changes include nystagmus, hand tremor, eyelid ptosis, dark circles under the eyes, and slurred or otherwise altered speech. Some sleep pattern disturbances are related to environmental stimuli or stressors that may be reported during the interview or detected by observing the person at sleep. If the person reports insomnia, the type of insomnia can be determined through the interview and observation as well as by sleep laboratory monitoring and observation.

Sleep pattern disturbances may be related to clinical problems, such as pain, which you may treat collaboratively with a physician.

Clinical Problems Related to Sleep and Rest

Narcolepsy

Narcolepsy is a sleep disorder characterized by the following:

- *"Sleep attacks":* Irresistible episodes of daytime sleepiness
- *Cataplexy:* A sudden loss of motor tone that may cause the person to fall
- *Sleep paralysis:* Skeletal muscle paralysis, which occurs during the transition from wakefulness to stage I
- *Hypnagogic hallucinations:* Nightmares

The cause is unknown but may be related to a central nervous system genetic defect that causes an uncontrollable REM sleep phase.

History

Involuntary daytime sleep attacks may begin in puberty. Most people with this problem have symptoms for about 15 years before the disorder is accurately diagnosed. The daytime sleep attacks are absolutely irresistible. Cataplexy, especially weak knees, is often precipitated by strong emotion, either positive or negative. Hypnagogic hallucinations or nightmares occur most often as the person falls asleep. Sleep paralysis may affect most skeletal muscles; it is frightening, because the person can neither move nor speak. However, the ability to move the eyes is retained and is usually sufficient to reverse the paralysis, as is someone touching the person or applying other external stimuli. Recovery occurs even if the person is left undisturbed. A small percentage of people who do not have narcolepsy may experience sleep paralysis for unknown reasons. Familial incidence of narcolepsy is 20 times that of the general population.

Sleep Laboratory Evaluation

In addition to the obvious signs of daytime sleep attacks, narcolepsy involves disturbed nighttime sleep as revealed through sleep laboratory evaluation. The person suffering from narcolepsy tends to enter REM sleep immediately after falling asleep. (Normally, 90 minutes of sleep elapses before the first REM phase.)

Sleep Apnea Syndrome

Temporary cessation of breathing during sleep for short periods of 10 seconds or so is referred to as sleep apnea. In sleep apnea syndrome, as many as 300 episodes of breathing cessation may occur during the sleep period. Most types of sleep apnea are classified as obstructive, or secondary to airway obstruction, which commonly results from enlarged adenoids or tonsils, or obesity. However, the airway is patent during the waking state. Sleep apnea has been linked to sudden infant death syndrome (SIDS).

History

Men over age 50 are most frequently affected. Obesity is a risk factor, especially if the person has a short, fat neck. The person usually seeks health care for hypersomnolence or EDS, indicating that the disturbance is interfering with his or her life-style. Unlike the sleep attacks associated with narcolepsy, the daytime sleepiness that accompanies sleep apnea is resistible. The person may report moving around or slapping himself or herself to stay awake.

Laboratory Evaluation

Sleeping partners of people with sleep apnea syndrome often report that the person stops breathing during sleep for 10 to 20 seconds. Loud snorts follow that increase in intensity until suddenly the person bolts upright in bed and resumes breathing, all without waking. Another possible manifestation is a pattern of irregular snoring. Such behavior is usually confirmed in the sleep laboratory. The person may exhibit typical symptoms of sleep deprivation, including increased irritability, decreased attention span, and impaired memory. The alveolar hypoventilation associated with apneic episodes may contribute to more serious sequelae, including cor pulmonale, pulmonary hypertension, and brain hypoxia.

Kleine–Levin Syndrome

Kleine–Levin syndrome, a rare hypersomnolence disorder unrelated to narcolepsy, is characterized by sleep attacks that last several hours to several days, three or four times a year. Eating patterns vary greatly; the person may gorge with food for several days and gain weight. Often the person suffers from depression or other psychological problems. Sleep laboratory evaluation reveals an otherwise essentially normal sleep pattern.

Nocturnal Myoclonus

Nocturnal myoclonus is a rare form of sleep pattern disturbance whereby the person is awakened by calf muscle spasms, which may occur as frequently as every 30 seconds. Excessive daytime sleepiness or waking feeling unrefreshed may be reported.

Parasomnias

The parasomnias include somnambulism (sleepwalking), pavor nocturnus (night terrors), nocturnal enuresis, talking in one's sleep, and bruxism (teeth grinding). These manifestations originate during non-REM sleep. Parasomnias, which primarily interfere with children's sleep and often appear together in the same child, have a familial tendency.

Somnambulism (Sleepwalking)

Somnambulism, or sleepwalking, occurs most often in children, and boys are affected more frequently than girls. The person usually cannot remember the sleepwalking episode and may not awaken if the episode lasts less than 4 minutes.

Sleepwalking occurs most often in the first third of the sleep period during stage III or IV non-REM sleep. The sleep EEG usually reveals that sleepwalking is preceded by a burst of high-voltage, low-frequency activity similar to that occurring in stage IV. A normal percentage of REM sleep is noted, indicating that the person experiences normal dreaming.

Pavor Nocturnus (Night Terrors)

Night terrors most often affect children younger than age 6. After sleeping a few hours, the child usually bolts up in bed, shakes and screams, and appears terrified, but is difficult to awaken. Children usually do not remember these episodes.

Night terrors occur predominantly in stage IV sleep. They may be treated by administering benzodiazepines, which are known to suppress stage IV sleep.

Nocturnal Enuresis (Bedwetting)

Nocturnal enuresis, or bedwetting, may be either primary or secondary. In primary enuresis, bedwetting has no physiologic basis and persists from birth to age 6 or older. In secondary enuresis, bedwetting occurs because of psychological factors. Nocturnal enuresis is primarily a childhood disorder, occurring especially in boys, although 1% to 2% of some sampled adult groups exhibited the disorder as well.

When assessing enuresis, interview the parent(s) as well as the child. Although the child is usually asleep when the bedwetting occurs, the parent may believe the accident is intentional. Ask the parents questions such as, "How do you deal with your child and the bedwetting?" and "Do you feel your child can control the bedwetting?" Sibling jealousy or fear of walking to the bathroom alone in the dark may contribute to the problem. Finally, discuss bedwetting with the child.

Nocturnal enuresis occurs most frequently during the first third of the sleep period, following the transition from stage IV to stage II sleep. Immediately before entering REM sleep, while still in stage II, the child urinates. The child will not usually maintain restful sleep in wet clothing or bed linens.

Sleep Talking

Usually, talking in one's sleep occurs during non-REM sleep and is associated with body movement. Sleep talking is not considered a disturbance except to someone sleeping in the same room.

Bruxism (Teeth Grinding)

Bruxism, or teeth grinding during sleep, occurs in 15% of the population. The teeth may become chipped, and the person may need to wear a nighttime mouth guard to protect the teeth. Bruxism usually occurs during stage II non-REM sleep.

ASSESSMENT PROFILE

• •

Mr. Butcher, a 52-year-old patient who had undergone coronary artery bypass graft surgery, had consented to be a subject in a study to identify sleep pattern characteristics in critical care settings. After Mr. Butcher recovered from general anesthesia, data were collected by continuous EEG recordings and behavioral observations to verify whether he was sleeping. In addition, data were collected about stimuli that could potentially disrupt sleep. Data collection was nearly complete. Mr. Butcher's condition was stable, and he was awaiting transfer to a general surgical ward.

Although comprehensive data analysis for all subjects in the study was to follow, the nurse researcher reviewed the data collected during the previous 48 hours, including the EEG recordings that correlated with the various sleep stages. The data indicated that Mr. Butcher had not entered a sleep state for the previous 32 hours, but rather, had been in a wakeful or aroused state, despite his sleep-like appearance. However, the nurse's charting revealed Mr. Butcher had "slept well throughout the night."

Mr. Butcher displayed a number of behaviors that the nursing staff attributed to the ICU environment, such as irritability, inability to concentrate, and mild confusion. For example, he could not state the day or time and had pulled intravenous lines and removed his oxygen cannula frequently during the previous 12 hours. When caregivers approached Mr. Butcher, he asked them to leave him alone so he could get a good night's sleep.

The nurse researcher discussed Mr. Butcher's sleep status with the nursing staff.

Profile Analysis

It was relatively easy for the nurses to diagnose Sleep pattern disturbance following recovery from heart surgery for Mr. Butcher, because the nurse researcher had documented the problem by EEG recording. Could the nurses have arrived at the same diagnosis without such data? Most experts agree that interviewing and observing provide reliable data about the sleep pattern. However, the diagnostic process involved requires a different cognitive approach than that required to analyze data generated by the EEG.

Identifying the Assessment Focus

The nurses caring for Mr. Butcher noted several significant cues, even before the nurse researcher shared data collected from the EEG. One nurse described her thinking as follows:

> This man had been in the ICU only 2 days but we had met previously when he visited the unit as part of his preoperative teaching. At that time he was a little anxious but seemed to be coping well. He talked freely, expressing his concerns and asking pertinent questions. After surgery, his behavior changed. He acted paranoid and confused—always picking at lines and equipment. I wanted to focus on problems that might have precipitated his behavior. My initial thoughts focused on several possibilities: Sleep pattern disturbance, Anxiety, Fear, Ineffective coping, and that vague problem

area called "ICU psychosis." I realized I needed more information before I could diagnose the problem. It was important to see if fear was the primary problem causing sleep disruption or to see if sleep disruption was the primary problem leading to paranoid behavior. I focused on making the correct differential diagnosis because I knew treatment would be influenced by the final diagnosis.

Pre-encounter Influences

Sleep deprivation in ICU patients is common, and nurses have begun to place greater emphasis on interventions to promote sleep in such high-risk people. In 1983, critical care nurses were surveyed in order to determine significant patient problems that could be addressed through nursing research. The survey revealed that critical care nursing research needed to focus on promoting sleep and preventing sleep deprivation in critically ill clients (Lewandowski and Kositsky, 1983).

The expertise and knowledge of nurses in the ICU influenced the types of problems they considered when they noticed behavior changes in Mr. Butcher. The stage of his medical treatment also influenced the direction of nursing assessment. Mr. Butcher was still receiving the type of care associated with multiple stimuli that could interfere with sleep. For example, every hour a nurse measured vital signs, took a pulmonary artery catheter reading, and measured urine output. Once every 4 hours, a nurse, surgeon, intern, or surgical resident performed a head-to-toe examination. Moreover, every 2 hours, Mr. Butcher was turned and positioned and asked to cough, deep breathe, and use the incentive inspirometer. Between 4 and 5 AM, blood specimens were collected; a chest radiograph was taken; a weight was obtained on the bedscale; and a bath and linen change were provided. Environmental stimuli during daytime and evening hours included bright lights, telephones, cardiac monitors, alarms, intravenous pumps, and ventilators, background talking, and hissing sounds from suction and oxygen equipment.

In addition, Mr. Butcher had experienced some postoperative pain and had required one transfusion of packed red blood cells. Not only could such stimuli interfere with sleep, but they could contribute to additional problems such as anxiety, fear, and ineffective coping.

Possible Nursing Diagnoses

The nursing diagnosis of Sleep pattern disturbance was tentatively established for Mr. Butcher based on his difficulty falling asleep, his mood alterations, and his statements concerning sleep loss. Even though there was strong evidence supporting this diagnosis, the nurses remained tentative. Other nursing diagnoses, especially Anxiety, Fear, and Ineffective coping, as characterized by mood alterations, needed to be considered.

Additional Data Gathering and Analysis

Additional data were analyzed to select or assign priority to possible nursing diagnoses. To establish a precise diagnosis, the nurses compared the data with defining characteristics and etiologic categories associated with each diagnosis being considered. Occasionally, more data collection was required to make such comparisons. For example,

Anxiety

Assess patient further for the following:

- *Risk factors:* Knowledge deficit, underlying fear, conflict, insecurity, ineffective coping
- *Manifestations:* Verbalized expectation of danger, signs of sympathetic nervous system activation, feelings of apprehensiveness or concern, increased verbalization, sleeping disturbances

Fear

Assess patient further for the following:

- *Risk factors:* Perceived external threat or danger, perceived inability to control events, knowledge deficit
- *Manifestations:* Describes the focus of threat or danger, verbalizes expectation of danger, increased verbalization, restlessness, signs of sympathetic nervous system activation

Ineffective Coping

Assess client further for the following:

- *Risk factors:* Knowledge deficit, personal vulnerability, situational crisis
- *Manifestations:* Verbalized inability to cope, inability

to solve problems, destructive behavior toward self and others, inappropriate use of defense mechanisms

Sleep Pattern Disturbance

Assess client further for the following:

- *Risk factors:* Environmental stimuli, pain, anxiety, absence of bedtime rituals, previous sleep pattern disturbances, medication effects, periods of interrupted sleep time
- *Manifestations:* Complaints of insomnia, irritability, progressive disorientation, restlessness

Final Nursing Diagnosis

By comparing information obtained from the patient with information associated with each diagnostic possibility, the nurses decided that Mr. Butcher was most likely suffering from sleep pattern disturbance. Further assessment was directed toward determining optimal interventions and evaluating interventions. The patient's usual sleep pattern and bedtime rituals were assessed so that as he became more physiologically stable, he could be encouraged to resume previous patterns.

Furthermore, factors that might inhibit sleep, such as excessive environmental stimuli and pain, were identified and modified. Within 48 hours, Mr. Butcher was fully oriented and stated that he was sleeping well. Early nursing intervention and subsequent transfer out of the intensive care unit contributed to resumption of previously functional sleep patterns.

Chapter 12   SUMMARY

Sleep and rest assessment should focus on the following:
- The person's concerns related to sleep quantity and quality
- Stimuli and states that promote or inhibit sleep, rest, and relaxation
- Psychological and physiologic indicators of adequate sleep or sleep deprivation

When assessing sleep and rest consider the following:
- Sleep deprivation symptoms are general; therefore the patient may not associate such symptoms with sleep pattern disturbances.
- Self-reports of sleep quantity and quality usually correlate closely with polysomnographic data.
- Sleep requirements vary among people. Sleep adequacy is evaluated relative to age-related norms and the client's perspective.
- Normal progression through sleep stages enhances sleep quality. At least 90 minutes is required for completion of a single sleep cycle.

Multiple information sources may be used. The data base should consist of the following:

The Health History
- Usual sleep pattern
- Altered sleep patterns

- Sleep and bedtime rituals
- Sleep environment
- Sleep position
- Factors that influence sleep
- Sleep pattern disturbance symptoms

Observations
- Facial appearance
- Speech patterns
- Gross motor movements and posture
- Cognitive functions
- Sleep patterns

Polysomnographic Data (when available)
- EEG
- EOG
- EMG
- Respiratory pattern analysis
- ECG
- Arterial hemoglobin saturation analysis

Sleep and rest assessment, based on these principles and methods, helps the nurse to identify defining characteristics and risk factors for the following nursing diagnoses:
    Sleep pattern disturbance
    Fatigue

RESEARCH *Hi*GHLIGHT

How accurate are people's descriptions of their own sleep patterns, especially compared with objective polysomnographic measures?

Effectively treating sleep pattern disturbances depends on accurately diagnosing the problem. Polysomnographic evaluation during sleep, which includes monitoring EEG, EMG, and EOG recordings, is usually considered the most accurate and objective way to assess sleep quality and quantity. However, such methods are time-consuming and costly to implement, and not all people are suitable candidates for sleep laboratory evaluation. Given such limitations, researchers have conducted studies to determine how accurate a person's descriptions of his or her sleep are, especially compared with objective polysomnographic measures.

In a preliminary study, a sleep researcher found that subjects tended to have definite opinions about their sleep patterns and stated with certainty whether they were good or poor sleepers. Based on such self-reports, the researcher studied two groups, "good" and "poor" sleepers, recruited from a college population. Each subject's sleep was monitored for two sleep periods while data were obtained by EEG, body temperature and skin resistance measurements, and other physiologic monitoring devices. The good sleepers reported that they fell asleep in less than 10 minutes and rarely had nighttime awakenings and, if they did, could easily fall asleep again. The poor sleepers reported that they needed at least 30 to 60 minutes to fall asleep and that they awakened frequently and had difficulty falling asleep again.

Physiologic monitoring during the study confirmed that good sleepers slept more than poor sleepers, thus confirming the subjects' self-reports about ease or difficulty in falling asleep. Good sleepers spent less time in stage II sleep and reached REM sleep earlier. Poor sleepers spent the same amount of time in stage IV deep sleep as good sleepers but took more time to reach this stage. Based on these findings, the researcher decided that subjects' subjective recall concerning sleep periods closely correlated with objective findings.[1]

What significance does the study have for health assessment?

Even though Sleep pattern disturbance is a problem within the domain of nursing practice, data collection using poly-somnographic methods is not considered a primary nursing function. The nurse relies more on data collection methods such as the interview and observation. A study such as this one indicates that interview data may be reliably used to characterize a person's sleep pattern. Therefore, defining characteristics for the diagnosis Sleep pattern disturbance, such as "patient reports not sleeping well" or "patient reports difficulty falling asleep," may be considered excellent indicators that the problem does exist.

Can these findings be applied to practice?

Researchers other than Monroe have studied the correlation of self-reports about sleep with objective measures in subjects with psychiatric and chronic illnesses and found that self-reports were not as reliable as Monroe's study indicates. For example, persons suffering depression tend to overestimate sleep pattern disturbances, stating that they did not obtain sufficient sleep when, in fact, they often slept more hours than healthy subjects (Samuel, 1964). On the other hand, persons with manic disorders underestimated their sleep pattern disturbances (Platman, 1970). Similarly, elderly persons suffering dementias tended to understand their sleep patterns inaccurately (Feinberg and associates, 1969). They often underestimated sleep time, indicating that such persons may have difficulty distinguishing between light sleep and wakefulness (alternating between light sleep and wakefulness characterizes the sleep pattern of elderly persons). Additionally, peoples' perceptions about time spent awake may be distorted. Therefore, the nurse should proceed with caution, especially with patient groups mentioned above. Some people, such as the young healthy subjects in Monroe's study, may accurately describe sleep pattern disturbances, but other people may not. Studies should be replicated with the same patient groups and others. Meanwhile, such findings should be cautiously applied to assessment.

REFERENCE

1. Monroe, L.J. (1967). Psychological and physiological differences between good and poor sleepers. *Journal of Abnormal Psychology, 72*(3), 255-264.

Related nursing diagnoses may be detected during sleep and rest assessment including problems contributing to sleep pattern disturbance:

Anxiety
Ineffective individual coping
Altered family processes
Fear
Dysfunctional grieving
Pain

Additionally, you should develop skill at detecting and monitoring the following clinical problems:

- Narcolepsy
- Sleep apnea syndrome
- Kleine–Levin syndrome
- Nocturnal myoclonus
- Parasomnias

✳ CRITICAL THINKING

Your ICU patient is a 53-year-old man who has a flail chest following an automobile accident. He is intubated and being ventilated mechanically. The nursing staff describes the patient as confused, combative, and agitated. He is kept sedated to control his behavior.

Learning Exercises

1. Plan how you would evaluate your patient's sleep and rest pattern. Given that he is sedated and intubated, determine how this would affect your assessment strategies.

2. One of your colleagues tells you that an assessment of this patient's sleep and rest pattern is irrelevant because there is nothing that you can do about an abnormal pattern. Explain how you would respond. Would you agree or disagree with your colleague? Explain why or why not.

3. Determine what observations you would want to make about this patient's surroundings that would be relevant to sleep and rest.

4. Interventions to improve this patient's sleep and rest cycles are implemented, including the provision of uninterrupted time with the lights dimmed and the room door closed. Propose how you would evaluate the effectiveness of these interventions.

BIBLIOGRAPHY

Assousa, S.N., & Wilson, N.D. Validation of Sleep Pattern Disturbance. In R.M. Carroll-Johnson (Ed.). *Classification of nursing diagnoses: Proceedings of the ninth conference.* Philadelphia: J.B. Lippincott.

Baekeland, F., & Hoy, P. (1971). Reported vs. recorded sleep characteristics. *Archives of General Psychiatry, 24* (6), 548–551.

Bahr, R.T. (1983). Sleep-wake patterns in the aged. *Journal of Gerontological Nursing, 9* (10), 534–539.

Barndt-Maglio, B. (1986). Sleep pattern disturbance. *Dimensions in Critical Care Nursing, 5* (6), 342–349.

Berger, R.J., & Oswald, I. (1962). Effects of sleep deprivation on behavior, subsequent sleep, and dreaming. *Journal of Mental Sciences, 108,* 457.

Beyerman, K. (1987). Etiologies of sleep pattern disturbance in hospitalized patients. In A.M. McLane (Ed.). *Classification of nursing diagnoses: Proceedings of the seventh national conference* (pp. 193–198). St. Louis: C.V. Mosby.

Closs, S. (1988). Assessment of sleep in hospitalized patients: A review of methods. *Journal of Advanced Nursing, 13* (4), 501–510.

Fass, G. (1971). Sleep, drugs, and dreams. *American Journal of Nursing, 71* (12), 2316–2320.

Feinberg, I., Braun, M., & Shulman, E. (1969). EEG sleep patterns in mental retardation. *Electroencephalography and Clinical Neurophysiology, 27,* 128–141.

Floyd, J.A. (1984). Interaction between personal sleep–wake rhythms and psychiatric hospital rest–activity schedule. *Nursing Research, 33* (5), 255–259.

Frensebner, B. (1983). Sleep deprivation in patients. *AORN Journal, 37* (1), 35–42.

Hartmann, E.L. (1973). *The functions of sleep.* New Haven: Yale University Press.

Hartmann, E.L. (1973). Sleep requirements: Long sleepers, short sleepers, variable sleepers, insomniacs. *Psychosomatics, 14,* 95–103.

Hayter, J. (1983). Sleep behaviors of older persons. *Nursing Research, 32* (4), 242–246.

Helton, M.C. et al. (1980). The correlation between sleep deprivation and the intensive care unit syndrome. *Heart and Lung, 9* (3), 464–468.

Hemenway, J.A. (1980). Sleep and the cardiac patient. *Heart and Lung, 9* (3), 453–463.

Hodgson, L.A. (1991). Why do we need sleep? Relating theory to nursing practice. *Journal of Advanced Nursing, 16* (12), 1503–1510.

Jensen, D.P., & Herr, K.A. (1993). Sleeplessness. *Nursing Clinics of North America, 28* (2), 385–405.

Johns, M.W. (1971). Methods for assessing human sleep. *Archives of Internal Medicine, 127* (3), 484–492.

Kales, A., & Kales, J. (1970). Evaluation, diagnosis, and treatment of clinical conditions related to sleep. *Journal of the American Medical Association, 213,* 2229–2235.

Kales, A., & Kales, J. (1974). Sleep disorders: Recent findings in the diagnosis and treatment of disturbed sleep. *New England Journal of Medicine, 290* (9), 487–498.

Kroenke, K. (1991). Chronic fatigue syndrome: Is it real? *Postgraduate Medicine 89* (2), 44–46, 49–50, 53.

Lewandowski, L.A., & Kotsitsky, A.M. (1983). Research priorities for critical care nursing: A study by the American Association of Critical-Care Nurses. *Heart and Lung, 12* (1), 35–44.

Luce, G.G. (1965). *Current research on sleep and dreams.* Bethesda, MD: United States Department of Health Education and Welfare (Pub. #1389).

McFadden, E., & Giblin, E. (1971). Sleep deprivation in patients having open heart surgery. *Nursing Research, 20* (3), 249–254.

McNeil, B.J., Padrick, K.P., & Wellman, J. (1986). I didn't sleep a wink. *American Journal of Nursing, 86* (1), 26–27.

Monroe, L.J. (1967). Psychological and physiological differences between good and poor sleepers. *Journal of Abnormal Psychology, 72* (3), 255–264.

Oswald, I. (1976). The function of sleep. *Postgraduate Medicine Journal, 52,* 15–18.

Oswald, I. (1980). *Sleep.* London: Penguin Books.

Parrott, C.P., & Hindmarch, I. (1980). The Leeds sleep evaluation questionnaire in psychopharmacological investigations: A review. *Psychopharmacology, 71,* 173–179.

Parsons, L.C., & VerBeek, D. (1982). Sleep awake patterns following cerebral concussion. *Nursing Research, 31* (5), 260–264.

Platman, S.R., & Fieve, R.R. (1970). Sleep, depression, and mania. *British Journal of Psychiatry, 116,* 219–220.

Richards, K. (1987). Techniques for measurement of sleep in critical care. *Focus on Critical Care, 14* (4), 34–40.

Rossi, G. (1980). Neural regulation of sleep. *Experientia, 36,* 20.

Saletu, B. (1975). Is the subjectively experienced quality of sleep related to objective sleep parameters? *Behavioral Biology, 13,* 433–444.

Samuel, J.G. (1964). Sleep disturbance in depressed patients: Objective and subjective measures. *British Journal of Psychiatry, 110,* 711–719.

Snyder-Halpern, R. (1985). The effect of critical care unit noise on patient sleep cycles. *Critical Care Quarterly, 7* (4), 41–50.

Tierney, L.M. (1989). Chronic fatigue syndrome: Current recommendations for diagnosis and management. *Consultant, 29* (3), 25–27, 31–32.

Woods, N.F. (1972). Patterns of sleep in postcardiotomy patients. *Nursing Research, 21* (4), 347–352.

Assessing Self-Concept

Examination Guidelines

Assessment Terms

Self-Concept

Self-Concept
Self-Esteem
Extant Self
Desired Self
Presenting Self

Locus of Control
Social Identity
Personal Identity
Body Image

INTRODUCTORY OVERVIEW

Self-concept is how a person views or defines himself or herself at a given time and can often be reflected in answers to such questions as, "Who am I? What am I?" Self-concept includes the person's view of their personality traits, social roles, and physical traits. For example, a person's self-concept may include a personality trait, such as "dependable," or a social role, such as "community leader." Self-concept is always evolving and is influenced by values, beliefs, interpersonal interactions, culture, and perceptions of how one appears to others.

Self-esteem, a part of self-concept, is a personal judgment about self-worth, value, and competence—in other words, how positively or negatively a person feels about self.

When self-concept is threatened or disrupted, such as when a person loses his or her job, people fight or defend to maintain their beliefs about themselves using defense mechanisms such as rationalization, displacement, or projection. For example, a person who lost his or her job might say, "I'm glad I don't work there anymore. It wasn't a very ethical place (rationalization)". If self-concept is threatened and defenses are not sufficient, stress increases and the person may experience personality disorganization, a loss of control, and a sense of powerlessness and helplessness.

Assessing a person's self-concept enables the nurse to make judgments about a person's feelings of adequacy in a given situation and any behaviors that might be associated with these feelings. This assessment may provide insight into other problems the person may have. For example, a cardiac rehabilitation patient may not participate in recuperation activities because of feelings of inadequacy or feelings that he or she has no control over the outcome (Fig. 13-1).

Jill Fuller and Jennifer Schaller-Ayers:
HEALTH ASSESSMENT: A NURSING APPROACH, Second Edition.
© 1990, 1994 by J. B. Lippincott Company.

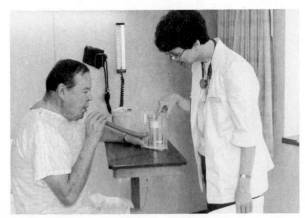

Figure 13-1. Patients will feel more in control if they can participate in their own care.

According to Coombs (1971), people "judge the value of their experience with helpers from the frame of reference of self-concept. What affects the self-concept seems relevant. What appears remote from it seems irrelevant." For example, self-concept influences a person's motivation to learn, so that people who perceive themselves as poor learners or who have a poor self-concept causing feelings of powerlessness or depression, may not respond to teaching interventions until their poor self-concepts are identified and altered.

Assessing a person's self-concept helps reveal how self-perceptions influence behavior and emotional responses. Such an assessment should involve identifying the person's thoughts and feelings about himself or herself; factors that have influenced self-concept development; threats to the person's self-concept; and the kind of responses demonstrated in the face of threats to the person's self-esteem.

Assessment Focus

Self-concept is evaluated by observing general appearance and body language; listening for statements about personal and social identity as well as statements indicating level of self-esteem; asking pertinent questions about self-concept; and interpreting results of questionnaires designed to measure self-perceptions.

Assessing self-concept can be especially difficult if the person uses defense mechanisms to conceal self. Therefore, special efforts should be made to establish rapport and encourage disclosure.

The overall assessment should focus on determining social identity and identifying self-descriptive labels or groups the person identifies with, the effect of life events on self-perception, level of self-esteem, and threats to self-concept (see display, Assessment Focus). A valid assessment depends on the person's ability and willingness to make self-disclosures.

Nursing Diagnoses

Nursing diagnoses that relate directly to disturbances in self-concept include the following:

Body image disturbance
Chronic low self-esteem
Situational low self-esteem
Personal identity disturbance
Self-esteem disturbance

Additional human responses to altered self-concept include the following:

Anxiety
Fear
Hopelessness
Powerlessness

RELATED NURSING DIAGNOSES

A person with self-concept dysfunctions is at high risk for other problems, such as the following:

Ineffective individual coping
Diversional activity deficit
Altered family processes
Altered health maintenance
Self-care deficit
Sexual dysfunction
Sleep pattern disturbance
Impaired social interaction
Spiritual distress (distress of the human spirit)

KNOWLEDGE BASE FOR ASSESSMENT
Self-Concept

According to Rosenberg, self-concept is "the totality of the individual's thoughts and feelings with reference to himself or herself as an object" (Rosenberg and Kaplan, 1982). Although theorists differ in the language they use to describe self-concept, nursing models of self-concept generally focus on the following four components: physical self (body image); social identity (role and role performance); personal identity (moral/ethical self, intellectual self, and emotional self); and self-esteem (Kim and Moritz, 1982). Each self-concept component provides a focus for assessment. A description of each component is expanded in the Health History section.

Rosenberg (1979) further identifies three broad areas of self-concept: the extant self, which refers to how the person views self; the desired self or self-ideal, which reflects how the person would like to view self; and the presenting self, or how the person shows self to others.

Extant Self. The person's concept of the extant self is his or her perception of actual self (the "real me") and includes social and personal identity and body image. You can never completely know the person's concept of the extant self, even if the assessment process is based on mutual trust and rapport. At best, certain feelings and emotions can be revealed only through self-disclosures or by overt signs such as body language or dress. The extant self is frequently obscured by various defense mechanisms. The per-

Assessment Focus **Self-Concept**

Assessment Goal	*Data Collection Methods*
	Selection of data collection methods is influenced by the patient's status, the depth of the assessment, and the nurse's skill and expertise. During screening evaluation, fewer methods may be used.
1. Identify aspects of the person's social identity.	*Interview and Observe* • Sociodemographic characteristics: age, gender, group memberships. • Self-disclosure statements reflecting social identity: How does the person respond to the question "Who am I?" or to the Twenty Statements Test?
2. Identify factors that contribute to the person's self-concept.	*Interview* • Social identity: What social affiliations help maintain and validate self-concept? • Significant life events: What aspects of the person's past have influenced the development of self-concept? *Observe* • Interactions with significant others. • Personal possessions: Are there personal objects symbolizing group or personal affiliations?
3. Identify material objects that may be extensions of the person's self-concept.	*Observe* • What references does the person make to material objects (equipment, prostheses)? • How does the person respond to these objects?
4. Identify the person's perceptions of self-worth.	*Interview and Observe* • How does the person feel abut his or her social identity? Personal identity? Physical self? • Self-disclosure statement: Do statements suggest self-approval or disapproval? • Congruence of behaviors with statements: Do behaviors contradict the person's statements about self? • What do the person's role performance and interpersonal relationships reveal about self-esteem? • What do self-drawings reveal about self-esteem? *Review the Results of Standardized Assessment Tools* • Rosenberg's Self-Esteem Scale. • Twenty Statements Test.
5. Identify actual or potential threats to the person's self-concept.	*Interview* • What are the individual's perceptions of threats to self-concept? *Observe* • Affective behaviors: Do the person's behaviors indicate anxiety or fear? • Threats in the person's environment: Are there threatening circumstances in the person's immediate environment? Can these threats be removed or modified?

son usually judges the extant self in relation to the desired self.

Desired Self. The person's concept of the desired self refers to his or her perceptions of the ideal self ("what I would like to be") and is a motivating force toward achieving goals or becoming a better person according to individually determined standards. Such standards, however, are often influenced by sociocultural ideals. In other words, what society dictates as desirable may influence the self-ideal. The desired self may be realistically or unrealistically conceived. The more unrealistic or the further the desired self is from the extant self, the greater the risk for poor self-esteem. However, some people learn to tolerate their human failings and maintain self-esteem. When assessing self-concept, you should be especially aware of the gap between extant self and desired self, providing the person does not actively conceal both.

Presenting Self. The most variable aspect of self-concept is the presenting self, which refers to how people want others to view them. The presenting self will vary, depending on who the person is interacting with, because different self-images are considered appropriate for different people or groups. For example, a person will project a different self-image when asked about himself or herself on a first date than when on a job interview. The presenting self is actually the person's self-report, or what the person is willing to divulge. The greatest assessment challenge is to judge the degree of correlation between self-report and actual self-concept. Unfortunately, strategies for enhancing such judgments are not well developed, and you may simply have to look for congruence as an indicator of the degree to which the presenting self correlates with the actual self-concept. For example, a person may report feeling self-confident, yet demonstrate behavior that indicates a need for excessive reassurance, thereby revealing a possible discrepancy between the presenting self and actual self-concept.

Self-Concept Development

Symbolic Interactionism. According to symbolic interactionism, self-concept evolves from infancy through old age. One of the most influential factors is the kind of interactions one has with others, such as parents, siblings, peers, authority figures, and the general sociocultural milieu. In other words, one often becomes what others expect.

Cooley (1902) is credited with being the first symbolic interactionist who formulated the idea of a "looking-glass self." According to this theory, self-concept is a reflection of one's perceptions about how one appears to others. Self-concept is formed in early childhood when an important person in the child's life exerts such influence that the child adopts that person's judgment of him or her. Therefore, a child who is consistently praised by the significant people in his or her life is more likely to develop a positive self-concept than one who is always criticized.

Mead (1934) expanded on Cooley's "looking-glass self" by stating that self-concept is not merely derived by interaction with significant others but also reflects a "generalized other." In other words, the entire sociocultural milieu influences self-perceptions.

Symbolic interactionist theory suggests that self-concept is a product of what a person *believes* others think of him or her regardless of what others may *actually* think. Any valid assessment of self-concept should be based on the person's perspective of self rather than on social labels or stereotypes.

Developmental Tasks. As a person grows and matures, skills and ability to perform different functions should increase. Different growth periods present specific developmental tasks or tests of strength and ability. The changes inherent in each crucial growth period present the person with developmental crises. Successfully passing through each developmental stage requires that developmental tasks be mastered and subsequent crises resolved in order to nurture a positive self-image. If developmental crises are not resolved, a negative self-concept may develop, and the ability to master subsequent developmental tasks may be impaired. Erikson's psychosocial stage theory of ego development (1963) provides a theoretical structure for assessing developmental aspects of self-concept. Additional guidelines for assessing a person's progression through various developmental stages are provided in Chapters 18, 19, and 20.

Self-Concept Stability

Despite the influences of interactions with others, the sociocultural milieu, and developmental stages, a person's self-concept is characterized by relative stability, which may be attributed in part to self-consistency. Driever (1976) defines self-consistency as that part of a person that strives to maintain a consistent self-organization and to avoid disequilibrium. Once an inner core of perception, or *phenomenal self,* is formed, the person has a personal frame of reference. The phenomenal self is stable and resistant to change, although the person may not be entirely satisfied with self-image.

The phenomenal self is established at a very young age when a person may not be aware of the variety of self-perceptions that can be incorporated into overall self-concept. Consequently, self-perceptions consisting of what the person believes others think of him or her becomes firmly embedded in the overall self-concept. Change may occur as a result of ongoing interactions or events, but resistance to such change is great. Nursing assumes that self-concept changes are possible, for without such an assumption, implementing many nursing interventions would be impossible. However, it is important to remember that changing a person's self-concept is a slow process.

Locus of Control. Personality characteristics or traits, which are stable features of a person, may also influence self-perception and account for a stable self-concept. One such characteristic influencing self-concept is suggested by the *locus of control* concept, a concept of social learning theory developed by Rotter (1966). According to this theory, locus of control refers to a relatively stable characteristic developed over time and influenced by social learning experiences. This concept reflects the person's perception that the cause of events or behaviors is either within or outside personal control regardless of the situation. The person is characterized by an internal locus of control if the belief is that what happens to him or her is largely the result of personal actions and choices. A person who believes that what happens to him or her is largely attributable to luck, fate, chance, or powerful people rather than him or herself has an external locus of control.

Locus of control characterizes one dimension of a person's self-perceptions. Because internal locus of control is associated with a positive self-concept, this aspect of a person's view of life should be evaluated when assessing self-concept.

Variables Affecting Self-Concept

The many factors that influence self-concept can be explained in terms of symbolic interaction theory, developmental theories, and personality theories. The following factors are most influential in the development of self-concept:

- Early bonding experiences
- Physical, cognitive, and interpersonal development and maturation
- Personality characteristics
- Culture
- Environment
- Socioeconomic status
- Historical perspective or the person's sense of a place in time (cohort effect)
- Physical attributes and capabilities, including present health status

- Interpersonal relationships
- Professional and personal roles

A Healthy Personality

A healthy personality is characterized by positive self-esteem, meaning that the person perceives self as valuable and worthwhile or has positive regard for himself or herself (Stanwyck, 1983). According to Jourard (1968), the term *healthy personality* is not equivalent to the term *normal personality,* which refers to people who play their roles suitably. Rather, a healthy personality is characterized by the ability to play roles satisfactorily and at the same time derive personal satisfaction from one's roles while continuing to grow (Dunn, 1961). The closer a person's extant self-concept is to the desired self-concept, the greater the person's self-esteem. You can effectively make judgments about whether or not a person has a healthy personality only by thoroughly evaluating self-perceptions and self-concept.

THE HEALTH HISTORY AND INTERVIEW

Data included as part of the health history should be helpful in making judgments about the following:

- Social identity
- Personal identity
- Body image
- Self-esteem

- Threats to self-concept
- Support systems

The history is compiled on the basis of reviewing records to identify medical concerns, illnesses, physical disabilities, or disfigurements that might be threats to self-concept. You should also determine whether or not the person is under the influence of consciousness-altering drugs (prescribed or nonprescribed). Of additional historical significance is the availability of family or significant others for support in times of crisis. The history is completed by interviewing the person about various aspects of self-concept.

Effective interviewing, which may be the primary data collection method to evaluate self-concept, incorporates principles of therapeutic communication discussed in Chapter 2 and requires a mutually trusting nurse–client relationship. You should be careful to avoid stereotyping or labeling the person because this might interfere with your abilities to be objective and listen well.

During the interview, you should phrase statements or questions in such a way as to elicit pertinent data directly. For example, you might say,

Tell me how you feel about yourself generally.
How would you describe yourself?
How has this illness (surgery, hospitalization) changed the way you feel about yourself?

The interview guide shown in the accompanying display may be used to direct the collection of appropriate data. Some practitioners use standardized diagnostic tools to further evaluate self-concept. The use of these tools is discussed in the next section of this chapter (see "Diagnostic Studies").

Interview Guide **Self-Concept**

Social Identity

Occupation _____
My family situation is best described as _____
Groups/clubs/affiliations important to me _____
People who know me would describe me as _____

Personal Identity

I would describe myself as _____
What I like best about myself _____
What I like least about myself _____

Body Image

My greatest physical (health) concern _____
What I like best about my body _____
What I like least about my body _____

Self-Esteem

How I would describe how I feel about myself _____

Threats to Self-Concept

Things that make me anxious/fearful/distressed _____

Although a structured interview enables you to obtain data pertaining to the separate components of the self-concept, it is important to relate the parts to one another and not to draw conclusions based on one component. How the person feels is more important than what you perceive as being important. For example, a young, physically active nurse who is interviewing a person with multiple physical disabilities may conclude that the person's body image is threatened. However, the person may have adapted to physical disabilities and feel much more threatened by a change in social identity or roles and relationships, such as may occur from being laid off from work. Therefore, it is important to determine how salient each area of self-concept is to the individual.

Once you have compiled a health history pertaining to self-concept, you should determine whether to proceed with additional observation and interaction. Additional guidelines for the examination of self-concept are found elsewhere in this chapter (see "Self-Concept Assessment").

Social Identity

Social identity includes sociodemographic characteristics such as age, gender, group membership (*e.g.,* minority group, religious affiliation, political affiliation), and cultural identity. Assessing social identity reveals the roles that are important to the person. Rosenberg and Kaplan (1982) associate social identity with self-concept for two reasons. First, social categories assigned from birth through old age provide a structure for a person's life experiences, which shape self-concept. Social labels may contribute to experiences such as prejudice, stereotyping, or discrimination, all of which profoundly influence and shape self-concept. Second, social labels also define how the person lives and what he or she does. For example, a physician and a migrant farm worker differ not only in what they do but also in the amount of social respect they command; both experiences influence self-concept. Rosenberg (1979) identifies the following six social identity categories:

- *Social status:* Universal classifications such as sex, age, family status, and occupation
- *Membership groups:* Voluntary association groups found within societies such as cultural, religious, sociopolitical, and fellowship groups, and special interest groups, such as Mothers Against Drunk Drivers
- *Social labels:* Labels conferred by a socially sanctioned agency or authority, such as *alcoholic, criminal, child abuser,* or *mentally incompetent*
- *Derived statuses:* Classification associated with personal history, such as a *Vietnam veteran, ex-convict, former num,* or r*eformed alcoholic*
- *Types or social types:* Socially defined perceptions, attitudes, or habits that characterize a person, such as *womanizer, hermit, intellectual,* or *ski bum.* Various subcultures may use their own terms for social types, such as *jock, narc, dead-head,* or *punk rocker.*
- *Personal identity:* In the social sense, a single, unique label, often as simple as the person's first name or nickname

Data related to social identity can be collected by asking the person direct, closed-ended, or open-ended questions:

Closed-Ended Questions

What is your name (age, occupation, religion, ethnic background)? What clubs or groups do you belong to?

Open-Ended Questions

Tell me about your family background. How would your friends (roommates, coworkers, boss) describe you?

Social identity may also be assessed by reviewing biographic data, available through patient records, and by listening for self-disclosure statements reflecting social identity categories, such as the following:

I'm a Yankees' fan.
I'm an alcoholic.
I'm a single parent.

Personal Identity

Bonham and Cheney (1983) describe four elements of personal identity: physical self, emotional self, moral/ethical self, and intellectual self. Physical self is discussed separately in the following section and reflects NANDA's classification, in which physical self is a distinct self-concept component.

In Rosenberg's schema (1979), personal identity refers to dispositions or inclinations to act in certain ways and becomes part of self-concept as a person becomes aware of such responses or tendencies.

Several categories of dispositions are frequently expressed as adjectives, such as attitudes (liberal, conservative); traits (stubborn, shy, compulsive); abilities (smart, gifted, expert); values (Christian, monogamous); habits or acts (reckless, anxious, nervous); and preferences.

During the interview, data collection is most productive if you use open-ended questions to elicit information about these abstract qualities:

How would you describe yourself as a person?

If the person has difficulty responding, you may help by asking questions such as, "Do you see yourself as happy or sad; shy or extroverted; industrious or lazy?"

The following questions may also be helpful to elicit data:

What do you like best (least) about yourself?
What achievements are you most proud of?
What would you change if you could?
How would you say your abilities compare to the average person?

More structured assessment tools such as the Twenty Statements Test and the Pier-Harris Self-Concept Scale may also be used to obtain a more thorough assessment of personal identity.

Body Image

Body image refers to a person's perceptions of personal physical characteristics, including physical attributes, functional abilities, sexuality, wellness–illness state, and appearance. Like other aspects of self-concept, body image develops and evolves over time. For the infant, body image involves sensorimotor experiences in which the body is not perceived as being separate from the surroundings. As a person ages, body image is increasingly influenced by sociocultural beliefs and values. Body image involves not only physical appearance and function, but also items associated with the body, such as clothing, jewelry, eyeglasses, pacemakers, and protheses. For hospitalized patients, equipment such as cardiac monitors, ventilators, and feeding tubes may be incorporated into body image. In addition to the physical self, body image involves the person's feelings about physical capabilities. This self-concept component is least stable and can readily be altered as a result of illness, hospitalization, or surgery.

Body image is assessed by observing, listening, and interviewing and by ascertaining what body parts or functions are most important to the person. For example, a pianist or artist may value his or her hands, whereas a runner may value leg strength. Teenagers may value overall mobility and physical attractiveness. In a clinical setting, body image can be threatened by invasive procedures or devices, such as intravenous lines. How the person reacts in such a situation may provide a clue to possible body image problems.

You should listen to self-disclosing statements about body image and descriptions and perceptions about machines. Machines that have been assigned names by the patient may be viewed as self-extensions (Fig. 13-2).

Open-ended interview questions may include the following:

> What concerns you most about your body?
> What do you like most (least) about your body?
> What physical feature would you like most to change?

Assessing a child's perception of body image may present a challenge because children may have difficulty ver-

balizing these perceptions. Encouraging the child to draw a self-portrait and then talking about the picture is one way to overcome this obstacle.

Self-Esteem

Self-esteem refers to how a person feels about the various components of self-concept, including social identity, personal identity, and body image. These perceptions may be reflected in statements of self-approval or disapproval. Negative evaluations may indicate actual or potential low self-esteem.

Reflections of self-esteem may be observed through body language, interpersonal relationships, negative talk about the self, and role performance. Open-ended questions based on statements the person has already made about self-image may be helpful. For example,

> You identify yourself as a traditional wife and mother. How important is this image to you?
> Now that you have different responsibilities in your work, would you say you have a positive or negative attitude about your present abilities?

Other, more general questions may be asked in relation to self-esteem:

> How do you feel about yourself as a person?
> How do you feel about your ability to deal with situations or events happening to you now?

If the responses indicate low self-esteem, the next step is to determine how long the problem has existed. Low self-esteem may be a basic feature of the person's psychological makeup, or it may be related to a specific situation.

You may more thoroughly assess a person's self-esteem by using assessment tools such as the Rosenberg Self-Esteem Scale (see the following section, "Diagnostic Studies"). You may also gain further insight by evaluating the person's locus of control. For example, persons who have an external locus of control are at greater risk for negative self-esteem.

Threats to Self-Concept

To identify threats to self-concept ask the person to respond to the following question:

> • What types of events or things about your present situation are most distressing (or unpleasant, threatening)?

Actual or potential threats to self-esteem are individually determined. What may threaten self-esteem in one person will have no effect on another. The person's statements can provide clues about possible vulnerability to self-image. Hirst and Metcalf (1984) list the following elements of self-esteem: roles, touch, meaningful relationships, sexuality, independence, and space. Actual or potential threats to any of these elements should be explored from the client's perspective.

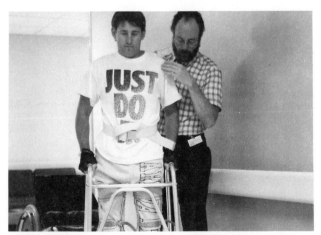

Figure 13–2. A walker may be viewed as a self-extension to patients who are regaining their mobility.

Roles. Roles contribute to self-concept and foster self-esteem. Because personal identity is often tied to one's role or roles in life, any change in role can pose possible threats to self-esteem. Significant role changes include job changes, relationship changes, bereavement, and inability to fulfill roles following illness or injury. The impact of any such changes should be evaluated to identify possible health problems.

As you interview, ask the person about any significant changes in their life or lifestyle.

Touch. According to Hirst and Metcalf (1984), touch is an element of self-esteem that conveys caring and acceptance by others. People who are denied physical contact can experience a diminished sense of self-worth. This problem may affect hospitalized patients who also suffer the added threat of separation from loved ones. Nurses can counter these adverse reactions by using touch as a form of therapy when delivering care.

Meaningful Relationships. Close relationships with others promote self-esteem by fostering feelings of importance and desirability. A person who experiences a lack or deterioration of meaningful relationships is at greater risk for altered self-concept. Inquire about the stability of important relationships.

Sexuality. Threats to sexuality or sexual identity threaten self-esteem (see Chap. 15). A healthy self-concept involves feeling attractive and desirable to others.

Independence. Independence and control over one's life are essential to one's sense of well-being. Loss of independence, such as entering a long-term health care facility, may threaten self-esteem.

Space. Invasion of one's territory, personal space, or privacy may also pose a threat to self-esteem. Generally, people with lower self-esteem require a greater amount of personal space than other people do.

DIAGNOSTIC STUDIES

Diagnostic assessment tools have been developed to measure certain aspects of self-concept. Some tools have limited use because they have not been extensively tested in clinical situations. In such cases, conclusive interpretation of the data obtained by using the tool may be difficult. Other tools may not be appropriate because they require too much time to administer or are not well accepted by the person being interviewed. Nevertheless, self-concept assessment tools may prove helpful and may guide you in determining the type of information you can elicit during related assessment processes, such as interviewing.

Twenty Statements Test. McGuire and Padawer-Singer (1982) point out that the structured approach to assessing self-concept may have limitations, especially when the person is asked to make self-evaluative statements, because the person may be forced to describe irrelevant self-concept dimensions. Their studies indicate that when people were asked to describe themselves, fewer than 10% of their statements dealt with self-evaluation, indicating that highly structured self-concept assessment may prevent spontaneity. One alternative that may help you to more accurately determine a person's relevant self-perceptions is the Twenty Statements Test (TST) developed by Kuhn and McPartland (1954).

The TST is an unstructured paper and pencil test in which the person is given a blank sheet of paper and asked to give 20 answers to the question, "Who am I?" within 12 minutes. The score is obtained by classifying each response according to a coding scheme. The code and response reflect the person's self-concept.

Locus of Control Scales. Locus of control may be evaluated by observing the person's behaviors or by administering objective tests, including Rotter's Internal-External (I-E) Scale (1966), the Health Locus of Control (HLC) Scale (Wallston & coworkers, 1976), or the Multidimensional Health Locus of Control (MHLC) Scale (Wallston and coworkers, 1978). Locus of control scales require the person to choose statements that reflect his or her perception of the cause of events. The person's responses are scored in a standardized manner, and judgments are made about the person's locus of control on the basis of this score. For example, the higher the score obtained on Rotter's I-E Scale, the more external the person's locus of control.

Rosenberg's Self-Esteem Scale. The Rosenberg Self-Esteem (RSE) Scale (1979) consists of 10 statements to which people are asked to strongly agree, agree, disagree, or strongly disagree (Display 13-1). Responses with the asterisks are associated with low self-esteem.

The Piers-Harris Self-Concept Scale. The Piers-Harris Self-Concept Scale (1969) measures self-concept in school-aged children. The child is asked to make a "yes" or "no" response to items such as the following: "I am a happy person"; "I am smart"; "I am often sad"; "I give up easily." The Piers-Harris Children's Self-Concept Scale is available through Western Psychological Services, 12031 Wilshire Blvd., Los Angeles, CA 90025.

NURSING OBSERVATIONS RELATED TO SELF-CONCEPT
Examination Focus

In the course of conducting a physical examination, a number of observations may be pertinent to self-concept. Any deformities or physical alterations should be noted and consideration given to the possible effects that physical alterations may have on self-concept. The general appearance of the person often provides important cues to self-concept and self-esteem.

General Appearance

General appearance represents only one dimension of assessment and should not be the only element used to judge self-concept. Appearance varies widely among people and

---

Display 13–1
Rosenberg's Self-Esteem Scale

The RSE is a 10-item Guttman scale with a Coefficient of Reproducibility of 92% and a Coefficient of Scalability of 72%. Respondents are asked to strongly agree, agree, disagree, or strongly disagree with the following items (asterisks represent low self-esteem responses):

1. On the whole, I am satisfied with myself.	SA	A	D*	SD*
2. At times I think I am no good at all.	SA*	A*	D	SD
3. I feel that I have a number of good qualities.	SA	A	D*	SD*
4. I am able to do things as well as most other people.	SA	A	D*	SD*
5. I feel I do not have much to be proud of.	SA*	A*	D	SD
6. I certainly feel useless at times.	SA*	A*	D	SD
7. I feel that I'm a person of worth, at least on an equal plane with others.	SA	A	D*	SD*
8. I wish I could have more respect for myself.	SA*	A*	D	SD
9. All in all, I am inclined to feel that I am a failure.	SA*	A*	D	SD
10. I take a positive attitude toward myself.	SA	A	D*	SD*

(After Rosenberg, M. [1979]. *Conceiving the self* [p. 291]. New York: Basic Books)

---

may be influenced by culture, economic status, or general state of health.

Self-Care. General grooming and hygiene may reflect a person's view of self. People with low self-esteem may neglect their self-care needs. Self-care deficits related to other causes such as physical immobility should be ruled out before such deficits are interpreted as being related to self-concept problems.

Dress. The way a person dresses may provide another clue to self-concept. For example, a person who dresses in a becoming style may have a positive self-image. On the other hand, a 45-year-old mother who dresses like her teenage daughter may be expressing an inability to accept her age or her role as mother.

Facial Expressions. Facial expressions can also provide cues about self-concept, especially expressions that contradict verbal statements. For example, if the person says that everything is fine but is crying and avoiding eye contact, further investigation is indicated. Various facial expressions may have several different meanings and should be carefully considered to avoid premature conclusions.

Frowns, grimaces, and startled looks may indicate misunderstanding, pain in listening, or sudden reaction to what is being discussed. Staring may indicate caring, disbelief, pleasure, or displeasure. Lack of eye contact may represent poor self-esteem or may be a culture-specific response. For example, people from Asian, Native American, and Arab cultures may consider direct eye contact aggressive and avert their eyes when interviewed.

Blushing, excessive perspiration, and pallor may indicate affective responses such as fear, anxiety, embarrassment, shock, or anger. Smirking or an insincere smile may indicate skepticism, disdain, or ridicule. A smile may depict warmth and joy, or it may be a sign of anxiety, especially when the smile is not appropriate. Tears may represent grief, pain, or joy—in essence, an outlet for intense emotion.

Posture. Postures that indicate low self-esteem include hanging one's head or staring at the ground, sitting in a slumped position, and letting the shoulders sag. A very rigid posture may indicate physical discomfort, a lack of receptivity, or a defensive attitude.

Body Movements and Touch. Restlessness or continual movement may be associated with anxiety or fear. Failure to touch or acknowledge a particular body area or part may indicate a body image disturbance. Recoiling from another person's touch may indicate a rejection of physical contact or an inability to express a sense of closeness with others.

Affective Responses. Affective responses such as anxiety, irritability, anger, or withdrawal may be cues indicating self-concept disturbances or associated responses such as powerlessness.

Associated Body System Alterations

Physical indicators may help you diagnose human responses to self-concept problems, especially those related to fear and anxiety. Physiologically, anxiety and fear are associated with sympathetic nervous system activation such as occurs with the stress response. Some related, observable body system alterations include cardiovascular, respiratory, musculoskeletal, and gastrointestinal signs (see Chap. 16).

Nursing Observations   *Self-Concept*

General Principles   Judgments about self-concept may be based on interview data, physical findings, and additional observations. You should observe the person's behaviors and interpret verbal statements to evaluate self-esteem and locus of control. This requires attentive listening and observation of behaviors during ongoing interaction.

Patient Preparation and Positioning   Interview the person in a quiet, comfortable, and private setting. As you interview, face the person and make eye contact. Avoid standing over the person or using defensive body postures such as folding your arms across your chest.

Examination and Documentation Focus
- Verbalizations about self
- Verbalizations and behaviors related to body image
- Verbalizations about ability to deal with events/perform roles
- Willingness to try new things
- Ability to make decisions
- Interactions with others

Examination Guidelines   *Self-Concept*

Procedure

1. EVALUATE SELF-ESTEEM.

   In order to make judgments about self-esteem, listen for self-negating verbalizations, observe the person's ability to perform his or her usual roles, and note characteristics of relationships with others. You may also conduct an interview using the guidelines presented previously in this chapter (see "The Health History").

   a. Actively listen for remarks indicating low self-esteem.

      Comments such as these are referred to as "Self-Negating Verbalizations."

   b. Actively listen for remarks indicating difficulty with role performance.

Clinical Significance

Statements indicating low self-esteem (Miller, 1992):

I feel I am no longer a good person.

I can't do anything anymore. Now I am good for nothing, useless.

I feel guilty and embarrassed when I have to ask for help.

I've lost my independence.

I've lost faith in myself.

Sometimes I feel my body has turned against me.

I don't like myself this way.

Self-negating behaviors (Miller, 1992):

Expresses self-blame

Expresses guilt over disease

Makes self-derogatory comments

Expresses negative attitude toward self (physical self, personal self)

Feels useless

Lacks self respect

Behaviors indicating difficulty with role performance (Miller, 1992):

Expresses having few accomplishments

Expresses doubts about ability to fulfill roles

Feels inferior; compares self to others

Feels own actions will have little effect on an outcome (feels ineffective)

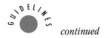
continued

Self-Concept

Procedure	Clinical Significance
	Feels insignificant
	Unable to take pride in accomplishing goals
	Unable to set goals
	Feels has failed in life's mission
	Lacks a sense of competence
	Statements indicating difficulty with role performance:
	I've never done anything important.
	I don't think I can do that.
	It seems like I'm the only one who hasn't done well.
	Nothing I can do will make a difference.
	I never seem to accomplish anything.
c. Note the manner in which the person interacts with others. Observe interactions with healthcare professionals, family, and groups.	Interaction indicators of low self-esteem include the following:
	Feels unworthy of nurses' time, care, attention
	Hesitant to ask for help
	Pessimistic
	Feels undeserving of praise
	Resentful of others who are well
	Lacks assertiveness
	Lacks self-confidence in one-to-one and/or group interactions
	Self-conscious
	Expresses a sense of worthlessness
2. EVALUATE BODY IMAGE.	
a. Determine whether or not the person has experienced a change in body structure or function. Survey for missing body parts or physical alterations. Listen for verbalizations of change in appearance or function.	
b. Note behaviors indicating an altered body image.	Behaviors indicating altered body image:
	Not looking at body part
	Hiding or overexposing body part
	Inability to estimate spatial relationship of body to environment
	Focus on past appearance or function
	Expresses fear of rejection
	Denial of change
	Expressions of helplessness or hopelessness
3. DETERMINE WHETHER OR NOT THE PERSON HAS AN INTERNAL OR EXTERNAL LOCUS OF CONTROL.	Internal locus of control is associated with a positive self-concept.
	A person with an internal locus of control believes that what happens to him or her is due to personal actions and choices. A person with an external locus of control believes that what happens to him or her is due to luck, fate, or other people.
Evaluate locus of control by observing behaviors and listening to statements the person makes about self and others.	Behavioral indicators of locus of control: See Table 13-1

Table 13–1. Locus of Control: Behavioral Indicators

	Internal	External
Role definition and satisfaction	More clearly defined, more satisfying	Less clearly defined, less satisfying
Relating to authority	Peer-like interactions	Passive-like interactions
Self-esteem	Higher or more stable self-esteem	Lower or less stable self-esteem
Responsibility for self-care	Active knowledge-seeking behavior	Do not actively seek information, accept what is given
Compliance with health care regimen	Manipulate regimen	Compliant
Confidence in abilities	Self-confident	Lack of self-confidence
Problem-solving abilities	More successful	Less successful
Goal-setting behavior	Realistic in goals set	Unrealistic
Level of motivation	Motivation	Tend toward helplessness at times
Involvement in decision-making	More involvement	Less involvement

(Miller, J.F. [1992]. Coping with chronic illness: Overcoming powerlessness [2nd ed.]. Philadelphia: F.A. Davis)

Documenting Self-Concept Assessment Findings

Document your observations related to self-concept with special attention to statements and behaviors indicating poor self-esteem or altered body image. It may be helpful to quote the person directly. A description of a person displaying a self-esteem disturbance might be as follows:

> Minimal eye contact or interaction with staff. States, "I feel useless." Does not participate in self-care. When asked to participate in bath stated, "I just can't do that now."

A self-esteem disturbance may also be indicated by expressions of guilt. This might be documented as follows:

> Children arrived today from other states. Visited only briefly with minimal conversation. After visit, stated, "If only I would have spent more time with my kids all these years I might not be so alone now."

A description of a person experiencing a change in body image might be as follows:

> Turns head away during all dressing changes. States it would be difficult for her to look at incision and physical changes at present. States, "Don't know if I'll ever be able to look at myself again."

NDx

Nursing Diagnoses Related to Self-Concept Assessment

Self-Esteem Disturbances

People with self-esteem disturbances do not necessarily respond in typical patterns (Carpenito, 1991). Some people may have self-esteem disturbances because of personal identity problems, whereas others may have intact personal identities but experience disruptions in social identity.

Once a diagnosis of Self-esteem disturbance has been established, you should further differentiate whether the problem is chronic or situational. People with chronic low self-esteem display a long-standing pattern of negative self-evaluation. In the case of situational low self-esteem, the person may have previously had positive self-esteem but because of a sudden loss or change, they are experiencing negative feelings about themselves.

Anxiety Versus Fear

Fear and anxiety both represent responses to altered self-concept. Making an accurate differential diagnosis between fear and anxiety is important, because nursing interventions are influenced by the diagnosis.

Fear and anxiety, as affective responses to danger, have some common features, including unpleasant feelings, and often accompanying bodily response, such as those associated with the stress response (see Chap. 16). Physical responses, however, vary among people. On a cognitive level, fear and anxiety can be recognized and verbally expressed. Emotional reactions to fear and anxiety are evident by affective behavior.

Generally, anxiety represents a more primitive response to threat. For example, an infant may respond to danger in an anxious rather than a fearful manner. Anxiety occurs when a threat is perceived but the person does not fully understand or cannot identify the source. Conversely, fear is a response to a clearly identifiable threat. Occasionally, a person may be able to identify the source of anxiety; therefore, anxiety does have a cognitive component. However, the cognitive component predominates in fear responses, whereas the emotional component predominates in anxiety.

Burke (1981) provides the following additional guidelines for differentiating fear and anxiety during assessment:

- *Use the "Of" test:* This assessment strategy involves asking whether or not the person has a fear *of* something.

If fear has an identifiable source, you should be able to analyze data and determine the source. For example, the person has a fear *of* pain, fear *of* losing control, fear *of* surgery. Anxiety, although related to some situation, is not always associated with a specific threat. Burke suggests asking, "Is the person anxious or does he have a fear of . . . ?"

- *Evaluate the immediacy and consistency of the threat:* Research indicates that fear is expressed immediately and consistently (Dunn, 1977). If behavioral responses to threats, such as crying, physical withdrawal, questioning, or aggression, are noted immediately on exposure to or mention of a particular threat, then the diagnosis is more likely to be fear. When the emotional or behavioral response is less predictable, consider anxiety.

In sum, fear is a response to an identifiable threat, whereas the specific threat is less obvious with anxiety. Carpenito (1991) suggests that fear and anxiety usually coexist, in which case you may consider writing *"Fear/Anxiety related to . . . "* as the diagnostic statement. In this case you should consider whether such a diagnosis is specific enough to direct nursing care.

Clinical Problems Related to Self-Concept Assessment

Assessment of self-concept provides indicators for nursing diagnoses but not for clinical problems. Alterations in self-concept, such as low self-esteem or body image disturbance, represent human responses and therefore would be considered nursing diagnoses rather than clinical problems. During your assessment, however, you should consider any clinical problems that may have an effect on self-concept. For example, trauma and disfigurement may threaten body image. Living with a chronic illness may threaten self-esteem.

ASSESSMENT PROFILE

* *

Elsie Johnson, a 71-year-old widow, was admitted to the orthopedic nursing service for treatment of a fractured femur believed to be secondary to bone metastasis. The patient's status was summarized as follows:

Physiologically stable with the left leg in Buck's traction (5 lbs). No reported pain. Vital signs: BP—136/82; HR—88; RR—18; T—36.6°C. Past medical–surgical history: left radical mastectomy 3 years ago followed by a right radical mastectomy 1 year ago for breast cancer; currently receiving cancer radiation therapy as an outpatient.

The nurse caring for Mrs. Johnson performed a routine head-to-toe physical examination, during which Mrs. Johnson asked her what the physician had meant when he asked her what she wanted done if her heart stopped. The nurse told Mrs. Johnson that the physician was trying to determine what her wishes were if her condition became life-threatening. In other words, did she want to be kept alive using life-support machines?

The nurse continued to talk with Mrs. Johnson, encouraging her to express her concerns. However, Mrs. Johnson said she felt confused and was not sure just how to respond. She explained that she had no family and was just beginning to become active and social again since her surgery. She could not understand why she was having physical problems again and decided not to think about the physician's questions any further.

During this interaction, the patient spoke calmly, maintaining eye contact with the nurse. She did not exhibit nonverbal signs of distress such as voice pitch changes, trembling, crying, or restlessness.

Based on this interaction, the nurse began to consider the possible nursing diagnoses of Anxiety, Powerlessness, *and Fear. Additional assessment of the patient's self-concept was indicated.*

Profile Analysis: Identifying the Assessment Focus

The nurse recognized several important cues during the initial interaction with Mrs. Johnson. The patient was concerned about her present health status, which had been improving but now appeared in jeopardy. She indicated confusion about her present status and avoided further discussion. Interestingly, she appeared calm, rather than acting angry, crying, or otherwise showing distress. The nurse was not sure how to interpret such cues, but decided further evaluation was indicated. Presently, the nurse believed that the patient was threatened by recent events, including hospitalization. The nurse described her thinking as follows:

I wanted to assess her situation further but wasn't sure how to proceed. I knew from report she had experienced multiple stressors associated with her illness and surgeries. Also, I knew her family support was limited but I couldn't say she had no other support systems until I obtained more data. Initially, I thought of problems in the area of stress and coping because the stressors seemed so obvious to me. But before I could pursue stress and coping, I felt I needed more information about her perceptions of recent events. Also, I was struck by her initial statements about decision-making regarding life support. It seemed like she might be upset about making such a decision or having it made for her. I needed to explore my impressions further with her and get at her perception of the situation. I decided to begin further assessment by focusing on self-concept, because it struck me her self-concept was threatened, and then evaluate stress and coping along with other areas.

Possible Nursing Diagnoses

The nurse focused additional data collection to support or rule out nursing diagnoses associated with altered self-concept, including Anxiety, Fear, Hopelessness, and Powerlessness.

Additional Data Gathering

The nurse initiated a focused interview aimed at further exploring Mrs. Johnson's self-concept and validating the initial perceptions. Mrs. Johnson repeatedly stated that she was not afraid of health changes or death, and that she had "come to terms with the inevitable" long ago. As she spoke, the nurse noted that her body language and behaviors remained congruent with what was being said. For example, her voice stayed calm, her body remained relaxed, and she did not cry. Based on these observations, the nurse ruled out fear as a possible nursing diagnosis.

The nurse initiated further discussion by asking, "Tell how you felt when the doctor asked what should be done

if your heart stopped?" Mrs. Johnson responded that she thought the question just a formality and that regardless of her wishes, others would decide what to do with her life. She explained that after lengthy treatment for cancer, she seldom felt authorized to make decisions about her health. By the second week of cancer therapy, she had assumed the role of passive, good, compliant patient. She described herself as never questioning medical judgments or decisions. However, she no longer wanted to assume this role now that she was feeling better and was able to resume some of her previous activities. But she stated, "What can I do? I want to live but who am I to say whether or not the doctors should be heroic?"

Final Nursing Diagnosis

Based on the nurse's observations, which were validated with the patient, a nursing diagnosis of Powerlessness was formulated. Specifically, the nurse observed that Mrs. Johnson felt she had no control over health care decisions. She was reluctant to make decisions she perceived to be out of her control. As a result, she was experiencing anxiety. Nursing interventions that would help her regain feelings of control and lessen threats to self-concept were planned.

Chapter 13 SUMMARY

Assessment of self-concept focuses on the following areas:
- The person's thoughts and feelings about self
- Factors influencing the development of self-concept
- Threats to self-concept
- A person's responses to threats to self-concept or low self-esteem

When assessing self-concept, you should consider the following factors:
- The presenting self may differ significantly from the extant self
- The person's concept of the extant self can be assessed only to the extent that the person is willing to share true self-perceptions
- Stereotyping or labeling the person will interfere with self-concept assessment
- Response patterns for self-esteem disturbances will vary

Cues should be analyzed in relation to meanings relevant to the person.
You should collect data pertaining to the self-concept pattern by the following methods:
- The interview, which focuses on social identity, personal identity, physical self, self-esteem, and threats to self-concept
- Nursing observations, including the person's self-disclosing statements, role performance, interpersonal relationships, general appearance, and affective responses

- Assessment tools (Twenty Statements Test, Rosenberg's Self-Esteem Scale, the Piers-Harris Self-Concept Scale, Rotter's I-E Scale)

Assessment of self-concept based on these principles and methods will help you identify defining characteristics and risk factors for the following nursing diagnoses:
> Anxiety
> Body image disturbance
> Fear
> Hopelessness
> Chronic low self-esteem
> Situational low self-esteem
> Personal identity disturbance
> Powerlessness
> Self-esteem disturbance

The following related nursing diagnoses may be detected during assessment, especially problems resulting from self-esteem disturbance:
> Ineffective individual coping
> Diversional activity deficit
> Altered family processes
> Altered health maintenance
> Self-care deficit
> Sexual dysfunction
> Sleep pattern disturbance
> Impaired social interaction
> Spiritual distress (distress of the human spirit)

RESEARCH *Hi*GHLIGHT

What influences women's self-esteem? How can nurses evaluate self-esteem of multirole women?

Self-esteem disturbance, Chronic low self-esteem, and Situational low self-esteem are diagnoses that address actual or potential problems related to negative beliefs about self. Self-esteem influences a person's total well-being and his or her ability to seek health care and promote well-being.

Concerned that most research about self-esteem has been biased toward the male perspective and that self-esteem is a factor in physical and mental health, Meisenhelder identified selected variables that influence women's feelings of self-worth and self-esteem. One hundred ninety-two married women with children were randomly selected and asked to participate in the study. A total of 163 women responded to the Rosenberg Self-Esteem Scale and were tested using two additional tools. The strongest predictor of self-esteem in a woman was her belief about her husband's perception of her. Women who worked full-time had higher self-esteem scores than women who worked part-time, but had scores similar to the scores of women who identified themselves as homemakers.

Homemakers generally described religious beliefs as promoting their self-esteem.[1]

What significance does the study have for health assessment?

If the nurse suspects a possible disturbance in self-esteem, then exploring the quality and quantity of the person's significant relationships may provide insight into etiological factors that may be amenable to nursing interventions. This study suggests that the nurse should focus on factors such as employment status and a woman's perceptions of her husband's perceptions of her when evaluating self-esteem.

Can the study's findings be applied to practice?

The results of this study suggest that significant others influence a woman's self-esteem. Additional research is necessary to determine if this is true of women unlike those in the study group; for example, unmarried women, women without children, or women from different socioeconomic or ethnic groups than the study group.

REFERENCE

1. Meisenhelder, J. (1986). Self-esteem in women: The influence of employment and perception of husbands' appraisals. *Image*, *18*(1), 8–14.

✳ CRITICAL THINKING

The assessment of self-concept is considered a crucial element of a holistic nursing assessment. It is through this type of assessment that the nurse begins to truly know the person who is the recipient of nursing care.

Learning Exercises

1. Propose a clinical situation in which understanding of a person's self-concept is meaningful.

2. Think of a person you know who has a healthy self-concept. Select and describe the indicators of a healthy self-concept in this person.

3. Think of a person you know who you believe has a negative self-concept. Select and describe the indicators of a negative self-concept in this person.

4. A nursing colleague tells you that assessment of self-concept is a luxury rather than a necessity in acute care clinical settings where patients require careful and constant monitoring of physiologic variables. Explain how you would respond.

5. Explain how knowing a person's locus of control might influence the discharge planning process.

6. Specify critical differences between self-concept and self-esteem.

BIBLIOGRAPHY

Bonham, P.A., & Cheney, P.A. (1983). Concept of self: A framework for nursing assessment. In P.L. Chinn (Ed.). *Advances in nursing theory development* (pp. 173–190). Rockville, MD: Aspen.

Bruss, C. (1988). Nursing diagnosis of hopelessness. *Journal of Psychosocial Nursing and Mental Health Services, 26* (3), 28–31, 38–39.

Burke, S.O. (1982). A developmental perspective on the nursing diagnoses of fear and anxiety. *Nursing Papers, 14* (2), 59–64.

Carpenito, L.J. (1993). *Handbook of nursing diagnosis* (5th ed.). Philadelphia: J.B. Lippincott.

Cooley, C.H. (1902). *Human nature and the social order.* New York: Scribner's.

Coombs, A. (1971). Self-concept: Product and producer of experience. In D. Avila, A. Coombs, & W. Purkey (Eds.). *Helping relationships.* Boston: Allyn and Bacon.

Driever, M.J. (1976). Theory of self concept. In C. Roy (Ed.). *Introduction to nursing: An adaptation model* (pp. 169–191). Englewood Cliffs, NJ: Prentice Hall.

Dunn, H.L. (1961). *High-level wellness.* Arlington, VA: R.W. Beatty Co.

Dunn, J. (1977). *Distress and comfort.* Cambridge: Harvard University Press.

Erikson, E.H. (1963). *Childhood and society* (2nd ed.). New York: W.W. Norton.

Gale, D. (1966). *Developmental behavior: A humanistic approach.* London: Collier-Macmillan.

Gordon, M. (1987). *Nursing diagnosis: Process and application* (2nd ed.). New York: McGraw-Hill.

Hirst, S.P., & Metcalf, B.J. (1984). Promoting self-esteem. *Gerontological Nursing, 10* (2), 72–77.

Jones, P., & Jakob, D.F. (1981). Nursing diagnosis: Differentiating fear and anxiety. *Nursing Papers, 13* (4), 20–29.

Jourard, S. (1968). Healthy personality and self-disclosure. In C. Gordon & K.J. Gergen (Eds.). *The self in social interaction. Vol 1: Classic and contemporary perspectives.* New York: John Wiley & Sons.

Kim, M.J., & Moritz, D.A. (Eds.). *Classification of nursing diagnoses: Proceedings of the third and fourth national conferences.* New York: McGraw-Hill.

Kuhn, M.H., & McPartland, T. (1954). An empirical investigation of self-attitudes. *American Sociology Review, 19,* 68–76.

LeMone, P. (1991). Analysis of a human phenomenon: Self-concept. *Nursing Diagnosis, 2* (3), 126–130.

Long, K. (1988). Use of the Piers-Harris self-concept scale with Indian children: Cultural considerations. *Nursing Research, 37* (1), 42–46.

McGuire, W.J., & Padawer-Singer, A. (1982). Trait salience in the spontaneous self-concept. In M. Rosenberg, & H.B. Kaplan (Eds.). *Social psychology of the self-concept.* Arlington Heights, IL: Harlan Davidson.

Mead, G.H. (1934). *Mind, self, and society.* Chicago: University of Chicago Press.

Miller, J.F. (1992). *Coping with chronic illness: Overcoming powerlessness* (2nd ed.). Philadelphia: F.A. Davis.

Piers, E.V., & Harris, D.B. (1969). *Piers-Harris Children's Self-Concept Scale (the way I feel about myself).* Nashville, TN: Counselor Recording and Tests.

Rosenberg, M. (1979). *Concerning the self.* New York: Basic Books.

Rosenberg, M., & Kaplan, H.B. (Eds.). (1982). *Social psychology of the self-concept.* Arlington Heights, IL: Harlan Davidson.

Rotter, J.B. (1966). Generalized expectancies for internal versus external control of reinforcement. *Psychological Monographs, 80* (1), 1–25.

Schroeder, P.S., & Miller, J.F. (1983). Qualitative study of locus of control in patients with peripheral vascular disease. In J.F. Miller. *Coping with chronic illness: Overcoming powerlessness* (pp. 149–161). Philadelphia: F.A. Davis.

Shrauger, J.S., & Schoeneman, T.J. (1979). Symbolic interactionist view of self-concept: Through the looking glass darkly. *Psychological Bulletin, 86* (3), 549–573.

Stanwyck, D.J. (1983). Self-esteem throughout the life span. *Family and Community Health, 6* (2), 11–28.

Wallston, B.S. et al. (1976). Development and validation of the health locus of control (HLC) scale. *Journal of Consulting and Clinical Psychology, 44,* 580–585.

Wallston, K.A., Wallston, B., & DeVellis, R. (1978). Development of the multidimensional health locus of control (MHLC) scales. *Health Education Monographs, 6,* 160–170.

Yocom, C.J. (1984). The differentiation of fear and anxiety. In M.J. Kim, G.K. McFarland, & A.M. McLane (Eds.). *Classification of nursing diagnoses: Proceedings of the fifth national conference.* St. Louis: C.V. Mosby.

Chapter

14 Assessing Roles and Relationships

Examination Guidelines

Roles and Relationships

Assessment Terms

Roles	Role Strain
Assigned Role	Family Structure
Achieved Role	Ecomap
Role Ambiguity	Communication Patterns
Role Overload	Punishment
Role Incompetence	Neglect
Role Bargaining	Abuse
Role Stress	

INTRODUCTORY OVERVIEW

In 1936, Ralph Linton identified roles as collective patterns of behavior socially prescribed within the social structure (Biddle and Thomas, 1966). More recently, Murray and Zentner (1993) have defined roles as patterns of behavior expected by others that are learned and performed in social settings. The individual performing the role uses perceived expectations and evaluations of others, and self-evaluation to modify behavior. Since the introduction of the role concept, researchers in the behavioral sciences have been concerned with roles and related conflict, strain, behavior, performance, competence, and stress. In nursing, roles and relationships are assessed to determine how people manage their particular roles with respect to expectations and social relationships.

Assessment Focus

Assessing role–relationship behavior involves collecting data on the quality and quantity of the roles and relationships of the client. Data collection includes considering the client's role conception, communication patterns, family and social interaction processes, and parenting abilities. Information is primarily collected through interview and observation.

The goals in assessing roles and relationship status include the following:

Jill Fuller and Jennifer Schaller-Ayers:
HEALTH ASSESSMENT: A NURSING APPROACH, Second Edition.
© 1990, 1994 by J. B. Lippincott Company.

- Identify the major roles and relationships with family, friends, and coworkers.
- Identify perceptions of roles.
- Determine the risk for role strain or response to role strain.
- Evaluate communication patterns between client and significant others.
- Identify factors restricting effective communication.
- Identify actual or potential dysfunction within the family.

The methods for collecting survey information are presented in the Assessment Focus display. The information collected can be analyzed to identify strengths or needs in-role–relationship behaviors or the need for an in-depth interview to identify possible problems that may arise in these areas. Conclusions must be based on an understanding that role behaviors and expectations vary from individual to individual, family to family, and culture to culture.

Nursing Diagnoses

The nursing diagnoses that address roles and relationship functions include the following:

Altered family processes
Altered parenting
Anticipatory grieving
Disturbances in role performance
Dysfunctional grieving
Impaired social interaction
Impaired verbal communication
Parental role conflict
Potential for altered parenting
Potential for violence
Social isolation

(Anticipatory and dysfunctional grieving are discussed in the framework of coping and stress; see Chap. 15.)

KNOWLEDGE BASE FOR ASSESSMENT

The assessment of roles and relationships requires an understanding of role theory, social interactions, communication, and family processes.

Role Theory

Role theory represents a collection of concepts and a variety of hypothetical formulations that predict how actors will perform in a given role, or under what circumstances certain types of behaviors can be expected. (Hardy and Conway, 1988, p. 65)

The term *role* has been borrowed from the theater and has been used to describe behaviors that are expected when an individual assumes a particular role. Throughout our lives we assume many roles, both ascribed (assigned) and achieved (acquired). Ascribed roles, such as those associated with gender, are usually determined at birth and are often influenced by society. Achieved roles, such as

professional or occupational status, are obtained through individual effort or competition. Roles such as husband, wife, mother, and father, are classified as ascribed, despite the fact that some effort may be necessary to obtain the status.

Each role has a corresponding set of behaviors or role expectations that are socially determined. People often fill several roles, ascribed as well as achieved; some of these roles may conflict with one another. Roles are learned in a continuous and cumulative process. Role behaviors of previous developmental stages prepare individuals for future role behaviors. Therefore, role behaviors from one age level to the next remain fairly consistent, and the individual builds a repertoire of behavioral responses to a variety of situational demands (Rosow, 1965). Role learning occurs as the result of assuming new roles or coping with role stress or role strain. In addition, role expectations can change as situations and society change, forcing people to manage several roles while attempting to maintain good health.

Problems experienced in managing role expectation can result in the following situations:

Role conflicts can occur when one or more role expectations compete against one another. For example, a working mother with a sick child may be conflicted about whether she should stay home or go to work. Obviously, she cannot be at both places and may have guilt feelings whatever her decision.

Role ambiguity may result when role expectations are not clearly identified within society or there is disagreement regarding role expectations. For example, adolescents are often unsure exactly what behavior is expected of them. Role ambiguity is characteristic of professional roles in which expectations are changing and disagreement exists regarding the direction of the change.

Role overload may occur when a number of roles and expectations are assumed or ascribed and there is insufficient time or energy to fulfill the obligations of all roles. For example, a single parent who works full time may perform all roles adequately until he or she returns to school and assumes the student role. The parent may be unable to find enough time or energy to meet all role expectations adequately.

Role incompetence may occur when the necessary skill or knowledge to fulfill role expectations is lacking. For example, a 14-year-old girl who becomes a mother may not have sufficient maturity or knowledge to care for a newborn.

Role bargaining refers to negotiation with others about acceptable role expectations. A family may abandon society's expectation about traditional responsibilities such as cooking, automobile maintenance, and child care to best meet the individual's and family's needs. For example, the father may become the primary caretaker of children and the mother may be the sole income-earner.

Role stress is a sociocultural situation in which role expectations and responsibilities are vague, conflicting, or unrealistic. Role stress is an attribute of the social system and not the individual (Hardy and Conway, 1989). *Role strain* is the individual's response to role stress and other role problems such as overload and conflict; the response can be distress such as anxiety and frustration. Role strain ultimately affects coping abilities (see Chap. 15).

Assessment Focus **Roles and Relationships**

Assessment Goal	Data Collection Methods
1. Describe the person's roles and relationships with family, friends, and work associates.	*Interview* • Role identification: How does the person perceive his or her roles? • Family composition: What is the nature of family roles and relationships? • Relationships outside the family: Who else is significant to the client? *Observe* • Drawings depicting the family unit (family diagram) and individual relationships (eco-map) • The person's interaction patterns with significant others
2. Identify the person's perceptions of role performance.	*Interview* • Role satisfaction/dissatisfaction: Is there evidence of role strain?
3. Evaluate communication modes between client and significant others.	*Interview and Observe* • Communication patterns
4. Identify factors restricting effective communication.	*Observe* • Capacities for verbal communication (language spoken, vocabulary, expressive ability, comprehension, hearing) • Capacities for nonverbal communication (writing, gestures)
5. Identify actual or potential dysfunction within the family.	*Interview and Observe the Family, Focusing on* • Individual perceptions of family relationships • Expressions of family problems or concerns • Family decision-making processes • Discipline patterns

The behaviors and attitudes that are associated with various roles are learned at home, in school, at work, and during interaction with others. When a person assumes a role for a length of time, role responsibilities become more refined and may increase. For example, role expectations of a 5-year-old child in school are different than role expectations of a 10-year-old. Similarly, a newly graduated nurse will not be expected to perform like a nurse who has been practicing for 6 years.

Social Interaction

Social interaction occurs when two or more people communicate. The characteristics of an interaction are influenced by the relationship between the parties. Relationships are influenced by role status and role hierarchy and can be classified as horizontal (equal), such as husband–wife, friend–friend, or vertical (unequal), such as parent–child, employer–employee, and physician–patient. Relationships are also influenced by culture; for example, some societies encourage a vertical relationship between husband and wife, or expect a parent–child relationship to progress from vertical to horizontal as the child matures.

The degree and depth of a social interaction are dependent upon the purpose of the interaction, and the degree of trust and familiarity between participants. Relationships between participants can be classified further according to type, such as therapeutic (see Chap. 1), familial, business, or social. Social relationships are formed primarily for plea-sure and companionship. No specific knowledge or skill is required, and neither person is responsible for the other. The strength of the relationship is dependent upon the amount of energy each party is willing to invest. In any given relationship, the people involved may value the association differently. The number of relationships and interactions people participate in varies greatly from person to person.

Communication

Communication, essential to all social interaction, involves sharing information or messages between a sender and receiver through a means of transmission, such as speech, art, writing, or body movements. During a communication exchange, a message is sent, received, and interpreted. Often more than one form of the message is exchanged; for example, with face-to-face exchanges, simultaneous verbal and nonverbal messages are sent and received. Communication can be either circular or linear (Fig. 14-1; Lancaster and Lancaster, 1982).

Nonverbal communication is equally important as verbal communication and includes touch, eye contact, facial expressions, silence, body movement, and posture. Nonverbal communication is more likely to be automatic and less repressed. Nonverbal communication can provide a more reliable insight into the individual's actual message. Verbal and nonverbal messages are either congruent or incongruent. Many characteristics of nonverbal communication are

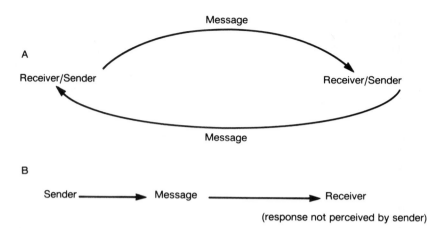

Figure 14–1. Communication patterns. In circular communication (A), receivers and senders transmit messages and return messages in response to messages received. In linear communication (B), one person sends a message to another, who receives it but does not respond.

culturally influenced. In the United States, for example, eye contact is important with face-to-face exchanges; however, some Native American cultures avoid eye contact. In certain Eastern cultures, a smile conceals emotions and unpleasant news and does not necessarily represent agreement with the message.

Assessing communication involves noting the message as well as related behaviors and influencing factors. The communication process is not static but changes in relation to family, social systems, and role expectations. Furthermore, as the number of persons involved in the interaction increases or decreases, the process changes. The communication process is influenced by factors such as environment; the type of relationship that exists between the sender and receiver; status of sender and receiver (emotional, physical, and cognitive); level of development of sender and receiver; culture; and past experiences. Assessing communication also includes assessing for the use of communication aids such as corrective lenses, hearing aids, electronic larynx, and word boards.

Family Process

Historically and culturally, the concept of family has had different meanings. In the United States, for example, a nuclear family usually includes a husband, wife, and children, whereas the extended family includes parents and siblings of the husband and wife. However, because of recent changes in roles, laws, economic opportunities, and lifestyles, alternate family configurations have come into existence. Multigenerational families in one home, which were common in the 19th century, have recently seen a resurgence. Today, a family can be defined as a living social system, usually sharing living quarters, with significant emotional bonds such as affection, interdependence, responsibility, or commitment (Levitt, 1982). Given this definition, two or more nonrelated, nonmarried adults with or without children who reside together may constitute a family. Essentially, members of a family can be anyone whom individuals mutually consider to be family members.

All families are organized to meet specific purposes or common goals. Some purposes or family functions are determined by society, such as education and socialization of children and nurturing and support of family members as

well as provision of clothing, shelter, and nourishment. Within a family system, family functions are not identical but are influenced by mutual expectation of members, repetitive and reciprocal patterns of behavior, roles, communication, power structure, boundaries, and individual capabilities. Within the family, roles determine task, influence communication and relationships, and define power (Phipps, 1980). Family roles may be either ascribed or achieved. Role expectations may be rigid or flexible, clear or vague, and complementary or conflicting. Some family roles may be dysfunctional, as reflected in such terms as scapegoat, martyr, and baby.

Family roles reflect values and determine behaviors, which in turn influence interactions and relationships. Unstable families tend to have covert, excessive, or ambivalent rules. Moreover, rules usually influence the roles family members are expected to perform. If a member fails to perform as expected, family stability is threatened. Punishment is an attempt to encourage conformity and ensure stability. The family unit usually depends on communication for function as well as stability. Family functioning can also be threatened by illnesses, abuse, divorce, or members leaving the family.

Parenting, a basic function of the *traditional* family involves the responsibility of physically and emotionally caring for dependent children. Parenting and family functioning is influenced by the ages of the dependent children. Society may remove children from their parents' care if such roles are unmet. On the other hand, society allows parents to relinquish their roles, rights, and responsibilities to others through adoption and guardianship.

Socialization of children refers to teaching children behaviors, values, and roles they must learn to survive and be effective within their society. In addition to families, day care centers, schools, and even the mass media play an important role in the socialization of children.

THE HEALTH HISTORY

During the interview, information is obtained about roles and relationships by observing the client's behavior and reactions and by interpreting statements and responses. Effective communication is crucial in assessing role functions and is dependent on a calm, nonjudgmental approach.

Being aware of the person's cultural background and family structure is also important to an understanding of role expectations and family functioning.

Although the individual is usually the focus of the actual delivery of health care, each person interacts with other family members and has role responsibilities within a particular family unit. The family is most effective when every member is functioning at an optimal level. Consequently, when roles and relationships are assessed, the entire family should be considered.

The following areas of role–relationship function should be evaluated during the interview:

Individual Roles

- Role perception
- Role satisfaction/dissatisfaction
- Role strain

Family Roles and Relationships

- Family composition and structure
- Family communication patterns
- Family problems or concerns
- Family decision-making process
- Discipline patterns

Social Relationships

- Individual social relationships
- Family social relationships
- Relationships with helping professionals

If the client does not report any problems with roles, family, or relationships, a screening assessment is indicated (see Interview Guide). However, a more comprehensive interview is indicated whenever a person reports role–relationship problems or is at high risk for problems, as re-flected in a family history of abuse, adolescent parenting, insufficient resources, or changes in family structure or roles.

Assessing roles and relationships during the interview involves listening to how the person describes interactions with family members as well as with health professionals. Body language and the family's verbal communication patterns are equally important. As the interview progresses, you can begin to identify the role–relationship pattern. It is important to remember that any interpretation of roles and relationships is subject to change as the person's situation changes.

Roles

Role Perception. To assess roles, ask the client to identify and discuss all pertinent roles and responsibilities. For example, a young woman may identify roles of wife, mother, housekeeper, child caregiver, meal manager, income earner, daughter, sister, and student. Inquire if the roles are realistic, excessive, or limited, and if there is sufficient time for rest and leisure. Does the client think the number of roles and responsibilities are appropriate? The number of roles a person can successfully fulfill is influenced by situations such as role complexity, disability, and illness. However, definitions of legitimate illnesses and role performances vary among societies. Furthermore, illness is associated with an expected sick role behavior that also varies culturally.

In some societies, a sick person is expected to express a desire to get well, comply with health regimens, and accept help. During periods of prolonged illnesses, other people may assume a client's role responsibilities. Some people who are sick refuse to assume the sick role, whereas others abuse the sick role, demonstrating little desire to get well.

Interview Guide **Roles–Relationship Pattern**

Roles

Describe your role with family/friends/coworkers? (wife/husband, son/daughter, sexual partner, scapegoat, confidant, boss, mentor, *etc.*): _____

Describe any pressures you associate with your roles: _____
_____

How has your health status altered your relationships with others? _____
_____

How are you preparing for your new role (parent, spouse, employee, resident, *etc.*)? _____
_____

Family/Relationships

Describe your family structure: _____

Do you live alone? _____ If no, with whom? _____

Who do you turn to for help? _____

How are decisions made concerning family/significant others? _____
_____

Any problems with:_____ communication _____ parenting _____ relatives _____ abuse _____ finances _____ martial
concerns _____ discipline

Both of these situations can cause difficulties and frustrations for health professionals and family members. Illness, whether acute or chronic, and trauma potentially can alter role perception, role capabilities, and family functioning.

Role Dissatisfaction. Role dissatisfaction can lead to *role strain,* a distressing state that can ultimately affect health. Role strain challenges a person's coping capabilities and can cause frustration, insecurity, fatigue, depression, or anxiety. If a role change is imminent or advisable, the person may need to discuss the change and impact it will have on well-being. Inquire as to the degree of frustration felt in each role and the degree to which this frustration is bothersome.

Role Strain. Many people experience role strain because of inadequate role preparation, rapid social change, and accelerated technology (Hardy and Conway, 1989). Even when a person is satisfied with his or her status associated with the role, strain can occur. How strain is resolved depends on available resources.

If role strain is identified, explore the potential causes and possible solutions. Possible resources include family support, role negotiation, education, and giving up nonessential roles. Assuming new roles because of birth or adoption of a child, divorce, or death is stressful. New roles involving jobs and promotions also create strain and tension. In such situations, a person needs to evaluate skills, knowledge, probable role expectations, and confidence in performing skills. Having a clear and realistic understanding of the new role will help in handling possible role strain. Locating available resources will help support a person who is assuming a new role.

Family Roles and Responsibilities

Family Composition and Structure. An integral part of family composition is organization or structure, which is usually influenced by culture. Many cultures have a patriarchal family structure, whereas others may be matriarchal or shared. To plan appropriate interventions, you should define the family structure and determine cultural expectations. The family structure has a strong influence upon decision making and primary authority within the family.

Western cultures include many different family types. Single parent, blended (step-family), same gender, and commuter (one parent lives out of the house part time) families are becoming more frequent. To clearly identify a client's family structure, consider diagramming the family unit (Fig. 14-2). The family structure diagram can be accomplished at the same time as the genogram (see Chap. 7). A written narrative may also be helpful if the structure is complex.

Identifying achieved roles within the family is also helpful when assessing composition and structure. For example, how many members are labeled as income-earners or identified as being the troublemakers? Such information may be added to the family diagram. Determining the composition of the family and the ages of its members also establishes a basis for assessing individual (see Chap. 17) and family developmental status. Duvall (1977) has identified eight stages of family development: marital, childbearing,

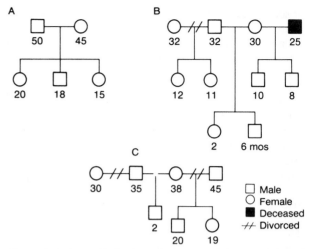

Figure 14–2. Possible family configurations include *(A)* a traditional nuclear family including a married couple and their three children; *(B)* a marriage between two people whose previous marriages ended by divorce or death, and who have children both from this marriage and the previous marriages; and *(C)* a family that includes an unmarried heterosexual couple, their child, and the woman's two children from a previous marriage. The numbers indicate peoples' ages.

preschool, school age, teenage, launching, middle age, and aging. Murray and Zenter (1993) have defined four developmental stages as establishment, expectant, parenthood, and parental disengagement. Awareness of stages of development alerts the nurse to developmental role transitions that can lead to role strain. However, not all families experience these developmental stages, which are based upon procreation and children's ages (*e.g.,* childless families).

Family Communication Patterns. Communication, the basis of all relationships, is accomplished by sending or receiving messages using spoken words, writing, or body language. If the client has a limited ability to speak, write, read, or move body parts, communication may be impaired. A person's ability to communicate verbally may be impaired by hearing loss, neurologic problems such as cerebral palsy or cerebrovascular accident, tracheostomy, stuttering, or inability to speak a second language. When communication is complicated by such impairments, families usually establish alternative methods of communicating. For example, children often translate for parents in health care settings. When one or more members cannot speak, the family may compensate by using sign language, word boards, or computers. You should identify any alternate means of communication used by family members.

One also needs to identify the nature and strength of relationships within the family. Do family members feel close to one another or distant? Inquire into the nature of communication. Are hostility and disapproval expressed more frequently than love and enjoyment? Can the client identify communication or relationship problems? Are these problems long-standing or a recent phenomenon as the result of illness or maturation transitions? Long-standing problems that were considered minor can worsen during times of transition.

Family Problems or Concerns. Socially, families have the responsibility to provide for the physical, emotional, and social well-being of every member. Because financial resources are necessary to satisfy many of these needs, housing and income should be evaluated in relationship to client needs. Outside resources such as food stamps and federally funded low-income housing are sometimes not used because family members are unaware of availability, do not know how to apply for such assistance, or are too proud to ask for help.

Families have numerous concerns that can become stressors and interfere with family health. Concerns may include relationships with in-laws, education of children, inadequate income to meet needs, unemployment or underemployment, disagreement on child rearing, substance abuse, environmental hazards, and religious/spiritual disagreements.

The health of all family members has a direct effect on the family and family members. The altered health status (whether it be short term or long term) of one family member affects all family members and alters the family process. If children of working parents become ill, for instance, then one parent may need to stay home, which could affect income and employment. The death of a family member or moderate to severe disability may cause role responsibilities to change, and other family members may need to assume new roles rapidly.

Yura and Walsh (1978) have developed a topology of family problems that classifies problems as (1) no apparent problems; (2) potential problems; (3) problems adequately handled by family; (4) problems that require intervention; (5) problems that require health professional intervention; (6) problems that require further data collection; and (7) temporary problems that involve short-term dependency that might occur during acute illness or death. In general, most family problems are brief in duration and can be adequately handled within the family.

Family Decision-Making Process. How families make decisions vary. In one family, a parent may have most of the authority; in another, family members may act as a unit in making most decisions. In some families, extended family members, such as uncles and brothers-in-law and family elders participate in making decisions that may range from naming a child to purchasing a house. Whether families react passively to situations or make decisions in order to control their lives is an important element to identify when assessing roles and relationships. It is also important to determine if family members are satisfied with their particular methods of making both minor and major decisions.

Discipline Patterns. For a family to function optimally, its members need to follow predetermined guidelines and rules. Generally, discipline involves parents teaching their children acceptable behavior, values, and attitudes, thereby giving children appropriate limitations. Punishment, a method of controlling undesirable behavior, relies on making a child feel guilty about a misdeed. Punishment may be verbal, physical, or restrictive. Extreme punishment is considered abuse. Abuse is a pattern of abnormal interactions that often result in physical, emotional, and/or sexual attacks.

Because methods of punishment reveal much about family relationships and beliefs about acceptable methods of discipline, assess the discipline and punishment patterns of families with dependent members. Consider if family rules are clear to everyone. Evaluate if behavior limits, expectations, and punishment patterns are consistent and appropriate for the child's age and developmental level. What type of punishment does the family use—is it physical such as spanking, behavior modification such as time-out, or emotional such as belittling? Also, is there a history of unexplained or vague injury accidents?

Assess adult family members for signs of abuse and abusive behavior. Next to children, women and elders are most at risk for abuse in the home. However, men can also be victims of abuse, as can people with developmental disabilities. Occasionally, adolescents abuse adults in their family.

Social Relationships

Individual Social Relationships. Individuals usually have numerous and varied relationships and interactions. When uncertainty exists about a client's social interactions, consider using a diagram, an *ecomap,* to present a graphic picture of the relationships and interactions of the client (Fig. 14-3). The ecomap allows the nurse and the client to assess the number of relationships and the quality of those relationships from the client's perspective.

A more comprehensive assessment of individual social relationships requires additional information, such as availability of a confidant, ability to maintain long-term relationships, ease of communication with others, and perception of others liking the client.

Family Social Relationships. The same criteria to evaluate individual relationships can be used to assess family social relationships. The focus of this assessment is not the relationship among family members but the relationship of

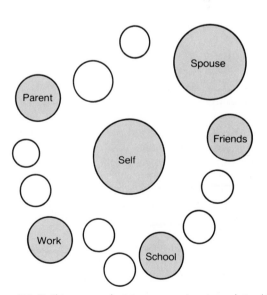

Figure 14-3. This ecomap depicting a person's various relationships is completed by labeling additional circles and drawing lines to show the nature of relationships. *Straight lines* indicate strong, positive relationships; *dotted lines* indicate weaker relationships; *slashed lines* represent strained relationships. The wider the line, the stronger the relationship.

the entire family with other individuals, other families, and agencies. As family size increases, the number of potential relationships increase. Within the family, there may be difference among members in the quantity and quality of a relationship with others. For example, parents may disapprove of the friends of a child.

Relationships with Helping Professionals. The relationship between the health provider and the client (individual or family) can influence the client's willingness to interact, plan, seek care, and adhere to mutually agreed health care plans. Determining whether the client is able to discuss problems with professionals is helpful. How much confidence does the client place in the professional? Also, does the client desire to be an active participant in making health care decisions and plans or is there an expectation that the health professional will tell the client what information is needed and what tasks are required? Assessing client expectations and validating findings with the client is helpful in establishing a therapeutic relationship (refer to Chap. 1).

DIAGNOSTIC STUDIES

There are no specific diagnostic studies for roles and relationships. Stress-related problems such as gastric ulcers and headaches may be symptoms of problems with roles and relationships. Communication problems such as poor articulation and aphasia can be detected by careful listening. Individuals with these problems should be referred to speech therapists/pathologists for follow-up and appropriate diagnosis. Communication can also be impaired by hearing and vision impairments (see Chap. 10 for appropriate diagnostic tests). Finally, radiographic tests such as x-rays may be of benefit to establish a history of physical abuse (multiple healed fractures).

NURSING OBSERVATIONS RELATED TO ROLES AND RELATIONSHIPS

A nurse makes observations for the role–relationship function during the entire contact with the client and client's family. Cues from other functions, such as problems with coping and stress, self-concept, and values and beliefs, can alert the nurse to potential problems within role–relationship function.

General Appearance

A person's appearance can provide many cues about the role–relationship pattern, alerting you to insufficient income, fatigue, recent physical injury, and difficulty communicating. Insufficient rest and signs of sleep deprivation may indicate excessive role responsibilities or role overload. Recent injury may be the result of an unsafe family environment or a family member's violence. Inappropriate or inadequate dress may indicate insufficient income. Inadequate dress and poor hygiene can be an indication of neglect, especially in young children and elders. The person's ability to communicate verbally and physically as well as knowledge of the dominant language can be determined within the first moments of contact.

Other observed behaviors can indicate other problem situations. For example, if a young mother brings her three preschool children with her to a clinic appointment for herself, it could indicate that she does not have sufficient funds to hire a babysitter or that she has few friends to help or limited extended support, or perhaps that she is too dependent on her children to separate from them.

Associated System Alterations

Stress and Coping. A stress-related problem such as duodenal ulcer, frequent headaches, and depression may be related to role strain. Ineffective coping may be the result of role ambiguity or insufficient knowledge or skill to perform a role.

Musculoskeletal and Integumentary Systems. Assessing the musculoskeletal and integumentary systems may reveal fractures and soft-tissue injuries in varying stages of healing. Inspection and palpation of these areas as well as any information provided by the client regarding musculoskeletal difficulties should alert you to the possibility of family violence. Muscle wasting or poor development may be the result of neglect, especially in the very young and very old. Palpation of an enlarged liver or needle track marks may indicate substance abuse. Recent unintentional loss of muscle mass may indicate role strain.

Nursing Observations ▐ *Roles and Relationships*

General Principles   Conclusions about roles and relationships are primarily based upon interview data. Observations are used to verify some interview data; however, observations need corresponding interview data to be accepted as factual. Individuals who are experiencing problems with stress and coping may also be experiencing role strain and problems or changes in relationships. Whenever the opportunity occurs, observe family interaction.

Preparation   Interview client in a quiet, comfortable, private area. Make eye contact as appropriate and provide enough private space for the person to feel comfortable. You should be at the same level as the client (i.e., if the client is sitting or lying, you should be sitting).

Examination and Documentation Focus	• Verbalization about roles • Observations about role strain • Verbalizations about relationships • Observations about interactions • Observations about communication ability • Observations for signs of physical abuse • Verbalizations about parenting • Observations about parenting skills

Examination Guidelines   *Roles and Relationships*

Procedure	Clinical Significance
1. EVALUATE ROLES.	
a. Actively listen to description of roles including:	
(1) Number of roles	Individuals are able to perform numerous roles; however, too many roles/responsibilities can result in role overload. Examples of statements regarding role overload may include expressions of insufficient time, reduced quality of work, or being overwhelmed.
(2) Role conflict	Role conflict occurs when role responsibilities compete for time or resources. Expression of role conflict may include one set of responsibilities interfering with another set of responsibilities, for example, "I don't get to spend enough time with my kids because of work."
(3) Role incompetence	Role incompetence occurs when the individual does not have sufficient knowledge or skill to adequately meet responsibilities. Expressions of role incompetence may include doubts about performance, feelings of failure, or inability to a good job.
(4) Role strain	Expressions that may indicate role strain include being overwhelmed, doubts about ability, feelings of inferiority in performing role, feelings of failing, not accomplishing anything, letting others down, lack of self confidence, not enough time, and insufficient knowledge or skill.
b. Observe for signs of role strain.	Physical signs of role strain might include fatigue, frequent headaches, depression, gastric and duodenal ulcers, anxiety, neglect of self, and physical illnesses.
2. EXAMINE RELATIONSHIPS.	
a. Actively listen for verbalization about family relationships.	Indicators of poor family relationships include the expression of frequent verbal hostility, physical violence, inability to talk with other members, lack of nurturing environment (needs are not met), and rigidity in family members and family rules.
b. Observe family interactions, noting: Who answers questions? What is pattern of communication? Who is silent? Who makes decisions? Are there signs of affection?	Behaviors indicating difficulty with family interaction may include expressions of anger when talking to one another; one individual answering all questions, even those directed to others; ignoring of family member(s) by others; lack of touching; belittling comments; evidence of physical violence; and little verbal interaction among members.
	Care must be taken not to make quick judgements. For example, some families have little physical contact such as touching and hugging; this does not always indicate a problem.
c. Actively listen about relationships with others and, when possible, observe interactions with others.	Expressions indicating difficulty with relationships include feelings of aloneness or loneliness; not being worthy of friends; lack of self-confidence in groups or in one-to-one relationships; feelings of inferiority; fear of groups of people; fear of meeting new people; and small support group. Observations of difficulty with relationships with others might include avoiding interactions; limited verbal communication; lack of eye contact; and allowing others to speak for self.

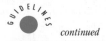

continued

Roles and Relationships

Procedure

3. OBSERVE COMMUNICATION SKILLS.

  a. Determine the individual's primary language and note language spoken to others.

  b. Determine level of language. Listen carefully to see if client uses simple or more complex words and sentences.

  c. Determine if there is any evidence of possible communication problems.

3. DETERMINE WHETHER THE INDIVIDUAL USES ANY COMMUNICATION AIDS SUCH AS CORRECTIVE LENSES, HEARING AIDS, ARTIFICIAL VOICE, WORD BOARD, OR COMPUTER.

4. OBSERVE FOR SIGNS OF PHYSICAL ABUSE.

5. EXAMINE PARENTING ROLE.

  a. Actively listen and observe for parental role adequacy.

Clinical Significance

The language primarily spoken may be the language the individual is most comfortable speaking.

When speaking to the client, utilize the same level of language to enhance understanding. Few clients know medical–nursing jargon.

Physical evidence of possible communication problems might include presence of tracheostomy, neck or facial surgery or post-surgery; hemiplegia indicating post-stroke; cerebral palsy, especially severe; and evidence of other neurologic problems such as Alzheimer's disease, parkinsonism, or post-traumatic brain damage.

If these are evident then encourage their use during the interview and physical examination.

Signs of physical abuse include bruising, especially between the elbows and knees; multiple injuries in various stages of healing; burn scars, especially those that are round and cigarette-sized; history of broken bones; reports of clumsiness; frequent falls; report of how injury occurred inconsistent with injury; history of using numerous different hospitals and physicians for injury treatment; and expressions indicating the victim is "bad" or deserving of injury. Individuals who perform acts of violence may demonstrate or express the following: low frustration tolerance; physical expressions of anger; chemical substance use; or history as an abuse victim.

Parents who are not having difficulty with the parenting role will express satisfaction with their role and pleasure with their children. Although they may have questions, generally they actively seek guidance from either professionals, books, or friends. Individuals having difficulty parenting may express the following: inadequacies in the role; frustration with parenting; anger with children; inappropriate discipline for child's age; dissatisfaction with child; conflict with other roles; and feelings of being overwhelmed and little or no time for self. Behaviors that may be observed include hitting children; inappropriate anger expressed; lack of touching; little or infrequent emotional support; and lack of nurturing. Children who are inappropriately parented may demonstrate the following: signs of physical violence; abusive behavior to others or to animals; inappropriate dress; unkempt appearance, poor hygiene; delay of physical and psychosocial development; clinging to or avoiding others; and malnourishment.

Documenting Assessment Data

Data from the role–relationship pattern may be documented as follows:

Example 1: Healthy Role–Relationship Pattern

Ms. W, aged 26, single mother of an 8-year-old child, was interviewed as part of a comprehensive assessment at a health maintenance organization. Documentation of the role–relationship pattern was as follows:

Denies any difficulty with identified roles of mother and waitress. Has numerous friends, two of whom she can confide in and discuss problems with. Has adequate child care, good relationship with daughter. Currently satisfied with life, thinking of returning to school to get high school diploma and possibly college degree. Talkative, expresses self freely and adequately, with appropriate affect.

These findings may be recorded in a problem-oriented record as follows:

S: Roles identified—mother, waitress; denies difficulty with these. Numerous friends, two of whom she can confide in and discuss problems with. Good relationship with 8-year-old child. Uses after-school day care for child. Satisfied with life. Thinking of getting high school diploma and college degree

O: Communicates easily, easy to understand, smiles when talking of child

A: Functional role–relationship pattern

P: Reassess in 1 year during routine screening. Check status regarding attending school and impact on current roles and life-style of family.

Example 2: Altered Role–Relationship Pattern

Mr. S, aged 67, had a stroke 2 days ago that affected his speech and resulted in left-sided paralysis. The discharge planning nurse documented the following about the role–relationship pattern:

Unable to speak, words garbled, speech therapy daily—to continue as outpatient two times per week after discharge. Becomes frustrated rapidly when trying to express self. Wife concerned about how they will manage, as husband pays all the bills, does yard work and most of the driving; she has arthritis, uses a walker, and depends on husband for assistance with household tasks. Will refer to public health nurse to evaluate home environment and needs before projected discharge.

These findings may be recorded in a problem-oriented record as follows:

S: Tries to communicate, garbled speech. Wife concerned how family will manage. Husband's roles: pay bills, yard work, driver, helps with household chores. Wife's activity limited, needs help, has arthritis.

O: Mr. S: Speech not understandable, speech therapy daily, to continue two times per week on discharge; left-sided paralysis, becomes frustrated after a few moments of trying to move or speak. Mrs. S: hand gnarled, uses walker.

A: Probable diagnoses: Mr. Smith—verbal communication impaired, related to recent neurologic insult. Both: role performance altered, related to recent illness of Mr. S. Family process altered related to recent debilitating illness of Mr. S.

P: Further data collection needed to support final diagnoses. Refer to public health nurse to evaluate home environment and needs before discharge. Visit in 2 days to note progress and additional concerns.

Example 3: Altered Role–Relationship Pattern

Mrs. P. is interviewed as part of a prenatal assessment. Her last menstrual period was 6 months ago. The nurse documented the role–relationship pattern as follows:

Married 18 months, EDC in 4 months, gravida 1. Husband in military—in Europe for 9 more months. Mrs. P from Korea, command of English fair. Has three friends who speak Korean and also have husbands in military. From large family, youngest child, little experience with child care. Misses sisters and parents in Korea, spends much of time watching TV to pass the time and learn English. Does

not drive, lives on base, has difficulty paying bills and managing money—husband previously assumed financial responsibilities.

These findings may be recorded in a problem-oriented record as follows:

S: Married 18 months, last menstrual period 6 months ago, gravida 1. Husband in military—in Europe for 9 more months. Mrs. P from Korea, has three friends who speak Korean and also have husbands in military. From large family, youngest child, misses sisters and parents, limited experience with child care, does not drive, lives on base, has difficulty paying bills and managing money—husband previously assumed responsibility. Spends much of time watching TV to pass time and learn English.

O: EDC 4 months, command of English fair, Western dress.

A: Possible: alteration of family process related to husband's absence; disturbance of role performance related to husband's absence; potential alteration in parenting related to lack of child care experience; impaired verbal communication and social interaction related to new cultural environment and English as a new second language.

P: Refer to public health nurse for follow-up and at-home data collection; refer to base social worker for assistance with money management. Confer with both in 10 days, schedule appointment with client in 2 weeks.

NDx

Nursing Diagnoses Related to Roles and Relationships

Altered Family Processes

Altered family process occurs when the family system that has been functioning effectively becomes unable to meet the needs of family members adequately, perform family responsibilities, or maintain communication for mutual growth and development. Ineffective family coping is the correct diagnosis for the family that has a history of inappropriate functioning (Carpenito, 1992).

History. The person reports an inability to communicate with other family members, disharmony between family members, disagreement in family about family rules, and is having difficulty adapting positively to a crisis that may be maturational, situational, or related to illness. Altered family process may occur any time a family member is hospitalized; leaves the family by death, divorce, or attending college; a new member enters the family by birth, adoption, or marriage; or there is a change in economic status such as unemployment, retirement, or obtaining employment.

Physical Examination Findings. The nurse may observe behaviors such as limited or no verbal exchanges between family members, self-blaming or blaming others, sudden outbursts of emotions, and verbal abuse. Family members may show physical evidence of Altered family process, such as weight loss or gain, alcohol and drug use, and stress-related conditions such as headaches, lack of sleep, and physical abuse.

Altered Parenting

Altered parenting is an actual inability by parents or caregivers to provide an environment that supports optimal physical and emotional growth and development of a dependent child.

History. An individual experiencing altered parenting may verbalize disappointment, resentment, or shame about a child; feelings of being an inadequate parent; or frustration with being a parent. There may be a documented history of numerous injuries that may be poorly explained.

Physical Examination Findings. The nurse may observe inappropriate parenting behaviors such as hitting, verbal abuse, and ignoring the child. Other observations may include lack of touching or holding, no eye contact, and hostility of child to the parent. The physical examination may reveal wounds in various stages of healing and poor correlation of how injury occurred between parent and child. In the hospitalized child, the parents may not visit or visit infrequently.

Potential for Altered Parenting

The nursing diagnosis Potential for altered parenting is used when significant risk factors are present that may interfere with the normal maturational process of adjustment to parenting. Risk factors may become evident during the prenatal period or during normal maturational transitions of the dependent child, such as from infant to toddler and school age to adolescent.

History. Individuals at high risk for alterations in parenting may be identified by verbalizations of own history of physical abuse, lack of good role model, unrealistic expectations of self, insufficient knowledge of child care, or feelings of social isolation.

Physical Examination Findings. The presence of physical or mental illness may interfere with the individual's ability to parent. The presence of physical or mental illness of the child may also interfere with the adult's ability to parent. Observations of problems in family process such as communication and support received within the family can increase the risk for alterations in parenting.

Disturbances in Role Performance

The nursing diagnosis Disturbances in role performance when there is a change, conflict, or denial of role responsibilities or when the individual is unable to fulfill role obligations.

History. The history includes any verbalization of difficulty or frustration with role responsibilities, such as an increase in the number of duties, forgetting to complete required tasks, or reports of conflicts between two or more roles, such as needing to attend two different meetings at the same time. The individual may also report a role but is unable to describe the responsibilities associated with it. With denial, the individual would not report a particular role.

Physical Examination Findings. Physical findings would be limited. Physical signs of stress may be evident (*e.g.,*

gastric and duodenal ulcers, headaches, and poor attention span). Denial of role may be evident in others; for example, in the parent who denies a parenting role, the child may have evidence of physical and psychosocial neglect.

Impaired Social Interaction

The nursing diagnosis Impaired social interactions is used when the individual experiences, perceives, or is at high risk for experiencing negative, insufficient, or unsatisfactory interactions with others. Interactions may be unsatisfactory because the individual is overwhelmed by numerous interactions that are considered superficial and time is not sufficient to have meaningful interactions.

History. The client may verbalize being uncomfortable in social interactions, avoiding people either individually or in groups, inability to have satisfying encounters with others, lack of friends or close confidants, and identification of few who can provide social support.

Physical Examination Findings. Individuals who have a mental illness such as schizophrenia and depression may have difficulty in sustaining social relationships and interactions. Findings may include physical evidence of panic or anxiety attacks during interactions with others, inappropriate communication pattern and content, or the lack of communication with others. Additionally, language barriers, visual and hearing deficits, impaired mobility, and speech impediments are physical findings that may contribute to impaired social interactions.

Impaired Verbal Communication

Impaired verbal communication occurs when the individual has a reduced, changed, or absent ability to use verbal communication. This nursing diagnosis may be situational. For example, an individual goes to a clinic where the providers do not speak his or her native language; this may not be a problem at another clinic where providers do speak that language.

History. The history from individuals with severe impaired communication may need to be obtained in writing or by a family member. A history of conditions such as cerebral palsy, cerebrovascular accident, and surgery for laryngeal cancer may be present. In children, there may not be a change in communication ability but delay or lack of verbal development. In individuals with a history of Alzheimer's disease, there may be nothing wrong with the ability to speak words; however, the content of the words is inappropriate. Individuals may verbalize frustration or inability to say certain sounds, speak the dominant language, and speak loud enough for others to hear.

Physical Examination Findings. Findings may include the presence of a tracheostomy, scars from laryngectomy, shortness of breath, cleft lip or palate, infected or inflamed throat, or polyps on the vocal cords. Diagnostic screening may identify difficulty with hearing or vision. Listening closely to the individual, you may document confusion, stuttering, slurring, inappropriate word use, incoherent speech, and the use of another language. You may also find that although the individual has a hearing aid, it is not used or it is malfunctioning.

Parental Role Conflict

The nursing diagnosis Parental role conflict is used when the parent is experiencing role confusion and conflict in response to crises experienced by one or both parents. The conflict can be between values/beliefs and societal expectation or between two or more role obligations. This diagnosis is used to describe a situation in which previously effectively functioning parents are having difficulty because of external factors such as illness. If not resolved, alteration in parenting may occur (Carpenito, 1992).

History. During the interview, parents with role conflict may express their concerns about changes in their roles. Verbalizations regarding frustration in not being able to meet their perceived responsibilities may be expressed. Parents may also report the occurrence of acute, chronic, or life-threatening illnesses/conditions of a family member that interfere with the ability to perform the parenting role as the parent desires.

Physical Examination Findings. The parent may verbalize feelings of guilt or inadequacy in meeting role obligations. If the parent needs to learn a new skill to provide care to a child, the parent may demonstrate poor technique and/or verbalize inability to perform skill. You may be able to observe feelings of fear, anger, anxiety, or frustration regarding the effect of illness, death, or separation on family process and ability to parent all children.

Potential for Violence

The potential for violence exists when the individual is at high risk for self- or other-directed physical aggression.

History. The history consists of reports or verbalizations of physical harm or attempts to harm self, others, or property. The individual may also report increased stress and difficulty handling stress.

Physical Examination Findings. The physical examination of the individual or others, such as children or spouse, may reveal wounds and bruises in various stages of healing, and x-rays may reveal old and new fractures. Other findings may include observations of low frustration level, verbal threats, and expressions of helplessness, hostility, and fear of loss of control. There may be evidence of drug and alcohol abuse. Body language may indicate intent to harm, such as rigid posture, tense facial expression, and clenched hands. Laboratory results may indicate a toxic response to drugs (prescription and others), altered electrolytes, presence of blood alcohol, and altered blood gases in individuals with potentially violent behavior.

Social Isolation

Social isolation is the individual's perception that contact with others is insufficient or nonexistent. It is the feeling of aloneness.

History. Because social isolation is subjective, most of the data are from the history. Some individuals desire very limited contact with people, whereas others need interaction with many people. Individuals with this diagnosis report a feeling of being alone or abandoned by others and a need for more contact with people. In elders, there is often a history of the spouse, friends, and family dying.

The individual may verbalize that he or she is the only one left.

Physical Examination Findings. There may be no physical findings. However, cues that may encourage you to explore this diagnosis include evidence of incontinence, anxiety attacks, reduced mobility, inability to speak the dominant language, physical handicaps, terminal illness, and a change from good health to poor health or increased illness symptoms.

Clinical Problems Related to Roles and Relationships

Assessment of roles and relationships provides indicators for nursing diagnoses; however, clinical problems are often associated with clinical problems in other assessment areas. For example, gastric ulcers are clinical problems in the elimination pattern, and fatigue is a clinical problem in the sleep–rest pattern. Ineffective coping is often a symptom of role strain. During your assessment, you should consider any clinical problems that may have an effect on roles and relationships.

Some clinical problems you may encounter primarily in roles and relationships include physical abuse, aphasia, tracheostomy, agrophobia, social isolation of elders, and adolescent parenting.

Physical Abuse

Physical abuse of an individual by another can occur at any age and with any gender; however, children, women, and elders are at higher risk than other groups. Signs of physical abuse include frequent trauma injuries from fists; objects such as electric cords, belts, and household items; and cigarettes (burns). The use of numerous physicians and different emergency rooms is also significant. Generally, the injury presented the explanation for the injury do not correspond. An atypical form of child abuse is *Munchausen syndrome by proxy.* The parent invents signs and symptoms of illnesses in the child and may induce some symptoms such as vomiting. The child is then subjected to numerous medical tests, hospitalization, and, in some situations, exploratory surgery.

Aphasia

Aphasia is a defect or loss of the ability to express one's self by speech or in writing or to comprehend the spoken language. Aphasia is the result of disease or injury to the speech center in the brain. *Broca's aphasia,* also known as expressive aphasia, often occurs as a result of a stroke. With this aphasia, the person can understand and knows what he or she wants to say but cannot find the correct words.

Tracheostomy

Tracheostomies interfere with the individual's ability to speak words. Air is diverted from the larynx, preventing the vocal cords from vibrating and making sounds. If not connected to a respirator, tracheostomies can be plugged by a finger or cork to allow the individual to speak. When temporarily closing the tracheostomy opening, you need to be observant for signs of respiratory distress.

Cancer of the Larynx

Generally, when cancer of the larynx occurs, the larynx is surgically removed. The individual may use an electronic device to simulate speaking. You need to listen very carefully, as the speech can be difficult to understand.

Agoraphobia

With agoraphobia, the most severe phobia, the individual fears open spaces, eventually becomes housebound, and all social interactions outside of the home stop. In the most severe forms, the individual cannot leave the house without experiencing a severe panic attack. If health care is needed outside of the home, the health professionals must also assist the individual in dealing with panic attacks.

Social Isolation Associated with Age

As an individual becomes very old and frail, social isolation often occurs as the result of loss of transportation, loss of mobility, and loss of friends to death. Some elders may seek medical care and hospitalization to avoid feelings of aloneness.

Adolescent Parenting

Adolescents, especially young adolescents, experience stress and role strain while attempting to parent an infant or child. The child may suffer from neglect and/or abuse because of the parent's lack of maturation and skill. Neglect can be purposeful or benign. Benign neglect occurs when individuals do not desire to neglect the child but are unaware they are causing harm.

ASSESSMENT PROFILE 1

• •

John, aged 34 years, lives with his parents and 17-year-old sister to save money. Six months ago, he learned that he has HIV (human immunodeficiency virus—the AIDS virus) antibodies. He chose not to tell his family, but he did advise his sexual partner. He is now hospitalized with pneumonia and has been told he has AIDS. When his family was informed of his diagnosis, they stopped visiting him. John's male lover continues to visit every other day but is now concerned about his own health and risks.

To assess John's role–relationship status, the nurse reviewed the available data and concluded that, in addition to other health problems, John was probably experiencing a problem with roles and relationships. The nurse based this judgment on the following data: John did not tell his family of his HIV status; when AIDS was diagnosed, John's family stopped visiting him; he lived with his family to save money and he had an alternative life-style; he recently learned that he has a life-threatening disease; and he maintains a relationship with a significant other who visits every other day but who is also concerned about his

own health and risks. After considering the initial data, the nurse identified the following possible diagnoses: Social isolation, Altered family process, and Altered role performance.

After identifying these possibilities, the nurse collected additional data to either support or reject the diagnoses. The nurse also considered alternative diagnoses. Once all the data were collected and analyzed, final diagnoses could be made. In this situation, the nurse made the final nursing diagnoses of Anticipatory grieving related to approaching death; Altered role performance related to increased dependency; Social isolation related to others' fear of AIDS; and Ineffective family coping: Disabling, related to nonacceptance of John's illness and life-style.

After careful data collection and analysis, the nurse concluded that the altered family process was related to the family's inability to cope with John's status, and that therefore the Ineffective family coping diagnosis was the most appropriate diagnosis. When John was discharged, his family refused to see him, so John moved into the home of his lover, where he died 10 months later.

ASSESSMENT PROFILE 2

• •

Karen, aged 25, is the mother of four children aged 6, 4, 3, and 1 years. She was divorced 6 months ago; her husband was abusive and refused to give her any money. She is receiving welfare while looking for work, and her former husband is not making child support payments. The children are underweight for their ages and heights. A public health nurse makes a home visit on a referral. While discussing discipline, Karen states, "Some days it's just too much with no money, all the pressure, the kids crying and

fighting. Spanking doesn't help. Sometimes, I think they are just being mean. I need some time for me."

When preparing for this home visit, the nurse reviewed the following data: name, age, height, and weight of each child, and Karen's name and marital status. Within the role–relationship pattern, the nurse decided to identify the focus as possible alteration in parenting based on the growth lag of the four children. Additional data collection supported this diagnosis and helped the nurse identify other possible diagnoses, such as Potential for violence related to stress (Karen), Altered role performance related to increased responsibilities as a single parent, and Altered family process related to recent divorce.

The nurse continued to visit the home and assess the role–relationship pattern. Data confirmed the diagnoses. However, within 3 months, the potential for violence was considered resolved after Karen began using a day care center 4 hours a week and developed new coping skills.

Karen was also considering returning to school to become a beautician so she would have a career skill. The other nursing diagnoses remained relevant, although they were revised as new data emerged. For example, Karen's decision to return to school would affect family processes, as well as her role performance and parenting behavior. Continuous data collection and analysis were indicated so that appropriate interventions could be added or modified to resolve problems.

ASSESSMENT PROFILE 3

● ●

Susan and Tom were both looking forward to spending time alone together now that both had retired and all the children had left home. Tom's father died 6 years ago; his mother now has terminal cancer and cannot live alone. Tom promised his father that he would always look after his mother. Tom's mother is moving into the spare bedroom at Susan and Tom's house next weekend. It has always been difficult for Susan to take care of sick people, even her children. Susan has contacted a home health agency to help provide care and has expressed some of her concerns and disappointments to the nurse.

In considering these circumstances, the nurse realizes that Susan, Tom, and Tom's mother will all assume new

roles and responsibilities, thereby altering the current family process. The nurse also considers that the stress of the move may have an adverse effect on Tom's mother. In addition, Susan and Tom may be grieving, not only for the mother's approaching death, but also for the loss of their chance to spend time alone together. The nurse is aware that information about the changes in roles and relationships should be gathered. The standard interview used by the agency does not include this type of information. Therefore, the nurse must ask additional questions and include the information in the record to ensure that any potential or actual dysfunctions related to roles and relationships will be identified.

Chapter 14 SUMMARY

Assessment of role and relationships focuses on the following:

- The person's perception of roles and relationships with family, friends, and associates
- The potential for role strain
- The functioning of relationships within a family
- The client's ability to express self

When assessing roles and relationships, you should consider the following:

- People assume many roles during the course of their lifetimes.
- Roles are either ascribed or achieved.
- Role strain can occur because of conflict, ambiguity, overload, and incompetence.
- Social interaction is influenced by the number of people interacting and the relationships of those people.
- Communication is verbal and nonverbal and is influenced by social interaction.
- The term *family* may be defined as a human group with significant emotional bonds, interdepenence, and (usually) shared housing.
- Family structure and role responsibilities are culturally influenced.

- Parenting involves the responsibility of providing physical and emotional care to minor children.

Methods for obtaining data about roles and relationships include the following:

The Interview
- Role perceptions
- Role satisfaction/dissatisfaction
- Role strain
- Family composition and structure
- Family relationships
- Family decision-making process
- Discipline patterns
- Relationships with helping professionals

Nursing Observations
- Signs of role strain
- Signs of family violence
- Interaction patterns between client and family members
- Discipline and decision-making process if observable
- Relationship with nurse
- Communication patterns
- Social relationships

RESEARCH *Hi*GHLIGHT

With the birth of a baby, do men and women in dual-employed families have similar experiences with transition to a new role?

The concept of role is abstract, and roles are not easily assessed. Often when individuals accept a new role, there is a redefining and a negotiation of all other roles. Nurses in clinical settings can assist adults with adjusting to the role of parent and provide support in redefining other roles. To better assist parents with this transition, nurses need to be able to assess and assist both parents.

In a qualitative study Wendy Hall studied how men and women redefined their roles upon the mother's return to work. There were significant differences in how both groups redefined their roles. Men monitored and limited role strain whereas women took on additional roles, experienced role strain, and then attempted to reduce strain.

In analyzing qualitative data from two studies, one with 8 women and another with 10 men, the author discovered that both men and women redefine their roles when the mother returns to work. Women often felt overwhelmed, whereas men felt their lives were difficult but not "out of control." Women attempted to reduce role strain by (in the following order) letting go of myths, setting priorities, organizing and planning, negotiating with spouses, establishing new expectations, and delegating responsibilities. On the other hand, men limited role strain from occurring by (in order) negotiating with spouses, changing expectations, establishing new responsibilities, organizing and planning, and compartmentalizing time. Women experienced more role strain than men because upon returning to work, women expected to fulfill all role obligations at the same level before returning to work plus work role obligations.

What significance does this study have for health assessment?

Women who return to work after the birth of an infant are at high risk for role strain. Assessing a woman's resources, knowledge of role expectations and skills, and ability to negotiate role obligations before the birth and return to work may assist women in limiting role strain. Hill suggests that unmet needs create role strain and increase the incidence of illness. By assessing roles, the nurse can identify issues that create role strain and assist families in managing multiple roles with parenting.

Can the study's findings be applied to practice?

By assessing roles and role transitions, nurses can assist individuals and families in identifying areas of potential role strain and developing of coping strategies to reduce role strain. Understanding that men and women approach roles and role transitions differently should assist nurses in assessing as well as planning interventions to assist with role strain.

These results indicate that role strain is a phenomenon that women experience when they return to work after the birth of an infant. Nurses can assist parents to prepare for and reduce role strain by providing information in prenatal courses, predicting areas of strain in a particular family, and planning interventions before the need arises. The nurse could use the postpartum hospital stay to provide information and identify community resources that may be of assistance. Occupational health nurses could be alert to increased health needs and potential of role strain in women returning to work after maternity leave.

The assessment of roles and relationships assists you in identifying defining characteristics (cues) for the following nursing diagnoses:
  Impaired verbal communication
  Altered parenting
  Anticipatory grieving
  Dysfunctional grieving
  Compromised parental role
  Altered parenting: Potential
  Altered role performance
  Impaired social interaction
  Social isolation
  Potential violence for: Self-directed or directed at
    others

Related nursing diagnoses may be identified during assessment of roles and relationships, such as the following:
  Impaired adjustment
  Anxiety
  Ineffective family coping
  Ineffective individual coping
  Fear
  Altered growth and development
  Altered health maintenance
  Identity adjustment
  Identity confusion
  Potential for injury
  Knowledge deficit
  Self-esteem disturbance
  Sleep pattern disturbance

✳ CRITICAL THINKING

You are a home health nurse visiting an elderly woman requiring dressing changes for a burn received from scalding water. One day before your visit, you received an anonymous phone call in which the caller stated that the woman was being abused by a family member.

Learning Exercises

1. Explain how you would discuss this anonymous phone call with the patient.

2. Specify additional observations you would make during a home visit to further evaluate this situation.

3. The patient tells you there is no truth to the caller's allegations, but you have reason to believe otherwise on the basis of physical signs of abuse. Determine and discuss what you would do next.

4. Explain how you would include the patient's family in the assessment of potential abuse.

BIBLIOGRAPHY

Biddle, B.J. & Thomas, E.J. (1979). *Role theory: Concepts and research*. New York: John Wiley & Sons.

Bramwell, L. & Whall, A. (1986). Effects of role clarity and empathy on support role performance and anxiety. *Nursing Research, 35* (5), 282–289.

Carpenito, L.J. (1993). *Nursing diagnosis: Application to clinical practice* (5th ed.). Philadelphia: J.B. Lippincott.

Corbin, J. & Strauss, A. (1984). Collaboration: Couples working together to manage chronic illness. *Image 26* (4), 109–115.

Duvall, E. (1977). *Marriage and family development* (5th ed.). Philadelphia: J.B. Lippincott.

Friedman, M. (1992). *Family nursing: Theory and assessment* (3rd ed.). Norwalk, CT: Appleton-Century-Crofts.

Hardy, M. & Conway, M. (1988). *Role theory: Perspectives for health professionals* (2nd ed.). Norwalk, CT: Appleton-Century-Crofts.

Hill, L. & Smith, N. (1989). *Self-care nursing* (2nd ed.). Englewood Cliffs, NJ: Prentice-Hall.

Hoff, L. (1984). *People in crisis* (2nd ed.). Menlo Park, CA: Addison-Wesley.

Lancaster, J. (1982). Communication as a tool for change. In J. Lancaster & W. Lancaster (Eds). *Concepts for advanced nursing practice: The nurse as a change agent* (pp. 109–131) St Louis: C.V. Mosby.

Leavitt, M. (1982). *Families at risk: Primary prevention in nursing practice*. Boston: Little, Brown & Co.

Marston, M. & Chambers, B. (1980). Development of family conceptual frameworks. In J. Miller & E. Janosik (Eds.). *Family focused care* (pp. 416–431). New York: McGraw-Hill.

Mays, R. (1988). Family stress and adaptation. *Nurse Practice, 13* (8), 52, 54, 56.

McBride, A. (1988). Mental health effects of women's multiple roles. *Image 20* (1), 41–47.

McLane, A. (Ed.). (1987). *Classification of nursing diagnoses: Proceedings of the seventh conference*. St. Louis: C.V. Mosby.

Mercer, R. (1985). The process of maternal role attainment over the first year. *Nursing research, 34,* 198–204.

Mikhail, J. (1988). Development of a family assessment and intervention protocol. *Critical Care Nurse, 8* (3), 114–118.

Moch, S. (1988). Promoting health with role reversal couples. *Journal of Community Health Nursing, 5* (3), 195–202.

Murry, R. & Huelshoetter, M. (1987). *Psychiatric mental health nursing: Giving emotional care* (2nd ed.). Norwalk, CT: Appleton & Lange.

Murray, R. & Zentner, J. (1993). *Nursing assessment and health promotion strategies through the lifespan* (5th ed.). Norwalk, CT: Appleton & Lange.

Payne, M. (1988). Utilizing role theory to assess the family with sudden disability. *Rehabilitation Nursing, 13* (4), 191–194.

Paynich, M. (1964). Cultural barriers to nurse communication. *American Journal of Nursing,* 1964 Feb; 64(2):87–90.

Pender, N. (1987). *Health promotion in nursing practice* (2nd ed.). Norwalk, CT: Appleton & Lange.

Phipps, L. (1980). Theoretical frameworks applicable to family care. In J. Miller & E. Janosik (Eds.). *Family-focused care*. New York: McGraw-Hill.

Rosow, I. (1965). Forms and functions of adult socialization. *Social Forces, 44,* 35–40.

Stanhope, M. & J. Lancaster. (1992). *Community health nursing: Process and practice for promoting health* (3rd ed.). St. Louis: C.V. Mosby.

Yura, H. & Walsh, M. (1978). *The nursing process* (3rd ed.). New York: Appleton-Century-Crofts.

Walker, L., H. Crain, & E. Thompson. (1986). Maternal role attainment and identity in the postpartum period: Stability and change. *Nursing Research, 35* (2), 68–71.

Watzlawich, P., Beavin, J. & D. Jackson. (1967). *Pragmatics of human communication*. New York: W. W. Norton.

Assessing Sexuality and Reproductive Function

Examination Guidelines

Female Genitals and Pelvic Structures

Breasts and Axillae

Measuring Fundal Height

Fetal Heart Auscultation

Male Genitals and Inguinal Area

Assessment Terms

Sex Role (Gender Role)

Sexual Response Patterns

Gender Identification

Infertility

Impotent

Masturbation

Menarche

Sexual Abuse

Sexual Assault

Sexually Transmitted Diseases (STDs)

Pap Smear

Fundal Palpation

Pawlik Palpation

Lateral Palpation

Leopold's Maneuver

Kegel's Exercises

Pregnancy-induced Hypertension (Toxemia)

Uterine Ballottement

Piskacek's Sign

Chadwick's Sign

Godell's Sign

Hegar's Sign

McDonald's Sign

Kyphosis

Cervical Lordosis

INTRODUCTORY OVERVIEW

Human sexuality, a complex phenomenon, is the behavioral presentation of sexual identity. It is influenced by lifelong attitudes and reflects individual perceptions of that identity. Although reproductive development and function are determined at conception, reproductive patterns are influenced by the individual's perception of maleness and femaleness and by social and cultural norms.

Until recently, the client's sexual and reproductive functions were not routinely assessed or considered essential components of a complete health history. Sexual assessment continues to be the most frequent function omitted from the health history. Such an omission is alarming because many illnesses, surgical procedures, physiologic aging processes, and medications affect sexual function and satisfaction.

Unfortunately, certain taboos against discussing sexuality have pervaded the Western health care fields. In the 1960s, Masters and Johnson's studies, which promoted an understanding of normal sexual responses in men and women, were initially rejected by publishers of

Jill Fuller and Jennifer Schaller-Ayers:
HEALTH ASSESSMENT: A NURSING APPROACH, Second Edition.
© 1990, 1994 by J. B. Lippincott Company.

obstetric and gynecology journals. Eventually, these studies were published in the *Western Journal of Surgery*.

The work of Masters and Johnson encouraged health professionals to assess their clients' sexuality and, when indicated, to initiate sexual counseling. Additional factors that open the subject to discussion include social forces such as the women's movement, the availability of reproductive control and abortion, and the prominence of sexually transmitted diseases (STD), including HIV disease (AIDS).

Sexual and reproductive functions are evaluated during health assessment in order to assist clients to express sexual or reproductive concerns, identify teaching needs, identify problems that need to be treated, and monitor normal development of reproductive structures and functions from birth to senescence.

Assessment Focus

Although human sexuality is now considered a legitimate focus of nursing practice, many nurses have not received the education required for effective sexual counseling. Logically, health assessment should be guided by actual or potential problems identified. However, because registered nurses without graduate education or other specialized training are not qualified to offer sexual counseling, the appropriateness of nurses assessing sexual behaviors is often questioned. Nevertheless, nurses are qualified to perform screening assessments and refer clients when the problem identified is beyond the nurse's scope of practice.

One approach to assessing sexual and reproductive functions is offered by the PLISSIT sexual health model, which was developed by psychologist Jack Annon (1976). The PLISSIT model establishes guidelines for assessment and interventions nurses with different levels of educational prep-

aration are qualified to perform. The model establishes a scale of complexity for client sexual problems, indicates the treatment suitable for each level of complexity, and indicates who is qualified to offer treatment.

PLISSIT is an acronym for four levels of therapeutic approach in dealing with sexual concerns of problems: permission, limited information, specific suggestions, and intensive therapy (Table 15-1). All professional nurses should have the educational foundation to assess sexual function to intervene at the first level of approach, giving permission to discuss sexual concerns and offering limited information. Therapeutic interventions involve providing specific factual information to deal with sexual problems. For example, the client may express uncertainty or may reveal misconception arising from myths about sexual matters. The client may express fears or uncertainties about suitable sexual behavior following illness or surgery, such as a myocardial infarction or a hysterectomy. A preadolescent girl may need information about menstruation and physical development. People with such concerns can benefit extensively from health teaching. More intensive assessment and therapy should be performed by advanced practitioners (see Table 15-1). However, all nurses should be able to identify clients who need this level of intervention and make appropriate referrals.

Concerns and problems related to reproductive structure and function should also be assessed to detect signs or symptoms of specific clinical problems such as genital infections, menstrual problems, physiologically related aging problems, or malignant processes involving reproductive organs. In these cases, appropriate referral for treatment should be made.

The assessment of sexual and reproductive function should focus on the following:

Table 15-1. PLISSIT Sexual Health Model*

	Professional Preparation Required[†]	Levels of Assessment	Levels of Therapeutic Intervention
Level 1	Professional nurse	Takes health history; screens for sexual functions and dysfunctions	Provides limited sex education, including information about sexual feelings, behaviors, and myths. Refers client to level 2 or 3 professional if necessary
Level 2	Professional nurse with postgraduate training in sex education and counseling	Takes sexual history	Provides sex education and counseling, including specific information about sex and sexuality; concise suggestions about sexual fears and adaptations to illness; and anticipatory guidance. Refers client to level 3 professional if necessary
Level 3	Professional nurse, physician, psychologist, or social worker who has received training as a sex therapist	Takes sexual problem history	Provides sex therapy: individual, group, or couple. Refers client to level 4 professional if necessary
Level 4	Masters prepared psychiatric nurse clinician, physician, or social worker who specializes in sex therapy	Takes psychiatric and psychosexual history	Eclectic approach: may provide intensive individual psychotherapy, sex therapy, or marital therapy

*Developed by Jack Annon, 1976.
†The more serious the client's sexual problem, the more advanced is the level of professional preparation required to treat the problem.
(Watts, R.J. [1979]. Dimensions of sexual health. American Journal of Nursing, 79(9), 1570)

Assessment Focus **Sexuality and Reproductive Function**

Assessment Goal	Data Collection Methods
1. Identify the person's immediate sexual concerns.	*Interview* • Screening questions related to sexual concerns: Screening questions indicate permission to discuss sexual concerns. • Sex roles and gender identification: Is the person satisfied with sex roles? • Sexual/reproductive knowledge base: Are there knowledge deficits in relation sexuality and reproduction? • Sexual performance and satisfaction: Does the client perceive problems? Is a referral needed?
2. Considering the person's developmental stage and health status, evaluate knowledge of sexual and reproductive functions.	*Interview and Observe* • Any component of the interview may reveal real or potential knowledge deficits: Does the client need anticipatory guidance? Are sexual myths or misinformation contributing to sexual dysfunction or psychological distress? • Observe the person's behaviors and statements made during the genital examination. Patient teaching and evaluation of knowledge base may take place during the examination.
3. Evaluate the effects of altered body structures, body functions, or body image on sexual function.	*Interview* • Any component of the interview may be relevant. • The interview may focus on the specific alterations in body structure, function, or image influencing sexuality. For example, you may ask a person taking medication known to affect sexual performance questions about sexual performance and satisfaction. • Self-concept (see Chap. 12): Has self-concept been altered?
4. Evaluate physical changes associated with reproductive development.	*Physical Examination* • Female genital and pelvic examination. • Male genital examination. • Breast examination.
5. Evaluate the physical changes of pregnancy.	*Physical Examination* • A head-to-toe examination is indicated with special attention to the abdomen and pelvis.
6. Identify problems related to sexuality, reproduction, or reproductive structures requiring patient referral to other care providers.	*Interview* • Any component of the interview may be relevant. *Physical Examination* • Genital and pelvic examination: Can contributing factors to sexual dysfunction be identified, such as chronic infections that cause pain during sexual relations? • Can clinical problems be identified, such as veneral disease or hernias?

• Identifying any immediate sexual concerns
• Evaluating the person's understanding of sexual and reproductive function
• Determining the stage of sexual development with associated and expected physical changes
• Identifying any sexual or reproductive problems that require referral to a specialist

The methods for collecting the data in each of these areas are outlined in the Assessment Focus display.

Nursing Diagnoses

The following nursing diagnoses are associated with sexual and reproductive function:

Altered sexuality patterns
Breast-feeding: ineffective and effective
Rape-trauma syndrome
    Rape-trauma syndrome: Compound reaction
    Rape-trauma syndrome: Silent reaction
Sexual dysfunction

Dysfunctions in sexual and reproductive function may be related to other health problems. Nursing diagnoses related to sexual and reproductive function include the following:

Altered family process
Altered role performance
Body image disturbance
Incontinence
Ineffective family coping
Ineffective individual coping
High risk for infection
Knowledge deficit
Spiritual distress

KNOWLEDGE BASE FOR ASSESSMENT

Sexuality

Sexuality refers to a person's perceptions, thoughts, feelings, and behaviors related to sexual identity and sexual interaction with others. Individuals who do not engage in sexual intercourse or coitus are sexual beings. Expressions of sexuality are not limited to sexual intercourse or coitus but include the manner in which people project themselves as sexual beings, and the way they respond to others as sexual beings.

Adult sexuality has been broadly classified as procreative or nonprocreative. Procreative expressions of sexuality are associated with childbearing. In women, these expressions cease with menopause. Nonprocreative sexuality refers to behaviors involving sexual satisfaction that are noted in persons of all ages, whether or not they are involved in sexual relationships with others.

Sexual Health

The World Health Organization defines sexual health as follows:

> The integration of the somatic, emotional, intellectual and social aspects of sexual being in ways that enhance personality, communication, and love. Every person has a right to receive information and to consider accepting sexual relationships for pleasure as well as for procreation.

Sexual health is promoted when the individual has the ability to enjoy and control sexual behavior and reproduction in harmony with personal and social values. There should be freedom from psychological factors such as fear, shame, and guilt that may inhibit sexual responses and sexual relationships. Also, physiologic factors such as organic disease, deficiencies, and disorders should not interfere with sexual and reproductive functions.

Gender Identity

Gender and gender identity are two different concepts. Gender is traditionally assigned at birth and is based on external genitalia ("It's a boy"). Gender identity is a sense of being male or female; it usually develops in children between the ages of 2 and 3 years ("I'm a girl"). Although gender and gender identity are generally in harmony, it is not unheard of for some men and women to feel "trapped" in the wrong gender body.

Sex Role (Gender Role)

Roles involve a set of expectations about a person's position in life (see Chap. 14 for a more thorough discussion of roles). Sex roles, based on gender, are assigned at birth. Assigning maleness or femaleness establishes expectations for appropriate role behaviors. In the United States, for example, girl babies are often dressed in pink, whereas boys are dressed in blue. Infant clothing for girls may be trimmed with flowers or laces, whereas clothing for boys is frequently adorned with athletic symbols such as footballs or with boats. Parents often choose names for newborns that are considered either boy or girl names. Because of these early attempts to establish a child's sex role on the basis of anatomy, sex roles are learned through socialization. Consequently, cultural norms, role models, personal values, sexual experiences, and other factors ultimately influence individual performance of the sex role.

During the 1960s, attention began to focus on the impact of negative influences associated with male and female roles in the United States. Stereotypical male behavior (masculine) expectations can be identified as aggressiveness, strength, dominance, endurance, toughness, and orientation to achievement. On the other hand, stereotypical female behavior (feminine) can be identified as submissive, delicate, passive, sensitive, and emotional (teary). Such stereotypes promoted myths about appropriate masculine and feminine behaviors, which may have a negative impact on both sexual and physical well-being.

Forrester (1986) has suggested that sex role stereotypes are a contributing factor to higher mortality rates and lower life expectancies in men than in women. For example, cardiovascular disease may be linked to type "A" behavior, which is described as aggressive, competitive behaviors. Also, because men have been told most of their developing years not to cry and to "act like a man," they may be more likely to ignore signs and symptoms of health problems and delay preventive or palliative health care. Traditionally, men receive less health care than women during their adult years, even when differences in life expectancy are considered.

Similarly, sex role stereotypes have had a negative impact on women. For example, the "super-mom" who attempts to do it all (*i.e.*, have a career and family) is placed under undue stress when attempting to perform *all* of her wife–mother sex role along with her career role. Also, women who have experienced menopause are often viewed (even by the women themselves) as having lost their feminine appeal; as a result, middle-aged women are at higher risk for depressive disorders and low self-esteem.

In the last 30 years, sex role expectations have been changing and have been open to negotiation. Men are beginning to be more active in traditional female roles such as nurturing and caregiving of small children. Women are also beginning to be more represented in traditional male roles such as corporate executive and politician. This blending of sex role behavior (androgynous role—possession of both masculine and feminine characteristics) is becoming more common and is becoming synonymous with health. Sex roles, even if changing, vary among people and may have a profound impact on sexuality and overall health.

Sexual Response Patterns

An understanding of normal sexual responses assists with identifying misconceptions and the need for information about sexual matters. For example, elderly men often believe that impotence accompanies the aging process. This myth is based on the misconception that certain physio-

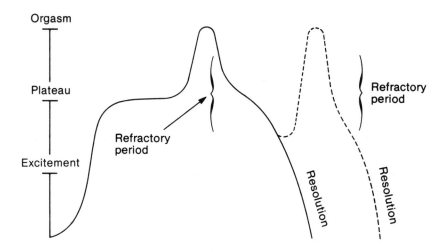

Figure 15-1. Male sexual response cycle.

logic changes associated with aging prevent sexual activi-ties. The changes that occur may alter sexual response but do not lead to impotence. Many adolescents believe that women do not ovulate for the first few years after menar-che. This myth could result in an undesired pregnancy. Be-cause sexual myths may cause unnecessary anxiety and/or unsafe sexual practices, identification and discussion of such myths should occur when assessing a person's sexual functions and beliefs.

THE SEXUAL RESPONSE CYCLE

The sexual response cycle reflects an interaction between sexual function, sexual identity, and sexual relationships. Masters and Johnson's (1970) studies during the 1960s re-vealed that response to sexual arousal was related to geni-tal tissue changes, extragenital changes, and subjective or feeling states. Sexual response cycles were identified for men and women (Figs. 15-1 and 15-2). The phases are ex-citement, plateau, orgasm, and resolution. Normal varia-tions were noted between men and women as well as among persons of the same gender. For example, some women experience multiple orgasms following sexual arousal and others do not reach orgasm at all.

Excitement. Sexual response is characterized by two main physiologic changes that begin during the excitement phase: vasocongestion and myotonia. *Vasocongestion,* the primary response to sexual stimulation, results from local-ized pooling of venous blood, occurs in response to erotic stimuli, and is influenced by steroid sex hormones. In men, penile erection and increased scrotal size are attributed to vasocongestion. Vasocongestion in women incudes en-largement of the clitoris, elongation of the clitoral shaft, and vaginal lubrication. Vaginal lubrication is the result of fluid transudating across vaginal mucous membranes. The Bartholin's glands secrete no lubrication during the excite-ment phase.

Myotonia involves an increase in muscular tension result-ing in involuntary muscle contractions that occur through-out the body. In men, the testes elevate in response to con-traction of the cremaster muscle and retraction of the spermatic cord. In women, irregular contractions of the vaginal vault occur, increasing the vaginal vault in width and length. The uterus may rise in response to muscle con-tractions in the surrounding tissues. Extragenital myotonic responses of both genders include nipple erection, tension of the long muscles of the arms and legs, and involuntary contraction of the abdominal and intercostal muscles.

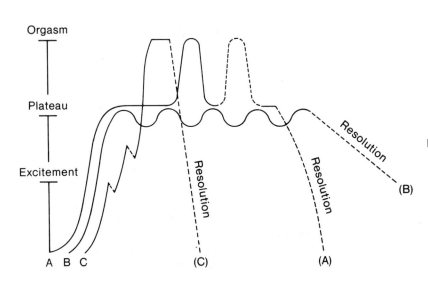

Figure 15-2. Female sexual response cycle.

The excitement phase may last from minutes to hours. Erotic stimuli may be psychic or sensory. For example, reading erotic literature, rubbing lotion on the body, smelling a particular fragrance, fantasizing, dreams, or giving verbal messages are stimuli capable of including excitement. Interpretation of erotic stimuli varies greatly among people. For instance, some people may be socially conditioned to find certain stimuli offensive rather than erotic.

The excitement phase may be interrupted by distracting stimuli such as a baby crying or the telephone ringing. Psychic stimuli, such as guilt feelings, anxiety, or stress, may also interrupt this phase. For men, distracting stimuli may cause loss of erection. The person may become anxious about sexual performance during the excitement phase, especially if he or she does not understand the effects of distracting stimuli on normal sexual function.

Plateau. The plateau phase follows excitement and is characterized by an increase in sexual tension as vasocongestion and myotonia intensify. A woman will experience increasing vasocongestion in the labia and lower vagina and retraction of the clitoris. Color changes secondary to vasocongestion may occur. The labia minora may change from pink to dark blue, indicating impending orgasm. The vagina continues to expand in length and width. Several drops of lubricant may be secreted from Bartholin's glands to augment vaginal lubrication. The plateau phase does not always lead to orgasmic resolution in women (see Fig. 15-2). Many factors, including the amount of sexual stimulation and psychological factors such as stress, can affect the nature of the plateau response.

During the plateau phase, the penis increases in circumference at the coronal ridge. The testes also continue to enlarge and are fully elevated just before ejaculation. The penis may have a bluish color change as vasocongestion continues. A small amount of mucoid lubricating fluid containing active spermatozoa, may be secreted from Cowper's glands. Typically, the plateau phase lasts from 30 seconds to 3 minutes.

Extragenial responses occur in both sexes. Breast engorgement and marked nipple erection may occur in both sexes. The skin may become flushed, a phenomenon sometimes referred to as "sex rash." Hyperventilation usually occurs toward the end of the plateau phase. Heart rates increase from 100 to 175 beats/minute. The average heart rate increases up to 120 beats/minute or more for relatively short periods of approximately 15 seconds. Systolic blood pressure may elevate 20 to 80 mm Hg, and diastolic pressure may increase by 10 to 40 mm Hg. Generally, men have higher blood pressure elevations during the plateau phase than women.

Orgasm. Orgasm involves the involuntary resolution of vasocongestion and muscle tension through a series of 5 to 12 muscle contractions. The contractions decrease in intensity and frequency during orgasm, which last from 3 to 15 seconds. Female orgasmic response is most intense in the area called the orgasmic platform, which includes the outer third of the vagina and labia minora. Male orgasmic contractions are felt most intensely along the penile urethra and help propel ejaculate. In men, the internal bladder sphincter is closed during ejaculation, preventing retrograde ejaculation into the bladder.

Extragenital responses parallel those occurring during plateau. Heart and respiratory rates increase, blood pressure elevates, there is involuntary muscle contraction, and skin flushing, and diaphoresis may occur.

Women may experience a series of orgasms with only brief returns to the plateau phase (see Fig. 15-2). Men generally require longer returns to the plateau phase before subsequent orgasms. Although individual responses are highly variable, the Kinsey studies (1965) indicated that only 15% of the population is capable of multiple orgasms (orgasms occurring within seconds or minutes of each other). Women are more likely to experience multiple orgasms than men; this tendency persists with age. However, men may experience more than one orgasm in a short time span provided that the sexual response cycle is reinitiated at the excitement phase.

Resolution. During the resolution phase, vasocongestion and myotonia dissipate entirely. If orgasm has not been achieved, the resolution phase will be longer. In women, genital organs gradually return to their normal positions, swelling subsides, and skin color returns to pre-excitement tones. In men, genital organs return to their pre-excitement size. Heart and respiration rates and blood pressure return to baseline levels.

During part of the resolution phase, the refractory period, men cannot be restimulated to orgasm. The length of the refractory period varies usually between 10 and 30 minutes.

Influencing Factor. Sexual response is an integrated biologic function involving the entire body, sexual identity, and sexual relationship. Anything affecting any one component can influence the sexual response cycle. Fear and pain are strong antagonists of sexual desire. Other factors, such as illness, medications, environmental changes, and emotional stimuli, can influence the sexual response cycle. If sexual desire is not perceived as appropriate or other behaviors more important, it is possible to diminish sexual response urges.

THE HEALTH HISTORY

Certain attitudes or assumptions on the part of the interviewer can act as barriers to obtaining a health history. These barriers should be overcome to ensure accurate collection of relevant data. It is important not to allow personal prejudices or aversions to develop toward the client or to inject your own values, morals, or beliefs into the discussion. Nor should the nurse assume that sexuality or sexual matters are not important to the client or that certain sexual behaviors are practiced or preferred. For instance, do not assume on the basis of appearance or stereotypes that a person is monogamous, homosexual, or asexual. Waterhouse and Metcalfe (1991) found that the overwhelming majority of clients (regardless of gender, age, educational level, and marital status) reported that nurses should discuss sexual concerns with clients.

Being sure of your own knowledge of sexual matters and making every effort to understand the views, perceptions, and language of the client will help open communication and will convey a professional attitude about the importance of sexual function in health promotion.

General Guidelines for Sexual History

Questions about sexuality should be incorporated into the initial interview. Frequently, this aspect of assessment is postponed until a sense of rapport exists between the client and the interviewer. Many people do need time to develop a trusting relationship with a nurse before they are comfortable discussing personal matters. However, including questions about sexuality in the initial interview conveys the message that sexuality is a natural part of life and has health implications in the same way that nutrition, elimination, and activity do. Introducing the subject early in the assessment process also gives the person permission to discuss any sexual concern or problems.

A screening interview may be sufficient to determine if any problems need to be discussed. The conversation can be prefaced with a statement concerning the importance of sexuality to healthy functioning or by noting that certain illnesses, medications, surgery, stress, or other factors may affect sexual functioning. The following screening questions may be appropriate to initiate a discussion:

> From what we have discussed so far, it appears that there have been many recent changes in your life-style. How has this affected your sexual activities?
> Sometimes people who have had surgery such as yours wonder about future sexual activity. What concerns or questions do you have about sex? What concerns do you think your partner has about resuming sexual activity?
> How has this illness affected your sexual functions?

Such introductory questions may encourage further discussion. On the other hand, the person may have no perceived sexual concerns to discuss or may be reluctant to continue the discussion because of embarrassment or discomfort. Whatever the response, it is wise to accept it and to invite further questions at a time when the client feels more comfortable about discussing such matters.

Privacy and Confidentiality. One reason people are reluctant to discuss sexual matters is the fear that their conversation will be overheard or divulged to others. To ensure privacy in the hospital setting, the interview should be conducted where other people, including roommates, will not overhear the conversation. Waiting until others have left the room or using a private conference room can avoid the possibility of embarrassment. The discussion should be initiated without family or sexual partners present. With the client's permission, the family or partners may be included during subsequent discussions or teaching sessions.

The interview on this subject should be conducted by one care provider rather than several. Asking a person to discuss intimate subjects repeatedly may cause anxiety, embarrassment, or guilt and is unnecessary. Ideally, one person should interview the client and share pertinent information with other care providers. Based on the person's response to initial sexuality screening questions, a decision should be made about who should initiate an in-depth interview, if indicated. For example, if the person states that impotence is a problem with his or her spouse but not with other partners, a referral may be made to a sex therapist.

If notes are recorded during the interview, the person may become concerned about confidentiality. Such concerns can be alleviated by stating at the beginning that parts of the interview are to be entered on the record and the reason for doing so. Requesting permission is also appropriate and may be phrased as follows: "It would be helpful to record some of your concerns in your health record. Is that okay with you?" If a referral seems in order, you might state, "A specialist in this clinic may be most helpful in answering some of your specific concerns about sexual relations. May I put some of our conversation in your record so that he or she can follow through?" Be careful to document only data necessary for ensuring continuity of care, ensuring the client's privacy.

Structure. Extensive guidelines and interview questions have been developed for obtaining and recording a sexual history. Usually, specialized professionals such as sex therapists will use a more structured lengthy approach. For the initial assessment and screening interview, questions about sexual matters should be kept to a minimum. The purpose of the screening interview is to identify any specific sexual concerns or problems and to determine if the client needs further information or referrals.

The need for more extensive questioning may be indicated by the presence of specific sexually related problems. For example, if the client you are interviewing is seeking treatment for a STD, it is essential to ask specific questions about his or her sexual partners and knowledge of disease transmission and prevention.

Beginning the Discussion. To initiate a more general discussion and to relieve anxiety, the conversation may be geared initially to clinically oriented and less sensitive topics. For example, cervical Pap smears may be discussed with a woman before discussing sexual intercourse. A discussion about nocturnal emissions could proceed a discussion about masturbation. If the sexuality interview is part of general history taking, then the interview can begin with less intimate questions, such as questions about work, family, or favorite pastimes.

Facilitating Communication. When asking questions about sexuality, phrase questions in a nonthreatening manner so as not to stir guilty feelings or resentment. You may preface certain questions in a specific way to indicate that the behavior is normal. Consider the following examples:

> Many people find masturbation a way to. . . .
> Many people feel uncomfortable discussing sexual problems. . . .
> It is not unusual to feel unsure about resuming sexual relations. . . .
> In Kinsey's study over half the men had at least one homosexual experience. . . .

Because the interview provides an opportunity to dispel sexual myths, questions should be phrased accordingly, as follows:

> Many people believe that withdrawing the penis from the vagina before ejaculation is an effective way to prevent pregnancy. Actually this is not true because sperm are released before ejaculation. What type of concerns do you have about preventing pregnancy?
> Some women mistakenly believe that they cannot resume sexual relations after a hysterectomy. How do you feel about sexual relations since your surgery?

Generally, questions that require a yes or no answer should be avoided. For example, "Are there any concerns about your sex life?" may elicit less information than a more open-

Interview Guide Sexuality and Reproductive Pattern

A structured interview guide may be used to facilitate data collection. The headings on this interview form correlate with major interview areas discussed in the text. Items may be deleted if deemed inappropriate for age or situation. Items should also be adapted to correlate with the developmental age and sexual activity of the individual. Remember that the very young or very old individual may be sexually active.

Sex Roles and Gender Identification

Gender _____

Sexual life-style (preference and activity) _____

Has any health problem or condition interfered with your ability to be a mother/father, wife/husband, daughter/son? _____
_____

What questions do you have with your sex roles or gender identification? _____
_____

Knowledge About Sexuality and Reproduction

Do you have any questions about reproduction or sexuality? _____
_____

People sometimes experience changes in sexual function with (name of illness/condition/injury); have you received any information about this? _____ What concerns do you have about this? _____
_____

People sometimes have questions about how their illness/condition/injury will affect sexual aspects of their lives; what type of concerns do you have? _____

Sexual Performance and Satisfaction

Are your sexual relationships satisfying to you? _____

Has anything changed that interferes with your ability to achieve satisfying sexual relationships? _____

What concerns do you have about your sexual performance? _____

Reproductive History

Both Genders

Method of family planning/birth control _____

Method for protection against sexually transmitted diseases _____

History of sexually transmitted diseases (STDs) _____
_____

Symptoms of STDs in sexual partners _____

Any pain or discomfort with intercourse? _____

Any history of sexual abuse? _____ Status of abuse and need for or currently in therapy _____

Male

Medical history: Endocrine disorders _____

Prostate problems (difficulty urinating) _____

History of genital/reproductive surgery _____

Perform monthly testicular self-examination (TSE)? _____

Any question about confidence to detect abnormal findings with TSE? _____

Female

Age at menarche _____

Menstrual pattern: interval between periods _____ duration of periods _____ amount and pattern of flow _____ last menstrual period _____

Associated discomforts: cramps _____ tension _____ pain _____ bloating/swelling _____ premenstrual syndrome _____

Describe discomforts _____

Pregnancy: number of pregnancies _____, number of live births _____, number of stillbirths _____, number of abortions/miscarriages _____

Any pregnancy or delivery complications? _____

Medical–surgical history: Endocrine disorders _____

Gynecologic surgeries _____

Last Pap smear date _____ Results _____

(continued)

Interview Guide Sexuality and Reproductive Pattern (continued)

Breasts: Last mammogram _____ Results _____
Perform monthly breast self-examination (BSE)? _____
Any question about confidence to detect abnormal findings with BSE? _____
_____
Detection of lump _____ Location, size _____
When found _____ Any changes during menstrual cycle? _____
Family history of breast cancer: Mother (age) _____
Sister (age) _____ Other relative _____
Breast surgery _____
Menopause: Onset _____ Any symptoms such as vaginal lubrication changes _____ mood changes _____
hot flashes _____
Describe (pattern, trigger, pattern of spread, degree of life-style disruption) _____
_____

ended question such as "Can you tell me how the accident has affected your sexual relations?"

Choosing Appropriate Terminology. Derogatory or judgmental terms should be avoided during the interview. Using terms such as promiscuous, unfaithful or inadequate may convey a judgmental attitude and may block further discussion. Using words such as wife, husband, or girl friend may also reflect incorrect assumptions. Using more general terms such as sexual partner or mate will help you maintain a more neutral approach.

Technical terms such as erection or orgasm may sound intimidating or may not be understood. On the other hand, slang terminology may be offensive or embarrassing. Finding a common ground for understanding or describing sexual activity will allow for a more natural flow of information. It is essential that the terms be clarified and understood. For example, a woman may state that her "bottom" feels itchy following sexual intercourse. Does bottom refer to rectum, vagina, or labia? A person may use slang to describe sexual practice. If the meaning is not clear to you, take a matter-of-fact approach, such as asking the person to explain the terms.

Even legitimate-sounding terms may need to be defined. For example, if a man reports that he is "impotent," it is important to determine if this means that he is unable to obtain an erection or if it means he has a problem only with certain partners or in certain circumstances. Perhaps he is referring to something totally different, such as infertility?

Children require a different approach because they use a special vocabulary to refer to sexual matters or genitalia. If a 5-year-old boy refers to his penis as "pee-pee," then you should use this term with him to ensure understanding. If necessary, the child's parents can help clarify and identify such terms.

Components of the Interview

An interview focused on sexual and reproductive function should emphasize the following general topics (see the Interview Guide):

- Sex roles and gender identification
- Knowledge about sexuality and reproduction
- Concerns about sexual performance and satisfaction
- A history related to the reproductive system

The circumstances of the interview will determine the topics discussed and the depth to which they are discussed. For example, interviewing a sexual assault victim entails an entirely different approach that will be discussed later in this chapter.

SEX ROLES AND GENDER IDENTIFICATION

Understanding the manner in which a person perceives his or her sex role contributes to a broader understanding of the person. For example, a married woman may perceive her sex role in terms of being a wife and mother. She may see herself as providing guidance and help to their children and giving and receiving emotional support and sexual companionship from her husband. Obviously, if she is hospitalized, especially for a prolonged period, these roles will be disrupted. Providing opportunities for her to fulfill these roles to some extent will help her cope. For example, during her husband's visits, privacy might be provided so that sexual and emotional intimacy can be expressed. Her children can be allowed to visit so that she can hold or kiss them or hear about their daily activities.

For many women, developmental milestones such as menarche, pregnancy, and menopause may threaten perceived sex roles. Both genders may feel threatened by relationship transitions, such as the loss of a lover through divorce, separation, or death. Because of stereotyped sex roles that emphasize invulnerability and strength, many men feel less masculine following life-threatening illnesses such as a myocardial infarction. Any illness or surgery involving reproductive organs, such as a vasectomy, hysterectomy, or prostate surgery may threaten sex roles. Finally, changes in body image following hair loss, mastectomy, ostomy surgery, amputation, or other disfigurements or disabilities may cause concern or conflict about sex roles and

Table 15–2. Physiologic Alterations, Sexual Function, and Teaching Needs

Sexual Activity Problems	Teaching Needs
Cancer and associated treatment (surgery, radiation, chemotherapy)	
Decreased physical energy	Fatigue and debilitation commonly alter libido and forms of sexual expression.
Fears about touching and causing harm	Alternative coital positions to avoid physical contact with painful surgical or radiation sites.
Fear of inducing bleeding if thrombocytopenic	Alternative forms of sexual expression.
Fear of infection if immunosuppressed	Good oral and perineal hygiene; "safe sex" practices.
	Avoid anal intercourse, which is associated with greater risk of abscess formation.
Body image disturbance	Depression is a common reaction to changes in body image and may alter libido.
	Full impact of mutilating surgery on body image may not be felt for 2 or 3 months.
Oral mucosa ulceration following chemotherapy or radiation	Avoid oral contact.
Anger	Anger secondary to cancer diagnosis may be directed toward healthy sexual partner.
Ostomy	
Concerns about stoma leakage, odors, and possible stoma damage during sexual activity	Empty stoma before sexual activity.
	Dietary means to control stoma discharge and odors.
	Sexual activity will not harm stoma.
Body image disturbance related to stoma	Open communication with sexual partner is important.
	Stoma can be covered during sexual activity.
Decreased physical energy and libido following ostomy surgery	May affect potency; may take several months after surgery to regain strength and functional abilities; alternate sexual positions may conserve energy.
Cardiovascular disorders	
Fear of additional cardiac damage	Resumption of sexual activity usually safe 5 to 8 weeks after MI (patient should consult physician).
	Symptoms indicating adverse cardiac response to intercourse: rapid heart and respiratory rates persisting 10 minutes after orgasm, or extreme fatigue the following day are indications to consult physician.
	Avoid intercourse immediately after large meals, excessive alcohol intake, in hot or humid weather, when extremely anxious or tired, or with unfamiliar partners.
Partner's fear of causing the other harm	A common response; open discussion of fears important.
Depression	Depression is a common post-MI response that may persist for several months; may adversely affect libido.
Spinal cord injury/multiple sclerosis	
Paralysis and weakness making sexual activity difficult and certain coital positions impossible	Alternate forms of sexual expression and alternate coital positions.
Inability to achieve or maintain an erection	Patients with upper motor neuron involvement have high percentage of reflexogenic erections (physically stimulated erections); psychogenic erections (stimulated by thought or emotion) are rare.
	Patients with lower motor neuron involvement have higher incidence of psychogenic erections and lower incidence of reflexogenic erections.
	Erectile ability after spinal cord injury is highly variable.
Loss of pelvic sensation (men and women)	Sexual enjoyment is often decreased; loss of sensation and pelvic vasocongestion may cause lack of orgasm.
Concerns about involuntary bowel or bladder emptying during sexual activity	Empty bowel or bladder before sexual activity; indwelling catheters may be removed before sexual activity or left in place (men can fold and tape catheter back along penis and wear a condom; women can tape catheter to one side). Good hygiene is important to reduce transmission of chronic urinary tract infections.

(continued)

Table 15–2. Physiologic Alterations, Sexual Function, and Teaching Needs (continued)

Sexual Activity Problems	Teaching Needs
Diabetes mellitus	
Males: erectile dysfunction Females: orgasmic dysfunction	Affects 50% males, 33% females Sexual desire usually remains constant. Increased foreplay may be helpful.
Frequent vaginitis interferes with sexual activity	Avoid pantyhose, wear cotton underwear, monitor vaginal pH; a water-soluble lubricant useful if dyspareunia present
Concerns about having children: fear of pregnancy for diabetic women related to higher stillbirth and risk of neonate health problems; for diabetic father, concerns about fertility—reduced sperm count and volume; and concerns of either parent for genetic transmission.	Adequate diabetic control and physician supervision should decrease risk of stillbirth and health problems. Genetic counseling may be helpful. Having intercourse on day of ovulation and abstaining before ovulation may increase chance of fertilization.

function, not only for the client but also for his or her partner.

The following approaches may be helpful when interviewing the client about usual sex roles and role transitions caused by events such as hospitalization, illness, or normal growth and development:

What does this surgery (illness, disability) mean to you as a woman (or man)?
How do you think this pregnancy will change you life or your feelings about yourself or family?
How do you think this illness (surgery) will alter your sexual functioning after you leave the hospital?
How do you expect your ability to function as a wife (husband, lover, mother, father) will change?

Further inquiries about the client's sexual life-style may be necessary if such information is considered important. Care must be taken to elicit this information in a nonjudgmental matter. Inquiring about a person's sexual lifestyle means asking about sexual activity and preferences such as heterosexual, homosexual, or bisexual orientation and whether he or she values monogamous relationships. Conflict can occur over sex roles. The perceived ideal sex role or socially dominant sex role may be very different from the perceived actual sex role. Such conflict may result in dissatisfaction with sex roles, or gender identification. In some cases, personal conflict about sex roles may require professional counseling.

KNOWLEDGE ABOUT SEXUALITY AND REPRODUCTION

Inadequate knowledge may contribute to sexual dysfunction; genital disease, including STDs; HIV disease; unwanted pregnancy; or anxiety about sexual functioning. Certain illnesses and physiologic alterations, such as cancer, ostomies, cardiovascular disease, diabetes mellitus, spinal cord injury, and multiple sclerosis, have sexual ramifications that necessitate patient teaching. The types of sexual problems and teaching needs associated with these disorders are presented in Table 15-2. Each person has unique needs and should be encouraged to express such needs. If additional information is needed, consultation with a specialist may be indicated.

CONCERNS ABOUT SEXUAL PERFORMANCE AND SATISFACTION

Sexual dysfunction often can be attributed to problems or dissatisfaction with sexual performance, which in turn may affect or be affected by other problems. For example, fatigue, anxiety, and depression can interfere with sexual performance or even sexual desire and should be discussed. The perception of poor sexual function may also reinforce a low self-concept ("I can't do anything right"). Medications and normal, healthy aging can also contribute to alterations in sexual performance (Display 15-1). Questions about such factors should be posed in a manner that will not suggest a problem where one does not exist. For example, it is not wise to say "Most men become impotent from this drug. Has this happened to you yet?" Rather, the question can be rephrased to allow for a more extensive response: "Some people, taking similar medications, experience changes in sexual function. What concerns do you have about this?"

REPRODUCTIVE HISTORY

Questions about reproductive history are usually directed toward women and concern such topics as onset of menarche, menstrual patterns, pregnancy, past medical and surgical problems, and menopause. The following areas are typically discussed with respect to a woman's reproductive history:

- Age at menarche
- Menstrual patterns (interval between periods; duration, amount, and pattern of flow; associated discomfort such as pain, cramping, tension, premenstrual syndrome; last menstrual period or last normal menstrual period)
- Pregnancy and contraception (types of contraception used; number of pregnancies and outcome of each; pregnancy or delivery complications; desired number of children)
- Medical–surgical history (endocrine disorders, STDs, gynecologic-breast surgery)
- Menopause (onset and pattern; hot flashes, including trigger, pattern of spread, degree of life-style disrup-

Display 15–1
Medication and Sexual Function

Alcohol

May release inhibitions and promote relaxation. May interfere with sexual function because it may act as central nervous system depressant, suppress motor activity, and induce diuresis.

Amyl Nitrate

Questionable effect on sexual function. May potentiate intensity of orgasm by genitourinary tract vasodilation and smooth muscle relaxation.

Antidepressants

(amitriptyline, desipramine, imipramine, nortriptyline, pargyline, phenelzine sulfate, protriptyline)
May interfere with sexual performance and libido because of central nervous system depression and peripheral blockade of nerve innervation of sex glands/organs.

Antihistamines

(chlorpheniramine, diphenhydramine, promethazine)
May have negative effect on sexual function due to blockade of parasympathetic innervation of sexual glands or organs.

Antihypertensives

(clonidine, methyldopa, beta-blockers, reserpine, trimethaphan)
May impair sexual performance by peripheral blockade of nerves involved in sexual function.

Antispasmodics

(glycopyrrolate methobromide, hexocyclium, methantheline, poldine)
May impair sexual performance by ganglionic blockade of nerves involved in sexual function.

Barbiturates

May impair sexual function secondary to central nervous system depression, suppression of motor activity, and hypnosis.

Caffeine

Questionable effect on sexual function; acts as central nervous system stimulant.

Cantharis (Spanish fly)

Considered an aphrodisiac by some although there is no basis for this claim; generally irritating and inflammatory to genitourinary tract mucosa; may result in systemic poisoning.

Cimetidine

Associated with reduced sperm counts (though still within the normal range), gynecomastia, and loss of libido or impotence (rare).

Diuretics

May interfere with sexual activity secondary to diuresis.

Lithium Carbonate

Specific effects questionable; may interfere with sexual function secondary to broad endocrine alterations and diuresis.

Narcotics and Psychoactive Drugs

(amphetamines, cocaine, heroin, LSD, marijuana, methadone, morphine)
May transiently enhance sexual function by releasing inhibitions, increasing suggestability, and promoting relaxation. May interfere with sexual function secondary to central nervous system depression, loss of libido, and impotence.

Sedatives and Tranquilizers

(chlordiazepoxide, chlorpromazine, diazepam, methaqualone, prochlorperazine, thioridazine)
May promote sexual function by relaxation. May interfere with sexual function secondary to central nervous system depression, blockade of autonomic innervation of sex glands or organs, suppression of hypothalamic and pituitary function.

Vitamin E

Questionable effects—promotes fertility in laboratory animals.

tion; vaginal lubrication changes; other changes; estrogen replacement therapy)

Interviewing Sexual Abuse or Assault Victims

Victims of sexual abuse or assault often experience extensive psychological and emotional trauma. The expression of the psychological trauma may be delayed for years if sexual abuse occurred during early childhood. The interview should be directed at eliciting specific details for medical and legal purposes. In addition, specialized crisis intervention techniques should be used to support the victim's feelings and associated behaviors. Generally, nurses who interview sex crime victims have received special education and are frequently available through emergency departments on a 24-hour, emergency basis. Understanding the basic interviewing principles will help the nurse who has initial contact with such victims. In general, the following principles are applicable:

- The most qualified available staff member should conduct the interview.
- The number of people who interview the victim should be kept to a minimum.
- The interview should be conducted before the physical examination.
- A quiet, private setting free from interruptions should be selected for the interview.
- Time should be taken to establish rapport with the victim and explain the purpose of the interview.
- According to institutional policy, you may have to ask about the following: characteristics and identity, if known, of the assailant; type of assaultive activity that took place, including orifices that were penetrated; time and place of the assault; threats made by the assailant; significant others the victim wants contacted; immediate emotional needs of the victim; and extent of any injuries.

Because of lack of maturity and vulnerability, any sexual activity with or without consent between a minor child and an adult (or other child significantly older than the minor child) is considered sexual abuse. Minor children cannot legally provide consent because they cannot fully understand the consequences of their consent. Mentally retarded adults, depending upon cognitive ability, may or may not be able to give consent, and are vulnerable to sexual abuse and assault. Violence is rarely needed to force children into sexual acts because they can be easily coaxed, bribed, enticed, or intimidated. Usually a child is told that such acts are part of a special game that must be kept secret. A secrecy pact is often made through threats or coercion. The abuser may say, for example, "If you tell anyone, I won't love you any more" or "If you tell anyone, I'll kill your mother."

In such cases, effective interviewing skills are needed to obtain information from the victim, who has already been told not to talk and who may feel shame and guilt. Additionally, children do not have the adult vocabulary to describe the abuser's actions. However, one should be suspicious when a child is sexually precocious in speech, mannerism, and dress. Special media such as drawing or playing with anatomically correct dolls may facilitate communication. Children may also be reluctant to discuss sexual abuse because the threat of being removed from the parents' care is greater than the threat of continued abuse. Children and mentally retarded adults may find such approaches helpful and less threatening when describing abusive acts. Important principles to keep in mind when interviewing sexually abused children and lower functioning mentally retarded adults include the following:

- Parents, other family members, or friends should not be present until it is certain that such persons are not the abuser. The parent's presence may heighten the child's feelings of guilt and shame.
- The parents and family members should be interviewed separately at the same time the child is interviewed. Parents need an opportunity to ventilate feelings and receive emotional support.
- Use sexual language comprehensible to the child's language development, preferably their own terms.
- Asking a child to draw pictures may be less threatening than asking him or her to describe incidents of sexual abuse. Encourage the child to draw himself or herself, the offender, and what happened, and to describe their drawings.
- Anatomically correct dolls may be used to encourage the child to describe the assault or assaults.

Victims of sexual assault may experience delayed reactions to the incident. Female adult incest survivors often seek professional help as adults because of relationship problems, depression, and substance abuse. Sexual assault victims may have problems with somatic symptoms and psychological and sexual functioning. Victims often report an absence or reduction of sexual feelings and desires following an attack. Other common emotional reactions include anger, fear, guilt, helplessness, feeling "dirty," numbness, and not wanting to be alone. In some cases, either peer or professional counseling is indicated.

The primary responsibility of the nurse is to identify manifestations of Rape trauma syndrome and to make appropriate referrals. It is also important to be aware that trauma from sexual assault can be a long-standing phenomenon that persists for months or years after the assault occurred. The victim may also have a short-term fear of pregnancy (pregnancy testing can be performed in less than 2 months after the assault) and the long-term fear of contracting HIV (AIDS) disease (an incubation period of several years). Equally important is the prompt, precise documentation of data; all of the victim's records as well as the professional staff are likely to be subpoenaed if there is a court case.

DIAGNOSTIC STUDIES

A complete sexuality assessment includes consideration of laboratory results, including Pap smear for women; testing for sexually transmitted diseases such as VDLR (Venereal Disease Research Laboratories), *gonorrhea* culture,

Table 15–3. Pap Smear Classification

Class I	Absence of atypical cells
Class II	Atypical cells but no evidence of malignancy
Class III	Suggestive but not conclusive for malignancy
Class IV	Strongly suggestive of malignancy
Class V	Conclusive for malignancy

Chlamydia culture, wet slide preparations, and HIV; sperm counts; mammogram for women; pregnancy tests; ultrasonography of uterus; and amniotic fluid analysis.

The Pap smear, more properly known as Papanicolaou smear, is a cytology test for cervical cancer. There are five levels of findings that range from cells that are not abnormal to those that are conclusive for malignancy (Table 15-3). For more conclusive testing, a cervical biopsy or colposcopy (a speculum with a magnifying lens) is used to examine the vagina and cervix. Viral, fungal, and parasitic conditions can also be identified with Pap smears.

Diagnostic testing of sexually transmitted diseases is usually performed in high-risk populations, in pregnant women (to protect the fetus), and in people applying for a marriage license (typically VDLR and, in some states, HIV). The *VDLR* is a blood test used to detect syphilis. Two blood tests (enzyme immunoassay [EIA]; if positive, then Western blot test) are used to diagnose HIV disease. Cultures from the cervix in women and meatus in men are used to detect gonorrhea and chlamydia. Wet preparations of vaginal secretions on a slide and viewed with a microscope are used to detect *Candida* (a fungus) and *Trichomonas* (a parasite).

Several tests are used to test for fertility. In men, the most simple test is a sperm count. The semen is tested for the amount of fluid and sperm present. Less than 20 million sperm/mL is considered low. The sperm are also assessed for mobility (initial and sustained), maturity, and abnormalities. For women, the least intrusive diagnostic test for fertility is monitoring *basal body temperature* each morning to determine if ovulation is occurring. When ovulation occurs, there is a drop and then a sharp increase in body temperature. The sperm can be tested to determine if the woman has developed antibodies that destroy the sperm. Other more elaborate diagnostic tests, such as laparoscopy, fluoroscopic x-rays of the uterus and fallopian tubes (hysterosalpingography), and endometrial biopsy, may be performed to assess the uterus and cervix, and to test for patency of the fallopian tubes. Other tests for endocrine abnormalities may be performed. The presence of infection, inflammation of the reproductive organs, or malnutrition can result in infertility.

Mammograms are x-rays of the breasts to detect the presence of tumors and cysts. Benign cysts are generally well defined and tend to be bilateral, whereas malignant tumors are irregular, poorly defined, and tend to be unilateral. Abnormalities can be detected with mammograms before they are palpable. Ultrasonography (ultrasounds are beamed into the tissue and reflected by body tissue) can also be used to detect breast abnormalities. This is usually performed after an abnormality is discovered on the mammogram.

Diagnostic tests routinely used in pregnancy include pregnancy tests and ultrasonography. Other screening tests, such as Pap smears, testing for sexually transmitted diseases, and blood tests such as a complete blood count are also routinely performed to establish health status. Amniocentesis may be performed if the woman is over 35 years old, if there is a history of genetic disorders, to determine lung maturity if caesarean section is required, and if there are any questions regarding the status of the fetus. *Home pregnancy tests* are readily available and are often used by women before they seek health care. Pregnancy tests measure the presence of human chorionic gonadotropin hormone, which is produced only in pregnant women by the trophoblast cells of placental tissue. *Ultrasonography* is used to confirm pregnancy, note fetal and placental position, detect abnormalities such as heart and neurotube defects, confirm gestation, and identify gender. The purpose of the *amniocentesis* is to remove amniotic fluid for analysis. This is done any time after 16 weeks' gestation. Amniotic fluid analysis can reveal chromosomal disorders such as Down syndrome, neurotube defects, inborn errors of metabolism, and lung maturity. *Chorionic villus sampling,* in which a sample of placental material is obtained and analyzed, can be performed from 9 to 12 weeks' gestation and provides information about the fetus at an earlier stage. Chorionic villus sampling provides most of the same information as amniocentesis, except it does not provide information about lung maturity.

THE PHYSICAL EXAMINATION

Assessment Focus and Overview

Generally speaking, the interview is helpful in providing information about the person's sexuality and sexual concerns. The physical assessment provides information about the status of reproductive organs. However, certain sexual dysfunctions may be related to changes in physical function. For example, cardiovascular or neurologic disorders may affect the sexual response cycle. Consequently, physical assessment findings can be used to support conclusions based on the interview data.

The following physical examination skills are most helpful when evaluating reproductive structures and functions:

- Breast examination
- Female genital and pelvic assessment
- Male genital assessment
- Rectal assessment (see Chap. 8)

Teaching breast and testicular self-examination techniques is considered part of health management (see Chap. 76). During pregnancy, breast tissue and other systems undergo predictable changes, which are discussed in this chapter (see Physical Changes During Pregnancy).

When STDs are detected, related areas such as the genitals, mouth, and rectum should be examined and specimens obtained for further laboratory analysis.

Associated Body System Alterations

Physical indicators from other assessment areas may assist you in diagnosing problems in the sexuality pattern. Some related body system alterations may be observable in the cardiovascular, respiratory, and musculoskeletal systems. Individuals who easily fatigue, have shortness of breath, or problems such as rheumatoid arthritis may have difficulty with sexual satisfaction. Individuals with new abdominal ostomies may fear leakage during sexual contact and avoid coitus. Para- and quadriplegics may fear loss of sexual ability and sexuality self-identity changes. Additionally, an individual with disfiguring injuries or surgeries may experience a change in sexual identity and fear being sexually repulsive to his or her mate.

ELIMINATION PROBLEMS RELATED TO PELVIC ALTERATIONS

Cystocele. A cystocele is caused by herniation of the posterior bladder wall into the vagina and is more common in multiparous women (see Chap. 9). Altered urinary elimination patterns are common and include urinary frequency, dysuria, stress and/or urgency incontinence. The woman may also report a feeling of vaginal fullness. Pelvic examination usually reveals a soft, reducible mass that bulges into the vagina and is accentuated by straining.

Rectocele. A rectocele is a rectovaginal hernia caused by rupture of the fibrous structures between the vagina and rectum, which usually occurs during childbirth. Altered bowel elimination patterns may be noted, including constipation, aggravated by hemorrhoids, anal fissures, and fecal lodgement in the rectocele pouch (see Chap. 9). The client may report vaginal or rectal fullness. The rectocele may be noted as a bulging perineum when the woman strains. Alternatively, a bulging lower, posterior portion of the vagina may be noted, often without using a speculum. A rectal examination will probably enable you to feel the rectal pouching.

FEMALE GENITALS AND PELVIC STRUCTURES

Anatomy and Physiology Overview

Examining the female reproductive structures involves the external genitals and internal structures.

External Genitals. Visible external genitalia include the mons pubis, labia majora, labia minora, clitoral prepuce, clitoral glans, urinary meatus, vaginal orifice, hymen, and perineum (Fig. 15-3). The labia can be separated to bring the clitoral glans, urinary meatus, and vaginal orifice into view. The appearance of female genitalia varies depending on the stage of growth and development, and individual differences. Therefore, graphic drawings or photos of female genitalia should be used as general guides.

The *mons pubis* is a fatty pad over the symphysis pubis and is usually covered with hair after puberty. However, hair may be sparsely distributed in women who shave this area and in older women.

Vulva is a term used to refer collectively to the following structures: labia major and minora, clitoral prepuce and glans, and vaginal orifice. The labia majora, also called the outer lips, are large folds of adipose tissue extending from the mons publis to the perineum. The outer surfaces are covered with hair after puberty, the inner surfaces are smooth and moist. The labia minora, or inner lips, are thin-

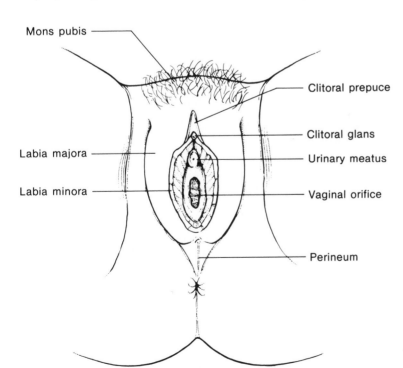

Figure 15–3. External female genitals.

ner skin folds that surround the vaginal and urethral openings. The boat-shaped area between the two labia minora is also known as the vestibule. The labia minor are very vascular and are subject to some degree of vasocongestion (vascular engorgement) during sexual arousal and pregnancy. Vascular engorgement may cause a variable increase in tissue size, which may persist even in an unaroused state; consequently, the labia minora may protrude between the labia majora. This occurs to a greater extent following childbirth, which causes concern for some women.

Just below the mons pubis is the *clitoral prepuce,* a small fold (or folds) of tissue covering the *clitoris.* The clitoris has three parts: the visible glans, a rounded structure varying in size; a body (corpus); and two bands of fibrous tissue, or

crura, that attach the structure to the pelvic bones. The clitoral structures contain many anastomosing blood vessels that become engorged during sexual arousal. Clitoral tissue has erectile properties and is homologous to the male penis.

The *urinary meatus* is located approximately midway between the clitoris and vaginal orifice. Although the sphincter-like structure is often represented as a small, circular, doughnut-shaped orifice on drawings and models, it is not easily visualized because it may blend with surrounding skin folds (see Fig. 15-3). In some cases, however, trauma from catheters, assault, or other factors may exaggerate the meatal opening. The meatus may be more visible if the skin is stretched with the fingers or if the woman bears down as though having a bowel movement. The

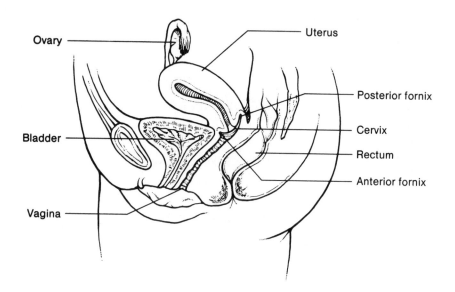

Figure 15–4. Internal female genital structures.

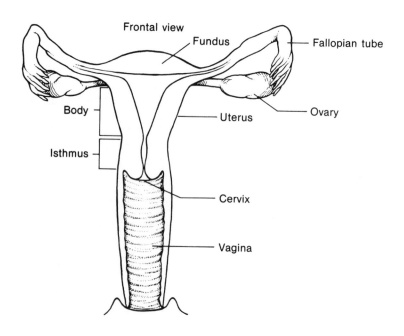

ducts of Skene's glands, on either side of the urinary meatus, may be visible if the margins of the meatus are gently spread apart.

The *vaginal orifice (vaginal introitus)* or opening may be partially occluded by a mucous membrane, the *hymen*. The hymen usually tears in response to trauma such as that associated with tampon use, sexual intercourse, or other vaginal penetrations. Occasionally, the hymen may be elastic enough to remain intact after penetration. The ruptured hymen shrinks in size and may appear as a fringe of skin around the vaginal opening. The ductal openings of Bartholin's glands, located on each side of the lower vaginal opening, secrete small amounts of mucoid lubrication during the plateau phase of sexual arousal and are rarely noted on examination.

The *perineum* refers to the area between the lower border of the vaginal opening and the rectum.

Internal Structures. The internal structures include the vagina, cervix, uterus, and adnexa.

The *vagina* is tubular, rugated, 11 to 15 cm long, and extends from the vaginal orifice to the uterus (Fig. 15-4). This structure is lined with mucous membrane composed of squamous epithelial cells, is surrounded by layers of longitudinal and circular muscles, and has a rich arterial and venous blood supply. When not aroused, the vagina is collapsed. A vaginal speculum may be used during the physical examination to distend the vaginal wall. The angle of the vagina is directed backward and then upward over the pelvic floor or slanted toward the small of the back. At the terminal end, the projection of the cervix produces the posterior, anterior, and two lateral fornices. Uterine structures may be palpated through the thin fornix walls.

The *cervix* is the lower neck of the uterus and projects into the terminal portion of the vagina. The cervical opening to the vagina, the *cervical os,* is visible when the vagina is examined with a speculum. A *nonparous cervical os,* which has not been dilated by childbirth, appears as a small, round depression. A *parous cervical os,* dilated by childbirth, will appear larger and irregularly shaped, usually as a slit. The *uterus* is an inverted pear-shaped, muscular organ oriented at a right angle to the vagina, or anteverted in most women, and located between the bladder and rectum. It is composed of the upper body of fundus, the isthmus, which is a narrower section between the fundus and the cervix. In some women, the uterus may be retroverted and the body of the uterus may be felt immediately above the posterior fornix. The *fallopian tubes,* each approximately 10 cm long, extend between the fundus and the ovaries and allow ova to pass into the uterus. The two *ovaries* are almond-shaped and vary in size among women, with the average size being 4 cm in length, 2 cm in width, and 2.5 cm thick. They are usually located near the lateral pelvic wall, in line with the anterosuperior iliac spines. The term *adnexa* refers collectively to the ovaries, fallopian tubes, and supporting muscles and ligaments.

Musculature. The three major groups of pelvic muscles include the superficial muscles, the urogenital diaphragm, and levator ani muscles (Fig. 15-5). Contractions of the pelvic muscles enhance orgasm and affect the ability to control urinary flow. The levator ani muscles are composed of several muscles that form a hammock-like support to the pelvic floor. Poor muscle tone in this area has been associated with urinary stress incontinence. People can be taught to exercise the levator ani muscles by voluntary contraction of these muscles as though stopping the flow of urine or tightening the anal sphincter (Kegel exercises). Not only do such exercises help control stress incontinence, but several weeks of toning may result in stronger orgasms.

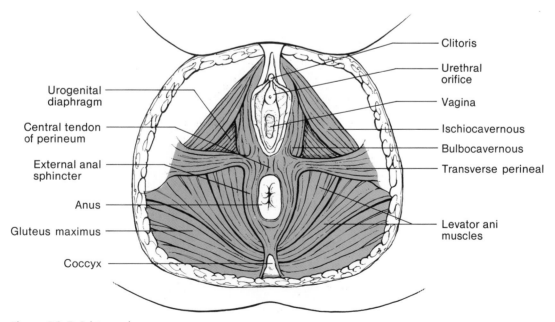

Figure 15–5. Pelvic muscles.

Physical Examination

Female Genitals and Pelvic Structures

General Principles

The female genital structures and pelvis are examined by inspection and palpation, using a vaginal speculum. At the beginning of the assessment both hands should be gloved. Later for bimanual palpation, the glove can be removed from the hand used for palpating the abdomen. The assessment begins with inspection of the external genitals and progresses to palpation of the vaginal opening, inspection of the vagina and cervix with the vaginal speculum, bimanual palpation to assess internal pelvic structures, and, in some cases, rectovaginal palpation.

Minimizing Anxiety

Women often have negative feelings about pelvic assessments and may even avoid recommended health screening practices such as Pap tests to detect cervical cancer because they dread the assessment. Some women feel anxious about the pelvic assessment because they have been taught that their genitals are unclean or shameful, or they fear the genitals emit embarrassing odors or secretions. Many women have adverse feelings about the pelvic assessment because they feel a loss of control during the procedure (Domar, 1986). Some women, because of cultural or personal beliefs, feel more comfortable with a woman performing the assessment than a man. In addition, they may view the lithotomy position as having a sexual implication, or the position may be associated with feelings of helplessness and vulnerability. The fact that the woman is usually draped during the examination prevents her from seeing what is being done. Lack of eye contact between the examiner and the woman may inhibit communication, causing feelings of depersonalization. Feelings of discomfort can be compounded by a lack of understanding about the procedure. Being aware of such fears and concerns allows you to reassure the woman by offering support and guidance and to provide a warm, friendly atmosphere.

Because women generally view the pelvic examination as something unpleasant to endure, you should make every effort to reduce this anxiety by providing adequate explanations and being as sensitive as possible. Begin explaining before the examination rather than after the woman is in the lithotomy position so she has an opportunity to anticipate what will happen and thereby maintain a sense of personal control. The purpose of the assessment, the basic steps of the procedure, and any associated discomfort should be described before the assessment. One way to help the woman understand the assessment is to give her a hand-held mirror so she can view her genitals as you explain anatomy, physiology, and the procedure (Fig. 15-6). Some women prefer not to view the assessment with a mirror; you should respect their decision.

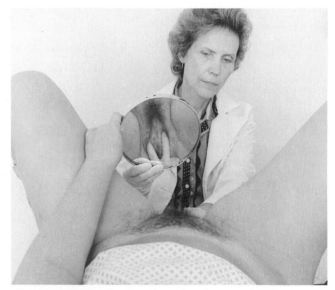

Figure 15–6. Use of a mirror during the pelvic examination.

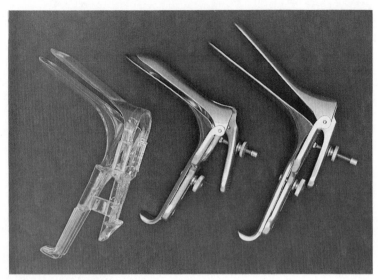

Figure 15–7. Vaginal specula.

Basic instructions for relaxing pelvic muscles during the assessment will help give the woman time to implement relaxation techniques. In addition, if she wishes to have someone present during the assessment, every effort should be made to accommodate this request. In the United States, male examiners often have a female associate present. Any conversation between the examiner and the associate should include the woman. Joking with the client or anyone else during the assessment may cause the woman to feel degraded or embarrassed.

Equipment

- Gloves: nonsterile, examination type
- Water-soluble lubricant (KY jelly, Lubrifax)
- Vaginal speculum
- Hand-held mirror
- Goose-neck lamp
- Glass slides, sterile cotton tip applicators, wooden spatulae, fixative (for specimens), culture media (if screening for STDs)

Vaginal Specula

The vaginal speculum is used to inspect the vagina and cervix. The speculum may be made of metal or disposable plastic. The plastic specula, although they are clear, are usually more uncomfortable. Specula vary in size and shape (see Fig. 15-7). Graves specula are somewhat larger than Pedersen specula, which are used if the vaginal orifice is very small. The speculum has two blades that are spread to open the vaginal orifice, and a level or screw device for opening and closing the blades. Proficiency in using the speculum can be gained by practicing opening and closing the blades.

Before the speculum is inserted, it is warmed by running the blades under warm water. The client's natural vaginal secretions are usually sufficient lubrication to allow the speculum to be inserted. If additional lubrication is necessary, warm water poured over the blades is usually sufficient. Lubricating cream, jellies, and lotions are not advisable because they interfere with specimen collection for analysis. Furthermore, such substances may irritate vaginal tissues.

Preparation and Positioning

Before the pelvic assessment, instruct the client to empty her bladder. Although the lithotomy position is uncomfortable, it is the most effective position for the pelvic assessment. Help the client into the lithotomy position by having her lie supine on the examining table. Place her feet in the stirrups to help support the legs. In some instances, for women in labor or with limited joint motion, stirrups are not used. Instead, a modified lithotomy position on a bed can be substituted. When stirrups are used, the buttocks should be at the edge of the examining table, with the knees dropped to the sides and the heels in the stirrups. You should be seated, facing the

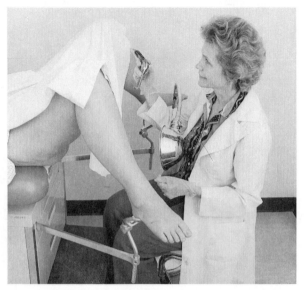

Figure 15–8. Pelvic examination: position of patient and examiner.

genitals, while inspecting and assessing with the speculum (Fig.15-8). During the last half of the assessment, you may stand to perform bimanual palpation.

Women may wear stockings or shoes and should be kept warm to prevent additional muscle tensing that could increase discomfort. The upper body should be covered either by the examining gown or street clothes, if other body parts are not being assessed. Tensing of the abdominal muscles can also be decreased by placing a small pillow or folded towel under her head and instructing her to place her arms at her side or folded across her chest. She should not lie with arms over her head.

The woman is draped by placing a small sheet over her legs and pushing the center of the drape down enough to provide eye contact between you and the client. You should observe facial expressions for signs of pain or anxiety. If the client prefers to watch or does not want a drape, the drape is eliminated.

Good lighting is essential, especially while inspecting the cervix. A goose-neck lamp at the end of the table is usually sufficient.

Hygiene Techniques

A water-soluble lubricant should be placed on the gloved fingers to facilitate vaginal penetration during the bimanual assessment. Ideally, the lubricant is dispensed from small, disposable tubes intended for single use that lower the risk of contamination of the lubricant. The lubricant is obtained from a large tube that is used repeatedly. The tube should be squeezed in a manner that allows lubricant to drop to the gloved fingers. The gloved fingers should not be placed against the opening of the tube, which could contaminate the contents.

The vagina should never be examined after the rectum unless you rewash your hands and change gloves. If a vaginal infection is present or suspected, gloves should be changed between the vaginal and rectal assessments to prevent inadvertent spread of infection to the rectum. After the examination, wipe any excess lubricant from the genitals with tissues, using firm strokes from the pubis to rectum. The woman may wish to wipe the area herself.

Examination and Documentation Focus

- *External genitals:* Color and pigmentation, contour and symmetry, discharge, lesions, masses, infestations
- *Vaginal structures:* Skin integrity, cervical contour and position, color, lesions or discharges of the cervix and vagina, vaginal muscle tone
- *Uterus:* Position, contour, and consistency; mobility; masses; pain or discomfort on palpation
- *Adnexa:* Size, contour, and consistency of the ovaries; masses; discomfort on palpation

Examination Guidelines *Female Genitals and Pelvic Structures*

Procedure

1. INSPECT THE EXTERNAL GENITALS.

   a. Help the client into lithotomy position. To prevent pelvic muscle tensing, touch the back of her thigh with the back of your hand before touching the genitals.

   b. Use the fingers of nondominant hand to gently spread the labia so the clitoris, urinary meatus, and vaginal opening are clearly visible. Note any skin lesions or discharge and pubic hair distribution and color.

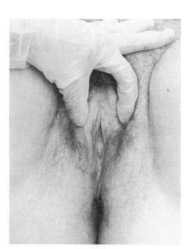

External genital inspection

2. PALPATE SKENE'S AND BARTHOLIN'S GLANDS.

   a. While spreading the labia with nondominant hand, insert the index finger of your other hand into the vagina. Palpate Skene's glands by gently exerting pressure against the anterior vaginal wall, moving your finger from inside to outside the vagina.

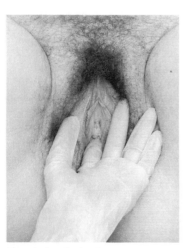

Skene's gland palpation

Clinical Significance

Normal Findings

The color of the labia minora varies from pale pink to red. Bluish or brown pigmentation may be noted. It should be slightly darker than the rest of the skin color, sometimes resembling lip color. The skin surrounding the labia should have pink or brown undertones. The labia majora usually appears symmetric, and the labia minora ranges in shape from triangular to semicircular. Edges of the labia minora appear smooth or irregular and may protrude through the labia majora.

Normal vaginal discharge: Odorless, nonirritating vaginal discharge is normal with appearance varying according to the menstrual cycle. Following menstruation, a slight, white discharge may be noted. Toward ovulation, a thin clear discharge usually occurs. Following ovulation, the discharge may again be thickened and appear white. Some women note changes in discharge or cervical mucus color and consistency, to estimate ovulation for either pregnancy or contraception purposes.

Deviations from Normal

Bright red skin color is abnormal and commonly associated with vaginal yeast infections. Abnormal vaginal discharge is strong smelling, discolored, or purulent and may be associated with vaginal itching. Genital lesions, masses, and lice infestations are abnormal.

Normal Findings

No discharge should be noted.

Deviations from Normal

Discharge from the urinary meatus with this maneuver is abnormal, and any discharge should be cultured.

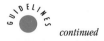
continued

Female Genitals and Pelvic Structures

Procedure

b. Palpate Bartholin's glands on each side of the posterior vaginal opening by placing your index finger inside the vagina at the lower lateral aspect and your thumb opposite the labia majora. Gently squeeze the skin between thumb and index finger.

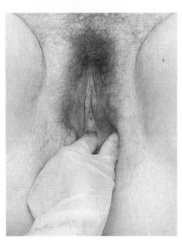

Bartholin's gland palpation

3. EVALUATE VAGINAL MUSCULATURE.

a. To evaluate muscle tone, insert your index finger 2–4 cm into the vagina; ask the woman to squeeze around your finger.

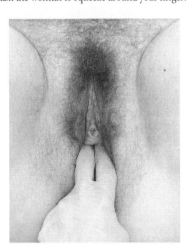

Evaluating vaginal musculature

b. Place your middle and index fingers at the lower border of the vaginal orifice and spread the labia majora by displacing the fingers laterally. Ask the woman to bear down so that you can inspect the vaginal orifice. Note any bulging, which may indicate cystocele or rectocele, and any release of urine.

Clinical Significance

Normal Findings

The glands and ducts should not be palpable.

Deviations from Normal

Discharge or discomfort may indicate inflammation of Bartholin's gland. Swelling is abnormal and may indicate a plugged duct.

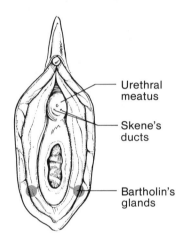

- Urethral meatus
- Skene's ducts
- Bartholin's glands

Normal Findings

Good vaginal muscle tone is indicated by the ability to tighten the vagina around the examiner's finger. Muscle tone is usually firmer in nulliparous women.

Normal Findings

You should feel no bulging.

Deviations from Normal

Cystocele: Herniation of the bladder into the vagina

Rectocele: Herniation of the rectal wall into the vagina

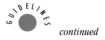

Female Genitals and Pelvic Structures

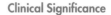

Procedure

Clinical Significance

4. INSERT THE VAGINAL SPECULUM.

   a. Open the vaginal orifice by placing your index and middle fingers just inside the lower vagina and gently press down.

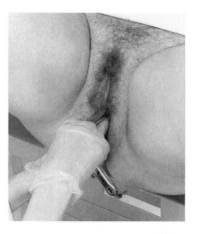

   b. Direct the closed, prewarmed speculum blades over your fingers into the vagina at a 45-degree angle, following the natural contour of the posterior vaginal wall. Insert the blades obliquely to minimize discomfort. Be careful not to scrape or pinch genital tissue or pull pubic hairs. Insertion may be difficult if the woman tenses the pelvic muscles. If this occurs, stop advancing the speculum momentarily and remind the woman to relax. Instruct her to take slow, deep breaths and exhale through slightly pursed lips in order to relax. Then continue advancing the speculum.

   c. When the speculum is inserted, remove your fingers holding the lower vagina open and gently rotate the speculum so the blades are oriented horizontally. Partially open the blades by pressing the speculum lever with your thumb.

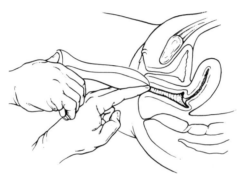

Vaginal speculum insertion

   d. Look through the open blades for the cervix. The cervix will be in full view if the blades are correctly located in the anterior and posterior fornices. If the cervix is not fully visible, slowly close the blades, withdraw the speculum slightly, and reinsert at a slightly different angle.

   e. Once the cervix is clearly visible, lock the blades in the open position by turning the thumbscrew (metal speculum) or completely depressing the lever (plastic speculum).

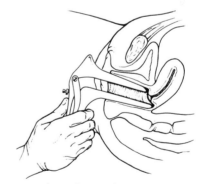

Vaginal speculum in place

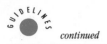

continued

Female Genitals and Pelvic Structures

Procedure

5. INSPECT THE CERVIX.

   a. Look through the open blades to inspect the cervix. Adjust external light source if necessary.

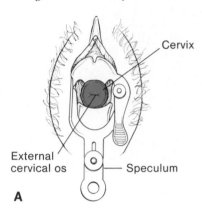

Cervix

External cervical os — Speculum

A

Nonparous external os

Parous external os

B

The cervix

6. OBTAIN CERVICAL SPECIMENS (OPTIONAL).

   Cervical specimens may be obtained for cytology evaluation (Pap smear), pathogen identification (gonorrhea culture), or fertility evaluation (postcoital, cervical mucus evaluation). Three techniques may be used to obtain specimen.

   a. The cervical scraping technique involves inserting a specially designed wooden spatula (Ayre spatula), through the open speculum blades. Place the spatula against the cervix and scrape by rotating the instrument 360 degrees against the cervical surface. Withdraw the instrument and smear both sides of the spatula end gently across a glass slide. Spray the specimen with a fixative solution.

Clinical Significance

Normal Findings

Shape and position: The cervix is a rounded structure, 3 to 4 cm in diameter, protruding about 2.5 cm into the vagina. The position of the cervix is determined by the configuration of the uterus. For example, in most women the cervix is directed posteriorly. However, when the uterus is retroverted, the cervix is directed anteriorly. Normally, the cervix appears midline rather than laterally displaced. The cervical os, or opening, appears as a small round depression in the nulliparous woman and as a flat slit in the parous woman.

Color: The cervix is usually pink and generally appears paler after menopause. In the pregnant woman, bluish pigmentation usually occurs by the sixth week. Oral contraceptives may cause dark pink to reddish cervical pigmentation.

Deviations from Normal

Cervix size: A cervix larger than 4 cm in diameter or a lateral diversion is abnormal and should be evaluated.

Lesions: Because the cervix may tear during childbirth, the parous woman may have cervical scarring from healed lacerations. Cervical lesions may indicate serious pathology or infections and should always be thoroughly evaluated. A relatively benign lesion, nabothian cysts, appear secondary to cervical gland duct obstruction. Such cysts may occur in groups as small, yellowish papules less than 1 cm in diameter. A string protruding from the cervical os usually indicates an intrauterine device (IUD) used for contraception.

Discharge: Colored or purulent discharge is abnormal. Bloody discharge except during menses is abnormal.

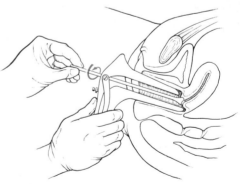

Cervical scraping with wooden spatula

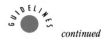

Female Genitals and Pelvic Structures

Procedure

b. The endocervical swab technique involves inserting a sterile, cotton-tipped applicator through the cervical os about 0.5 cm. Rotate the applicator 360 degrees with your fingers and leave the applicator tip in place several seconds to allow saturation. Withdraw the applicator and gently brush the speculum across a glass slide and spray with a fixative.

c. The vaginal pool technique is performed with the wooden spatula. Insert the spatula through the speculum blades to the posterior fornix. Scrape this area; remove the spatula; transfer the material to glass slide and spray with a fixative.

Clinical Significance

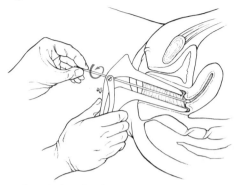

Endocervical swab technique

Normal Findings

Vaginal appearance: The walls of the vagina appear pinkish in color with rugae, ridge-like structures caused by folding of the mucous membranes. Normal vaginal secretions may give the vagina a shiny or wet appearance. The walls may be pale pink with fewer rugae in post menopausal women.

Deviations from Normal

Discharge: Any discharge other than clear or white-creamy and thin should be described according to color, consistency, amount, and appearance.

Vagina: A pale vagina may indicate anemia. A red vagina is indicative of an inflammation process and should be evaluated.

7. INSPECT THE VAGINA.

Inspect the walls of the vagina as you remove the vaginal speculum. Release the locking device that holds the speculum open, being careful to manually hold the speculum open as you begin to withdraw. Removing a partially open speculum may cause pain or pinch tissue if the blades are suddenly snapped shut at the vaginal opening. Once the cervix is no longer visible, allow the speculum to close slowly so that the blades are completely closed when the speculum is withdrawn through the vaginal opening.

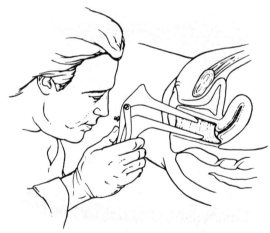

Vaginal inspection while withdrawing the speculum

8. PALPATE THE VAGINA AND CERVIX.

a. While standing, use your index and middle fingers, which are gloved and lubricated, to palpate the vagina.

b. Insert your fingers, following the natural vaginal contour, by exerting slight posterior pressure. Hold your thumb abducted and flex the other fingers. If the vaginal opening is very small, you can use one finger.

c. Palpate the vaginal wall and note nodules, masses, or tenderness. Palpate the cervix and note position, mobility, consistency, and tenderness.

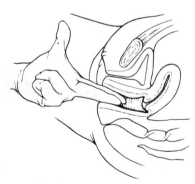

Vaginal palpation

Normal Findings

The cervix is firm, like the tip of the nose, and mobile.

Deviations from Normal

Palpable masses are abnormal. Do not mistake vaginal rugae for masses. Any tenderness or immobility of the cervix should be evaluated.

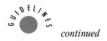

continued

Female Genitals and Pelvic Structures

Procedure

9. BIMANUALLY PALPATE THE PELVIC STRUCTURES.

   a. Remain standing with the index and middle fingers in the vagina.

   b. Place your other hand, which now may be ungloved, on the client's abdomen between the umbilicus and symphysis pubis.

   c. Use two hands to "trap" deeper pelvis structures, making palpation possible.

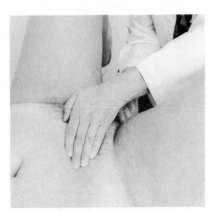

Bimanual palpation: Pelvic structures

d. Palpate the uterus by pressing the abdominal hand downward toward the vaginal hand, which is held firmly in the vagina, by exerting slight pressure against the perineum with your flexed, outside fingers. The uterus should be palpable just above the symphysis pubis. Palpate the anterior wall and fundus of the uterus and note any masses or tenderness.

Clinical Significance

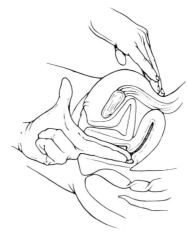

Bimanual palpation: Uterus

Normal Findings

The uterus is pear-shaped, firm, and smooth. The uterus should be slightly mobile when pressure is applied. The uterus of a nonpregnant woman is 7–8 cm long and 5 cm wide across the body of fundus. Slight discomfort secondary to muscle tensing may be noted with palpation.

Deviations from Normal

Masses, sharp pain, cramping, or enlarged nonpregnant uterus.

Retroverted uterus: A retroverted uterus is usually not palpable with this approach.

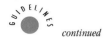
continued

Female Genitals and Pelvic Structures

Procedure

e. Move the vaginal fingers toward the left, lateral fornix and rotate this hand so that your palm is facing upward. Move the abdominal hand to the left lower quadrant. The ovary and adnexa, which are not always palpable, are now trapped between your two hands for evaluation. Use the vaginal hand for palpation. Press the abdominal hand toward the vaginal hand. Note any masses or tenderness as well as ovary size if palpable. Repeat on the right side.

Clinical Significance
Normal Findings
The fallopian tubes are usually not palpable. The ovaries may or may not be palpable and should feel small, firm, almond-shaped, mobile, and smooth, without masses. Slight discomfort on palpation is common.

Deviations from Normal
Palpation of ovaries larger than 6 cm, irregular or round shaped, pain on palpation.

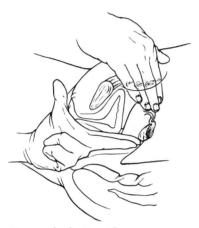

Bimanual palpation: Adnexa

10. PALPATE THE UTERUS AND ADNEXA USING THE RECTOVAGINAL APPROACH (OPTIONAL).

   a. Remove your fingers from the vagina and change the glove. A glove change guards against possible contamination of the rectum with vaginal secretions. Deep breathing helps to relax the anal sphincter.

   b. Lubricate the index and middle fingers of your newly gloved hand. Explain the procedure and ask the client to use relaxation breathing. Tell her she may feel sensations associated with having a bowel movement.

   c. Insert your index finger into the vagina and your middle finger into the rectum. Keep your index finger against the cervix so the rectal finger does not mistake the cervix for a rectal wall mass.

   d. Repeat the maneuvers used during bimanual palpation to evaluate the uterus and adnexa. With this technique, use the rectal finger to palpate the uterus and adnexa.

11. COMPLETE THE EXAMINATION.

   Remove your fingers and wipe perineum, using front-to-back strokes. Help the woman out of the stirrups and provide additional tissues for cleansing.

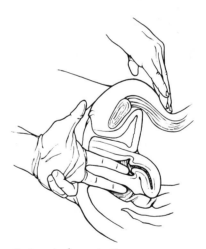

Rectovaginal examination

Documenting Female Genital and Pelvic Examination Findings

Example 1: Normal Findings

Ms. K, aged 33, had a pelvic assessment and Pap smear as part of the routine health assessment. The assessment findings were normal and were recorded as follows:

> External genitals and vagina moist, pink, without lesions or discharge. Cervical specimen for Pap obtained by endocervical swab. No visible cystocele or rectocele. Bimanual exam reveals no palpable masses, no tenderness: uterus midline, mobile, and anteverted.

The same findings may be summarized in the following problem-oriented format:

- S: Denies vaginal itching, pain, or discharge. Nonparous; uses barrier contraception—satisfied with method; regular menstrual periods with LMP 15 days ago. Here for annual Pap smear. All previous smears normal; no family history of pelvic cancer.
- O: External genitals and vagina moist, pink, without lesions or discharge. Nonparous cervical os, pink, midline with trace for clear discharge. Cervical specimen for Pap obtained by endocervical swab. No visible cystocele or rectocele. Bimanual exam reveals no palpable masses or tenderness. Uterus midline, mobile, and anteverted.
- A: Normal genital pelvic assessment.
- P: Follow up with routine exams. Notify about Pap results.

Example 2: Vulvovaginitis

Mrs.L., aged 23, had a genital–pelvic assessment after noticing vaginal itching and discharge. The findings were abnormal and were recorded as follows:

> Vulva and vagina erythematous, covered with patchy white, thick exudate. Parous cervical os, midline without discharge. Bimanual palpation reveals no masses; marked tenderness over right adnexa.

The same findings may be summarized in a problem-oriented format as follows:

- S: Reports intense vaginal pruritus accompanied by thick white discharge for 1 week. Denies history of similar problem, recent use of antibiotics, and diabetes mellitus. Taking oral contraceptives for 2 years.
- O: Vulva and vagina erythematous and covered with patchy, thick, white exudate. Parous cervical os midline without discharge. Bimanual palpation reveals no masses; marked tenderness over right adnexa.
- A: Vulvovaginitis—suspect monilial vaginitis.
- P: Refer to physician for confirmation and treatment. Instruct about administration of vaginal suppositories. Discuss risk factors for monilial vaginitis. Instruct to return if treatment ineffective.

Nursing Diagnoses Related to Female Genitals and Pelvic Structures

Currently, three nursing diagnoses in the sexuality pattern are related to assessment of the female genitals and pelvic structures: Rape-trauma syndromes, Altered sexuality pattern, and Sexual dysfunction. Nursing diagnoses from other functional patterns such as High risk for infection, Health-seeking behavior, Knowledge deficit, and Pain may also be appropriate depending upon examination findings.

Rape-Trauma Syndromes

The nursing diagnosis of Rape-trauma syndrome is appropriately used when an individual experiences a forced sexual assault against one's will and without consent. Sexual assault can be either vaginal, anal, oral, or a combination of any. The reaction to rape has short- and long-term implications. The nursing diagnosis Rape-trauma syndrome: compound reaction is noted when an individual after a rape event also experiences the reactivation of previous physical or psychosocial problems, or a reliance upon drugs and alcohol. The nursing diagnosis Rape-trauma syndrome: silent reaction is used when the individual exhibits signs and symptoms of rape trauma but does not tell anyone about the event. If the assault is recent, you may wish to refer this individual to another nurse or health professional with additional education.

History.   The individual may or may not report a sexual assault. During the acute phase of the rape-trauma syndrome, the individual may report gastrointestinal upset, genitourinary discomfort, and skeletal muscle discomfort. Verbalization of other responses may include insomnia, fear, anger, guilt, panic attacks, change in sexual behavior, and a distrust of others of the same gender as the rapist. Long-term effects of the rape may continue if resolution does not occur. In these situations, the individual may report phobias, nightmares, anxiety, and depression.

Physical Examination Findings.   Recent rape victims should be examined by an individual with expertise in rape victim examinations for legal purposes (see discussion on interviewing sexual abuse or assault victims in this chapter). Observe injuries such as ecchymoses, lacerations, and abrasions in recent victims. Observe emotional status and responses as well. After the initial examination, victims may avoid, refuse, or experience increased discomfort during future genital and pelvic examinations.

Altered Sexuality Pattern

The nursing diagnosis Altered sexuality is utilized when the individual experiences or is at risk of experiencing a change in sexual health or is concerned with her own sexuality.

History.   During the health history or during the examination, the individual may verbalize concerns about possible or actual difficulties, limitations, or changes in sexual behavior. Verbalizations about these concerns may be about fear of pregnancy or sexually transmitted diseases, concern about infertility, effects of new or worsening health problems or conditions (such as pregnancy, cancer, paraplegia, and multiple sclerosis), change in sexual response or reaction of partner, or sexual orientation or identity.

Physical Examination Findings. The individual's perception of the existence or probability of a problem may have more significance than physical findings. You may discover the presence or absence of pregnancy or sexually transmitted diseases, which may either reassure or distress the woman. Observing the individual during a discussion of sexuality may provide information about the presence of depression, withdrawn behavior, and low self-esteem.

Sexual Dysfunction

The nursing diagnosis Sexual dysfunction is used for the individual who is experiencing or is at high risk for experiencing a change in sexual function that is perceived as undesirable. The individual experiences a dissatisfaction with sexuality.

History. During the health history or during the physical examination, the individual may verbalize problems with sexuality, difficulty in fulfilling the sex (gender) role, inability to achieve sexual satisfaction, alteration in relationship with significant partner(s), or value/belief conflicts with others regarding sexual expression and practice.

Physical Examination Findings. There may be no direct genital or pelvic structure findings for this diagnosis; however, the woman who is unable to get into a lithotomy position because of discomfort or hip mobility restriction may experience difficulty in traditional sexual intercourse positions. Other physical findings that may indicate the necessity of different positions include pregnancy, abdominal obesity, and spinal cord injuries. The presence of Foley catheters may interfere with satisfaction. While examining the vagina, you may note excessive dryness or inflammation that can be a cause of pain during coitus.

Clinical Problems Related to Female Genital and Pelvic Assessment

Sexually Transmitted Diseases

Many organisms are transmitted by sexual contact. A person who contracts an STD may or may not have multiple sexual partners. For example, trichomonal infections may develop in the vagina when the normal vaginal flora is altered. A male sex partner of a woman with trichomonal infections may become infected but have no symptoms and therefore may not receive treatment. The woman may then be reinfected by the partner, meaning that the disease is sexually transmissible even in sexually monogamous relationships. Table 15-4 summarizes clinical features of major STDs. Often, clinical findings differ between genders because of anatomic differences in reproductive organs.

Gonorrhea

Gonorrhea, also called clap, is caused by the *Neisseria gonorrhoea* bacterium. The organism invades and inflames the columnar and transitional epithelium of the urethra, cervix, fallopian tubes, and Skene's and Bartholin's glands. Because the disease rarely affects the vulva, vagina, or uterus, many women are asymptomatic during the acute phase. In some women, the condition is first diagnosed when their male partner is treated for the disease.

In symptomatic women, gonorrhea has variable courses. Usually cervicitis develops. Symptoms range from slightly increased vaginal discharge to purulent discharge, urethritis, inflammation of Skene's and Bartholin's glands, and acute salpingitis, or pelvic inflammatory disease (PID). The diagnosis may be confirmed by isolating the gonococcus. A culture specimen should be obtained and applied to a Thayer–Martin culture medium.

Additional findings include discharge or tenderness during palpation of Skene's or Bartholin's glands. Salpingitis is indicated during bimanual pelvic palpation if cervical movement or adnexa palpation causes marked pain. Rectal infection may be characterized by rectal pain, itching, and purulent discharge.

Systemic manifestations include fever, prostration, and abdominal tenderness and guarding accompanying acute salpingitis; leukocytosis with left shift, nausea, and vomiting; gouty arthritis; and skin lesions. Fallopian tube damage may cause infertility.

Syphilis

Less common than gonorrhea, syphilis is caused by sexual transmission of the bacterium *Treponema pallidum*. If untreated, the disease is disseminated through the blood stream, ultimately affecting all body systems. The disease has five stages: incubation, primary, latency, secondary, and tertiary. Incubation and primary syphilis are noted by a primary lesion, called a chancre, a painless, ulcerated papule up to 2 cm in diameter. In women, the chancre most commonly occurs on the cervix or vagina and heals spontaneously within weeks. Regional lymph node involvement may cause enlargement and swelling of inguinal lymph nodes at this stage. Primary and secondary stages are separated by an asymptomatic latency period.

Secondary syphilis is characterized by systemic manifestations, especially the development of lesions on the skin and mucous membranes. These lesions are usually rash-like, bilateral, and symmetric. The hallmark of tertiary syphilis is the gumma lesion, a granulomatous lesion affecting the skin, bones, and viscera. Syphilis bacteria do not grow on routine culture media; therefore, the disease is diagnosed based on chancre appearance and serologic testing (VDLR).

Herpes

The *herpes simplex virus type 2 (HSV-2)* is most often implicated in genital infections, although HSV-1 may also be the infective agent. In both cases, similar genital lesions may be noted. The lesions are a grouping of small vesicles that eventually rupture and may ulcerate. Intense pain and itching are usually reported. Lesions usually heal in 4 to 6 weeks. In women, genital lesions are commonly distributed on the cervix, labia, vagina, and clitoris. Sexually transmitted herpes lesions may also occur in the mouth and anus.

(Text continues on pg. 471)

Table 15–4. Sexually Transmitted Diseases

Etiology and Incidence	Clinical Presentation	Diagnosis	Therapy	Complications
Syphilis: *Treponema pallidum* (spirochete)				
40,452 cases were reported in 1991. Highest reported case rates are in age group 20–24. Early syphilis increasing among women of childbearing age.	Incubation–10–90 days *Primary syphilis:* Classical chancre is painless, eroded lesion with a raised, indurated border. Atypical lesions common; multiple lesions may occur. Extragenital chancres may appear. Unilateral or bilateral lymphadenopathy may accompany. *Secondary syphilis:* Highly variable cutaneous and mucous membrane lesions, alopecia, generalized lymphadenopathy, mild cold symptoms.	Demonstration of *T. pallidum* from exudate of primary or secondary lesions by dark-field microscopy is definitive. Typical lesions (with or without the presence of treponemes) and a reactive (positive) reagent test result for syphilis (VDRL or RPR). FAT/ABS or MHA-TP can confirm questionable reagent test results. If the initial reagent test result is nonreactive, repeat test 1 wk, 1 mo, and 3 mo later.	*For early syphilis* (less than 1 yr duration): Benzathine penicillin G, 2.4 million units IM at 1st visit. Or aqueous procaine penicillin G, 4.8 million units total (600,000 units IM daily for 8 days). Or tetracycline HCl, 500 mg PO q.i.d. for 15 days. Or erythromycin, 500 mg q.i.d. for 15 days. *More than 1 yr duration:* Benzathine penicillin G, 2.4 million units IM 1 time/wk for 3 successive wk.	Complications at all stages are secondary to gumma lesions. Gummas, resulting from treponemal tissue invasion, are granulomatous lesions with necrotic centers. Gummas occur in visceral, cardiovascular, and nervous tissue. Associated clinical manifestations during late syphilis include the following: *Visceral gummas:* Alterations in liver, esophagus, stomach, intestines *Cardiovascular gummas:* Aortic valve incompetence, aneurysms, coronary artery disease *Neurologic gummas:* General paresis: dementia, euphoria, mania, depression, schizoid reactions. Argyll Robertson pupils, optic nerve atrophy *Tabes dorsalis:* Loss of sensation, locomotor ataxia, incontinence, constipation, pain or sensory disturbance, swelling joints secondary to posterior column invasion (Charcot's arthropathy), pathologic fractures *Congenital syphilis:* Fetus affected—crippling blindness, facial abnormalities, deafness, abortion, stillbirth
Gonorrhea: *Neisseria gonorrhoeae*				
586,638 cases reported in 1991. Highest reported case rates are in age group 20–24. First among reported communicable diseases in United States.	Incubation—Male: 3–30 days. Female: 3 days–indefinite time. Men have dysuria, frequency, and urethral discharge that is usually purulent and often more severe in the morning. Women experience vaginal discharge and cystitis. 10%–40% of men and about 10%–80% of women have no symptoms.	Presumptive identification—Microscopic identification of typical gram-negative, intracellular diplococci on direct smear of urethral exudate from men. Because sensitivity is low in females, smears *cannot* be substituted for culture or positive oxidase reaction of typical colonies from specimen obtained from anterior urethra, endocervix, anal canal, or oral pharynx and inoculated on selective media.	Aqueous procaine penicillin G, 4.8 million units IM at 2 sites with probenecid, 1 gm PO. Or tetracycline HCl, 0.5 gm PO q.i.d. for 5 days, 10 gm total. Or ampicillin, 3.5 gm. Or amoxicillin, 3 gm, either with probenecid, 1 gm PO. Reculture 3 to 5 days after therapy is completed. For penicillinase-producing *N. gonorrhoeae*, treat with spectinomycin, 2 gm IM. Or cefoxitin, 2 gm IM plus probenecid, 1 gm PO; single dose of 9 tablets trimethoprim sulfamethoxazole (for pharyngeal infection) for 5 days.	*In both sexes:* Primary gonococcal infections may affect the pharynx, conjunctivae, and anus. May cause blindness in infants infected at birth. Disseminated infections may result in meningitis, sepicemia, arthritis, and endocarditis. *In men:* Epididymitis Urethral stricture Prostatitis *In women:* Inflammation of Skene's or Bartholin's glands Pelvic inflammatory disease Tubo-ovarian abscesses

(continued)

Table 15–4. Sexually Transmitted Diseases (continued)

Etiology and Incidence	Clinical Presentation	Diagnosis	Therapy	Complications
Genital Herpes (Herpes Genitalis): Herpes simplex virus, types I and II				
300,000–500,000 new cases reported annually. Highest reported cases found in 20–29-year-olds. (10%–50% of genital herpes infection found to be type I.)	Incubation—Virus is dormant for a period lasting from 3 days to years. Virus migrates along sensory nerves into dorsal root ganglia, remaining inactive, nonreplicating until reactivated. Multiple shallow vesicles, lesions, or crusts occur on genital area, including buttocks and inner thighs. Inguinal adenopathy, dysuria, local pain, edema, fever are more severe with primary infections. Initial infection lasts 7–10 days; recurrent infection, 3–10 days.	Clinical appearance of herpetic lesions, Pap smears from lesions, stained to show multinucleated giant cells with intranuclear inclusion bodies (40% sensitivity). Tissue culture most definitive test.	No known cure. Symptoms may be relieved by warm baths, topical anesthetic, and systemic analgesic, and acyclovir ointment 5%. Apply sufficient quantities to cover all lesions every 3 hr 6 times a day for 7 days. Therapy should be instituted as early as possible after onset of signs and symptoms. (*Note:* Acyclovir has not been found to prevent recurrences and has not been tested in pregnant and lactating women.) Acyclovir IV may be prescribed.	Neonatal herpes infection Associated risk of cervical cancer Neuralgia, meningitis Ascending myelitis Urethral stricture Lymphatic suppuration
Chlamydia: *Chlamydia trachomatis*				
Estimated to be 2–4 million cases per year. Caused by *Chlamydia trachomatis* bacteria. Usually affects adolescents and young adults, especially those with multiple sex partners. Most common STD in the United States.	Frequently asymptomatic. Women may experience yellowish endocervical discharge, dysuria, acute salpingitis. Men may experience nonspecific urethritis (NGU; see discussion in this table).	Isolation of *C. trachomatis* on culture or antigen detection. Very difficult to diagnose.	Doxyciline Hyclate (Vibramycin) 100 mg PO b.i.d. for 7 days. *Or* tetracycline 500 mg PO q.i.d. for 7 days. *Or* erythromycin 500 mg PO q.i.d. for 7 days.	*Women:* Pelvic inflammatory disease (PID), which increases risk for sterility and ectopic pregnancies. Can develop chronic PID. If pregnant, risk of spontaneous abortion, stillbirth, and postpartum fever. *Men:* See NGU
Nongonococcal Urethritis (Nonspecific Urethritis, NSU, NGU)				
Chlamydia trachomatis—Estimated cause in 40% of cases. Ureaplasma urealyticum—Estimated cause in 40% of cases. Other etiological agents—*Trichomonas vaginalis*, *Candida albicans*, HSV, coliform bacteria: Estimated cause in 10%–20% of cases. Age distribution parallels that of other STDs, notably gonorrhea. Recurrences very common.	Incubation period—Appears to exceed 10 days in half of cases. Urethral discharge varies from profusely purulent to slightly mucoid. Dysuria may or may not be present. Some men may have asymptomatic infection; women asymptomatic; often appears following gonorrheal infection (postgonococcal urethritis) in 30% of treated infections.	Clinical picture of dysuria or urethral discharge with greater than or equal to 4 polymorphonuclear leukocytes on urethral smear negative for intracellular *N gonorrhoeae* and negative culture for gonorrhea on modified Thayer-Martin medium. Chlamydia trachomatis difficult to diagnose.	Tetracycline, 500 mg q.i.d. for 7 days. *Or* erythromycin, 500 mg q.i.d. for 7 days. *Or* Doxycycline, 100 mg PO b.i.d. for 7 days.	Epididymitis Sterility Prostatitis Proctitis Urethral strictures Neonatal ophthalmia or pneumonia
Vulvovaginitis: *Gardernerella Vaginalis* (Formerly *Corynebacterium vaginale* or *Haemophilus vaginalis*)				
Cultured from 23%–96% of women with vaginitis. Recovered from 0%–52% of asymptomatic women.	Nondescript thick or thin, occasionally frothy vaginal discharge, usually gray-white. Punctate hemorrhages and vulvar irritation are occasionally seen. 10%–40% of culture-positive patients have no symptoms. Foul, fishy amine odor.	Clinical picture, microscopic examination, or culture. Gram stain or KOH wet mount of vaginal exudate may show tiny, gram-negative coccobacilli ("clue cells") adhering to vaginal epithelial cells and the presence of white cells, though specificity of this finding is low.	Metronidazole, 500 mg PO b.i.d. for 7 days. Alternative regimen: Ampicillin, 500 mg PO 4 times a day for 7 days—less effective but suggested for pregnant women.	None

(continued)

Table 15–4. Sexually Transmitted Diseases (continued)

Etiology and Incidence	Clinical Presentation	Diagnosis	Therapy	Complications
Candidiasis (Moniliasis): *Candida albicans*				
Saprophytic in the oropharyngeal and gastrointestinal tracts in 25%–50% of the population and in the vagina of 25%–50% of asymptomatic women.	Vulva is usually erythematous and edematous. Vaginal discharge, may be thick and white, resembling cottage cheese. Occasionally discharge is thin and watery. Satellite lesions may spread to the groin. Many women have no symptoms. Male sexual partners may develop balanitis or cutaneous lesions on penis.	Microscopic examination of gram-stained smears of introital or vaginal wall scrapings. Microscopic examination of KOH wet mount of vaginal discharge. Culture on Sabouraud's modified agar.	Nystatin vaginal suppositories b.i.d. for 7 to 14 days or Miconazole vaginal cream q.d. for 7 days. (now available in nonprescription form)	Increased risk of neonatal thrush
Trichomoniasis: *Trichomonas vaginalis*				
Prevalence ranges from as low as 5% of private gynecologic patients to as high as 50%–75% of prostitutes. Colonization rates are higher among women than men.	Incubation period unknown. From no signs or symptoms to excoriation, edema, and pruritis of external genitalia and frothy, foul-smelling, greenish-gray vaginal discharge. Punctate hemorrhages and granular appearance of vagina and cervix yield classic strawberry appearance of trichomonal cervicitis. Postcoital bleeding may occur. Most men are asymptomatic, though some may present with urethritis.	Microscopic examination of wet mount of vaginal discharge. Pap smears may show the parasite. Culture methods are available.	Oral metronidazole, 2 gm PO stat or 250 mg t.i.d. for 7 days.	Epididymitis (rare) Prostatitis (rare)
Human Immunodeficiency Virus (HIV, previously and currently known as AIDS—Acquired immunodeficiency syndrome)				
43,389 new cases of AIDS in 1991. Total of 218,301 known cases of AIDS (final stage of HIV disease) in the U.S. through March 1992. Caused by human immunodeficiency viruses 1 and 2. Median interval between HIV infection and onset of final stage (AIDS) is nearly 10 years. High-risk groups include homosexual men, IV drug users, bisexual men, fetus of infected mother, and sexual partners of high-risk groups.	*Early:* May be asymptomatic with serologic conversion from HIV negative to positive. *Mid:* Reduced resistance to diseases, malaise, fatigue, and enlarged lymph nodes—especially of groin and axilla. *Late:* Compromised immune system, opportunistic diseases such as *Pneumocystis carinii* penumonia (PCP), tuberculosis, and esophageal candidiasis.	Serologic testing: Enzyme immunoassay (EIA); if positive then Western blot test for HIV-1; if negative then Western blot test for HIV-2; if either Western blot positive, then diagnosis of HIV disease. Can be diagnosed without serologic testing if diagnosis of conditions such as Kaposi sarcoma, PCP, candidiasis of esophagus, or T-helper lymphocyte count < 400/mm³ in high-risk group. Serologic testing preferred method for diagnosis.	Currently no cure. Azidothymidine (AZT) is currently being given to individuals with HIV disease. Initial dose 200 mg every 4 hours for 1 month, then 100 mg every 4 hours thereafter. AZT is thought to delay onset of the end stage of HIV (AIDS) and to prolong life. Other medications are currently being tested. Individuals also use other medications to prevent/control/cure symptoms associated with opportunistic infections and other conditions.	Death is the most severe complication; as of March 1992, 141,223 individuals in the U.S. had died from HIV. Other complications include blindness, dementia, muscle wasting, PCP, Kaposi sarcoma, and tuberculosis.

(Adapted from Centers for Disease Control. [1989.] 1989 sexually transmitted diseases treatment guidelines. Morbidity and Mortality Weekly Report, S-8, 1–43; Centers for Disease Control. [1990]. Reports on HIV/AIDS: January–December 1989 (PB90–117235GDJ); Centers for Disease Control. [1990]. Case definition for public health surveillance. Morbidity and Mortality Weekly Report, 39 (RR–13); Centers for Disease Control. [1992]. Summary: Cases of specific notifiable diseses. Morbidity and Mortality Weekly Report, 40 (50 & 51), 893–898)

Venereal Warts

Warts occurring on the genitalia and perineal area are known as *condyloma acuminata*, a human papillomavirus (HPV). Rarely, venereal warts occur prior to puberty or after menopause. The dry, wartlike growths may appear on the vulva, vagina, cervix, or rectum. They may occur singularly or in clusters large enough to occlude the vagina. They are highly infectious and can be transferred to a fetus during a vaginal delivery.

Vaginitis

Vaginitis is a general term referring to infections characterized by vaginal discharge. Organisms causing vaginitis may originate from several sources, including normal vaginal flora, the large intestine (as a result of cross contamination), and exogenous sources, including sexual transmission.

The most common cause of altered vaginal flora is douching, which causes the normally acidic ph to become more alkaline. Antibiotic therapy and diabetes mellitus can also alter the normal vaginal flora and predispose a woman to infection.

General assessment findings related to vaginitis include odorous vaginal discharge, genital pruritus, dyspareunia (painful intercourse), and dysuria. Multiple infections may be noted.

Trichomonas caused by the *Trichomonas vaginalis* organism is easily transmitted between sexual partners but is endogenous and may cause infections in persons who do not contract it through sexual activity. The vaginal discharge is watery, yellow, or yellow-green. The organisms are easily identified under the microscope by placing a few drops of vaginal discharge on a glass slide and applying normal saline. Genital examination may reveal erythematous mucous membranes, and reddened papules may be noted on the cervix and vaginal walls.

Candida albicans is a yeast organism that is part of the natural vaginal flora. However, certain conditions such as taking oral contraceptives, receiving antibiotic or corticosteroid therapy, pregnancy, and poorly controlled diabetes mellitus, predispose women to this type of infection. Candida infections are characterized by intense genital pruritus and a thick, white, curd-like vaginal discharge. The genitals appear bright red and are covered with whitish exudate.

Atrophic vaginitis, an inflammation of the vaginal walls associated with estrogen deficiency, occurs most frequently in postmenopausal women. The vaginal walls become thin, and accompanying pH changes may predispose women to bacterial infections. Vaginal discharge, if present, may be mucoid and occasionally flecked with blood. Vaginal inspection reveals a smooth, thin, and glistening vaginal mucosa unless infection is present, in which case the vaginal walls appear red.

BREASTS AND AXILLAE

The examination of the breast and axillae is the same for men and women. Because the woman has more breast tissue, this discussion is female-oriented.

Anatomy and Physiology Overview

The breasts are paired, modified sebaceous glands located between the second and sixth ribs and between the sternal border and the midaxillary line on the anterior chest wall. A nipple, surrounded by the areola, is centrally located on each breast.

The breast is composed of glandular tissue, fibrous tissue, and retromammary and subcutaneous fat. The variation in breast size is a result of the amount of fat present. The amount of glandular tissue is about the same in all women and is organized into some 12 to 25 lobes in a circular pattern around the nipple. These lobes are composed of lobules containing acini, the milk-producing glands. The lobes have a duct that terminate on the nipple (Fig. 15-9). Most of the glandular tissue occurs in the upper lateral quadrant of the breast. A portion of the glandular tissue, known as the tail of Spence, extends toward the ax-

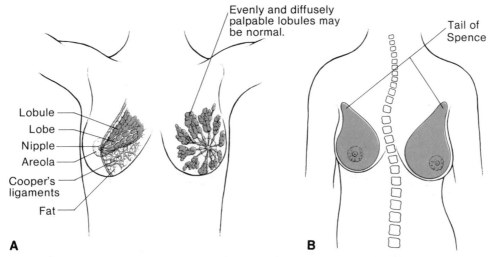

Figure 15–9. Female breast anatomy. *(A)* Internal tissues and support structures. *(B)* Tail of Spence extends to support axilla. Note normal asymmetry of breasts due to scoliosis.

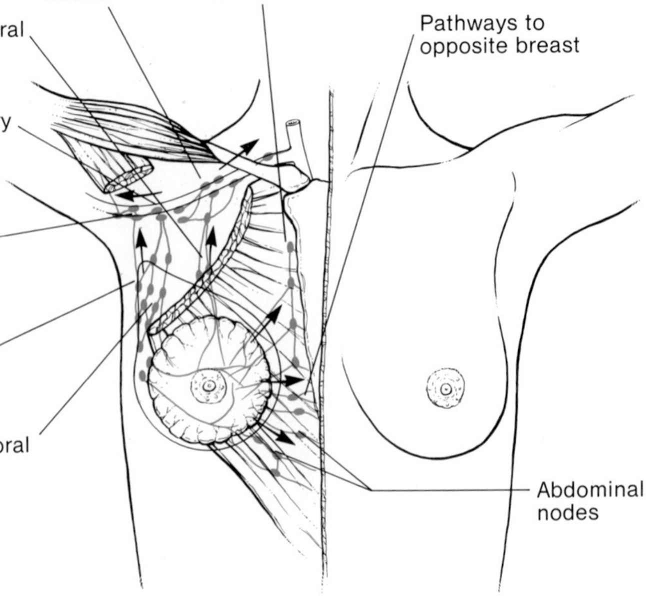

Figure 15-10. Lymphatic drainage of the breast. *Arrows* indicate direction of lymph flow.

illa. The breasts also contain fibrous tissue or Cooper's ligaments, which connect the skin and fascia to the pectoralis muscle.

Although breasts are usually symmetric, slight variation in shape between the breasts is normal. Breast size in a woman may vary with age, menstrual cycle, and pregnancy. Breasts should be fairly mobile, and the skin should be the same as that of the abdomen.

The areolae are pigmented areas surrounding each nipple. Color may vary from pink to brown and may change during pregnancy. The size of the areolae vary greatly, may

enlarge during pregnancy and remain enlarged. Montgomery's tubercles, sebaceous glands, are found within the areolae. Nipples are projectile tissue that contain the ducts from the glandular milk-producing tissue. Nipples are the same or a little darker in color as the areolae, and generally "point" up and laterally.

The breast contains several lymph node groups (Fig. 15-10). Most but not all of the lymph drains toward the axilla. The lymphatic system within and proximal to the breasts frequently serves as a vehicle for the spread of cancer.

Physical Examination   *Breasts and Axillae*

General Principles

The breast examination has two components—inspection and palpation—that are performed with the client in sitting and supine positions. The chest and breast must be completely exposed for inspection. You should provide appropriate explanations during the breast examination. Cold hands can interfere with the client's comfort and with the interpretation of examination findings.

Landmarks

The breast can be described using two mapping methods: the clock and the quadrant. In the clock method, the breast is compared to the face of a clock with the nipple at the center. Lesions or other findings should be located by their position on the clock face such as 11 o'clock or 2 o'clock.

The quadrant method divides the breast into four areas: upper inner, upper outer (including the tail of Spence), lower outer, and lower inner. Horizontal and vertical lines cross at the nipple (Fig. 15-11).

Male Breasts

The male breast examination is essentially the same as the female breast examination. The breast should feel flat and smooth, and glandular breast tissue should not be present. Gynecomastia, enlargement of the male breast, has multiple causes, such as drugs, illnesses, and pubertal changes. This condition should receive prompt attention if the enlargement is a recent development. Size and shape of male breast vary according to body structure and fat distribution. The axillae are evaluated in men as in women.

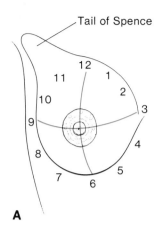

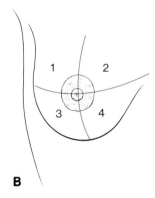

Figure 15-11. Breast examination landmarks. *(A)* Breast clock landmarks, including tail of Spence; *(B)* breast quadrants.

Examination and Documentation Focus
- Size, shape, symmetry
- Skin color, texture, lesions, and vascular patterns of skin
- Tissue quality
- Breast lymphatics
- Nipple discharge

Examination Guidelines   *Breasts and Axillae*

Perform breast inspection with the person in five different positions: seated with arms at side, with arms over head, leaning over, with hands pressed onto hips, and supine. Inspecting the breast in these five positions enables you to assess the quality of fibrous tissue stretching limits, to determine if any part of the breast is fixed, and to detect asymmetry or decrease in breast mobility as positions are changed.

Procedure

1. OBSERVE BREASTS WITH THE PERSON IN THE FOLLOWING POSITIONS:

   a. *Seated with arms at side.* Ask the person to sit comfortably with both arms at the side. Observe breasts for symmetry, size, shape, skin color, texture, vascular patterns, presence of moles, nevi, lesions, and visible lymph nodes. Note direction and symmetry of nipples and any discharge.

   If you detect abnormalities, ask the person when the finding was first noted and whether there have been any past evaluations or treatment. Inspect the breast from different angles and positions.

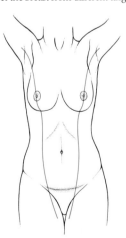

Milk lines

Clinical Significance

Normal Findings

Breast size and shape may vary according to age and body type, but breasts should be symmetric. Slight asymmetry may be normal if not a recent development. The nipples should look the same on each breast and point slightly up and laterally. Inverted nipples may be congenital and are insignificant if the condition existed before puberty. However, inverted nipples may make breast-feeding difficult. Note the exact location of any supernumerary nipples (extra congenital nipples found along milk lines from the axilla to the groin). During movement, breast size and shape should remain symmetric.

Normal skin color: Skin color should be the same on each breast and similar to that of the abdomen. Areolae should be pink to brown. Nipples and Montgomery tubercles may be slightly darker than areolae. There may be a few hair follicles around the areolae.

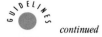
continued

Breasts and Axillae

Procedure

b. *Arms over head.* Ask the person to raise both arms over the head and continue to inspect the breasts.

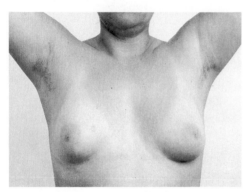

Breast examination: Arms over head

c. *Leaning over.* Ask the person to lean over. You may need to support the person's arms to help with balance. If preferred, the person may stand and lean over. Continue to inspect the breasts.

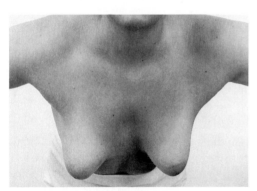

Breast examination: Leaning over

d. *Pressing hands onto hips.* Ask the person to place hands on hips and press in. An alternate method is for the person to put palms together and press to cause the pectoral muscles to contract. Inspect as before.

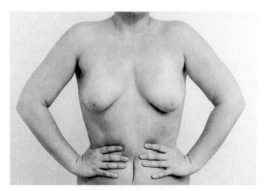

Breast examination: Pressing hands onto hips

Clinical Significance

Normal vascular patterns on the skin: Vascular patterns should be symmetric. Vascular patterns may be difficult to note on dark-skinned persons. Increased vascularity, indicated by bluish or reddish hues, may occur during pregnancy. Such vascular changes should be symmetric and diffuse.

Deviations from Normal

Skin lesions: The breast should be without lesions; however, moles and nevi are common. The breasts are susceptible to the same lesions as the rest of the skin.

Change in breast size/shape: A unilateral change in size, shape, or symmetry of the breast is abnormal. When the arms are raised or lowered or when the client is lying down or leaning over, any change in symmetry may be the result of a mass or lesion restricting the stretching ability of the ligaments. Note whether one breast seems to be fixed to the chest wall or shortens or bulges with movement.

Nipples: Recent nipple inversion is abnormal and is a sign of retraction. Bright red nipples and areola may be an indication of Paget's Disease (See display, "Deviations from Normal Breast Findings").

(continued)

Deviations from Normal Breast Findings

Retraction Signs

- Signs include skin dimpling, creasing, or changes in the contour of the breast or nipple
- Secondary to fibrosis or scar tissue formation in the breast
- Retractions signs may appear only with position changes or with breast palpation.

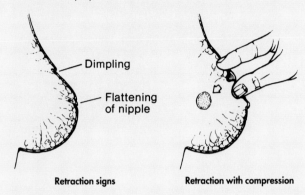

Retraction signs   **Retraction with compression**

Breast Cancer Mass (Malignant Tumor)

(See Chapter 6 for risk factors)
- Usually occurs as a single mass (lump) in one breast
- Usually nontender
- Irregular shape
- Firm, hard, embedded in surrounding tissue
- Referral and biopsy indicated for definitive diagnosis

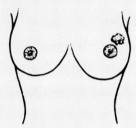

Breast cancer mass

Breast Cyst (Benign Mass of Fibrocystic Disease)

- Occur as single or multiple lumps in one or both breasts
- Usually tender (omitting caffeine reduces tenderness); tenderness increases during premenstrual period
- Round shape
- Soft or firm, mobile
- Referral and biopsy indicated for definitive diagnosis, especially for first mass; later masses may be evaluated over time by a specialist

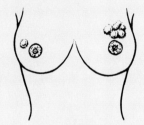

Breast cysts

Fibroadenoma (Benign Breast Lump)

- Usually occurs as a single mass in women aged 15–35 years
- Usually nontender
- May be round or lobular
- Firm, mobile, and not fixed to breast tissue or chest wall
- No premenstrual changes
- Referral and biopsy indicated for definitive diagnosis

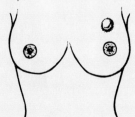

Fibroadenoma

Increased Venous Prominence

- Associated with breast cancer if unilateral
- Unilateral localized increase in venous pattern associated with malignant tumors
- Normal with breast enlargement associated with pregnancy and lactation if bilateral and bilateral symmetry

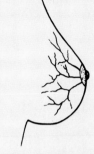

Increased venous prominence

Peau d'Orange (Edema)

- Associated with breast cancer
- Caused by interference with lymphatic drainage
- Breast skin has "orange peel" appearance
- Skin pores enlarge
- May be noted on the areola
- Skin becomes thick, hard, immobile
- Skin discoloration may occur

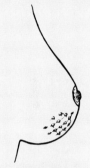

Peau d'orange

Nipple Inversion

- Considered normal if long-standing
- Associated with fibrosis and malignancy if recent development

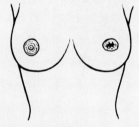

Nipple inversion

Acute Mastitis (Inflammation of the Breasts)

- Associated with lactation but may occur at any age
- Nipple cracks or abrasions noted
- Breast skin reddened and warm to touch
- Tenderness
- Systemic signs include fever and increased pulse

Paget's Disease (Malignancy of Mammary Ducts)

- Early signs: Erythema of nipple and areola
- Late signs: Thickening, scaling, and erosion of the nipple and areola

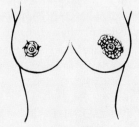

Paget's disease

G U I D E L I N E S *continued*   ***Breasts and Axillae***

Procedure

2. PALPATE THE BREASTS AND AXILLAE WITH THE PERSON IN A SITTING POSITION (Option—see procedure for palpation in the supine position).

   The sitting position is optional unless the person reports an abnormal finding, has a history of breast abnormalities, has a high risk for breast cancer (family history), or has pendulous breasts.

   a. Bimanually palpate pendulous breast. Use one hand to support the inferior side of the breast while palpating the breast with the dominant hand, moving from the chest wall toward and including the nipple.

   b. Palpate the axillae while the muscles are relaxed. To relax the muscles, adduct and support the person's arm on top of your arm. Place the hand of the arm that is supporting the client's arm in the axillae with the dominant hand on the anterior surface of the chest. Most of the lymphatic drainage of the breast is toward the axillae. Locate the nodes of the axillae according to their anatomic position. Evaluate the nodes by rolling the soft tissue against the chest wall and between your hands. Examine the anterior, posterior, medial, and lateral aspects of the axillae. Bimanually palpate the anterior aspect of the axillae to obtain access to the nodes near the pectoralis muscle. Also palpate the subclavian and supraclavicular nodes.

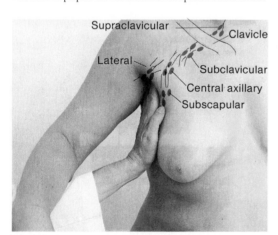

Axillae nodes: Palpatory areas

3. INSPECT AND PALPATE THE BREASTS WITH THE PERSON IN THE SUPINE POSITION.

   a. Position the person on the examination table in the supine position. Place the arm on the same side as the breast being examined comfortably over and behind the person's head. For women with moderate to large breasts, place a folded towel or small pillow under the shoulder and upper back to displace tissue evenly. Inspect each breast.

Clinical Significance

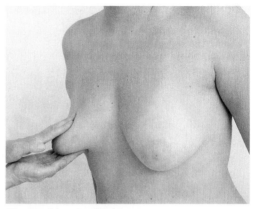

Bimanual breast palpation

Normal Findings

Lymph nodes should not be palpable.

Deviations from Normal

Palpable axillary nodes are abnormal. If palpated, note size, consistency, mobility, and tenderness.

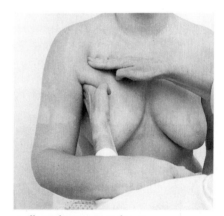

Axillae palpation: Seated position

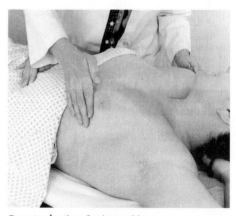

Breast palpation: Supine position

continued　　　　　　　　　　　　　　**Breasts and Axillae**

Procedure

b. Palpate to evaluate tissue texture and detect masses. Light palpation is followed by deep palpation. With deep palpation the breast tissue is compressed against the chest wall. Palpate all four quadrants and the tail of Spence. When palpating use the distal finger pads, the fingers held together, and move the fingers in a circular motion without lifting until the assessment is complete. Use a systematic approach to help ensure a consistent and complete evaluation. Begin palpation at the same location on both breasts. Use the clockwise, spoke, or horizontal or vertical lines approach. If person reports abnormal findings in one breast or inspection reveals possible problem with one breast, begin palpation in the nonsuspected breast.

Clinical Significance

Starting palpation on the nonsuspected breast allows for better comparison and evaluation of possible abnormalities.

Normal Findings

Breast tissue should be smooth, elastic, soft, and easily moved. During palpation, the normal breast feels glandular and lumpy. The lumpiness is the result of glandular tissues, lobes, fat, and connecting fibers. The closer to menstrual period, the more lumpy the breast may feel. Generally, the breast is not uniform in quality, but the two breasts are symmetrically uniform. A firm ridge, which is normal, may be noted along each breast between the 4 and 8 o'clock positions. Nipples should be smooth and may become erect during palpation.

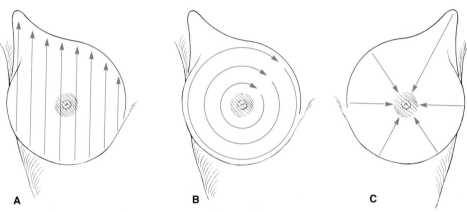

A　　　　　　　　　**B**　　　　　　　　　**C**

(A) Vertical lines approach; (B) clockwise approach; (C) spoke approach

Give special attention to the upper outer quadrant and the tail of Spence, as most breast changes develop in the upper outer quadrant and the tail of Spence.

c. Palpate the areola for underlying masses, and compress the skin around the nipple to assess for masses and discharge. If you note discharge, compress the breast along the suspected ducts to identify the lobe producing the discharge. Note color, consistency, and odor of discharge.

Deviations from Normal

Palpation of any unusual masses or notation of differences in quality and quantity of breast tissue between breasts.

Normal Findings

There should be no discharge for the nipple of a nonstimulated breast. A milky discharge (galactorrhea) may be normal during pregnancy and lactation; near or during the menstrual period; during sexual breast stimulation; as a side effect of some psychotropic drugs; and as a symptom of either hyper- or hypothyroidism.

Deviations from Normal

Any bloody nipple discharge should be considered the result of cancer until proved differently. Any discharge other than noted in normal findings should be evaluated and possibly cultured.

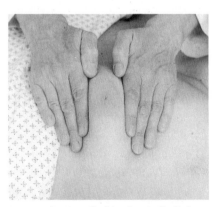

Breast palpation: Checking for nipple discharge

Documenting Breast and Axilla Examination Findings

Record breast examination findings carefully so that comparison with subsequent findings will be meaningful and reliable. Any changes noted by the client should also be recorded. If a breast lump is discovered, document the following characteristics:

- Location using clock orientation or quadrants, and distance from nipple in centimeters
- Size (length and width), in centimeters
- Shape
- Consistency (soft, hard, rubbery)
- Discreteness (are borders easy to distinguish from surrounding tissue?)
- Mobility
- Skin color over the lump
- Tenderness to palpation
- Any retraction signs

If a lymph node in the axillary area or any other area is palpated, document the following:

- Location
- Size
- Contour
- Consistency
- Discreteness
- Mobility
- Tenderness

Example 1: Normal Breast Assessment

Ms. M, aged 29, had a breast assessment when she came to the clinic for contraception and a cervical Pap smear. The examination results were normal and recorded as follows.

States she performs monthly breast self-examination (BSE) and has noted no changes, lumps, or tenderness except for a few days prior to menses. No palpable masses; no nipple discharge. No palpable axillary or supraclavicular nodes.

The same findings may be summarized in a problem-oriented format as follows:

S: Performs monthly BSE; no lumps or changes noted; slight breast tenderness a few days prior to menses every month.
O: Breasts symmetric with intact skin; no dimpling or edema. No symmetry changes in breast shape with movement. No palpable masses; no nipple discharge; no palpable axillary or supraclavicular nodes.
A: Practices and understands appropriate health screening activities; breast assessment within normal limits.
P: Reinforce appropriateness of BSE; advise next professional breast exam should be in 3 years unless changes noted with BSE; consider baseline mammogram in 5 years.

Example 2: Breast Masses

Mrs. C, aged 40, reported to the clinic for a breast assessment after she found a single lump in her left breast. The assessment findings were recorded as follows:

Breasts symmetric with no visible masses, slight dimpling noted in upper outer quadrant when hands pressed on hips. No complaints of tenderness. No masses noted on palpation of right breast. In upper outer quadrant at 11 o'clock and 6 cm from nipple, firm mass, nonmobile, difficult-to-distinguish borders approximately 0.5 by 0.25 cm, slight retraction with compression.

The same findings may be summarized in a problem-oriented format as follows:

S: Performs BSE every 3 to 4 months, found mass in left breast, upper outer quadrant, 3 days ago. Denies tenderness. LMP 10 days ago. No family history of breast cancer. No baseline mammogram.
O: Right breast—no visible or palpable masses, no changes in symmetry with movement, no dimpling. Vascularity symmetric bilateral. Left breast—slight dimpling upper outer quadrant only when hands pressing on hips; on palpation, noted firm mass in upper outer quadrant at 11 o'clock and 6 cm from nipple, nonmobile, difficult-to-distinguish borders approximately 0.5 by 0.25 cm, slight retraction with compression.
A: Abnormal breast assessment, need to rule out malignancy
P: Refer to physician for diagnostic testing and treatment. Follow up with phone call in 2 days.

NDx

Nursing Diagnoses Related to Breast and Axilla Examination

No nursing diagnoses within the sexuality pattern are directly related to the breast and axilla examination. Appropriate nursing diagnoses from the nutrition and metabolism pattern may include Altered tissue integrity and Impaired skin integrity.

Women who are having difficulty with breast-feeding may perceive themselves as not meeting sex role obligations. Additionally, women post mastectomy may have difficulty with sexual identity and worry about their own sexual attractiveness to their partner. A discussion of sexuality nursing diagnoses related to the breast and axilla is in the section for genital and pelvic structures.

Effective Breast-Feeding

The nursing diagnosis Effective breast-feeding is used when both the woman and infant exhibit proficiency and satisfaction with the breast-feeding process.

History. Verbalizations by the breast-feeding woman that indicate effective breast-feeding include satisfaction with breast-feeding, infant content after feeding, and regular breast-feeding times.

Physical Examination Findings. Observations indicating effective breast-feeding include effective maternal–infant communication patterns and signs of oxytocin release (let-down reflex when infant cries). Physical findings may include appropriate weight for age of infant and strong sucking reflex.

Ineffective Breast-Feeding

This nursing diagnosis is used when the woman or infant or child experiences dissatisfaction or difficulty with the breast-feeding process.

History. For Ineffective breast-feeding, the woman may report difficulty or lack of satisfaction with breast-feeding, sore nipples, and/or insufficient milk for infant. She may report that the infant is fussy shortly after feeding, has poor sucking, and does not like to nurse.

Physical Examination Findings. Nipples may be sore to touch, cracked, or inverted. There may be no signs of oxytocin release (let-down reflex), and breast may not be engorged just prior to regular feeding. The woman may show signs of insufficient nutrition and fluid intake (see Chap. 8). Infant may not be gaining weight for age. When possible, observe the breast-feeding event and note the following: Does the woman appear uncomfortable or tense? How is infant sucking? Is sucking sustained? Is each breast emptied at feeding? Does infant resist sucking?

Clinical Problems Related to Breasts and Axillae

Clinical problems related to breasts and axillae generally are related to the integumentary system, the lymphatic system, and glandular tissue. Problems include breast cancer, fibrocystic and fibroadenoma disease, nipple inversion, and mastitis. These clinical problems are illustrated in the previous display, "Deviations from Normal Breast Findings."

ASSESSMENT OF PHYSICAL CHANGES DURING PREGNANCY

Anatomy and Physiology Overview

Observable physical changes occur throughout pregnancy, especially in the skin, breasts, abdomen, and pelvis. Less noticeable changes occur in other body systems, including the cardiovascular, gastrointestinal, genitourinary, respiratory, and musculoskeletal systems. Physical assessment of the pregnant woman is similar to that of other people and requires only occasional modification of technique.

Prenatal assessment involves periodic evaluation throughout pregnancy. Although the frequency of professional assessments depends on the person, the following schedule for clinic visits is generally recommended:

- First 28 weeks: every 3–4 weeks
- Last 12 weeks: every 1–2 weeks

At each prenatal visit, the following aspects of maternal and fetal health are evaluated:

- Weight
- Blood pressure
- Glucose and protein in the urine
- Fluid retention (edema)
- The height of the fundus
- The position of the fetus (Leopold's maneuvers)
- Fetal heart sounds

Other evaluations are conducted as needed and include the following:

- A complete head-to-toe physical assessment at the first prenatal visit
- Pelvic assessments at the first prenatal visit and during the last trimester
- Evaluation and measurement of the bony pelvis at the first prenatal visit and again at 32 to 36 weeks
- Specific examinations indicated by the condition of the mother or the fetus, such as abdominal ultrasound, amniocentesis, or antibody titers (some serologic testing may be required by state law)

Pregnancy is confirmed on the basis of characteristic subjective symptoms, physical signs, and laboratory values. Signs and symptoms are grouped into categories called presumptive signs, probable signs, and positive signs.

Presumptive signs of pregnancy include symptoms reported by the woman such as the following:

- Amenorrhea 10 days or more past the date the menstrual period was expected to begin
- Morning sickness (nausea or vomiting persisting 3 weeks or more past the missed period)
- Tingling, soreness, or heaviness of the breasts

Probable signs of pregnancy include many physical assessment findings, including the following:

- Uterine enlargement
- Hegar's sign (softening of the uterine isthmus)
- Piskacek's sign (asymmetric enlargement of one uterine cornua)
- Chadwick's sign (bluish pigmentation of the vagina and cervix)
- Godell's sign (cervical softening)
- Internal ballottement of the uterus
- Urine or serum that is positive for human chorionic gonadotropin (HCG). The urine test for HCG can be done at home with an over-the-counter pregnancy test kit.

Positive signs of pregnancy confirm the presence of a fetus and include the following:

- Auscultation of a fetal heartbeat
- Palpation of fetal movement
- Identification of fetal parts by x-ray or ultrasound

Display 15–2
Integumentary Changes During Pregnancy

Changes	*Clinical Significance/Cause*

1. COLOR AND PIGMENTATION
   a. Month 2 through term: generalized hyperpigmentation develops, especially over the bony prominences and breast nipples and areola.
   b. Week 16 through term: *linea nigra,* a brownish-black line of pigment extending from the umbilicus to the pubic bone, may appear.
   c. Chloasma, mottled hyperpigmentation over the cheeks and forehead, may develop (called the "mask of pregnancy").
	Changes in the color and pigmentation of the skin during pregnancy are associated with an increased blood level of melanocyte-stimulating hormone. The resulting hyperpigmentation is benign, although body image may be altered.

2. MOISTURE Increased perspiration (especially during the first trimester)	Secondary to an increased output of the exocrine glands
3. THICKNESS Gum hypertrophy	Secondary to proliferation of blood vessels in oral mucosa
4. TURGOR AND MOBILITY a. Localized edema or ankle edema	Usually not considered pathologic, secondary to an increase in venous pressure in the lower extremities
b. Generalized edema	Caused by sodium and water retention secondary to elevated levels of steroid hormones
5. VASCULAR ALTERATIONS Palmar erythema; spider nevi over the face, chest, or abdomen	Secondary to the effects of estrogen and usually insignificant except for possible effects on body image
6. SKIN LESIONS Striae gravidarum (stretch marks) especially over breasts, abdomen, and thighs	Caused by stretching of the skin as weight is gained and fetus grows; pink or red during pregnancy and turning silvery white after delivery

INTEGUMENTARY CHANGES DURING PREGNANCY

Skin changes during pregnancy are common and include changes in color and pigmentation, moisture, thickness, turgor, and vascularity. The degree to which these changes occur varies from woman to woman and from pregnancy to pregnancy. Some women become alarmed by the changes and need to be reassured about why the changes occur, when they will occur, and how long they will last.

The skin assessment is performed in the same manner for pregnant women as other people. Skin is assessed by inspection and palpation. See Display 15-2 for integumentary changes related to pregnancy.

BREAST CHANGES DURING PREGNANCY

Breast changes are normal during pregnancy and include changes in size, shape, color, vascularity, and tissue quality. If the woman intends to breast-feed, her understanding and feelings about breast-feeding should be explored during the third trimester. The nipples would also be assessed to determine if they are everted or inverted. If the nipples are inverted, the woman should be shown how to roll the nipple to promote eversion. You should ascertain if she is toughening the nipples (preparing the nipples to withstand infant suckling) by methods such as rubbing them vigorously with a rough, dry washcloth. Breast self-examinations should be practiced during pregnancy (see Chap. 6 for detailed breast self-examination techniques). Changes that occur in the breasts during pregnancy are highlighted in Display 15-3.

GENITAL AND PELVIC CHANGES DURING PREGNANCY

Changes in the genitals and pelvis are noted throughout pregnancy and include alteration in the appearance of the genitals, vagina, and cervix, and changes in the consistency of the cervix and uterus. Some of these alterations help establish the confirmation of pregnancy, and others are monitored as indicators of normal fetal growth and development. Generally, the pelvic assessment is conducted in the same manner for pregnant and nonpregnant women. Special variations in the technique of bimanual palpation may be required to elicit pregnancy signs. For example, Hegar's sign, occurring after 6 weeks, is a softening of the uterine isthmus. This change is detected by bimanual pelvic palpa-

---

Display 15–3
Breast Changes During Pregnancy

Changes	*Clinical Significance/Causes*
1. SIZE AND SHAPE Month 2 through term and lactation: breast and nipple enlargement	Accompanies the increase in glandular and ductal tissue occurring because of hormonal influences, and later because of milk production.
2. SKIN COLOR Hyperpigmentation of the nipple and areolae; the areolae may increase in size; secondary areola may develop	Secondary to increased levels of melanocyte-stimulating hormone
3. VASCULARITY Venous engorgement of the breasts; venous patterns should remain bilaterally symmetric	Causes the breast to appear larger; caused by the venous pressure increases in pregnancy. The venous engorged breast may feel slightly warmer than surrounding skin and may be tender.
4. TISSUE QUALITY Increased nodularity	The breast may feel generally lumpy as glandular and ductal tissue become more prominent during pregnancy. Other breast lumps should be considered and ruled out.
5. LESIONS Striae gravidarum	Secondary to skin stretching as breasts enlarge
6. DISCHARGE Week 16 though term: Colostrum may be secreted from the nipples. Amount secreted increases in third trimester.	Colostrum, a yellowish premilk fluid, is secreted from the mammary glands. Milk is secreted 49 to 96 hours after delivery.

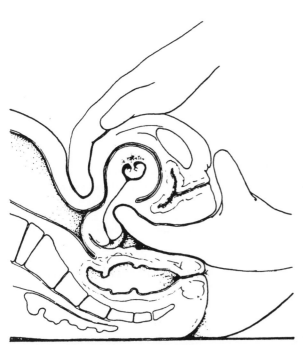

Figure 15-12. Bimanual palpation: Hegar's sign.

tion. Place two fingers of the vaginal examining hand in the anterior vaginal fornix in front of the cervix. Use the abdominal palpating hand to compress the uterus slightly above the symphysis pubis so that the isthmus is trapped between both hands (Fig. 15-12). Display 15-4 highlights changes that occur to the pelvic structures and genitals during pregnancy.

Advanced nurse practitioners and nurse midwives learn additional assessment techniques to determine pelvic configuration and size. Such techniques are discussed in most maternity textbooks.

MISCELLANEOUS PHYSICAL CHANGES DURING PREGNANCY

Miscellaneous changes occur throughout the body during pregnancy. These include changes in the mobility, weight, vital signs, and hair distribution. These changes are outlined in Display 15-5.

ABDOMINAL CHANGES DURING PREGNANCY

The abdomen is evaluated at regular intervals during pregnancy to determine fetal growth and development, gestational age, fetal position, and fetal lie.

Display 15–4
Genital and Pelvic Changes During Pregnancy

Changes

Clinical Significance/Causes

1. GENITAL PIGMENTATION
   May note hyperpigmentation of labia or vulva

   Secondary to increased levels of melanocyte-stimulating hormone during pregnancy

2. VAGINAL DISCHARGE
   Moderate to profuse thick, clear, odorless mucus is present from 6 weeks through term

   Discharge is associated with the increased vascularity of the vagina.
   Leukorrhea may be noted and represents discharge secondary to hypertrophied cervical glands.
   Any bloody or excessive watery discharge may represent impending termination of pregnancy.

3. VAGINAL WALLS
   a. Rugae become more pronounced.
   b. Vaginal tissue becomes more edematous.
   c. Vaginal skin develops a bluish pigmentation (Chadwick's sign).

   Caused by increase in vaginal vascularity

4. CERVIX
   a. By 6–8 weeks, the cervix has a bluish pigmentation (Chadwick's sign).

   Secondary to increased vascularity and venous congestion

   b. By 5–6 weeks the cervix softens (Goodell's sign).

   Secondary to increased vascularity

5. UTERUS
   a. After 6 weeks, Piskacek's sign appears (asymmetric uterine enlargement).

   Related to rapid uterine enlargement at site of ovum implantation

   b. By 6–8 weeks, Hegar's sign appears (softening of the uterine isthmus).

   Secondary to increased vascularity

   c. After 6 weeks, McDonald's sign appears (cervix and uterus may be flexed at junction during bimanual palpation).

   Secondary to increased vascularity

   d. After 16 weeks, uterine ballottement is possible.

Display 15–5
Miscellaneous Physical Changes During Pregnancy

Findings

Clinical Significance/Causes

1. POSTURE
   a. Increased lumbar lordosis
   b. Increased dorsal kyphosis and cervical lordosis

   The expanding uterus contributes to lumbar lordosis. These changes represent compensation for lumbar lordosis and are necessary to maintain center of gravity.

2. GAIT
   Waddling gait

   Secondary to postural alterations and slight instability of the pelvis

3. WEIGHT
   Progressive weight gain; optimal weight gain is 24 to 28 pounds. First 28 weeks' gain should be about one half a pound a week; after 28 weeks about 1 pound per week.

   Secondary to fetal growth, maternal fat storage, and maternal water retention

(continued)

Display 15–5
Miscellaneous Physical Changes During Pregnancy (continued)

Findings	*Clinical Significance/Causes*
4. VITAL SIGNS	
a. Heart rate may increase slightly above baseline.	Secondary to increased blood volume and increased oxygen consumption
b. Systolic blood pressure usually unchanged; diastolic may decrease slightly. In last trimester there may be a slight fall.	A decreased peripheral vascular resistance alters the diastolic blood pressure
c. Respiratory rate may increase, and after 7 months thoracic breathing replaces abdominal breathing.	Secondary to increased oxygen consumption and breathing pattern changes due to displacement of the diaphragm by the growing fetus
5. HEART SOUNDS	
A physiologic systolic murmur (grade II/VI) may be heard during the third trimester. Apical pulse may be displaced laterally about 1 cm.	Results from increased blood flow secondary to an increased blood volume. Displacement is result of fetal growth.
6. HAIR	
Loss or straightening of scalp hair; increased facial or abdominal hair	Secondary to increased amounts of androgens and corticotrophic hormones
7. REDUCED PERISTALSIS	Secondary to relaxation of the muscles of the large intestines

Physical Examination

The Pregnant Woman

Measuring Fundal Height

The term *fundus* refers to the body of the pregnant uterus. During pregnancy, the height of the fundus is measured at each prenatal visit to evaluate fetal growth. The height of the fundus correlates with gestational age (Fig. 15-13). Equipment needed for this examination is a measuring tape in centimeters.

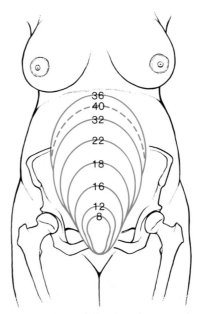

Figure 15–13. Fundal height and gestational age.

Fetal Heart Auscultation

Fetal heart tones are an indicator of the health of the fetus throughout pregnancy beginning at about 10 weeks, when heart sounds are first detected by Doppler flow devices. After 16 weeks, heart tones may be detected by the fetoscope. The intensity of fetal heart sounds varies depending on the position of the fetus.

Leopold's Maneuvers

Leopold's maneuvers consist of four abdominal palpation techniques for determining fetal position and lie. The fetal lie can be longitudinal (fetal spine fairly parallel to mother), transverse (fetal spine somewhat perpendicular to mother's spine), and oblique (fetal lie is between longitudinal and transverse). Leopold's maneuvers are performed routinely after 26 weeks' gestation, when the fetal parts are more discernible.

Examination Guidelines   *Measuring Fundal Height*

Procedure

1. Prior to 13 weeks of gestational age, the height of the fundus is evaluated by bimanual pelvic examination.

2. After 13 weeks:

   a. The fundus is palpable with one hand over the abdomen. With the woman supine, place your fingers over the abdomen as shown in the figure. Start to palpate from above the point where you expect the fundus to be palpable; then progressively palpate downward. Estimate and record the distance between the symphysis pubis and the fundus in centimeters.

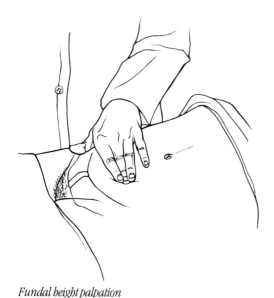

Fundal height palpation

Clinical Significance

This procedure is not usually performed by a professional nurse without additional training, such as a certified nurse midwife and nurse practitioners.

Normal Findings

When you note a change in tissue consistency from soft to firm, you have palpated the fundus. Slight measurement variations may occur with different examiners. Nevertheless, progressive increases of approximately 1 cm per week in fundal height until week 37–40 then a decrease. Increasing size is associated with fetal growth. A decrease in fundal height at 37–40 weeks associated with pelvic engagement of presenting part.

Deviations from Normal

Excessive uterine growth may indicate more than one fetus, excessive amniotic fluid, or a very large fetus. Excessive amniotic fluid is often associated with congenital anomalies, and a very large fetus is associated with maternal diabetes mellitus. A stoppage of growth may indicate fetal death, whereas slow uterine growth may indicate incorrect calculation of gestation. Ultrasound of the uterus is indicated with unusual uterine growth.

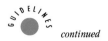

continued **Measuring Fundal Height**

Procedure

b. When the fundus expands above the umbilicus, the height of the fundus may be measured with a tape measure. Place the end of the tape measure at the top of the symphysis pubis and measure the distance in centimeters to the height of the fundus.

Clinical Significance

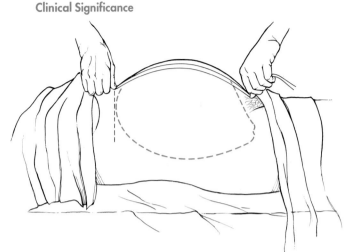

Fundal height measurement

Examination Guidelines   *Fetal Heart Auscultation*

Procedure

Generally, heart sounds are auscultated by placing the fetoscope over the area between the symphysis pubis and umbilicus. Occasionally, heart tones are heard slightly above the umbilicus.

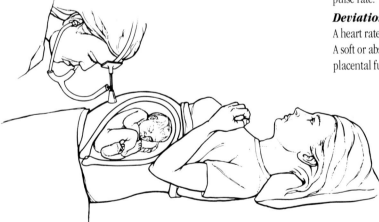

Fetal heart auscultation

Clinical Significance

Normal Findings

Fetal heart rates are between 120 and 160 beats/minute. A uterine bruit (also called uterine souffle), representing increased uterine blood flow, is a normal variation and will occur at the same pulse rate as the woman's pulse rate.

Deviations from Normal

A heart rate lower than 120 or greater than 160 may indicate fetal distress. A soft or absent uterine bruit may indicate poor uterine blood flow and placental function.

Examination Guidelines   *Abdominal Palpation*

Procedure

1. Assist the woman into a supine position on the examining table. Tensing of the abdominal muscles may be minimized by slightly flexing the knees and supporting them with a pillow.

2. Begin with *fundal palpation* to determine what fetal part occupies the fundus. Stand beside the woman, facing her head. Place both hands on top of the fundus and palpate to determine which fetal part is present.

Clinical Significance

The buttocks of the fetus, the most frequently presented part, will feel soft and slightly irregular with limited side to side mobility. The head will feel firm, hard, and round and be more freely moveable.

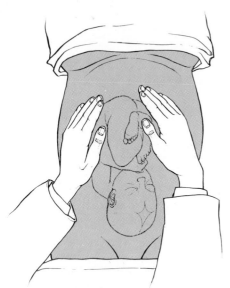

First Leopold's maneuver: Fundal palpation

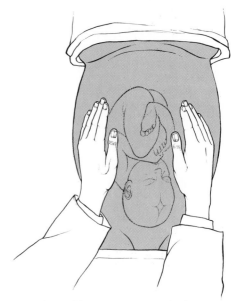

Second Leopold's maneuver: Lateral palpation

3. Next determine the position of the spine by *lateral palpation*. Move your hands from the fundus to the sides of the adbomen. Support one side of the fetus with one hand while using your other hand to palpate the opposite side of the uterus. Then palpate the other side of the adbomen in a similar fashion.

The fetal spine will feel bony and continuous, whereas the limbs will feel irregular or nodular.

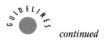

continued

Abdominal Palpation

Procedure

4. The third maneuver, called *Pawlik palpation,* determines what fetal part lies over the pelvic inlet. Place your right hand just above the symphysis pubis. Then grasp the skin firmly between your thumb and third finger.

Clinical Significance

A nonengaged head is palpable as a moveable, round, hard, smooth mass. If the head is engaged, you may feel a shoulder as a bony, nonmoveable nodule.

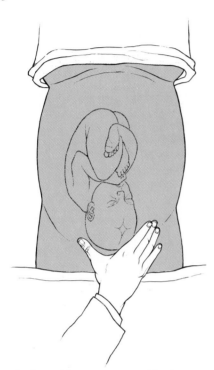

Third Leopold's maneuver: Pawlik palpation

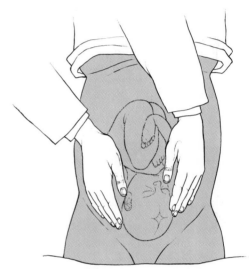

Fourth Leopold's maneuver: Deep pelvic palpation

5. Finally, perform *deep pelvic palpation* to determine the position of the head (cephalic prominence). Change position to face the woman's feet. Place both hands over the neck of the uterus just above the pelvic inlet. Ask the woman to inhale deeply and exhale slowly. During exhalation, apply pressure to each side of the uterine neck.

6. During palpation you may note occasional abdominal movement.

7. Abdominal muscle tone may seem to be reduced from the nonpregnant state.

If the presenting part is engaged, one hand will descend further than the other. Cephalic prominence refers to that part of the fetal head preventing hand descent. If the head is flexed, the prominence of the forehead is most likely. If the head is extended, the occiput will be prominent.

The abdominal movement is fetal movement and is felt especially after 6 months.

Reduced muscle tone is expected secondary to separation of the rectus abdominal muscle by the expanding uterus.

Documenting Measurement of Fundal Height

Example 1: Normal Findings

J. A., 6 months pregnant, returns to the clinic for a regular visit. Findings are recorded as follows:

   S: Now wearing maternity outfits—most of clothing no longer fits

   O: Has gained 3 pounds since last visit, fundal height 24 cm

   A: Fundal height growth and weight gain appropriate

   P: Return in 4 weeks for follow-up and repeat measurements

Example 2: Abnormal Findings

S. S., 4 months pregnant, returns to the clinic for a regular visit. Abnormal findings are recorded as follows:

   S: Now wearing maternity outfits—most of clothes do not fit; with last pregnancy, did not change over until 6 to 7 months

   O: Has gained 4 pounds since last visit, fundal height at umbilicus, believe possibility of two different fetal heart sounds

   A: Possibility of more than one fetus

   P: To be seen by certified nurse midwife in 1 week, will follow up at that time

Documenting Fetal Heart Auscultation

Example 1: Normal Findings

Suzanne, 6 months pregnant, comes to the clinic for a regular visit. Findings are recorded as follows:

   S: No data

   O: Fetal heart sounds 144/minute, and strong, Uterine bruit 74/minute heard in right upper outer quadrant of uterus

   A: Appropriate fetal heart rate

   P: Return in 1 month and repeat.

Example 2: Abnormal Findings

Diane, 7 months pregnant, comes to clinic for regular appointment. Abnormal findings are recorded as follows:

   S: Last felt fetus move 1 week ago; prior to that, movement infrequent

   O: Unable to hear fetal heart sounds or uterine bruit where last heard; fundal height 2 cm less than 4 weeks ago

   A: Suspect possibility of fetal demise

   P: Refer to physician for immediate follow-up and diagnosis

Documenting Abdominal Palpation During Pregnancy

Example 1

   S: Feels "butt" under ribs

   O: Nonengaged head presenting to pelvic outlet, spine along left side of uterus, feet palpated on right side

   A: Left, occipital, transverse position

   P: Assess in 3 weeks for engagement

Example 2

   S: Last baby was breech

   O: 30 weeks' gestation, fetal spine parallel to maternal spine, head palpated at fundus, nonengaged fetus

   A: Breech presentation

   P: Recheck position at next appointment in 3 weeks. Advise nurse midwife of findings today.

NDx

Nursing Diagnoses Related to Special Examinations for Pregnancy

Pregnancy is a time of great adjustment (physical as well as psychosocial) for the woman and her partner. Nursing diagnoses from other functional areas would include Altered nutrition (see Chap. 8), Health-seeking behavior (see Chap. 7), Fatigue (see Chap. 10), Sleep pattern disturbance (see Chap. 12), Altered family process and Potential for altered parenting (see Chap. 14), Spiritual distress (see Chap. 17), and Ineffective individual and family coping (see Chap. 16).

Pregnancy can also alter or challenge perceptions regarding sexuality. Nursing diagnoses in the sexuality pattern that apply to pregnant women include Rape-trauma syndromes, Sexual dysfunction, and Altered sexual patterns. A discussion of these diagnoses are included in the section on female genitals and pelvic structures in this chapter. Characteristics unique to pregnancy for these diagnoses are addressed here.

Rape-Trauma Syndromes

Pregnancy may be an outcome of the rape event. This can place an additional burden upon the woman: Should the pregnancy be aborted, or should the infant be placed for adoption or kept in the family? The stresses that normally occur after rape are compounded by the necessity of this decision.

Sexual Dysfunction and Altered Sexuality Patterns

During pregnancy, many factors can affect sexual functioning. There may be a fear of damage to the fetus or breast leakage with coitus, fatigue, cultural beliefs regarding coitus and pregnancy, changes in sexual drive and satisfaction, and discomfort (dyspareunia) during coitus with traditional positions. Sexual identity confusion is common during pregnancy and in the postpartum period (Carpenito, 1992). Sexual partners may also affect the woman's perception of her own sexuality. The partner may also fear hurting the fetus or the pregnant woman. If the pregnancy was unplanned, both partners may experience feelings of guilt.

Clinical Problems Related to Pregnancy

During pregnancy, women can experience any clinical problem they could have when not pregnant. The risks and occurrences of sexually transmitted diseases are the same for the pregnant woman as the nonpregnant woman. (Refer to the discussion of sexually transmitted diseases and women in this chapter).

Clinical problems related solely to pregnant women include pregnancy-induced hypertension (toxemia), fetal demise, and fetal presentation other than occipital. Pregnancy-induced hypertension is the only disease of pregnancy and can be life-threatening to the fetus and woman. This problem generally occurs after 24 weeks' gestation and is characterized by a systolic blood pressure over 140 mm Hg or a 30 mm Hg rise above the usual reading in two measurements at least 6 hours apart, and a diastolic pressure of 90 mm Hg or a 15 mm Hg rise above the usual reading in two measurements at least 6 hours apart. In addition, the woman will have protein in her urine, excessive weight gain, and edema of her face or hands. In the later stages of toxemia, convulsions and death can occur. This condition is considered a medical emergency, and the woman should be seen by a specialist immediately.

Fetal demise can occur for numerous reasons and often results in a natural abortion (miscarriage). Some times a natural abortion does not occur and a therapeutic abortion must be performed. Mummification of the fetus can occur if the fetus is not aborted. Cardinal signs of fetal demise include no fetal heart sound, no fetal movement, and no growth or decreasing fundal size. With natural abortions, signs and symptoms include increased vaginal secretions, vaginal spotting or bleeding, and uterine contractions before fetal survivability.

Fetal presentations other than occipital are not of great concern until engagement occurs. The fetus can and does change position. Fetal positions that can cause trauma for the woman and fetus include breech (buttock) and shoulder presentation. With breech presentation, the buttock is engaged; if the fetus delivered vaginally, the legs and feet are generally delivered with the body and the head is last. Shoulder presentation can cause the most difficulty, and generally the fetus is delivered by caesarean section. With shoulder presentation, the shoulder is in the pelvic outlet and the body lies horizontally (transverse lie) in the uterus. The health professional that is to deliver the fetus should be advised of all presentations that are not occipital.

MALE GENITALS AND INGUINAL AREA
Anatomy and Physiology Overview

Physical assessment of the male reproductive system involves assessing the penis, scrotum, and the groin area for lymphatic integrity and herniating masses. The prostate gland, an internal structure that contributes to seminal fluid formation, should be evaluated during the rectal examination (see Chap. 8).

EXTERNAL GENITALS

The visible external reproductive structures include the penis, urinary meatus, and scrotum. The *penis* is a hairless, cylindrical organ that is normally flaccid, except during sexual arousal. The *glans penis* is the bulbous end of the penis. In an uncircumcised man, the glans may be partially or completely covered by a loose fold of skin called the *foreskin* or *prepuce* (Fig. 15-14). The *coronal ridge* or *corona* forms the border between the glans penis and the penile shaft. The *frenulum,* a fold of tissue between the glans and shaft that joins the foreskin to the glans, is extremely sensitive to erotic stimuli. The urethral opening, located near the ventral tip of the penis, appears as a small, horizontal slit. Tyson's glands are modified sebaceous glands located around the corona and on either side of the

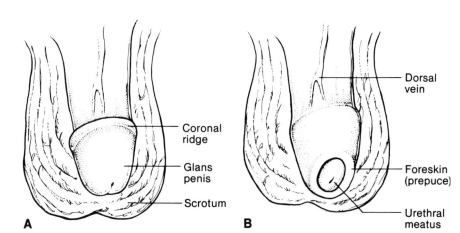

Figure 15-14. External male genitals. *(A)* Circumcised; *(B)* uncircumcised.

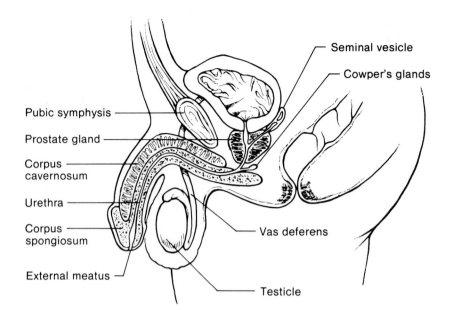

Figure 15–15. Internal male genitals.

Labels on figure: Seminal vesicle / Cowper's glands / Pubic symphysis / Prostate gland / Corpus cavernosum / Urethra / Corpus spongiosum / External meatus / Vas deferens / Testicle

frenulum. Secretions from the glands are one of the components of smegma, an odorous, cheese-like material that becomes a bacterial growth medium if not removed.

The penis has three columns of erectile properties secondary to vascular engorgement: the *corpus spongiosum,* which surrounds the urethra, and the *left* and *right corpus cavernosum,* which are located along the dorsal half of the penis and terminating at the glans.

The *scrotum* is the pendulous sac of tissue behind the penis that holds the testicles. The scrotal skin, which has a darker pigment than surrounding skin, is hair covered with a medium ridge or *raphe* extending from the base of the penis to the anus. The raphe divides the scrotal sac into two sections. The left side of the scrotum usually hangs slightly lower than the right because the spermatic cord is longer in the left testicle. The cremasteric or dartos muscle surrounds the testicles and spermatic cord. These muscles contract in response to cold, causing the scrotum to appear smaller than usual.

INTERNAL STRUCTURES

The internal male genitalia are designed for sperm production and propulsion as well as urinary excretion. Sperm form in the *testes,* enter the coiled tubules of the *epididymis,* and are propelled by muscle contraction through the *vas deferens* and *ejaculatory duct,* and through the *prostate gland.* During ejaculation, sperm leave the prostate and pass through the urethra and urinary meatus (Fig. 15-15). *Cowper's glands,* located near the prostate, are homologous to female Bartholin glands and secrete mucus into the sperm during sexual arousal. Additional secretions are produced by the *seminal vesicles.*

THE INGUINAL AREA

The term *inguinal* refers to the groin region. Several inguinal structures are routinely assessed as part of the male genital examination. The *inguinal ligament* is an important assessment landmark that extends from the anterior iliac

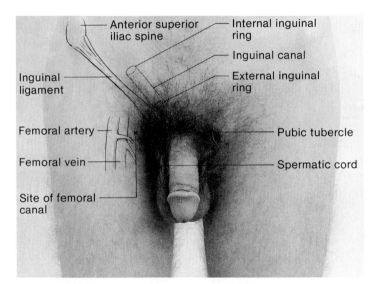

Figure 15–16. Male inguinal structures.

Labels on figure: Anterior superior iliac spine / Internal inguinal ring / Inguinal canal / External inguinal ring / Inguinal ligament / Femoral artery / Femoral vein / Pubic tubercle / Spermatic cord / Site of femoral canal

spine to the pubic tubercle. Above and parallel to the inguinal ligament is the *inguinal canal,* which carries the spermatic cord (Fig. 15-16). The distal opening of the inguinal canal is called the *external inguinal ring,* a structure accessible to palpation. Occasionally, because of weakness in the abdominal wall, the visceral contents protrude through the inguinal canal and, in some cases, extend through the external inguinal ring to the scrotum. This is called an *inguinal hernia.*

The femoral canal, although not generally palpable, represents another potential route for herniation. The femoral canal lies below the inguinal ligament, medial to the femoral artery. Lymphatic chains are located below the inguinal ligament and medial to the femoral vein.

Physical Examination   *Penis, Scrotum, and Inguinal Areas*

General Principles

Assessment techniques for assessing the male genitals and inguinal region include inspection and palpation.

Minimizing Anxiety

Generally, men have less concerns about the sexual implications of the genital examination than women, and they usually do not feel as depersonalized or degraded by this facet of the assessment process. Sociocultural factors may influence attitudes in that many men feel comfortable being examined by male physicians and are accustomed to nudity in locker rooms. However, some men may feel anxious about the assessment, especially if a rectal assessment is performed in conjunction with genital assessment.

Some men may experience an erection during the assessment, which can be a source of embarrassment. Should this occur, the assessment should continue and the client reassured that this is a normal physiologic response to genital palpation.

Female nurses may feel anxious about assessing male genitals and may convey their embarrassment to the client. Working through your own feelings and discussing them with colleagues may help build confidence and self-assurance in performing this assessment.

Equipment

• Gloves: nonsterile, examination type
• Flashlight

Using Gloves

Both hands should be gloved during the assessment. Gloves offer protection from inadvertent exposure if an infection is present. Gloves should be changed before the rectal assessment to avoid cross-contamination in the case of genital infections.

Preparation and Positioning

The client should stand for the assessment so that the inguinal area can be palpated easily. You should be seated, facing the client's genitals. The client may wear an examining gown that is easily lifted during the assessment.

Assessment and Documentation Focus

• Penis: skin color and pigmentation, skin lesions, masses, or discharge; discharge from urinary meatus
• Scrotum: skin integrity, consistency of testicles, epididymis, and vas deferens
• Inguinal area: bulges, masses

Examination Guidelines   *Male Genitals and Inguinal Area*

Procedure	Clinical Significance

1. INSPECT AND PALPATE THE PENIS.
 	
  a. Ask client to expose genitals by lifting gown.
 	
  b. Inspect penis and note skin integrity of glans, foreskin, and shaft. If the client is uncircumcised, ask him to retract the foreskin so that you can inspect the underlying area. Inspect the base of the penis and pubic hair; note any signs of infestation.
	Normal Findings
	
	The size and shape of the penis normally vary considerably among adult men but are often a source of concern. Although penis size may vary considerably in the flaccid state, considerably less size variation exists in the erect penis. The glans penis varies in size and shape and may appear rounded, broad, or even pointed. Assist the client to understand normal variations if he expresses concern.

Male Genitals and Inguinal Area

Procedure

c. Inspect the urinary meatus by grasping the glans between your thumb and forefinger and gently squeezing to expose the meatus.

If the client reports a history of discharge from the urethra but none is revealed by the above maneuver, ask him to milk the shaft of the penis from the base to the tip with his fingers.

d. Palpate the shaft of the penis between your thumb and forefinger, noting any masses or tenderness (optional in the young asymptomatic boy or man).

2. INSPECT AND PALPATE THE SCROTUM.

a. Displace the penis to one side or ask the client to do so, in order to inspect the scrotum. Lift the scrotal sac and inspect the posterior side. Note skin integrity. If the scrotum is enlarged, place a flashlight next to the scrotum and observe for transillumination of the scrotum.

Clinical Significance

Smegma is a normal discharge that may accumulate on the penis, especially beneath the foreskin of the uncircumcised male who does not thoroughly clean the area. Smegma results from Tyson gland secretions and appears as a thick, white, cheeselike substance. Accumulated smegma may convert into a bacterial growth medium.

Deviations from Normal

A ventral curvature (chordee) of the penis shaft is abnormal and is the result of a fibrous band of tissue constricting the penis.

Normal Findings

Normally, the urinary meatus is free of drainage and discharge.

Deviations from Normal

Any discharge noted with this maneuver is abnormal and should be cultured. Any time the meatus is not found centered on the glans it should be noted. The meatus can be found on the shaft of the penis; this is known as *hypospadias.*

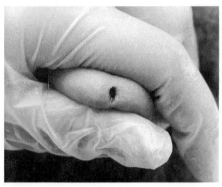

Inspecting the urinary meatus

Normal Findings

Masses should not be palpable along the shaft of the penis. The penis is not normally tender to palpation and should not be tender when the glans is squeezed gently to assess the urinary meatus.

Normal Findings

Scrotal size and shape vary considerably, and this may cause anxiety in men who believe the sexual myth that a large scrotum is associated with virility. Some scrotal sacs hang below the penis, whereas others are above. The left side of the scrotum is usually lower than the right. The scrotum is held high and appears smaller in size when scrotal muscles contract in response to fear or cold. Scrotal skin has scattered hairs. The skin should be thin and rugated, causing a wrinkled appearance.

Deviations from Normal

Lesions should be noted as abnormal. The absence of rugated skin, red color, warmth to touch, and an enlarged scrotum indicate inflammation and possibly infection. An enlarged scrotum that is not red may indicate excessive fluid or a mass in the scrotum. A scrotum that is enlarged with fluid except for blood will transilluminate. A scrotum enlarged by a mass such as intestines or tumor will not transilluminate.

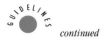
continued

Male Genitals and Inguinal Area

Procedure

b. Palpate one scrotal compartment at a time by grasping the scrotum between your thumb and forefinger. Gently squeeze to detect the testicle, remembering that this maneuver may be slightly painful.

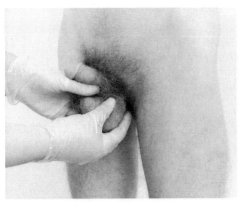
Scrotal palpation

c. Palpate the epididymis by grasping the posterior portion of the scrotum between your thumb and forefinger and feeling for a firm, comma-like structure. If not found in the posterior portion, it may be found in the anterolateral or anterior areas of the testes.

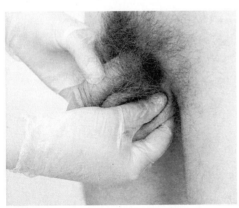
Palpating the epididymis

d. Finally, palpate the vas deferens by moving your thumb and forefinger from the epididymis to the vas in an anterior direction. Palpate the inguinal ring.

Clinical Significance

Normal Findings

Two testicles that feel ovoid, smooth, and homogeneous in consistency should be palpable through the thin scrotal skin. The testicles should be freely moveable, equal in size, and slightly sensitive to compression.

Deviations from Normal

Any inconsistency of homogeneity between the two testes should be evaluated. *Any mass should be referred immediately, since testicular cancer metastasizes rapidly.*

Normal Findings

The epididymis should be firm. In 7% of males the epididymis is located in the anterolateral or anterior portions of the testes.

Deviations from Normal

A nonfirm or very tender epididymis may indicate inflammation.

Normal Findings

The vas should feel cord-like and move freely. The epididymis should be discrete, smooth, nontender, and without masses. The vas deferens should feel like smooth cords and are moveable and nontender.

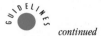

continued

Male Genitals and Inguinal Area

Procedure

3. INSPECT FOR INGUINAL AND FEMORAL HERNIAS.

   a. Inspect the inguinal area and note any bulges. Ask the client to bear down so you can detect any bulges.

   b. Palpate the area overlying the femoral canal with and without the client bearing down.

   c. Palpate the skin overlying the superficial inguinal lymph nodes, noting enlargement and mobility of palpable nodes.

Clinical Significance

Normal Findings

Bulges should not be noted on the skin overlying the inguinal and femoral canal or during coughing or straining.

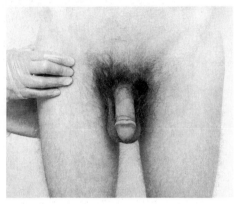

Femoral canal palpation

4. PALPATE THE INGUINAL CANAL.

   To palpate the right inguinal canal, approach the client from the right side. Palpate the inguinal canal by invaginating the loose scrotal skin with your right index finger at the bottom of the scrotal sac. Follow the spermatic cord with your finger to the external inguinal ring, a triangular, slitlike opening. If the inguinal ring is large enough, continue advancing your finger along the inguinal canal. Ask the client to cough or bear down. Repeat the procedure on the left side.

Normal Findings

You should not feel a bulge in the inguinal canal or a mass moving down the canal when the client coughs or bears down.

Deviations from Normal

Palpable masses in the inguinal canal may represent hernias. See display for types of hernias in the inguinal–femoral area.

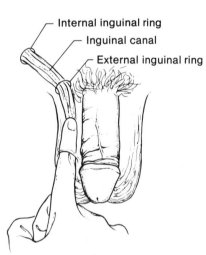

- Internal inguinal ring
- Inguinal canal
- External inguinal ring

Inguinal canal palpation

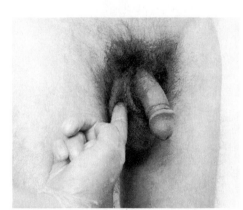

Inguinal canal palpation

Inguinal and Femoral Hernias

Indirect Inguinal Hernias

An indirect inguinal hernia is a herniation through the inguinal canal. The hernia may be felt with the fingertip as a bulge in the canal or may extend beyond the canal into the scrotum. Indirect inguinal hernias may be detected by inserting your index finger into the inguinal canal.

Direct Inguinal Hernia

A direct inguinal hernia does not travel through the inguinal canal; rather, the hernia sac protrudes anteriorly through the abdominal wall. During inguinal canal palpation, the hernia displaces the examining finger forward. Alternatively, a direct hernia may be felt as a bulge between the thumb and forefinger when palpating the skin around the external canal as the person bears down. Direct inguinal hernias rarely descend into the scrotum.

Femoral Hernia

A femoral hernia may be detected below the inguinal ligament and medial to the femoral pulse as a visible or palpable bulge. Femoral hernias are more common in women.

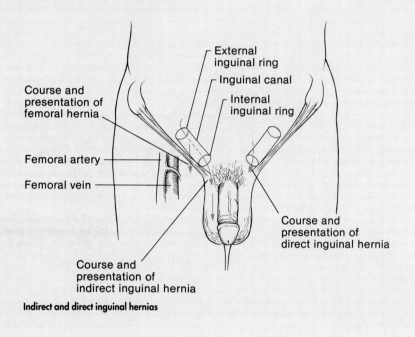

Indirect and direct inguinal hernias

Documenting Male Genital and Inguinal Examination Findings

Example 1: Normal Findings

Mr. L, aged 26, had a complete physical assessment, including genital and hernia assessment. The findings were normal and recorded as follows:

External genital skin smooth without lesions or discharge. Testes descended and equal size, scrotal contents smooth, nontender to palpation. No palpable masses in inguinal or femoral canals.

These same findings may be recorded in a problem-oriented format as follows:

S: Denies genital lesions, dysuria, or urethral discharge
O: External genital skin smooth; no lesions or discharge. Testes descended and equal size, scrotal contents smooth, nontender to palpation. No palpable masses in inguinal or femoral canals.
A: Normal male genitals, no inguinal or femoral hernias
P: Evaluate teaching needs regarding TSE, STDs, reproductive management. Routine annual follow-up.

Example 2: Suspected Inguinal Hernia

Mr. B., aged 45, had an inguinal assessment in an occupational health clinic. He had recently been treated for low back pain. The findings were abnormal and recorded as follows:

No visible inguinal masses. Small, firm mass palpated in right inguinal canal with Valsalva maneuver. Nonpalpable when relaxed.

These findings may be recorded in a problem-oriented format as follows:

S: Job responsibilities include heavy lifting. Denies genitourinary problems such as dysuria, lesions, or urethral discharge.

O: No visible inguinal masses. Small, firm mass palpated in right inguinal canal with Valsalva maneuver. Not palpable when relaxed.

A: Suspect indirect inguinal hernia.

P: Evaluate teaching needs regarding hernia complications and preventive treatment—proper body mechanics while lifting. Refer to physician.

Example 3: Genital Skin Lesions

Mr. M, aged 18, came to the student health clinic for evaluation and treatment of genital skin lesions. The physical assessment findings were recorded as follows:

Nut-like particles on shaft of pubic hair concentrated at base of penis and scattered on pubic hair of scrotum. No lice or other parasites noted. Small cluster of multiple vesicles noted at base of penis. Skin otherwise intact. Reports of burning at lesion sites and generalized genital area itching.

NDx

Nursing Diagnoses Related to Male Genital and Inguinal Examination

Currently, three nursing diagnoses in the sexuality pattern are related to assessment of the male genitals and inguinal area: Rape-trauma syndromes, Altered sexuality pattern, and Sexual dysfunction. Nursing diagnoses from other functional patterns, such as High risk for infection, Health-seeking behavior, Knowledge deficit, and Pain, may also be appropriate depending upon examination findings.

See the discussion of sexuality-pattern nursing diagnoses in the section on nursing diagnoses related to female genitals in this chapter. Characteristics unique to men for these diagnoses are considered here.

Rape-Trauma Syndromes

Although rape occurs more frequently to women, men also experience rape. Those men at higher risk are adolescents and younger men in abusive situations, and adult men in prison or jails. Men are generally subjected to anal penetration and sometimes oral. The male response to rape is similar to the female response.

Sexual Dysfunction and Altered Sexual Pattern

In addition to the problems experienced by women, men may report difficulty attaining or sustaining an erection and ejaculation problems, including premature, retarded, and retrograde ejaculation. The nature of these problems may be psychogenic, or disease- or medication-related. In male diabetics, erection problems are common. Men with erection and ejaculation problems should be assessed by a specialist.

Clinical Problems Related to Male Genital and Inguinal Examination

Sexually Transmitted Diseases

Gonorrhea

Although the clinical course and presentation of the disease vary, men with gonorrhea, unlike women, are seldom asymptomatic. Usual symptoms are related to urinary elimination and appear early as the organism invades the urethra. The man may report urgency, frequency, burning, and a serous or purulent urethral discharge. Within a week of exposure, the discharge may become profuse, yellow, and blood-tinged. The discharge should be cultured on a Thayer-Martin medium to identify the organism. Rectal infection may be noted in homosexual men and is associated with rectal pain and burning as well as purulent discharge. Infection of the oropharynx should not be overlooked. Untreated gonorrhea affects the epididymis, prostate, and periurethral glands, causing acute inflammation.

Syphilis

As with women, untreated syphilis in men advances through five stages (see p. 467). During early stages, a syphilitic chancre appears, usually on the glans penis or shaft. The chancre is a round, ulcerated papule that may be palpable with a gloved hand as a firm, hard mass. For those who engage in oral or anal intercourse, the chancre may be found near the mouth or anus.

Herpes

Genital herpes presents as a cluster of small painful vesicles on the penis, which eventually rupture and heal. Recurrence is common. Viral shedding, even when vesicles are not present, can infect others during intercourse.

Genital Warts

In men, warts appear on the penis as a single lesion or multiple elongated lesions. Occasionally, the warts proliferate to the extent that they appear as large cauliflower-like lesions. They may heal spontaneously or may undergo malignant transformation.

Nonspecific Urethritis

Affecting only men, nonspecific urethritis refers to urethritis from which specific organisms such as Gonococcus cannot be isolated. In many cases, *Chlamydia* may be the responsible organism. Men with nonspecific urethritis are usually sexually active with multiple partners. With physical assessment, a urethral discharge may be noted, ranging from a slight watery discharge to a copious, purulent discharge. The infection may spontaneously resolve within 8 weeks, although recurrences are common.

Phimosis

In phimosis, the foreskin of an uncircumcised man cannot be retracted because of stenosis. Circumcision is indicated.

Carcinoma of the Penis

Malignant lesions are noted more often in uncircumcised men. The lesion, often covered by the foreskin, appears as a hard, nontender nodule.

Scrotum Abnormalities

Hydrocele. A hydrocele is a collection of fluid in the tunica vaginalis of the testicle. This abnormality is associated with many clinical conditions that involve inadequate fluid reabsorption, including local inflammation and injury, cirrhosis, congestive heart failure, and testicular tumor. On physical assessment, the scrotum is enlarged, and if transuluminated with a penlight, transmits light. Hydroceles are usually painless until large enough to create excessive pressure or scrotal pulling.

Varicocele. A varicocele is a mass of varicose veins in the scrotum, usually around the spermatic cord. The mass is palpable, feels like a "bag of worms," and may dissipate after the client has been supine. It usually appears at puberty.

Scrotal Edema. The scrotal skin can become edematous; palpation causes pitting. With any generalized edema associated with such conditions as congestive heart failure, scrotal edema is common.

Testicular Cancer. Any palpable mass or nodules on the testicles should be suspected of malignancy. The testicular self-examination should be taught to adolescent men as a means of early detection (see Chap. 6). Tumor masses are often painless.

Epididymitis. Epididymitis may result from the spread of an STD or from an infected prostate or urethra. The scrotum is usually diffusely tender, edematous, and erythematous. Localized scrotal pain may be noted, especially during palpation.

Torsion of the Spermatic Cord. Torsion is an axial rotation or twisting of testicle on the spermatic cord. A mass is felt anterior to the testicle. Extremely painful, the scrotum may become edematous and erythematous. This condition is considered a surgical emergency because of obstructed circulation and eventual infarction of the testicle. It occurs most frequently in adolescents.

ASSESSMENT PROFILE 1

● ●

Ben, aged 52, was recently discharged from the hospital after an acute myocardial infarction. Although he had suffered no serious complications, his illness had frightened him. Before his discharge, many health care providers discussed his recovery with him and assessed his teaching needs in relation to diet, exercise, medications, and gradual resumption of work activities. Because no one had addressed sexual concerns, Ben decided that sexual activity must be forbidden.

Profile Analysis

Ben has the potential for sexual dysfunction because the following risk factor is present: He is uninformed about sexual function following acute myocardial infarction. Moreover, Ben's health care providers have failed to elicit this important cue, so his potential problem has not been diagnosed and preventive measures have not been initiated.

Several factors may have contributed to failure to diagnose the problem. Factors that may have influenced assessment and, ultimately, diagnosis include the following:

1. *Failure to perceive sexual functions as part of the nursing domain.* The profile indicates that many other functions were evaluated before Ben's discharge, but sexual functions were not. Possibly, sexuality assessment was not a usual part of the data collected by nurses at this institution. Such an omission may prevent the nurse from asking a simple screening question such as, "What concerns do you have about sex following this illness?" Failure to ask the question could indicate that sexual matters were not a nursing concern.

2. *Failure to use pre-encounter patient data to notice the possibility of sexuality problems.* According to Car-

nevali and coworkers (1984), pre-encounter patient data, such as age, sex, and medical diagnosis, may be used to narrow or direct data collection. In other words, on the basis of pre-encounter data, the nurse may decide on probable diagnoses and focus data collection by looking for cues to confirm these diagnoses. It is well documented in nursing and medical literature that middle-aged men often have sexual concerns following acute myocardial infarction. Therefore, the nurse should assess the sexual concerns of such patients even though the patients may not initiate the discussion. Failure to use pertinent pre-encounter data may indicate a deficit in the nurse's knowledge base about acute myocardial infarction.

3. *Failure to extract meaning from the available cues.* Often the most meaningful cues are those that indicate well-known signs or symptoms of specific problems. Other cues may be more elusive or may be perceived by the nurse as unreliable, particularly if cues do not correlate with textbook representations of a problem. For example, the most obvious cues indicating actual or potential sexual dysfunction include the defining characteristics for this nursing diagnosis specified by NANDA. Apparently, Ben did not reveal any such signs or symptoms to health care providers. However, other cues were significant. Ben had risk factors for sexual dysfunction, including a major health problem—acute myocardial infarction. Ben's failure to discuss sexual concerns may serve as an indicator of potential sexual dysfunction. Furthermore, knowledge of possible sexual partners (in this case, Ben's spouse) and observation of their interactions should have provided additional cues related to sexual dysfunction.

ASSESSMENT PROFILE 2

• •

Betsy, aged 11, came to the community health clinic for a physical examination that was required for summer camp. During the interview, the nurse discovered that no one had discussed menstruation with Betsy.

Profile Analysis

The community health nurse assessing Betsy believed that sexuality assessment was a component of comprehensive health assessment for people of all ages. Based on Betsy's age and sex, the nurse was able to ask pertinent questions to elicit data about her sexual and reproductive functions. The nurse used a screening question to invite Betsy to discuss sexual and reproductive functioning: "Betsy, you are beginning to develop as a young woman and within the next year or two, will begin menstruating. Has anyone ever talked with you about what that means?" The nurse's belief that a client's sexuality and reproductive concerns are nursing concerns, and the nurse's knowledge of pre-encounter data about sexuality teaching needs for this age group, influenced the assessment process.

ASSESSMENT PROFILE 3

• •

Paul, aged 35, was recovering from diabetic ketoacidosis. He thought that the stress he had suffered after terminating an intimate relationship had contributed to the diabetic crisis. He also wondered if his recent impotence had been caused by insulin. When the nurse attempted to discuss sexual aspects of his disease with him, Paul denied having any problems because he thought the nurse would not understand that his sexual partners were usually men.

Profile Analysis

Paul is unlikely to discuss sexual aspects of his disease with health care providers that he perceives might be judgmental about his sexual life-style. The nurse should initiate the topic of sexuality again even though no prior concerns were expressed. If a trusting relationship has developed between nurse and patient, information is more likely to be shared. At all times, avoid judgmental language such as, "How has this illness affected your relationships with *women?*"

ASSESSMENT PROFILE 4

• •

Anna, aged 64, was recovering from a radical mastectomy. She was an attractive woman who enjoyed dressing fashionably, trying different hair styles, and using cosmetics. A widow, Anna was devoted to her children and grandchildren. After surgery, Anna became depressed and withdrawn and finally told the nurse that even though she had no desire to remarry, she felt she had lost her sexual identity. "Even an old widow like myself needs to feel like a woman," she cried.

Profile Analysis

Identifying the Problem. The nurses caring for Anna recognized cues indicating a potential problem with sexual health. Additionally, the diagnostic process was influenced by pre-encounter knowledge.

Pre-encounter Knowledge. Anna was receiving care from the professional staff of a surgical oncology unit. The nurses realized that most cancer surgery, especially if disfiguring, threatens body image. Furthermore, they knew that body image influences sexuality, regardless of a person's age. Sexual health is especially threatened when cancer surgery affects organs such as breasts.

Although younger patients often express concerns related to sexual performance and procreative functions, the older patient is also concerned with feeling like and being perceived by others as a sexual being. Both body image and sexuality contribute to a person's overall self-concept (see Chap. 12). On the basis of this knowledge, the nurses realized that because Anna had had a mastectomy, she was at greater risk of developing an altered body image, an altered sexuality, and an altered self-concept. Therefore, they collected data relevant to such diagnostic possibilities. The nurses considered the following questions: What does this surgery mean to Anna? How does she perceive self and body in this situation? What body parts have the greatest importance for the self-concept?

Cues in the Profile. The following cue indicated that Anna was at risk for self-concept alterations: loss of a body part (breast) by surgery. A subjective indicator of this problem was Anna's statement: "Even an old widow like myself needs to feel like a woman." Other cues suggesting strengths that might promote recovery included strong family ties and Anna's previously healthy body image, as manifested by her pride in her appearance. Additionally, the nurses noted that Anna was widowed and stated she had no desire to remarry. This cue suggested that Anna was not concerned with the immediate reaction of a sexual partner to her changed appearance. However, they would need to validate this inference with Anna.

Possible Nursing Diagnoses

One of Anna's nurses describes her thoughts leading to a definitive nursing diagnosis:

> Anna kept making references to her sexual identity or feelings about being a woman, so I first considered a diagnosis related to sexual dysfunction. Knowing that radical surgery can be an etiologic factor also influenced my diagnosis. She wanted confirmation of her sexual desirability, which is a defining characteristic for sexual dysfunction. My first diagnosis was sexual dysfunction related to radical surgery.
>
> Then I began to ask why her sexual health was threatened. It seemed to make more sense to focus nursing intervention on the underlying factors threatening sexuality, in which case, a more spe-

cific diagnosis was needed. I began to consider the diagnosis *Body image disturbance,* and reevaluated the data with this diagnosis in mind. She indicated that she now views herself differently, a cue consistent with this diagnosis; she had lost a body part, which can be an etiologic factor, and she showed signs of grieving (depression, withdrawal, and weeping) as well as negative feelings about her body, which are associated defining characteristics. It seemed to me that we should focus on the Body image disturbance, keeping in mind that failure to resolve this problem could alter sexual health.

Final Nursing Diagnosis

The definitive nursing diagnosis, Body image disturbance related to loss of body part, was recorded on the nursing care plan and interventions and outcomes were formulated.

Prognosis

Planning interventions required further assessment. Assessment focused on factors known to influence adaptation to body image alterations, including the reactions of significant others and the patient's interpretation of such reactions; the meaning of the body change to the patient; and the patient's coping style and ability.

Chapter 15 SUMMARY

Sexuality and reproductive function assessment focuses on the following:
- The person's concerns related to sexual and reproductive functions
- The person's sexual and reproductive teaching needs
- Identification of sexual or reproductive problems requiring nursing intervention or referral
- Evaluation of reproductive growth and development

When assessing sexuality and reproductive functions, you should consider the following:
- A trusting, nonjudgmental nurse–client relationship facilitates the assessment process.
- Data collection is initiated by giving the person permission to discuss sexual concerns.
- Sexuality assessment is important regardless of the person's age, marital status, sexual activities, or physical status.
- Your own values or personal beliefs may influence assessment, especially when they conflict with the client's.
- Some sexual problems should be treated by health professionals with more advanced training than nurses. You should facilitate appropriate referrals.

Data sources for assessment of sexuality and reproduction include the following:

The Interview
The interview may be limited to granting permission to discuss sexual topics, or it may focus on specific topics, such as the following:
- Sexual roles and gender identification
- Sexuality and reproduction knowledge base

- Sexual performance and satisfaction concerns
- Reproductive history

Nursing Observations
- Interactions with significant others
- Breast examination
- Female genital and pelvic examination or male genital examination
- Rectal examination

Sexuality and reproductive function assessment, based on these principles and methods, enables you to identify defining characteristics that may be present for the following nursing diagnoses:
   Ineffective breast-feeding
   Rape-trauma syndrome
      Rape-trauma syndrome: compound reaction
      Rape-trauma syndrome: silent reaction
   Sexual dysfunction
   Altered patterns, sexuality

Related nursing diagnoses may be identified, especially Body image disturbance.
   Additionally, you will develop skill at detecting and monitoring the following clinical problems:
   Sexually transmitted diseases
   Vaginitis
   Pelvic structure alterations
   Malignant processes involving reproductive organs
   Hernias
   Scrotal abnormalities

Finally, you will develop skill at monitoring the health status of pregnant women.

RESEARCH *Hi*GHLIGHT

What type of questions do women ask after receiving abnormal Papanicolaou test results?

As nurses, we often inform individuals of abnormal diagnostic tests. Often these findings are unexpected. Weiner (1985, cited in this study) and other theorists suggest that individuals seek to find causes for these unexpected events. Clients often ask questions such as "Why me?".

Diane Lauver, Andrea Barsevick, and Mary Rubin believed that there was a need to understand affective and behavioral responses to unexplained Pap smear results. The literature reviewed for this study suggested that 17% to 44% of women with abnormal Pap results do not seek prompt follow-up. It was not know if attempts to discover causes for results resulted in prompt or delayed care seeking.[1]

Participants for this study came from a university hospital medical center; 118 women were interviewed. Most of the women were African-Americans, single, had at least one pregnancy, were working or going to school, and had at least a high school education. Open-ended questions were used to ask women about their Pap results. Of those who participated, 72 asked one or more questions about the results, but only 39 asked about possible causes. Another 13% asked about the seriousness of the findings. Fifty-five women expressed being worried, frightened, and scared. The study's findings did not support a relationship between seeking causes for unexpected Pap results and delayed or prompt follow-up.

What significance does this study have for health assessment?

When providing information to individuals about diagnostic tests performed during a health assessment, the nurse should be prepared to answer questions not only about the findings but also about probable causes (if known), and to provide emotional support. The nurse may need to ask if the individual has any questions or concerns about the results. In this study people had misconceptions regarding possible causes. Exploring concerns and correcting misinformation can relieve unnecessary worry and concern for the client.

Can the study's findings be applied to practice?

Although nurses do not always report abnormal results to clients, they often have contact with clients after receiving abnormal results. Abnormal results may be simply corrected by increasing nutrients, such as vitamin C and potassium, or may be perceived as life threatening, such as a positive HIV test or breast cancer. Being prepared to ask open-ended questions about concerns clients have and to supply correct information and emotional support as needed improves the care provided to clients.

REFERENCE

1. Lauver, D., Barsevick, A., & Rubin, M. (1990). Spontaneous causal searching and adjustment to abnormal Papanicolaou test results. *Nursing Research, 38* (5), 305–308.

✸ CRITICAL THINKING

Historically, nurses did not venture into the assessment of sexuality and sexual functions with patients, but since the publication of Masters and Johnson's work on human sexuality in the 1960s, the assessment of sexuality has become increasingly sanctioned. The 1990s are a time of public emphasis on issues relating to sexuality and reproductive functions, including the AIDS epidemic, abortion, and homosexuality. Health professionals have an increasing need to obtain accurate data about sexual and reproductive functioning.

Learning Exercises

1. Develop some guidelines to determine when a screening assessment of sexuality is indicated over a comprehensive assessment.

2. Explain how health problems can affect sexuality.

3. Explain how you would put a client at ease during an assessment of sexuality.

4. Identify and describe a situation in which you would feel uncomfortable assessing sexual functions. Evaluate and discuss your reasons for feeling uncomfortable.

BIBLIOGRAPHY

Aiken, M. (1990). Documenting sexual abuse in prepubertal girls. *MCN, 15* (5), 176–177.

Andrews, J. (1992). How we do it: Sexual assault aftercare instructions. *Journal of Emergency Nursing, 18* (2), 152–157.

Annon, J.S. (1976). The PLISSIT Model: A proposed conceptual scheme for the treatment of sexual problems. *Journal of Sex Education and Therapy, 2,* 1–15.

Becker, J.V., et al. (1984). Sexual problems of sexual assault survivors. *Women and Health, 9* (4), 5–20.

Bem, S.L. (1981). Gender schema theory: A cognitive account of sex-typing. *Psychological Review, 88* (4), 354–364.

Bobak, I.M., & Jensen, M.D. (1991). *Essentials of maternity care* (3rd ed.). St. Louis: C.V. Mosby.

Brink, P. (1987). Cultural aspects of sexuality. *Holistic Nursing Practice, 1* (4), 12–20.

Bullard, D.G., & Knight, S.E. (Eds). (1981). *Sexuality and physical disability: Personal perspectives.* St. Louis: C.V. Mosby.

Carnevali, D.L. et al. (1993). *Diagnostic reasoning in nursing* (3rd ed.). Philadelphia: J.B. Lippincott.

Carpenito, L. (1993). *Nursing diagnosis: Application to clinical practice* (5th ed.). Philadelphia: J.B. Lippincott.

Castiglia, P. (1991). Sexual abuse of children. *Journal of Pediatric Health Care, 4* (2), 91–93.

Chapman, J., & Sughrue, J. (1987). A model for sexual assessment and intervention. *Health Care for Women International, 8* (1), 87–99.

Comfort, A. (1972). Refractory period after ejaculation. *Lancet, 1*:1075.

Domar, A.D. (1986). Psychologic aspects of the pelvic exam: Individual needs and physician involvement. *Women and Health, 10* (4), 75–90.

Fogel, C., Fogel, L., & Woods, N.F. (1981). *Health care of women.* St. Louis: C.V. Mosby.

Forrester, D.A. (1986). Myths of masculinity: Impact upon men's health. *Nursing Clinics of North America, 21* (1), 15–23.

Friend, R. (1987). Sexual identity and human diversity: Implications for nursing practice. *Holistic Nursing Practice, 1* (4), 21–41.

Heinrich, L. (1987). Care of the female rape victim. *Nurse Practitioner, 12* (11), 9–10.

Hogan, R. (1985). *Human sexuality: A nursing perspective* (2nd ed.). Norwalk, CT: Appleton-Century-Crofts.

Holmes, K.K., & Mardh, P.A. (Eds.). (1983). *International perspectives on neglected sexually transmitted diseases.* New York: McGraw-Hill.

Kelley, S.J. (1985). Interviewing the sexually abused child: Principles and techniques. *Journal of Emergency Nursing, 11* (5), 234–241.

Kinsey, A.C., et al. (1965). *Sexual behavior in the human female.* New York: Pocket Books.

Kinsey, A.C., Pomeroy, W.B., Martin, C.E. (1948). *Sexual behavior in the human male.* Philadelphia: W.B. Saunders.

Lasater, S. (1988). Testicular cancer: A nursing perspective of diagnosis and treatment. *Journal of Urological Nursing, 7* (1), 329–349.

Masters, W., & Johnson, V. (1970). *Human sexual inadequacy.* Boston: Little, Brown.

Nettles-Carlson, B. (1989). Early detection of breast cancer. *Journal of Obstetric, Gynecologic, and Neonatal Nursing, 18* (5), 373–381.

Nolan, J.W. (1986). Developmental concerns and the health of midlife women. *Nursing Clinics of North America, 21* (1), 151–159.

Paul, E.A., & O'Neill, J.S. (1983). A sexual health model for nursing intervention. *Issues in Health Care for Women, 4* (2/3), 115–125.

Pritchard, J.A., & MacDonald, P.C. (1980). *William's obstetrics.* New York: Appleton-Century-Crofts.

Schifeling, D., & Hamblin, J. (1991). Early diagnosis of breast cancer: Universal screening is essential. *Postgraduate Medicine, 89* (3), 55–62.

Siemens, S., & Brandzel, R.C. (1982). *Sexuality: Nursing assessment and intervention.* Philadelphia: J.B. Lippincott.

Spence, J.T., & Helmrich, R.L. Androgyny versus gender schema: A comment on Bem's gender schema theory. *Psychological Review, 88* (4), 365–368.

State, D. (1991). Nipple discharge in women: Is it cause for concern? *Postgraduate Medicine, 89* (3), 65–68.

Waterhouse, J., & Metclife, M. (1991). Attitudes toward nurses discussing sexual concerns with patients. *Journal of Advanced Nursing, 16,* 1048–1054.

Watts, R.J. (1979). Dimensions of sexual health. *American Journal of Nursing, 79* (9), 1568–1572.

Willson, J.R., Carrington, F.R., & Ledger, W.J. (1991). *Obstetrics and gynecology* (9th ed.). St. Louis: C.V. Mosby.

Wilson, P. (1991). Testicular, prostate and penile cancers in primary care settings: The importance of early detection. *Nurse Practitioner, 16* (11), 18–26.

Woods, N.F. (1984). *Human sexuality in health and illness* (3rd ed.). St. Louis: C.V. Mosby.

Woods, N.F. (1987). Toward a holistic perspective of human sexuality: Alterations in sexual health and nursing diagnoses. *Holistic Nursing Practice, 1* (4), 1–11.

Woods, N.F., & Mandetta, A.F. (1976). Sexuality in the baccalaureate nursing curriculum. *Nursing Forum, 15* (3), 294–313.

World Health Organization. (1975). *Education and treatment in human sexuality: The training of health professionals.* WHO Technical Report Series 572.

Assessing Stress and Stress Responses

Stress Response

Suicide Potential

Assessment Terms

Stress
Stress Response
Positive Stress (Eustress)
Negative Stress (Distress)
Coping
Tension Reduction
Problem Resolution
Defense Mechanisms
Intrapsychic Processes

Denial
Displacement
Projection
Rationalization
Regression
Repression
Suppression
Crisis
Suicide Ideation

INTRODUCTORY OVERVIEW

Stress, as defined by Lazarus (1966), is the disruption of meaning or smooth functioning in a person's life that results in harm, loss, or challenge to that person. People respond to stress in a variety of ways. Responses can be cognitive (involving mental capacities), affective (involving emotional/psychological aspects), and physical. Some people may respond to stress with feelings of tension or anguish, others may interpret stress as normal and something to be endured, and still others might learn a new skill that helps them adapt to the new situation. Selye (1976) emphasized that stress is inevitable and that stress can affect a person's health either positively or negatively. Positive stress, which Selye calls *eustress*, is associated with adaptation and is necessary for growth and development. An example of positive stress might be the initial pressures and anxiousness felt by an individual when promoted into a new job with added responsibilities. Another example is the normal anxiousness of adolescents as they strive to be accepted by their peers and the opposite sex.

In contrast, negative stress, called *distress*, is potentially harmful and may exhaust one's ability to adapt. In the example above, the positive stress might turn into negative stress if the newly promoted individual realizes that the new boss requires that he works 60 hours a week and meanwhile, at home, his wife is expecting a third child, is having a difficult pregnancy, and he faces time and energy demands at home to

Jill Fuller and Jennifer Schaller-Ayers:
HEALTH ASSESSMENT: A NURSING APPROACH, Second Edition.
© 1990, 1994 by J. B. Lippincott Company.

help out with the other young children in the evenings and weekends.

Stress may interfere with a person's abilities to meet basic needs, function on the job, or solve daily problems. Negative stress can become excessive and cumulative. It can build up over time, spanning several different events or problems, and become overwhelming to the individual and reach a crisis stage. Such unresolved negative stress can adversely affect individuals both physically and emotionally. It can contribute to serious illness such as hypertension, coronary artery disease, and peptic ulcer in addition to unpleasant feelings of powerlessness, helplessness, or fear. In worst cases, unresolved negative stress can lead to despondency, depression, or even suicide.

Coping is one way humans react to stress and how they attempt to solve their problems in order to restore the meaning or eliminate the disruption to their lives. Coping strategies can be negative or positive and can be successful or unsuccessful. An example of a negative coping strategy might be to avoid problems through abuse of drugs or alcohol. In contrast, a positive coping strategy might be to take specific actions to solve a particular problem. Types of coping strategies are discussed in more detail in a later section.

Clearly, stress and stress response have a great effect on health and the quality of life. Therefore the nurse's evaluation of an individual's health status should always include stress and stress responses. Assessment involves a careful analysis of events or situations precipitating stress, the person's perceptions of the event or situation, and the person's responses to it.

Assessment Focus

The assessment of stress and stress responses focuses on the following:

- Identifying situations that precipitate stress
- Understanding the meaning of the stressful situation to the individual
- Identifying the person's strengths and coping skills
- Identifying responses to stress
- Recognizing signs of crisis or threats to safety brought on by stress

The methods for collecting information on each of these topics are outlined in the Assessment Focus display.

In any assessment of stress or coping, the nurse should always keep in mind that the primary purpose is to understand the meaning of the stressful situation or event to the individual. How the individual perceives or interprets the stressful event greatly influences his or her choices of reaction and coping strategies. For example, a woman who is 68 years old, still very physically active and mobile, still able to drive a car and get out of the house will certainly grieve and feel lonely over the death of her husband of 47 years. In contrast, a woman who is 75 years old, disabled, and unable to walk without assistance may not only grieve over the loss of her husband as a companion and loved one, but she may perceive her situation as hopeless and fear that she may not be able to survive without the help of her husband. Each woman's choice of coping strategies or options to alleviate the stress carries a perceived meaning to the individual as well. For example, selling a home of 40 years and moving into a retirement community might be a good option for the first widow described because it would offer her a place to meet many people her age and have planned activities to get her involved. That same option might seem frightening to the second woman who is physically disabled, and she might desperately fear leaving the familiar surroundings of her home and having to depend on "strangers" for assistance. Before making judgments as to whether a person's method of coping is good or bad, effective or ineffective, the nurse should fully understand what motivated the person to use such methods of coping. The nurse should be able to answer the following questions:

Why did the person choose this behavior over another?
What role did personal values (such as autonomy) play in the selection of this behavior?
Which options are possible for this person?
Which options are not possible?

During this process of trying to understand why a person reacted or responded in a certain way, it is important that nurses do not allow their own values to bias the evaluation process. For example, the second woman described previously may choose to quit eating and taking her medication in hope that she can die too rather than be without her husband. Although this option may seem unacceptable to the nurse or she may think it bizarre, she should not let her bias or feelings influence her understanding of the meaning of this choice to the individual.

Nursing Diagnoses

Nursing diagnoses associated with stress and stress responses include the following:

Ineffective individual coping
Defensive coping
Ineffective denial
Decisional conflict (specify)
Anticipatory grieving
Dysfunctional grieving

Diagnoses pertaining to family coping (Ineffective family coping) are discussed more thoroughly in the chapter on roles and relationships (see Chap. 14).

Grieving is a normal process that a person uses to adapt to a significant loss, whether the loss pertains to a person, an animal, a role, or a valuable function. In addition to grieving for the loss of a loved one, a person may also grieve the loss of a home, job, or health. Grieving is a complex emotional response, incorporating numerous and varied coping strategies. Because grieving represents a specific stressful experience, nursing diagnoses pertaining to grieving are listed here.

Nursing diagnoses related to grieving may also be evaluated in relation to roles and relationships, in which case the emphasis is on evaluating the meaning of terminating significant relationships and roles.

Assessment Focus **Stress and Stress Responses**

Assessment Goal	Data Collection Methods
1. Identify the stressors confronting the person.	*Interview* • Nature of the stressors. *Review Questionnaire Data* • Social Readjustment Rating Scale • Everyday Hassles Scale: Can additional data pertaining to stress and coping be obtained by using questionnaires? Can questionnaire items be used to direct the interview?
2. Identify the person's perception of actual and potential stressors.	*Interview* • Nature of the stressors. • Stressors and stress perception: How does the person's perception of the stressor influence the stress response? • Evaluate self-concept (see Chap. 13): Do personality traits exist that influence the person's perception of the stressor (especially locus of control)?
3. Identify potential stressors confronting the person to provide anticipatory guidance.	*Observation* • Potential stressors in the environment. • Potential stressors associated with various health and illness states. What are the typical stressors that might be expected?
4. Identify specific coping strategies that are used by the person.	*Interview* • Coping strategies: What coping strategies can be identified by interviewing the person? *Review Questionnaire Data* • Jaloweic Coping Scale: Can additional data pertaining to coping strategies be obtained by using questionnaires? Can questionnaire items be used to direct the interview? *Observation and Interpretation* • Behaviors. • Statements made by the client: Does observation of behaviors and statements indicate the use of specific defense mechanisms or other coping strategies?
5. Determine the effectiveness of stress management.	*Interview* • Stressor perception. • Stress resolution. *Observation* • Physical responses: Stress has physiologic manifestations. Can possible effects of stress be noted by examining different body systems? • Cognitive processes: Have thought processes and the ability to solve problems been adversely affected by stress? • Self-care abilities: Have self-care abilities been compromised because stress is not managed effectively?
6. Recognize the stress response called *crisis.*	*Interview* • Any part of the interview may reveal cues indicating crisis. *Observation* • Behaviors and statements: Do cues in the person's behavior indicate crisis, or suicidal behaviors or ideation?

RELATED NURSING DIAGNOSES

Other nursing diagnoses related to the assessment of stress and stress responses include the following:

Impaired adjustment
Fear
Hopelessness
Post-trauma response
Powerlessness
Rape-trauma syndrome
Altered self-concept
Spiritual distress (distress of the human spirit)
Potential for Violence: Self-directed or directed at others

KNOWLEDGE BASE FOR ASSESSMENT

To assess stress and stress responses, it is helpful to first understand the nature of stressors, physical responses to stress, and what is meant by coping.

Stressors

Selye (1976) refers to stressors as alarming stimuli that arouse the body from a resting state into a state of readiness to combat or deal with the stressor. This initial response is the alarm phase of the stress response. Physiologically, stressors activate the hypothalamic–pituitary–adrenal axis, thereby stimulating hormones and other substances that enable a person to initiate a psychophysiologic stress response.

Stress responses vary among persons, because stress is initiated not only by a stressor but also by the person's perception of the stressor. For example, divorce and remarriage may be perceived as more threatening by someone who has been married for 35 years than by someone who has been divorced and married four times. One person may be aware of the inner strength that exists to deal with a stressor, whereas another person might perceive the stressor only in terms of the threat it poses. This difference in perception explains why potential stressors do not necessarily evoke a predictable and equal stress response in all people.

Lazarus (1966) has labeled this perceptual element the *cognitive appraisal* of the stressor, which is a process of evaluating the stressor and determining the potential threat it presents. A person usually evaluates a potential stressor and concludes that the event is (1) irrelevant, (2) benign or positive, or (3) stressful. Stressful events are commonly viewed as threats, losses, or challenges. Significantly, cognitive appraisal supports the premise that stress is psychologically, socially, and spiritually oriented as well as physiologically oriented. Cognitive appraisal has important nursing implications in that nursing intervention may help a person alter his or her perception of stress.

Stressors are classified by Guzzetta and Forsyth (1979) as physiologic, psychological, environmental, and sociocultural (Display 16-1). Although discrete categories of stressors are suggested by this classification, in reality the categories may overlap.

Stress may be initiated by both positive and negative life events. For example, marriage, the birth of a child, and the start of a new job are usually viewed as positive events that provide an opportunity for growth, enjoyment, and further

---

Display 16–1
Classification of Stressors*

Physiologic

Trauma
Surgery
Radiation
Body chemistry alterations (drugs, hormones, abnormal secretions, dietary, poisons)
Infectious processes (bacterial, viral, fungal)
Pain
Sleep deprivation or fatigue

Environmental

Pollutants
Urbanization
Changes in physical environment (relocation, hospitalization, poverty, incarceration)
Sensory deprivation
Sensory overload
Loss of privacy
Frightening or unpleasant noises, odors
Untidy surroundings

Psychological

Distressing emotions (fear, anxiety)
Psychological distress (helplessness, powerlessness, loneliness, poor self-esteem, lack of motivation)

Sociocultural

Change
Financial status
Vocational pressures
Family dysfunction
Difficulty with developmental tasks
Child rearing
Aging
Retirement
Religious beliefs

*Physiological stressors disturb primarily tissue systems; the other categories of stressors are evaluated cognitively before stressor recognition occurs.

(After Guzzetta, C.E., & Forsyth, G.L. [1979]. Nursing diagnostic pilot study: Psychophysiologic stress. *Advances in Nursing Science,* 2[10], 27–44)

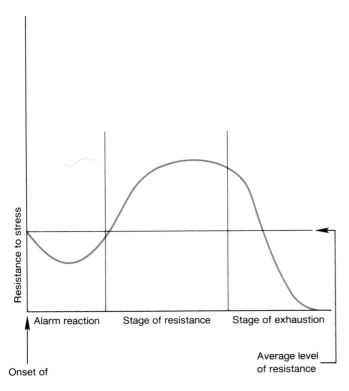

Figure 16–1. The general adaptation syndrome.

development. They also create negative stress, however, because they involve change, added responsibility, and adjustment.

The nature of the stressor should be assessed to determine appropriate nursing interventions to facilitate coping. For example, stress caused by severe pain from traumatic injury may not be resolved by coping strategies such as distraction.

Stress Response

Stress is a psychophysiologic response to demands or stressors. Selye (1976) characterized the stress response as an adaptive mechanism that restores a person's balance or equilibrium. Adaptation may potentiate personal growth and stress tolerance. If the stress response continues unabated and coping is ineffective, however, other outcomes are possible, including crisis, chronic stress or tension, and exhaustion or death. The adaptive mechanisms, also known as the general adaptation syndrome (GAS), are initiated when the sympathetic nervous system is aroused by a stressor. The GAS consists of three stages: (1) the alarm reaction, (2) the stage of resistance, and (3) the stage of exhaustion (Fig. 16-1). Alarm is the body's first response in preparing to deal with a stressor. The stage of resistance represents the point in the stress response when coping mechanisms may be used to alleviate stress. If stress is not relieved, exhaustion or even death may result. Chronic stress may contribute to disease by forcing the body into a constant state of tension. In fact, some authorities believe that most diseases can be linked to psychophysiologic stress (Selye, 1976; 1980).

The neuroendocrine and sympathetic nervous system activity associated with the stress response can result in signs and symptoms that may be detected during assessment (see "Nursing Observations Related to Stress and Stress Responses"). Responses to stress also include emotions, behaviors, and cognitive alterations (see "Stress Response Assessment"). Coping may also be viewed as a response to stress, because coping is what a person does about a disruption of meaning or smooth functioning.

Coping

Coping is defined by Weisman (1979) as follows: "what one does about a problem in order to bring about relief, reward, quiescence, and equilibrium . . . what one does or does not do about that problem, constitutes how one copes." Coping, as a distress-relieving process, may lead to one of two outcomes: problem resolution or tension reduction. Both problem resolution and tension reduction are adaptive in the sense that both approaches involve an active process enabling the person to adjust to the environment (Pollock, 1984; 1986). Each method represents a different level of adaptation, with problem resolution generally viewed as more adaptive.

Tension reduction involves coping strategies that provide some type of distraction to relieve the preoccupation with the stressor. Common negative examples include overeating, ingesting alcohol, and using drugs. A positive example is engaging in exercise or a fitness-program to redirect one's attention. Tension reduction may be an intermediate process eventually leading to problem resolution, or it may be the only coping outcome. In the previously mentioned negative examples, the effectiveness of the coping mechanisms are questionable, and the resulting behaviors may be viewed as maladaptive. As an intermediate process, tension reduction is employed to reduce stress to a more manageable level (Weisman, 1979). Subsequently, the stress is resolved, and the coping process may be viewed as contributing to a higher level of adaptation.

Lazarus (1966) defined coping as cognitive and behavioral processes used to deal with threats. This definition offers no distinction between coping and defending. In contrast, Weisman (1979) views coping and defending as two different processes that may occur, to some extent, simultaneously. According to Weisman, coping is a response to a recognized problem, whereas defending is a response to some unknown or unspecified concerns. Defending may occur as a reflex or autonomic response, as would happen when the sympathetic nervous system prepares a person for fight or flight, or it may involve psychic processes of defense, such as denial, regression, and repression. Once the instigating problem is understood, defending mechanisms become coping responses. Health care providers occasionally have the tendency to label coping strategies of which they do not approve as defense mechanisms, implying that such responses are an inferior way of dealing with stressors.

Coping Strategies

Coping strategies are specific techniques used to deal with a stressor and its consequences. Coping styles are typical, habitual patterns of behavior that a person prefers to use in dealing with stress. Several coping strategies, such as information seeking, physical activity, eating, or smoking, may contribute to the overall coping style. Coping style is influenced by multiple factors including personality traits, resources available to the person, and past outcomes experienced from different coping strategies.

Most people attempt to cope with stressors by using strategies directed toward problem solving or tension reduction. Problem solving involves dealing directly with the stressful situation or stressor. Tension reduction involves employing behaviors or thoughts to lessen unpleasant emotions associated with a stressor. Problem solving and tension reduction are embodied in the four coping modes identified by Lazarus and Launier (1978): direct action, information seeking, intrapsychic mode, and action inhibition.

Direct Action. Direct action includes the common coping strategy, fight or flight. The role of the sympathetic nervous system is paramount in preparing the body systems for this type of action. The body provides additional oxygen to the skeletal muscles, which facilitates the actions of the appropriate muscles for either fleeing or fighting; the bronchioles of the lungs dilate, allowing more oxygen to enter the body; the heart beats more forcefully to deliver the oxygen to the skeletal muscles; and glucose levels rise in response to the need for fuel for the activities of fight or flight.

Direct action may also involve goal-directed, problem-solving approaches to a situation, such as beginning a diet or joining an exercise class to resolve the stressor of poor self-esteem related to obesity. Using these approaches, the person confronts and acts on the stressor.

Information Seeking. Generally, information seeking is a cognitive coping strategy applied to dealing with potential stressors as well as existing stressors. It involves considering the potential stressor and associated unpleasant sensations and then developing advance strategies to deal with these sensations. Information seeking may help eliminate frightening misconceptions about the stressor and may be useful when information about the potential stressor's sensations are provided in advance. For example, the sensations associated with abdominal surgery include feeling incisional pain after surgery, fatigue with minimal activity, and cramping from abdominal gas. Providing this information preoperatively may help the patient in coping with the stress of surgery.

The process of providing information, also referred to as providing preparatory sensory information, represents a nursing intervention to promote coping based on the need for information seeking. Whether or not this method of coping is more effective than any other method has not yet been decided.

Intrapsychic Mode. The intrapsychic processes involve directing one's attention to other considerations. This coping strategy, which includes defense mechanisms, helps reduce the tension and anxiety associated with a stressor and involves distractions, such as daydreaming or fantasizing. Many "psychological" coping mechanisms are intrapsychic in nature, including the defense mechanisms of displacement, projection, suppression, repression, rationalization, regression, and denial.

Intrapsychic processes may be viewed as either effective or ineffective coping strategies. Intrapsychic defensive processes may provide a reprieve from the overstimulating and exhausting aspects of stress, allowing the person's energy to be directed toward developing other, more effective and long-term coping mechanisms.

Prolonged use of intrapsychic processes may encourage continual avoidance of stressors or denial, with no attempt at resolving the threats or problems. For example, many people use denial following various diagnoses such as cancer or myocardial infarction. Denial is also recognized as an aspect of the coping process observed with bereavement. Often, using denial temporarily eliminates intense negative effects of the stressor until the person is able to develop effective coping strategies.

Action Inhibition. When using this coping strategy, a person will refrain from activities that are impulsive, dangerous, or embarrassing. For example, some people may cope by acting out behaviors such as driving recklessly or initiating an argument. Action inhibition may be used to prevent such impractical behavior.

Effective Coping

Regardless of the coping strategy employed, effective coping is manifested by high levels of adaptation to stress or the development of stress tolerance. Effective coping has the following results (Visotsky and associates, 1961):

- Distress is maintained within manageable limits.
- Hope and encouragement are generated.
- A sense of personal worth is maintained.
- Relationships with significant others are maintained or restored.
- Prospects for physical recovery are enhanced.
- Prospects for favorable situations (interpersonal, social, and economic) are enhanced.

Coping effectiveness varies greatly among people and may be influenced by the following factors (Cohen, 1981; Kobasa, 1979; Selye, 1976):

- *Number of stressors confronting a person:* In the presence of multiple stressors, stress may be perceived as an insurmountable obstacle, and crisis may result.
- *Access to social or financial support resources.* People with such resources usually perceive themselves as more able to cope.
- *Stressor duration:* Chronic exposure to stressors predisposes a person to chronic stress or tension.
- *Stressor intensity:* An intense stressor may be perceived as insurmountable and may precipitate crisis.
- *Past experience with stressors:* If the person has coped successfully in the past, the stressor may be perceived as less threatening.
- *Personality:* Certain people are more stress resistant— especially those who view change as a challenge and believe they can influence events.

Crisis

Crisis occurs when the person feels overwhelmed by stressors and unable to resolve the problem (Aquilera and Messick, 1980). It is an acute, self-limiting state that is usually resolved within a period of 4 to 6 weeks. Although crisis may be associated with major disorganization of the personality, it is also viewed as a potential growth process. People in crisis may be more willing to accept help toward developing effective coping skills. Crisis intervention processes have been developed, based on crisis theory, to help people move through crisis and achieve the same levels of stress adaptation as existed before the crisis (Infante, 1982).

Fink (1967) identified four observable crisis stages that may be recognized during health assessment:

- *Shock (stress):* Stressors are perceived as overwhelming. The person may experience powerlessness, anxiety, and altered thought processes.
- *Defensive retreat:* Attempts are made to maintain usual structures, often by employing coping strategies to reduce tension and to reorganize one's thoughts. Being challenged at this stage may result in anger because it interferes with coping attempts.
- *Acknowledgment:* The person can no longer be distracted from the overwhelming stress. Feelings of hopelessness and powerlessness may be strong, and suicide may be considered. Thought processes are altered as perceptions must become more reality oriented.
- *Adaptation and change:* New or pre-crisis structures are established, and the person gains a feeling of con-

trol and increasing self-worth. Thought processes return to normal.

THE HEALTH HISTORY AND INTERVIEW

An assessment of what is stressful and a person's responses to stress begins by asking the person to describe stressful events or situations encountered presently or in the past. How specific stressors are perceived by the individual also should be explored. These aspects of the health history are usually established by interviewing the person. You should also review the person's medical diagnosis and prognosis, the quality of significant relationships, and social or work history to gain insights about stress and coping.

Some people find it difficult to discuss stress and coping. Whether or not the person responds to direct questioning during the interview may depend on what coping mechanism is being used to handle stress, as well as the stage of the stress reaction. For example, a person who is using denial* as a coping mechanism may offer little relevant information about his or her problems. Not every person will be ready to discuss stressors and coping at the moment the subject is raised in the interview. Even in the absence of denial, people may be reluctant to express their anxiety about the problems that confront them, or they may have difficulty openly discussing their coping methods. Drug and alcohol use are examples of coping mechanisms that people may be reluctant to discuss.

Injecting one's personal bias into the situation may interfere with objective evaluation of the person's statements and should be avoided. Keeping an open mind will provide an opportunity to evaluate fairly and rationally all coping mechanisms employed by the person.

Data obtained by eliciting a health history pertaining to stress and coping should help you make judgments about the following:

- *Stressors:* Identification of events or situations in the person's life that may result in stress
- *Perception of stressors:* The individual's perception and interpretation of stressful events or situations
- *Coping with stress:* How the person responds to stress. Personal strengths and options that might influence coping are also identified.

The Interview Guide shown in the accompanying display may be used to direct the collection of appropriate data. Some practitioners administer standardized tests to identify stress and stress responses. The use of these tools is discussed in the next section of this chapter (see "Diagnostic Studies").

Once you have identified indicators for stress, you should initiate a more thorough evaluation of the person's response to stress (see "Stress Response Assessment"). Such an evaluation is based on additional observation and interaction with the person.

---

*Denial may be considered a coping mechanism or a defense mechanism. It is commonly discussed in nursing literature as the latter. Weisman (1979) considers denial a phase of coping.

Interview Guide **Stress and Stress Responses**

A structured interview guide may be used to facilitate data collection. The headings provided on this screening interview form correlate with major interview areas discussed in the text and may be deleted when creating forms to record data in practice settings.

Stressors

Major changes/losses in the past year _____
Situations that cause stress: At the present time _____
                                          In the past _____

Perception of Stressors/Stress

What does this problem/stressor/loss mean to you? _____
Have stressful situations been good or bad for you? _____
How have stressful situations affected you? (physically and emotionally) _____

Coping Strategies

How do you relieve tension and deal with stress?

Talk to others _____   Try to solve the problem _____   Blame someone else for the problem _____
Try to forget _____   Try to relieve tension with alcohol _____   Seek help _____
Do something to get mind off problems _____   drugs _____ overeating _____   Other (describe) _____
Pray _____   Go to sleep _____   _____
Do nothing _____   Accept the situation _____   _____
Is there someone you rely on to help you solve problems? _____
Is there something the nurse can do to make hospitalization (clinic visits, home visits, *etc.*) less stressful? _____

Resolution of Stress

Do you usually solve your problems? _____
Do the methods you just described for relieving tension usually help? _____

Stressor Identification

To identify events or situations precipitating stress, ask the person questions such as the following:

What is causing you stress or problems now?
How stressful is this hospitalization for you?
What is changing in your life now?
Tell me about any losses you have experienced lately.

Some people easily recognize and discuss stressors, whereas some maintain that nothing ever bothers them, even when stress is apparent. Recognizing problems and talking about them is usually necessary before the person can learn to develop effective coping strategies. Understanding the nature of the stressors enables the nurse and the patient to plan appropriate interventions. For example, a person who is scheduled for coronary artery bypass surgery may be faced with fear of the unknown. Preoperative teaching (preparatory sensory information) would be an appropriate nursing intervention aimed at providing information and encouraging coping. If the stressor is tension from conflict with a coworker, problem-solving strategies or assertiveness techniques may promote effective coping.

Researchers have found that different groups of patients experience different types of stressors. The groups studied by nurses include people who have had a myocardial infarction, those who are undergoing hemodialysis for chronic renal failure, and those recently admitted to long-

term and short-term nursing care facilities (see the Research Highlight at the end of this chapter). Knowing the nature of potential stressors in these types of situations, as well as others, is one means of anticipating possible problems and psychological reactions.

In addition to interviewing, formal assessment tools, such as the Social Readjustment Rating Scale (SRRS) developed by Holmes and Rahe (1967), and the Everyday Hassles Scale (EHS) developed by Lazarus (1981), may be used to help identify and rank everyday stressful events (see "Diagnostic Studies").

Stress Perception

In order to better understand what the client might view as stressful and what might help, you need to evaluate the individual's perceptions of stressful events or situations. The personal meaning of a stressful situation to the individual will influence what coping options are realistic or possible. A person's perception of stress is influenced by several factors, such as other concurrent events, the person's feelings about ability to cope, and the degree of distress experienced.

Problems may arise if the person perceives the stressor to be especially intense, is dealing with multiple stressors, or questions his or her ability to deal with the situation.

Determining the number of stressors confronting a person at once is important, because more effort to adapt is needed when multiple stressors are present. Take the example of a woman who cries uncontrollably because her dinner tray is served cold—an event that hardly seems to warrant such an extreme reaction. Consider, however, what had happened to her before this time. She had been embarrassed earlier in the day by an episode of fecal incontinence, followed by three unsuccessful and painful attempts at restarting an IV, an unrelenting headache, fear about her prognosis, and an overdrawn notice from the bank. The cold tray, a seemingly insignificant event, became overwhelming when added to all of these other stressful occurrences.

When dealing with many stressful events, a person may be asked to rate the stressors, from the most distressing to the least distressing. The nurse and client can then establish priorities for developing coping strategies. For example, a person may state that the financial aspects of hospitalization are more distressing than the physical symptoms of illness. A lack of knowledge about options available for financial assistance may contribute to the sense of stress. Providing the necessary information, often in collaboration with the social worker, may represent one appropriate nursing intervention to solve the problem and thus enhance coping. The meaning that events have for the client must be assessed to help in establishing effective coping strategies.

Interview with the intent to determine the meaning of the stressful situation to the client. Some general questions that might be helpful include the following:

> What does this situation mean to you?
> What is the most upsetting problem you face as a result of this situation? Least upsetting?
> Do you feel like you can cope with this situation?

You may have determined from the person's history that health problems exist. To explore the client's perceptions of these problems, you may ask the following types of questions:

> How do you feel about your health?
> What are the major problems of this illness (*i.e.,* unpleasant symptoms, complications, treatments and medications)?
> What are the major problems of getting older?
> Earlier you told me you have difficulty sleeping. What do you think is interfering with sleep?

You may want to explore how a person perceives a stressful situation in relation to personal safety and security or personal control over events. Questions such as the following may be helpful:

> What frightens you or makes you feel uneasy about this situation?
> What persisting thoughts do you have?
> How do you feel when you cannot control some of these distressing feelings?
> How have your feelings toward yourself changed?

A person's surroundings can also elicit a stress response, especially in unfamiliar settings such as the hospital. Environmental stressors include unfamiliar sights, smells, or sounds; changes in daily routine; lack of privacy, heat, or cold; and sensory deprivation or overload. The person's perception of environmental stressors may be elicited with the following questions:

> What frightens or annoys you in this setting?
> In what way does this setting affect your life-style and usual routines?
> In which types of surroundings are you most comfortable?

You may identify stressful events related to family relations, career, financial concerns, and religion. Sample questions may include the following:

> How would you describe your relationship with your spouse (or children, parents, girlfriend, boyfriend, *etc.*)?
> How has this situation (*e.g.,* illness) affected your family?
> How do present circumstances in your life interfere with work or school?
> How would this situation be affected by a change in your financial state?

Coping with Stress

Determine how the person typically responds to stress, including what methods are used to reduce tension.

The manner in which a person has dealt with particular stressors in the past may have an influence on how he or she responds to similar situations. Successful experiences in the past will enhance successful coping in the present. Conversely, unsuccessful coping on one occasion may have an adverse effect on self-esteem and create self-doubt about dealing with a similar situation in the present. If prior coping strategies have been effective in relieving stress, these strategies should be supported and continued. If the past methods of coping have been dysfunctional, however, alternative coping strategies should be explored.

The following questions may help elicit data to determine prior methods of dealing with stressful events:

> Has anything like this ever happened to you before? Tell me how you responded. How did you feel about your response?
> What would change about the way you usually deal with this problem?

If a stressful experience is presently being addressed, ask the person how he or she will deal with that problem. Stay nonjudgmental as you listen to understand why choices are being made and why they may be perceived as right, given the circumstances.

You may use a more direct approach if you want to identify specific ways of dealing with stress. Ask the person, "How do you relieve tension or deal with stress?" Present options, such as those listed here adapted from Weisman and Worden (1979), and ask if each coping strategy does or does not apply to a particular stressful situation:

- Seek more information about the situation (rational-intellectual).
- Talk with others to relieve distress (shared concern).
- Laugh it off; make light of the situation (reversal of effect).
- Try to forget; put it out of mind (suppression).
- Do other activities for distraction (displacement).
- Take firm action based on present understanding (confrontation).
- Accept, but find something favorable in the situation (redefinition).

- Submit to and accept the inevitable (fatalism).
- Do something—anything—however reckless or impractical (acting out).
- Negotiate feasible alternatives (problem solving).
- Reduce tension by drinking, overeating, or drugs (tension reduction).
- Withdraw socially into isolation (stimulus reduction).
- Blame someone or something (disowning responsibility).
- Seek direction from an authority and comply (compliance).
- Blame self, sacrifice, or atone (self-pity).

Look for particular strengths the person has that might help him or her deal with stress. For example, determine whether the person feels "in control" of life.

People with an internal locus of control, who see themselves as active participants in determining their fate, tend to cope positively with stress. Conversely, those with an external locus of control, who perceive themselves as passive victims of events, may respond differently (Ewig, cited in Miller, 1983).

Different coping processes are associated with each personality type. Those who are self-reliant or "internal" tend to use active coping strategies such as problem-solving, whereas those who feel controlled by forces outside themselves, or "externals," display more passive or defensive behaviors. Characteristics associated with each of these personality types are listed in Display 16-2. Determining a person's locus of control can serve as a guide to assessing his or her coping style.

Identify the person's support system (family, friends, clergy) and determine how helpful they would be in dealing with stress. A person's social support systems such as family and other social contacts can serve as valuable coping resources. Support given by significant others helps a person develop a stable emotional state (Norbeck, 1981). It helps to determine if the person has turned to others, such as a clergyman, social worker, nurse, marriage counselor, or psychologist, in times of need. A person who has done so will probably be willing to accept support from others when such situations arise. If such support systems are absent or unavailable, the nurse can provide emotional support, cognitive assistance, and social reinforcement (Panzarine, 1985).

DIAGNOSTIC STUDIES

Diagnostic tools may be used to measure stress and stress responses. The diagnostic evaluation of stress may include the administration of questionnaires or surveys to deter-

---

Display 16–2
Coping Behaviors Associated With Internal and External Locus of Control

"Internals" showed more problem-solving, active coping behaviors associated with effective coping, whereas "externals" tended to show passive or defensive behaviors associated with ineffective coping.

Internal

- Is active in self-care.
  Examples: Helps others recognize self-care strides. Boasts of ability. Plans for care needs. Makes suggestions to health workers.
- Interacts socially.
  Example: Shows active interest in others and helps them solve problems.
- Sets goals.
  Examples: Modifies environment. Plans for safety needs. Uses problem-solving skills.
- Seeks information.
  Examples: Asks specific, relevant questions. Reads about condition.
- Shares perceptions of self as being important.
  Example: Describes positive role as strong person in family.
- Deliberately uses prayer to provide strength.
- Uses purposeful distraction.

External

- Is passive and dependent.
  Example: Sleeping more than usual.
- Has little or no interest in acquiring self-care skills.
- Demonstrates social withdrawal (isolation).
- Focuses on unrealistic cures.
- Refuses therapies that increase mobility (*e.g.,* physical therapy).
- Expresses verbally that nothing more can be done.

(After Miller, J.F. [1992]. *Coping with chronic illness* (2nd ed.). Philadelphia: F.A. Davis)

Display 16–3
Holmes and Rahe's Social Readjustment Scale

The person selects from the scale life events that have occurred during the past year. Add the stress unit values associated with each event to determine the final score.

Life Event	Stress Unit Value	Life Event	Stress Unit Value
Death of spouse	100	Children leaving home	29
Divorce	73	Trouble with in-laws	29
Marital separation	65	Outstanding personal achievement	28
Jail term	63	Spouse begins or stops work	26
Death of close family member	63	Begin or end school	26
Personal injury or illness	53	Change in living conditions	25
Marriage	50	Revision of personal habits	24
Fired at work	47	Trouble with boss	23
Marital reconciliation	45	Change in work hours or conditions	20
Retirement	45	Move or change in residence	20
Change in health of family member	44	Change in schools	20
Pregnancy	40	Change in recreation	19
Sexual difficulties	39	Change in church activities	19
Gain of new family member	39	Change in social activities	18
Business readjustment	39	Mortgage or loan less than $10,000	17
Change in financial status	38	Change in sleeping habits	16
Death of close friend	37	Change in number of family gatherings	15
Change to different line of work	36	Change in eating habits	15
Arguments with spouse	35	Vacation	13
Mortgage or loan more than $10,000	31	Christmas	12
Foreclosure of mortgage or loan	30	Minor law violations	11
Change in responsibilities at work	29		

Score interpretation:

150–199	Mild stress
200–299	Medium stress
300+	High stress: Associated with high rates of illness

(Adapted from Holmes, T.H., & Rahe, R.H. [1967]. The social readjustment rating scale. *Journal of Psychosomatic Research, 11*[2], 213–218)

mine the magnitude and type of stress experienced by the respondent.

The Social Readjustment Rating Scale. The Social Readjustment Rating Scale (SRRS) developed by Holmes and Rahe (1967) is a diagnostic tool designed to identify stressors and quantify the degree of stress a person is experiencing. The SRRS presents a list of major stressful life events and assigns a numerical stress quotient to each event (see Display 16-3). The stress quotients are added to provide a score indicating mild, medium, or high levels of stress. The score may be used to predict the person's susceptibility to illness.

Although the SRRS has received wide recognition since it was first introduced, some researchers challenge its reliability. Thorson and Thorson (1986) question the general application of the scale to all age groups, because older people may perceive and deal with stress differently than younger people do. Also, the tool does not take into account sociocultural background and personality, even though these factors may greatly influence the way a person perceives stress. Similarly, Baker and colleagues (1985) believe that some events listed on the SRRS are irrelevant to certain groups, such as the chronically mental ill, who tend to perceive a different set of life events as stressful.

The Everyday Hassles Scale. Lazarus' Everyday Hassles Scale (EHS) lists, in rank order, items associated with stress and behaviors and feelings that promote well-being (Display 16-4). The EHS emphasizes common, everyday irritants that contribute significantly to stress levels, especially if positive stimuli or events do not occur to buffer the stressor effects. Similar concerns have been raised for the Everyday Hassles Scale as were noted for the Social Read-

Display 16–4
Lazarus's Everyday Hassles Scale

The following scale rank-orders "hassles," which contribute to stress, and "uplifts," which contribute positively to stress management, as evaluated in several middle-aged groups. The nurse may determine the person's hassles and uplifts for purposes of providing anticipatory guidance. Individual person may perceive hassles and uplifts differently from the groups studied by Lazarus.

Hassles (Rank Ordered)

1. Feeling concern about weight
2. Worrying about health of a family member
3. Worrying about rising cost of living
4. Dealing with home maintenance
5. Having too many things to do
6. Misplacing or losing things
7. Doing yard work or outside home maintenance
8. Worrying about property, investment, or taxes
9. Worrying about crime
10. Feeling concern about physical appearance

Uplifts (Rank Ordered)

1. Relating well to spouse or lover
2. Relating well with friends
3. Completing a task
4. Feeling healthy
5. Getting enough sleep
6. Eating out
7. Meeting responsibilities
8. Visiting, telephoning, or writing someone
9. Spending time with family
10. Home pleasing to you

(Adapted from Lazarus, R.S. [1981]. Little hazards can be hazardous to your health. *Psychology Today, 15*[7], 58–62)

justment Scale. However, such tools are still useful for assessment if their limitations are recognized and considered.

The Stress Audit. The Stress Audit, developed by Miller, Smith, and Mehler (1991), is a self-administered questionnaire designed to assess experienced and anticipated stressful events. Unlike most tools, the Stress Audit focuses on stressful events anticipated in the future as well as situations from the past. The tool also identifies stress symptoms and responses to stress. The person's overall vulnerability to stress is also identified.

NURSING OBSERVATIONS RELATED TO STRESS AND STRESS RESPONSES
Examination Focus

Physiologic responses occur in reaction to stress, and physical indicators may be observed during an examination. Physical manifestations may provide an indication of the intensity and effects of stress.

Stressors activate the sympathetic nervous system and the hypothalamic–pituitary–adrenal axis, resulting in physiologic alterations that may be observed during the physical examination (Fig. 16-2). When the hypothalamus activates the stress response, corticotropine-releasing factor is secreted, which in turn influences the secretion of adrenocorticotropic hormone (ACTH) from the anterior pituitary gland. Then, ACTH stimulates the cortex of the adrenal gland to secrete cortisol and aldosterone into the blood stream. These hormones cause changes that may be ob-

served during assessment and include increased blood pressure, decreased urinary output, and laboratory changes such as increased blood sugar. Stressors and cognitive appraisal of the stressor may also stimulate the sympathetic nervous system, releasing the catecholamines norepinephrine and epinephrine into the blood stream. The catecholamines may cause signs and symptoms such as increased heart rate, elevated blood pressure, dilated pupils, and constricted coronary vessels, with resultant chest pain and chest palpitations. Psychological reactions, such as anxiety, interact with the physiologic changes, such as increased heart rate, which may create even more anxiety.

Observing a person for signs of stress includes noting sympathetic nervous system activity and adrenal cortex activity. The physiologic signs of stress, however, are highly variable among people. Absence of elevated blood pressure or a rapid heart rate does not indicate the absence of stress. Often, the signs and symptoms of stress become more apparent through interviewing the person and interpreting how he or she perceives the stressor.

General Appearance and Surroundings

A person's general appearance may or may not be affected by stress. Some people may display signs of tension such as anxious or alarmed facial expressions, restlessness, or excessive activity. Others may appear calm.

As you survey the person, you should also survey the person's environment. Note what would be considered threatening or disturbing in the person's surroundings. In a health care setting, consider the person's response to

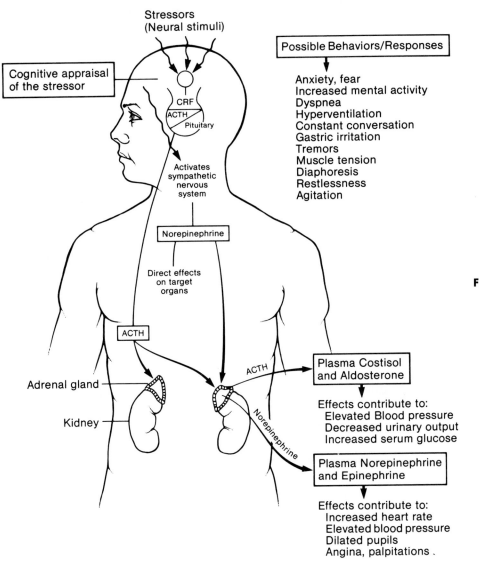

Figure 16–2. The stress response.

equipment, different people, and room furnishings. Any change in a person's normal environment may be perceived as stressful.

Associated Body System Alterations

Cardiovascular System. When the sympathetic nervous system is activated during stress, norepinephrine is released, producing the following effects on the cardiovascular system:

- Increased heart rate
- Increased force of myocardial contractions
- Vasoconstriction in the skin, viscera, and kidneys
- Increased myocardial oxygen consumption

The signs and symptoms that may result from these physiologic changes include the following:

- Increased resting heart rate (more than 10 beats/minute faster)
- Increased systolic blood pressure

- Cardiac dysrhythmias such as premature ventricular contractions and premature auricular contractions
- Electrocardiographic changes indicating cardiac ischemia
- Chest pain sensations or palpitations
- Headache (migraine)
- Ischemic pain (angina; Raynaud's syndrome)

(*Note:* A person with underlying cardiovascular system disease is more likely to exhibit these signs and symptoms during periods of stress.)

Respiratory System. Norepinephrine secretion during stress can lead to bronchiolar dilation, although this physiologic response is difficult to evaluate by physical examination techniques. A more discernible response to anxiety is an increase in respirations. Hyperventilation may occur with a subjective feeling of "air hunger." The effects of stress on the immune system may be associated with an increased incidence of upper respiratory infections.

Gastrointestinal System. Sympathetic nervous system activity usually inhibits gastrointestinal tract motility. Nevertheless, stress is often associated with nausea, vomiting, and increased peristaltic activity. The exact physiologic mechanism is unclear but may be related to cerebral activation of the vagus nerve. Increased peristalsis is associated with increased bowel sounds and an increased number of bowel movements per day. Excessive secretion of hydrochloric acid in the stomach in response to stress also contributes to nausea, abdominal pain, and ulcer formation.

Musculoskeletal System. Muscle tone may increase in response to stress. The person may appear tense and hold the extremities in a taut, nonrelaxed position. Low-back pain may be an associated symptom. Tremor may occur, especially in the hands, along with restlessness and fidgety movements.

Integumentary System. The skin may become diaphoretic in response to stress, a reaction that represents vasoactive changes in the subcutaneous vessels. Moist skin may be limited to the palms and face, or may be generalized. Skin lesions, including herpes, eczema, and dermatitis, may recur during periods of stress.

Nursing Observations   *Stress Response*

General Principles

Stress responses are highly variable among individuals and include cognitive, affective, and physical responses. Cognitive responses include mental processes, such as having thoughts about the stressful event or thoughts of problem solving. Affective responses consist of emotions or psychological responses such as crying, anxiety, or anger. The manner in which a person copes with stress is also evaluated as a response to stress. The person's responses to stress may indicate the types of interventions that are appropriate. For example, a person who is denying obvious problems will usually not benefit from problem-solving strategies until the denial has been addressed.

Some assessment of stress responses may be achieved during the interview process (discussed earlier in this chapter). Assessment is also based on observation and continuing interaction with the person as they experience stress. The nurse should be empathetic and supportive in order to encourage more honest disclosure related to stress and coping.

Preparation for Assessment

No special preparation of the person is required for the nurse to observe stress responses. Observations of this nature should be continuous and ongoing as nursing care is provided.

Examination and Documentation Focus

- Physical indicators of stress
- Cognitive indicators of stress
- Affective responses to stress
- Indicators of defensive coping
- Overall safety

Examination Guidelines   *Stress Response*

Procedure

1. EVALUATE THE PERSON'S EXPERIENCE WITH RESPECT TO THE STAGES OF THE GENERAL ADAPTATION SYNDROME (ALARM, RESISTANCE, EXHAUSTION).

Clinical Significance

Responses to stress and patterns of coping vary, depending on the stage of the stress reaction (*e.g.,* alarm vs. resistance).

Alarm Stage Indicators: Sense of panic, hypervigilance, feelings of being "nervous" or "jittery," hyperactivity, preoccupation with frightening images, ineffective problem solving or decision making, stereotyped thinking.

The alarm stage may persist for days or weeks after initial contact with the stressor. Problem solving may be impaired as the person directs mental energies toward detecting possible threats and as emotions interfere with memory, reasoning, and judgment.

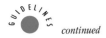 *continued*

Stress Response

Procedure	Clinical Significance

Procedure

2. NOTE COGNITIVE RESPONSES TO STRESS.

Clinical Significance

Cognitive Indicators of Stress: Decreased perceptual ability, narrowing of focus, thought disorganization, decreased problem-solving abilities, impaired decision making.

Cognitive Indicators of Stress Reduction: Increased participation in decision making and problem solving.

3. NOTE MOTOR RESPONSES TO STRESS.
Motor responses are highly variable among individuals.

Motor Indicators of Stress: Skeletal muscle tension, restlessness, constant movement of a body part.

4. NOTE AFFECTIVE RESPONSES TO STRESS.

Affective Indicators of Stress: Feeling overwhelmed, helplessness, loss of control, anxiety, guilt, anger, low self-esteem.

Affective Indicators of Decreasing Stress: Ability to express doubts, fears, and concerns; increased self-esteem.

5. IDENTIFY DISTRESSING PHYSICAL SYMPTOMS OR BEHAVIORS RELATED TO STRESS.

Physical/Behavioral Indicators of Stress: Nausea, insomnia, fatigue, too much sleep, anorexia, overeating, gastrointestinal pain, headache, backache, neck or back pain, chest pain.

6. LOOK FOR SIGNS OF DEFENSIVE COPING.

Defending is a means of protecting against an unspecified problem. The defensive response, however, avoids the problem; it does not solve it.

Recognition of defensive coping may be the first indication that a person is experiencing a threat to a stressor because other signs of stress may be masked.

Defensive Behaviors: Denial, displacement, projection, rationalization, regression (dependence), repression, suppression (see Display 16-5).

Display 16–5
Defensive Behaviors

- *Denial.* Consciously or unconsciously ignoring symptoms and avoiding discussion about a stressor to allay anxiety and reduce stress. (*Example:* The patient states, "It's only gas," when in fact he or she has had a myocardial infarction. Failure to follow activity restrictions after an illness or injury may represent denial.)
- *Displacement.* Unconsciously transferring emotional feelings from the actual stressor to a substitute. (*Example:* "None of you knows anything about taking care of sick people.")
- *Projection.* Attributing personal ideas or characteristics to others. (*Example:* "My wife thinks I am going to die.")

- *Rationalization.* Justifying behaviors or decisions to maintain self-respect and eliminate guilt. (*Example:* "I am glad I didn't get promoted because I would have had to work extra hours.")
- *Regression or Dependence.* Adopting behaviors used at an earlier level of emotional development. (*Example:* "I cannot give myself a bath. Will you do that for me?")
- *Repression.* Involuntarily blocking painful thoughts or memories from consciousness. (*Example:* "I do not remember yelling at you.")
- *Suppression.* Consciously and deliberately dismissing thoughts or feelings. (*Example:* "I do not want to talk about my illness; it would only upset me.")

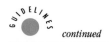

continued

Stress Response

Procedure

Avoid abrupt confrontation when first recognizing signs of defensive coping.

Clinical Significance

Defensive mechanisms are protective and may actually promote eventual development of adaptive coping behaviors. Abruptly removing a defense mechanism can predispose the person to a severe stress reaction when the defense is penetrated and no other coping strategies have been developed. However, some defensive behaviors are potentially harmful, and the defense may need to be penetrated. For example, a person who denies having had a myocardial infarction and persists in being fully ambulatory even though such activity is potentially dangerous may need to be confronted about the severity of the illness.

7. EVALUATE BASIC SAFETY.

Determine whether the person is meeting basic needs.

If the person is in physical danger, the nurse should take steps to assure physical safety.

Consider whether the person is in enough control to drive safely.

Evaluate suicide risk (see next section).

Nursing Observations

Suicide Potential

Suicide or suicide attempts may be a person's response to stress or crisis states. The greatest suicide risks occur in the following groups: alcoholics, adolescents, elderly persons, accident-prone persons, those with a history of previous suicide attempts, minority groups, police, and physicians (McClean, 1983).

When evaluating suicide potential, consider the following risk factors:

- *Age:* Suicide is the third leading cause of death in the age group of 15 to 24 years. Elderly persons (especially those in the eighth decade of life) are at higher risk for suicide. The suicide rate for elderly men is four times the national suicide rate.
- *Sex:* Men commit suicide more often than women by a ratio of 3:1. Most male suicides occur after age 45 years.
  Women attempt suicide more often than men by a ratio of 3:1. Most female suicides occur after age 55 years.
- *Recent loss:* Loss of loved ones, social status, health, independence, income, employment (especially if elderly person)—all may precipitate a suicidal crisis.
- *Drug and alcohol abuse:* Drug and alcohol abuse may precipitate suicide or be considered a type of passive suicide.
- *Social isolation:* Those who live alone or who have never married are at greater risk.
- *Depression:* You should be especially concerned if the person exhibits the triad of hopelessness, helplessness, and worthlessness.
- *Previous suicide attempts:* Evaluate seriousness of attempts in terms of lethality and intent.

General Principles

Assess suicide risk by interviewing the person, listening to statements for suicide ideation, and observing behaviors and appearance.

The quickest and most direct assessment method is to interview the person. Although a person may not volunteer an intent to commit suicide, he or she may discuss it when asked. Questioning should be conducted in a direct but caring manner. For example, it is better to ask the person, "Are you thinking of taking your own life?" than to say, "You would not harm yourself, would you?"

Establish rapport. Be empathetic by carefully listening to the person and being supportive. Avoid using language that is accusatory.

Examination and Documentation Focus

- Intent and suicide ideation
- Plan
- Means
- Previous attempts
- Additional risk factors

Examination Guidelines *Suicide Potential*

Procedure	Clinical Significance
1. DETERMINE INTENT.	
Ask the person if he or she has, or has had, suicidal thoughts.	Expression of suicide thoughts is referred to clinically as "suicide ideation."
Ask the person if he or she is currently contemplating suicide.	Direct questioning is usually most effective.
Listen for statements such as the following:	Statements may indicate that the person has made a decision to attempt suicide.
"They'll be sorry when I'm gone."	
"I'm such a burden."	
"I don't deserve to live anymore."	
Verbal statements may be less direct, such as:	
"Everything's okay now."	
"I've finally found the solutions to my problems."	
Look for behaviors that are out of character for the person. For example, someone who has been depressed may suddenly appear cheerful and animated and talk about the future. The person may give away prized possessions, suddenly decide to write a will, or contact friends and relatives as though saying goodbye. Behaviors associated with depression, such as sleep disturbances, use of drugs or alcohol, and feelings of hopelessness, are also significant.	Behaviors are more difficult to analyze in terms of suicide intent but may be the only clue. Not all of these behaviors indicate a suicide threat, but further assessment is always warranted.
2. DETERMINE WHETHER THE PERSON HAS A PLAN FOR HOW TO COMMIT SUICIDE.	If the person has a plan, suicide risk increases.
Ask the person questions such as the following:	
"How would you take your own life?"	
"When would you do it?"	
3. EVALUATE MEANS.	
Determine whether or not the person has the means to carry out the plan. Ask questions such as the following:	A person with a plan and the means to carry out the plan is considered high risk for suicide.
"Do you have a gun? How would you get a gun?"	If the means is highly lethal, the preson should be considered high risk for suicide.
"Do you have the sleeping pills?"	
4. NOTE PREVIOUS ATTEMPTS.	
Determine whether the person has a history of suicide attempts. If so, identify method.	
5. NOTE ADDITIONAL RISK FACTORS.	
Observe whether the person is under the effects of drugs or alcohol.	Drugs and alcohol may alter judgment and increase the risk of suicidal behavior.
Ask the person if he or she has been or is being abused (physically, emotionally, or sexually).	Abuse may be an indicator of a poor social support system. Having an unsatisfactory support system increases suicide risk.

Documenting Stress Response and Suicidal Potential

Document your observations with special attention to (1) observations you make regarding degree of vigilance, problem solving, judgment, and decision-making abilities, and (2) statements and behaviors indicating poor self-esteem, feelings of helplessness, defensive coping behaviors, or suicide ideation. It may be helpful to quote the person directly. A description of a person displaying defensive coping might be as follows:

> Does not verbalize reason for hospitalization. Physician discussed with him earlier. Continues to state, "I'm here for a couple of routine tests and I wouldn't be here at all if my kids weren't such worriers."

A description of a person displaying low self-esteem might be as follows:

> Does not initiate conversation. Keeps head lowered when talking to others. Participates minimally in activities and only after persuasion from staff. Told roommate, "I'm no use to anybody anymore."

A description of a person showing a decreased stress reaction might be as follows:

> Discussing discharge and return to family and work. States she wants to continue with outpatient physical therapy. Talks about accident. Appearance well-groomed. Less dependent on staff for assistance with ADLs.

A description of a person with suicide ideation might be as follows:

> States "Life just isn't worth it anymore." Denies having plan for suicide but states he has stockpiled approximately 40 "downers."

NDx

Nursing Diagnoses Related to Stress and Stress Responses

Nursing diagnoses addressing coping include the following: Ineffective individual coping, Defensive coping, and Ineffective denial. Benner and Wrubel (1989) question the use of terms such as *effective* or *ineffective coping* or *defensive coping,* which bring to mind a dichotomy of "good" coping versus "bad" coping. According to Benner and Wrubel, the use of this terminology suggests that someone outside the stressful situation, such as the nurse, has a clearer view and can pass judgment on whether the person is coping effectively. They go on to say that this approach might cause the nurse to fail to consider the individual's interpretation of the stressful situation. They suggest that the nurse focus on understanding personal meanings and why a particular way of coping may have been right for the person at the time. Although Benner and Wrubel discourage the use of terms such as *effective* or *ineffective coping,* such diagnoses are considered clinically useful by others. Ineffective coping is officially recognized as a nursing diagnosis.

Ineffective Individual Coping

Ineffective individual coping is a state of inadequate response to stressors because of lack of physical, psychological, and behavioral resources necessary to promote effective coping strategies. Dysfunctional coping behavior is not the same as a single instance of overreacting to a stressor, but rather represents a prolonged and debilitating pattern of ineffective coping.

Dysfunctional coping is identified if the person fails to adapt to a stressor within a 3- to 6-month period. Failure to adapt is manifested as follows:

- Persistence of distressing symptoms such as depression or anxiety
- Impaired social functioning such as drunken or reckless driving, abusive behavior toward others, failure to obey the law, truancy
- Inadequate performance on the job or at school or excessive procrastination

Other dysfunctional behaviors include self-destructive behavior, overuse of defense mechanisms, and verbalizing an inability to cope.

Dysfunctional or Anticipatory Grieving

Grieving, a normal process of coping, is the response to an actual or perceived loss of a person, object, function, status, or relationship. Grieving may also be anticipatory, in response to the realization of a future loss. If grieving is *dysfunctional,* more active intervention may be indicated.

Normal grieving consists of four stages: shock and disbelief, awareness, restitution, and resolution. Assessment is focused on evaluating the person's progress through the grief stages:

- *Shock and disbelief:* The person may feel numb to all unpleasant emotions or deny that the loss has occurred. Denial represents a defense mechanism used to alleviate the intense feelings precipitated by the loss.
- *Awareness:* The person may become increasingly and painfully aware of the reality of the loss and may express anger toward others. This coping mechanism is a form of displacement, or the unconscious transfer of feelings to others.
- *Restitution:* In this stage, the person begins to mourn the loss.
- *Resolution:* Finally, the person resolves the loss by using intrapsychic methods and, perhaps, becoming less preoccupied with the loss. The stage may last for many months.

Post-trauma Response

Trauma is the occurrence of extraordinary life events such as war, rape or other assault, natural disasters, accidents, or catastrophic illness. The trauma victim has usually been exposed to multiple stressors directly associated with the traumatic event, not to mention threats to life and safety, and increased feelings of vulnerability. Assessing a person who has experienced trauma includes evaluating coping mechanisms as well as the need for crisis intervention or other forms of emotional support. In the period immediately following the trauma, the person may use various defense mechanisms such as denial, regression, and suppression as a defense against overwhelming and possibly unknown threats. The use of such defense mechanisms in this phase is a normal stage of the post-trauma response.

stress has been linked to coronary artery disease, hypertension, and cardiac dysrhythmias. In the pulmonary system, stress is associated with asthmatic reactions. Stress affects the gastrointestinal system by contributing to ulcers, irritable bowel syndrome, diarrhea, nausea and vomiting, and ulcerative colitis. Stress may affect sexual functions, resulting in impotence or frigidity. Stress-related skin disorders include eczema and acne. Additionally, stress has been linked to headache, backache, and immunosuppression.

Clinical Problems Related to Stress and Stress Responses

Stress is believed to be an etiologic factor in a number of illnesses and conditions. In the cardiovascular system,

ASSESSMENT PROFILE

Tim Jensen, aged 38 years, believed that he was too young to be in the hospital for a bleeding ulcer. He thought this disease occurred only in people who were excessive drinkers or who had been overworked for years. It seemed like the older men he was acquainted with inevitably had either heart attacks or ulcers. Although he did not drink alcohol, he had a stressful job selling real estate and worked long hours. He had been experiencing heartburn for the last 6 years, used antacid tablets frequently, and was slightly overweight. His diet included soda and processed foods, because he was rarely home at his family's usual mealtime, and his relaxation activities included smoking marijuana. Tim believed the recurring heartburn, or what the physician had called an ulcer, was due to being overweight. After receiving a blood transfusion and ulcer medication, Tim signed himself out of the hospital. After all, he could not close any real estate deals and keep up with his competitors while lying in a hospital bed.

Mr. Jensen's medical diagnosis was hemorrhagic peptic ulcer, a stress-related illness. Peptic ulcers have been described as a 20th-century disease, especially in men under age 50 years. The pathogenesis of peptic ulcer is related to hypersecretion of hydrochloric acid and high concentrations of corticosteroids, which are associated with long-term stress and anxiety. Recognizing and modifying stress are important nursing concerns.

Profile Analysis

Many people seeking health care are confronted by significant stressors and demonstrate various responses. The nurse evaluates stress and responses to stress to identify nursing intervention needs.

Mr. Jensen showed signs of significant stress. Although the nurses caring for him following his hospital admission for hemorrhagic peptic ulcer identified stress, Mr. Jensen's decision to refuse health care prevented immediate nursing care.

Identifying the Assessment Focus

Once Mr. Jensen's physiologic status was stabilized, the nurses caring for him began evaluating stressors and stress perceptions. The decision to evaluate this area was based on knowledge of the role of stress in the disease etiology. Furthermore, Mr. Jensen's nutritional patterns were targeted for priority assessment because dysfunctional eating behaviors, often a response to stress, can further potentiate ulcer formation by adversely affecting digestion.

Assessment of Mr. Jensen's stress response focused on identifying what he perceived to be the stressful conditions in his life and his usual methods of coping with them.

Possible Nursing Diagnoses

Nursing diagnoses of Ineffective individual coping, Defensive coping, and Ineffective denial were tentatively established for Mr. Jensen based on the following cues the nurses had detected since his hospital admission:

- Destructive self-behavior. He repeatedly stated he would leave the hospital against medical advice, saying, "Dying might be better than not making a living."
- Denial of obvious health problems. He continued to attribute gastrointestinal symptoms to "just a little gas" rather than ulcer disease.
- Inability to ask for help.

Additional Data Gathering and Analysis

The nursing diagnoses prompted further investigation. Specifically, the nurses needed to identify etiologic or contributing factors. Important factors to consider and evaluate further included career and financial concerns as well as Mr. Jensen's usual coping strategies. A more thorough assessment was planned to identify or rule out other stressors such as strained family relationships, poor self-esteem, sleep loss, and health concerns.

Additionally, Mr. Jensen's use of denial and other attempts at coping warranted further investigation and analysis. The ulcer pain represents a stressor that Mr. Jensen may not have accepted; therefore, he chose to deny the significance of the pain. Rather than interpreting his pain as a signal of illness, he chose to reduce emotional distress by attributing the pain to being overweight. Although using denial is not always harmful, continually using such a mechanism represents an ineffective coping strategy. Furthermore, Mr. Jensen coped with tension by using drugs. Inasmuch as denial evades dealing with the cause of the symptoms, drugs only temporarily induced relaxation. Mr. Jensen's coping strategies may not be effective for dealing with stress.

Chapter 16 SUMMARY

Assessment of stress and stress responses should focus on the following:

- Identifying situations that precipitate stress
- Understanding the meaning of the stressful situation to the individual
- Identifying the person's strengths and coping skills
- Identifying responses to stress
- Recognizing signs of crisis or threats to safety brought on by stress

The nurse should remember several principles when assessing stress and stress responses:

- Assessment of stress and stress responses is optimal when nurse and client have an open and trusting relationship.
- Stressors vary among people because stressors are interpreted from each person's perspective.
- Individual responses to stress are varied and are influenced by personal values, culture, perception, socioeconomic resources, and past experience with the stressor.
- Physiologic signs of stress are varied and are usually not as reliable as information obtained by client interview and observation.
- Coping should be judged in terms of distress reduction and adaptation. Nurses should take not to judge coping strategies with respect to their own personal values.
- Many different coping strategies may facilitate effective coping, including the temporary use of defense mechanisms.
- Crisis or suicide ideation detected during assessment represents an emergency situation in need of immediate intervention.

Most of the information needed to evaluate stress and stress responses is collected by interview and observation. Specific assessment methods include the following:

Interview to Identify
- Stressors
- Perception of the stressors
- Coping strategies

Use of Assessment Tools
- Social Readjustment Rating Scale
- Everyday Hassles Scale
- The Stress Audit

Nursing Observations
- Body system indicators of stress
- Behavioral responses
- Affective responses

Assessment of stress and stress responses, based on these principles and methods, helps the nurse identify defining characteristics that might be present for the following nursing diagnoses and problems:

Ineffective individual coping
Defensive coping
Ineffective denial
Anticipatory grieving
Dysfunctional grieving
Post-trauma response
Impaired adjustment
Hopelessness
Altered self-concept
Fear
Powerlessness
Spiritual distress (distress of the human spirit)
Potential for violence: Self-directed or directed at others
Rape trauma syndrome

RESEARCH *Hi*GHLIGHT

What types of stressors affect different patient groups?

Nurses need to assess the nature of stressors confronting a person before planning and implementing interventions to support coping. Assessment may be facilitated by anticipating the types of stressors the person is or will be facing. Moreover, knowing typical stressors might provide insight about stressor prevention or reduction. The following summaries discuss research aimed at identifying specific stressors in three different client groups.

In one study, acute myocardial infarction patients experienced different stressors at different stages of hospitalization. One phase of a larger study concerned with psychophysiological stress examined the nature of stressors that might be present during hospitalization of patients with acute myocardial infarctions. The researchers iden- *tified 50 stressors believed to be predominant for such patients (see box). Then, five coronary care unit (CCU) patients with a diagnosis of acute myocardial infarction were assessed (by patient and family interview, physical examination, observation of chart and nursing care plan entries, and interviewing staff) to determine the specific stressors each encountered. Each patient was assessed shortly after CCU admission, following transfer from CCU, and just before hospital discharge.*

Study results showed that 31 out of 50 (60%) of the stressors existed for the five-subject sample. The nature of stressors changed over time. While the patients were in CCU, stressors were predominantly physiological and environmental, such as loss of rapid eye movement (REM) sleep, related heart complications, lack of privacy, and

Stressors Identified by Patients After Acute Myocardial Infarction

This list represents stressors identified by the researchers before the study. At least 1 of the 50 stressors listed was identified by each subject in the study.

Physiologic

Acute myocardial insult
Severity of illness
Related heart complications
Severity of symptoms
Previous history of heart disease
Other coexisting illness
Other complications
Rapid eye movement sleep deprivation
Other

Psychological

Fear of death
Fear of hospital procedures
Weakness
Altered body image
Loneliness
Powerlessness
Helplessness
Hopelessness
Loss of virility
Transfer from coronary care unit
Other

Environmental

Observation of cardiac arrest
Observation of other procedures
Lack of structure; boredom

Lack of privacy
Sensory deprivation/overload
Inability to sleep
Untidy surroundings
Unpleasant odors
Frightening noises
Multiple sounds
Lack of windows/clocks
Frightening machines
Restricted visitation
Altered daily routine
Other

Sociocultural

Age
Social class
Financial Status
Ethnic origin
Religious beliefs
Education
Fear of family reaction
Family conflicts
Concern for self
Concern for family
Interpretation of symptoms
Loss of peer respect
Inability to work
Other beliefs/attitudes
Other

(Guzzetta, C.E., & Forsyth, G.L. [1979]. Nursing diagnostic pilot study. Psychophysiologic stress. Advances in Nursing Science, *2[10], 27–44)*

(continued)

RESEARCH *Hi*GHLIGHT

What types of stressors affect different patient groups? (continued)

frightening machines and noises. Before hospital discharge, however, stressors were mainly psychological and sociocultural, such as alterations in body image, feelings of hopelessness, inability to work, and financial concerns. The researchers recommended that larger groups of similar subjects be studied to identify, label, and validate the nature of stressors.[1]

Another study found that fluid limitation, muscle cramps, fatigue, and uncertainty about the future were predominant, treatment-related stressors for hemodialysis patients. Researchers studied 35 patients undergoing hemodialysis to identify common stressors and related coping patterns. After reviewing the literature, a list of potential stressors was compiled and presented to nurses who cared for the patients as well as the patients themselves for validity. Nurse experts were asked to classify stressors as physiological or psychological. Revisions were made, and the patients were asked to determine the relative impact of the stressors. Additionally, patients were asked to identify predominant stressors not included on the original list (see table). The patients used the Jaloweic Coping Scale to assess coping strategies associated with each stressor. Table 16-2 lists stressors perceived by the patients in decreasing order of occurrence, with fluid limitations being cited most frequently. Problem-oriented coping methods were used more often than affective methods by this group. Optimism and controlling the situation were reported most often as preferred coping strategies.[2]

A third study indicated that stressors associated with institutionalization in elderly clients often represent changes related to the social milieu and aging. Phillips conducted taped interviews of institutionalized elderly persons in both long- and short-term care settings. Analysis revealed 13 separate categories of stressors for the patients (see box). Unfortunately, research methods leading to these conclusions are not discussed, so research critique and use is limited. Display 16-8 is included to illustrate similarities and differences among stressors in this group compared to previously cited studies.[3]

What significance do the studies have for health assessment?

The studies identify specific stressors for different patient groups. Assessment is facilitated by anticipating particular stressors. Additionally, the studies suggest that stressors have numerous forms, are derived from multiple sources, and may not be immediately apparent from a screening assessment.

Hemodialysis Stressors: Rank Ordering of 29 Stressors According to Frequency of Occurrence by 35 Hemodialysis Patients

Stressor	Class	Rank
Limitation of fluid	PS	1.0
Muscle cramps	P	2.5
Fatigue	P	2.5
Uncertainty concerning the future	PS	4.5
Limitation of food	PS	4.5
Interference in job	PS	6.0
Itching	P	9.0
Limitation of physical activities	PS	9.0
Changes in bodily appearance	PS	9.0
Arterial and venous stick	P	12.0
Nausea and vomiting	P	12.0
Length of treatment	PS	12.0
Limit on time and place for vacation	PS	12.0
Dependency on staff members	PS	12.0
Decrease in social life	PS	16.0
Changes in family responsibilities	PS	16.0
Cost factors	PS	16.0
Loss of bodily function	PS	18.0
Decrease in sexual drive	PS	19.5
Stiffening of joints	P	19.5
Limited to styles of clothing	PS	21.5
Dependency on physicians	PS	21.5
Transportation to and from the unit	PS	23.5
Frequent hospital admissions	PS	23.5
Sleep disturbances	PS	25.0
Reversal in family role with spouse	PS	26.5
Fear of being alone	PS	26.5
Reversal in family role with the children	PS	28.5
Decreased ability to procreate	PS	28.5

PS, psychosocial stressor; P, physiological stressor.
(Baldree, K.S., Murphy, S.P., & Powers, M.J. [1982]. Stress identification and coping patterns in patients on hemodialysis. Nursing Research, 31[2], 107–112)

The studies are also significant from an intervention standpoint because a person's descriptions of stressors may be used as a basis for anticipatory guidance. For example, machine noises, which may be frightening to the CCU patient, can be discussed before the patient's exposure to unfamiliar sounds.

Can the studies' findings be applied to practice?

The nurse could use the lists of stressors identified by the researchers to guide health assessment with minimal risk to patients. The greatest risk involved would be to assume that most people similar to those targeted in the studies

(continued)

RESEARCH *Hi*GHLIGHT

What types of stressors affect different patient groups? (continued)

experience exactly the same stressors. Guzzetta and Forsyth studied only five myocardial infarction patients, all of whom were men. It would be erroneous to say that this group is representative of all patients experiencing myocardial infarction. Similarly, patients may differ in other respects that may alter their stressor perception. For example, newly admitted nursing home patients may enter institutions where special care is taken to reduce certain stressors such as those identified by Phillips.

All the studies should be repeated using the same research design before final judgments are made about accuracy and applicability of findings.

Has the assessment and diagnosis of denial in coronary care patients been accurate?

Denial was identified by Hackett and associates in the early 1970s as a common coping strategy used by patients in the immediate period following acute myocardial infarction. This basic finding, although enlightening, did not contain many implications for nursing practice. Hackett then correlated denial in myocardial infarction patients with a better survival rate in the early days following hospital admission. In other words, patients who used denial more often survived myocardial infarction than those patients who

had immediately acknowledged and accepted the illness. This finding would imply that nurses should support the patient's use of denial in this particular situation. For example, the nurse could avoid talking to these patients about their illness.

Other researchers challenged Hackett's finding that denial was commonly used by patients following an acute myocardial infarction, relating lack of conversation about the illness to anxiety, fear, or the desire not to reveal their feelings to nurses. The following research summary illustrates one such challenge.

CCU patients were interviewed to determine what emotions they were experiencing and what coping strategies they were using. Nineteen CCU patients with a diagnosis of cardiovascular disease were interviewed, using open-ended questions to elicit information about preadmission symptoms, the patient's perceptions of what the symptoms meant, and the patient's perceptions of any life-style changes resulting from the symptoms. The tape-recorded interviews were analyzed for content indicating anxiety or denial, using two methods: interpretation by a psychoanalyst and rating by the G-G Content Analysis Scales. Few patient statements were found to reflect denial. The patients commonly experienced anxiety and

---

Stressors of Institutionalized Elderly Persons

- *Threats to life and health:* Client's apprehension about fate, whether in the form of the fear of death following acute trauma or surgery, the fear of permanent disability, or the fear of the dying process.
- *Discomforts:* The physical complaints of the client in regard to pain, cold, fatigue, poor food, lack of care, *etc.;* Client's apprehension regarding ability to regulate discomforts and being assured staff will attend to discomforts.
- *Loss of a means of subsistence:* Client's concern about economic conditions in general, economic conditions of significant others, own economic conditions, and economic concerns about illness.
- *Deprivation of intimacy:* Loss of physical closeness, sexual satisfaction, close affiliations, and friendships.
- *Enforced idleness:* Client's concern about inability to perform usual tasks, engage in necessary tasks for survival, such as cooking and shopping, and engage in recreational activities.
- *Restriction of movement:* Physical immobility, monotony of daily encounters, and the absence of personal privacy.

- *Isolation:* Separation of client from usual environment, and acquaintances or friends, and perception that care-givers are uncaring.
- *Threats to family structure:* Fear of loss of family status or family role, and realization of failing health and loss of resources of close family members.
- *Capricious behavior of those in charge:* Client's perception that care-givers are unpredictable.
- *Propaganda:* Client's lack of accurate information about status, feeling that information is being withheld, and pressure to do something not wanted or believed.
- *Awareness of personal degeneration:* Client's awareness of own physical and mental failings.
- *Rejection:* Feelings of being forgotten, or significant others not caring, and perception of the ridicule and dislike of others.
- *Unknown duration:* Feelings that the confinement will never end and that time drags.

(Adapted from Wolanin, M.O., & Phillips, L.R. [1981]. Confusion: Prevention and care [p. 273]. St. Louis: C.V. Mosby)

(continued)

RESEARCH *Hi*GHLIGHT

What types of stressors affect different patient groups? (continued)

would openly discuss their problems if given the opportunity. Discussing problems represents a problem-oriented approach to coping rather than the tension-reduction approach that denial indicates. The researchers concluded that CCU patients actively cope, and that nurses should provide these patients with opportunities and open-ended interviews to discuss their concerns.

What significance do the studies have for health assessment?

Hackett's studies and recommendations may influence some nurses to be reluctant to discuss stressors openly with CCU patients so as not to disrupt defense mechanisms. The nurse's own perceptions may influence the assessment findings. A patient may be diagnosed as using denial because the nurse assumes and fails to investigate further. Thomas and colleagues suggest that if nurses took the time to develop an open and trusting relationship needed to facilitate more accurate assessment, an entirely different perspective might be gained about the client's stress perception and response. The assessment of such patients should be ongoing and proceed simultaneously with fostering of a trusting nurse-patient relationship

Can the studies' findings be applied to practice?

At this point, Thomas and colleagues are using the research process to challenge accepted practices and theories about how patients cope with stress. Before making definite recommendations for nursing practice, researchers should repeat these studies. Additional studies will provide insight into these patients' actual coping mechanisms and emotional reactions.

REFERENCES

1. Guzzetta, C.E., & Forsyth, G.F. (1979). Nursing diagnostic pilot study: Psychophysiologic stress. *Advances in Nursing Science, 2*(10), 27–44.
2. Baldree, K.S., Murphy, S.P., & Powers, M.J. (1982). Stress identification and coping patterns in patients on hemodialysis. *Nursing Research, 31*(2), 107–112.
3. Phillips, L.R. (1976). The imprisonment model. Unpublished manuscript, University of Arizona. Cited in M.O. Wolanin & L.R. Phillips. (1981). *Confusion: Prevention and care.* St. Louis: C.V. Mosby.
4. Thomas, S.A. et al. (1983). Denial in coronary care patients: An objective reassessment. *Heart & Lung, 12*(1), 74–80.
5. Hackett, T.P., Cassem, N.H., & Wishnie, H. (1968). Psychological hazards of coronary care unit. *New England Journal of Medicine, 279*(25), 1365–1370.
6. Hackett, T.P., & Cassem, N.H. (1974). Development of a quantitative rating scale to assess denial. *Journal of Psychosomatic Research, 18*, 93–100.

✴ CRITICAL THINKING

A 66-year-old man has been recently diagnosed with a terminal illness. His prognosis is poor. His personal physician has just completed a thorough and frank discussion with him regarding his condition.

Learning Exercises

1. Describe how would you begin to evaluate this man's response to this information. Create a script of the first few sentences you might say in this situation.

2. Select and describe several barriers that might interfere with communication between the nurse and the patient at this time. Explain how you would overcome each barrier.

3. Explain how defensive coping can be assessed. Describe what it might look like in this person.

4. Describe how you would differentiate stress from crisis.

BIBLIOGRAPHY

Aquilera, D.C., & Messick, J. (1980). *Crisis intervention: Theory and methodology.* St. Louis: C.V. Mosby.

Baker, F., et al. (1985). The impact of life events on chronic mental patients. *Hospital and Community Psychiatry, 36* (3), 299–301.

Baldree, K.S., Murphy, S.P., & Powers, M.J. (1982). Identification of coping patterns in patients on hemodialysis. *Nursing Research, 31* (2), 107–112.

Benner, P., & Wrubel, J. (1989). *The primacy of caring: Stress and coping in health and illness.* Menlo Park, CA: Addison-Wesley.

Carpenito, L.J. (1993). *Handbook of nursing diagnosis* (5th ed.). Philadelphia: J.B. Lippincott.

Clark, S. (1987). Nursing diagnosis: Ineffective coping. I. A theoretical framework. *Heart and Lung, 16* (6), 670–676.

Clark, S. (1987). Nursing diagnosis: Ineffective coping. II. Planning care. *Heart and Lung, 16* (6), 677–685.

Clarke, M. (1984). Stress and coping: Constructs for nursing. *Journal of Advanced Nursing, 9* (1), 3–13.

Cohen, F. (1981). Stress and bodily illness. *Psychiatric Clinics of North America, 4,* 269–286.

Cole, M., & Vincent, K. (1987). Psychiatric-mental health assessment: A new look at the concept. *Archives of Psychiatric Nursing, 1* (4), 258–263.

Fink, S.L. (1967). Crisis and motivation: A theoretical model. *Archives of Physical Medicine and Rehabilitation, 48,* 592–597.

Green, B., et al. (1989). A conceptual framework for post-traumatic stress syndromes among survivor groups. In C.R. Figley (Ed.). *Trauma and its wake.* New York: Brunner/Mazel.

Guzzetta, C.E., & Forsyth, G.L. (1979). Nursing diagnostic pilot study: Psychophysiologic stress. *Advances in Nursing Science, 2* (10), 27–44.

Haan, N. (1977). *Coping and defending: Process of self-environment organization.* New York: Academic Press.

Hatton, C., & Valente, S. (1984). *Suicide: Assessment and intervention* (2nd ed.). Norwalk, CT: Appleton-Century-Crofts.

Holmes, T.H., & Rahe, R.H. (1967). The social readjustment rating scale. *Journal of Psychosomatic Research, 11* (2), 213–218.

Hoover, R.M., & Parnell, P.K. (1984). Stress and coping. *Journal of Psychosocial Nursing, 22* (6), 17–22.

Infante, M.S. (1982). *Crisis theory: A framework for nursing practice.* Reston, VA: Reston Publishing.

Jalowiec, A., & Powers, M.J. (1981). Stress and coping in hypertensive and emergency room patients. *Nursing Research, 30* (1), 10–15.

Kobasa, S.C. (1979). Stressful life events, personality, and health: An inquiry into hardiness. *Journal of Personal and Social Psychology, 37* (1), 1–11.

Lazarus, R.S. (1966). *Psychological stress and the coping process.* New York: McGraw-Hill.

Lazarus, R.S. (1981). Little hassles can be hazardous to your health. *Psychology Today, 15* (7), 58–62.

Lazarus, R.S., & Launier, R. (1978). Stress-related transactions between person and environment. In L.A. Pervin & M. Lewis (Eds.). *Perspectives in interactional psychology* (pp. 287–327). New York: Plenum Press.

Levine, S. (1971). Stress and behavior. *Scientific American, 224,* 26–31.

McClean, L. (1983). Guilt and fear of self-destruction. In J. Haber et al. (Eds.). *Comprehensive psychiatric nursing* (2nd ed., pp. 557–597). New York: McGraw-Hill.

Mellick, E., et al. (1992). Suicide among elderly white men: Development of a profile. *Journal of Psychosocial Nursing and Mental Health, 30* (2), 29–34.

Miller, J.F. (1992). *Coping with chronic illness: Overcoming powerlessness* (2nd ed.). Philadelphia: F.A. Davis.

Miller, L.H., Smith, A.D., & Mehler, B.L. (1991). *The stress audit.* Brookline, MA: Biobehavioral Associates.

Norbeck, J.S. (1981). Social support: A model for clinical research and application. *Advances in Nursing Science, 3* (7), 43–58.

Panzarine, S. (1985). Coping: Conceptual and methodological issues. *Advances in Nursing Science, 7* (4), 49–57.

Pellitier, L.R., & Cousins, A. (1984). Clinical assessment of the suicidal patient in the emergency department. *Emergency Nursing, 10* (1), 40–43.

Phillips, L.R. (1976). The imprisonment model. University of Arizona: Unpublished manuscript.

Pollock, S.E. (1984). The stress response. *Critical Care Quarterly, 6* (4), 1–14.

Pollock, S.E. (1986). Human responses to chronic illness: Physiologic and psychosocial adaptation. *Nursing Research, 35* (2), 90–95.

Roberts, J., et al. (1987). Coping revisited: The relation between appraised seriousness of an event, coping responses, and adjustment to illness. *Nursing Papers, 19* (3), 45–54.

Selye, H. (1976). *The stress of life* (2nd ed.). New York: McGraw-Hill.

Selye, H. (1974). *Stress in health and disease.* Boston: Butterworth.

Selye, H. (1974). *Stress without distress.* Philadelphia: J.B. Lippincott.

Selye, H. (Ed.). (1980). *Selye's guide to stress research, Vol 1.* New York: Van Nostrand Reinhold.

Thorson, J.A., & Thorson, J.R. (1986). How accurate are stress scales? *Journal of Gerontological Nursing, 12* (1), 21–24.

Vincent, K.G. (1985). The validation of a nursing diagnosis: A nurse consensus survey. *Nursing Clinics of North America, 20* (4), 631–640.

Weisman, A.D. (1979). *Coping with cancer.* New York: McGraw-Hill.

Weisman, A.D., & Worden, J.W. (1976–77). The existential plight in cancer: Significance of the first 100 days. *International Journal of Psychiatry in Medicine, 7* (1), 1–15.

Westreich, L. (1991). Assessing an adult patient's suicide risk: What primary care physicians need to know. *Postgraduate Medicine, 90* (4), 59–62.

Chapter 17

Assessing Values and Beliefs

Values and Beliefs

Values
Beliefs
Culture
Cultural Sensitivity
Dimensions of Orientation
Ethnicity
Race

Folk Remedies
Spirituality
Religiosity
Spiritual/Religious Beliefs
Faith
Philosophy of Life

INTRODUCTORY OVERVIEW

In a society with more than 270 subcultures and 1200 religious groups, nurses need to be aware of cultural and religious beliefs and values. People of all ages and backgrounds may face situations or crises that cause them to question the meaning and value of life. How these experiences are viewed may be influenced by the cultural and spiritual beliefs and values of the client and nurse.

Values and beliefs greatly influence a person's attitudes and moral outlook, which help guide behavior and establish life goals. A value is defined as "an effective disposition toward a person, object, or idea" (Steel and Harmon, 1979). Values are utilized in decision making and generally persist over a long time period. Beliefs are "a special class of attitudes in which the cognitive component is based more on faith than fact. They represent a personal confidence in the validity of some idea, person, or object" (Steel and Harmon, 1979).

The values and beliefs of an individual are influenced and shaped by one's culture. The values of a culture and the beliefs and values of an individual guide and influence individuals in forming goals, opinions, and decisions every day. Values and beliefs influence health-related decisions, health practices and priorities, and behavior in life-threatening situations. Behaviors that initially seem inappropriate or illogical to an observer may be logically explained once the values and beliefs of the individual are examined.

A value and belief system is the basis of a person's philosophy of life, whether conscious or unconscious, religious or secular. Such a phi-

Jill Fuller and Jennifer Schaller-Ayers:
HEALTH ASSESSMENT: A NURSING APPROACH, Second Edition.
© 1990, 1994 by J. B. Lippincott Company.

losophy is intimately connected with spirituality. Spirituality is a complex abstract concept. After a literature review and concept analysis, Julia Emblems (1992) defined spirituality as a personal life principle that animates the transcendent quality of a relationship with God or god being. Each person's spirituality is highly variable, individualistic, and ever-changing.

The pattern of a person's values and beliefs is closely related to his or her self-concept, coping abilities, stress tolerance, and role-relationship behaviors. Values and beliefs must be considered in the assessment process to provide holistic care that takes into account not only the physical needs of a client but the emotional and psychological needs as well. Understanding a client's values and beliefs also helps the health professional to understand the client's health-related decisions and to plan coping strategies and interventions that support those values and beliefs.

When providing care to people from different cultures, subcultures, and religious groups, it is important to avoid generalizing. Although particular values and beliefs may be associated with a certain group of people, they are not necessarily the values and beliefs of each member of that group. When assessing clients from different cultural or religious groups, you should try to learn as much as possible about the individual's values and beliefs, and what impact they may have on his or her health.

Nurse's Self-Assessment of Values and Beliefs

Awareness of possible conflicts in value–belief systems between yourself and a client is only possible if you understand your own values, beliefs, and spirituality. Nurses who evaluate their own life philosophies, values, and beliefs may be less vulnerable to stressors. If you understand your own spirituality, you will be more comfortable discussing the meaning of life and death with clients. It is difficult to provide holistic care and promote spiritual well-being if you are unaware of your own value and belief system and lack spiritual well-being.

Nurses should assess and question their own spirituality to gain and maintain the necessary reserves to assist clients in facing spiritual crises and to maintain their own well-being. The purpose of questioning beliefs is not to determine whether they are good or bad, but rather to determine how beliefs influence one's behavior and relationships with others. Spiritual assessment is one of the most omitted assessments in health care. Nurses need to know how to assess and support clients' spiritual needs. Supporting clients' spiritual needs can be done by the nurse or by others such as ministers and rabbis when the nurse is unsure of the need or the need is beyond his or her abilities and/or resources.

Assessment Focus

An essential component in assessing values and beliefs is to identify person's values and beliefs and their effect on the person's health, and to identify any areas that might conflict with the health care system providing care.

The purposes for assessing values and beliefs are as follows:

- Identify the person's cultural and ethnic background and the degree to which traditional ethnic values are maintained.
- Identify the person's values and beliefs about life, death, health, illness, and spirituality.
- Determine if the person's values and beliefs are in conflict with those of the health care system providing care.
- Identify culturally based health practices.
- Recognize any evidence of spiritual distress.

The methods for collecting this information are described in the Assessment Focus display.

Nursing Diagnosis

The main nursing diagnosis related to values and beliefs is Spiritual distress (distress of the human spirit).

RELATED NURSING DIAGNOSES

A person with spiritual distress is at high risk for other problems, such as the following:

Anxiety
Decisional conflict
Dysfunctional grieving
Hopelessness
Impaired social interaction
Ineffective individual coping
Personal identity disturbance
Self-esteem disturbance
Sleep pattern disturbance

KNOWLEDGE BASE FOR ASSESSMENT

Culture, spirituality, values, and beliefs are closely interrelated and must be considered together during the assessment process. These factors can greatly influence the outcome of treatment and the success of nursing interventions. Often these factors are not assessed by the nurse unless a problem occurs, such as the person does not comply with the established regimen or is unable to make a decision. It is important for the nurse to know how variables such as culture, values, and spirituality affect health and health behaviors.

Culture

Every person's definition of health, optimal health, and illness, and communication patterns are influenced to some extent by cultural background. Culture is socially inherited and represents a complex system of values, beliefs,

Assessment Focus **Values and Beliefs**

Assessment Goal	Data Collection Methods
1. Identify the person's cultural and ethnic background to promote the development of a realistic treatment plan.	*Interview* • Affiliation with particular ethnic group or dominant culture • Ethnic background and customs practiced *Observe* • Note cues to culture and use of folk remedies.
2. Identify the person's values and beliefs about life, death, health, illness, and spirituality.	*Interview and Observe* • Philosophy of life • Spiritual beliefs and values • Use of symbols or rituals • Meaning of health and illness
3. Determine if the person's values and beliefs are in conflict with the values of the providing health care system.	*Interview and Observe* • Note congruence (or lack of) between belief/value system of client and health system.
4. Identify culturally based health practices.	*Interview* • Validate health practices influenced by culture and spiritual belief system. • Determine cultural influences on diet. • Validate time focus, nature of humans, control of own health.
5. Recognize any evidence of spiritual distress.	*Interview and Observe* • Note any conflicts with beliefs and values or any questioning of belief system. • Note conflict between beliefs and values with prescribed health regimen. • Note use of folk remedies. • Adequacy of spirituality support

customs, rituals, taboos (laws), and norms shared by a group of people. Although cultures are always evolving, changes are often slow. Even though a person may not be totally influenced by all aspects of his or her culture, the influence of culture on a person's behaviors and a person's interpretation of the others' behaviors is inevitable and usually discernible.

The definitions listed in Display 17-1 may be used to further illustrate important aspects of culture.

CULTURAL SENSITIVITY

Being aware of a person's cultural background is important in assessing values and beliefs and in determining a plan of care. More important is determining the degree to which people identify with their ethnic heritage. Nurses should be careful not to stereotype individuals into a particular ethnic group because of their last name or physical appearance, as these factors are often not accurate indicators. Asian–Americans or Hispanic–Americans may identify more with the culture of the United States than they do with their foreign ethnic heritage (Fig. 17-1). Also, individuals adopted as infants in another country may know nothing of their birth culture. Avoiding cultural blindness, ethnocentrism, cultural imposition, and stereotyping is crucial in providing effective care (see Display 17-1 for definitions).

Because the United States and Canada are nations inhabited by native and immigrant peoples from numerous places, nurses frequently encounter clients from different ethnic groups. It is not unusual for nurses to encounter health beliefs and practices that differ or conflict with their own beliefs and practices. Therefore, it is essential that the nurse be sensitive to persons from different cultures and

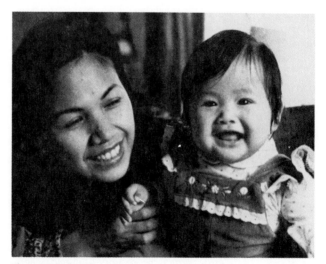

Figure 17-1. The entrance of Mexican-Americans into politics, new perspectives on their culture, and new opportunities have helped Mexican-American families come out of isolation into the "American" society.

Display 17–1
Definitions Related to Culture

Enculturation: The process of passing culture from one generation to another. Enculturation is accomplished through socialization.

Aculturation: The process of minimizing cultural differences when a member or members of one culture are a minority within another. Generally, members of the minority culture adapt. The majority culture, however, may adopt some aspects of the minority culture. For example, foods of other cultures ("ethnic" foods) are easily assimilated into American culture.

Ethnocentrism: The belief that a particular way of life and culture are superior to other ways.

Cultural blindness: Ignoring cultural differences and interacting as if no differences exist.

Culture shock: Immobilization and disorientation of a person that results from the awareness that the behaviors, values, and beliefs of others in the community are different from his or her own. For example, a particular gesture may have different meanings in different cultures, which may inhibit interaction and intensify culture shock.

Culture conflict: Occurs when persons from two different cultures are aware of their cultural differences and feel threatened by the differences.

Cultural imposition: The belief that everyone in a society must conform to the dominant culture.

Cultural relativity: The belief that all cultures are equal; no culture is better than another.

Subculture: A group that has a set of behaviors, values, and beliefs different from those of the dominant group. Also called an *ethnic* or *minority* group.

Ethnicity: Belonging to an identified cultural or ethnic group.

Stereotype: Assumption that all people in an ethnic group or race are the same, and ignoring differences and uniqueness among individuals.

Race: A biologic term referring to physical features and inherited traits. Race is not necessarily related to culture.

---

adapt intervention strategies to deliver effective, efficient care and avoid misunderstanding. Practicing cultural sensitivity includes (1) using nursing interventions based on the client's culture rather than on stereotypes; (2) understanding implications of culturally specific health beliefs and attitudes; (3) incorporating folk health practices when possible; and (4) acting as an advocate for a person of another culture who has been denied quality care (Clark, 1984).

Cultures share similar components in the shaping of values and beliefs. Five dimensions of orientation basic to all cultures have been identified as the nature of human beings, relationship between human beings and nature, time focus, purpose of life, and relationship with others (Klucknoln, 1961).

Nature of Human Beings. Some cultures view people as basically good; others as basically evil but having a potential for good, or as a combination of good and evil. In the United States, the dominant view is that human beings are both good and evil and are able to practice self-control in the interest of promoting good. Subcultures may reflect more polarized viewpoints; for example, the Appalachian subculture (individuals from the mountainous and coal mining areas of Georgia, Tennessee, North Carolina, and the Virginias) views human beings as essentially evil, and the Society of Friends, which represents Quaker beliefs, views human beings as good (Spector, 1993).

Relationship Between Humans and Nature. Cultural groups vary in their views as to how much control people have over their surroundings. Some groups believe that people have no control over the environment, whereas others believe they can eventually master the environment. In the middle are groups that believe in living harmoniously with nature.

Time Focus. All cultures have ideas about the past, present, and future. In the United States, however, the dominant culture is oriented to the future, whereas many Native American and Hispanic subcultures believe in concentrating on the present. The traditional Chinese subculture emphasizes the past.

Purpose of Life. Views about the purpose of life are closely identified with values. Cultural expectations of the dominant culture in the United States include continual achievement. Subcultures such as the Hispanic and Appalachian peoples place a higher value on personal development.

Relationship to Others. Interpersonal relations are influenced by cultural values. Views about relationships may be linear, collateral, or individualistic. Linear relationships emphasize the family and extended family; group goals take precedence over individual goals, and continuity through generations is important. An example of a linear relationship is a closely knit Korean family that may include several generations. Individuals work toward family goals and often have joint ownership in a family business in which everyone is employed. The needs of the family business often take precedence over individual goals. Collateral relationships also emphasize family and group goals, but the valued family unit is nuclear, and in some groups the people are the same age. Collateral relationships exist in kibbutzim in Israel and in some communes in which the individual is responsible to the group and the group is responsible to the individual. Within individualistic relationships, individual goals take precedence, and autonomy and self-responsibility are highly valued. In the United States, individualistic relationships are the most frequent.

Interpersonal relations and role expectations within the family are also influenced and defined by cultural values. Family structure and decision-making power are often prescribed. In the United States, family structure, prescribed roles, and relationships have seen a dramatic change in the last 25 years, and there appears to be no dominant pattern. Male dominance remains common in Hispanic and fundamentally religious families, however. The importance of extended families is common among Native American and Amish families. For some ethnic groups, such as Vietnamese and Koreans, the family may be the only social network for its members. For a more detailed discussion of roles and relationships, see Chapter 14, "Assessing Roles and Relationships."

CULTURE AND HEALTH

Cultural values influence an individual's behavior, beliefs, and attitudes about health and illness. In the United States, people place a high value on youth, health, and personal responsibility. When illness occurs, people tend to look to themselves, the environment, or other people for a cause. In the Appalachian subculture, however, in which people believe they have little control over what happens to them, other forces, such as fate and God's will, are considered responsible for illnesses.

Cultural beliefs include commonly held knowledge, opinions, trust, and faith about nature, relationships, self-worth, and purpose. Such beliefs influence the definitions of health and illness, and thus shape behavior. Health and illness are culturally and subjectively determined. What may be considered an illness in one culture may be considered a gift in another culture. For example, a person who reports seeing and talking with invisible people may be considered mentally ill in the United States; however, in another culture, this same person may be respected for such special powers. Individuals and families also evaluate how ill a person is to determine what activities should or should not be allowed.

How Various Cultures Define Health and Illness. Definitions of health vary from culture to culture. Rachel Spector (1991) has documented definitions from numerous cultural groups. Some examples follow:

- *Chinese:* Health is a state of spiritual and physical harmony with nature; the human body is a gift from ancestors and must be adequately maintained.
- *Hispanic:* Health is a reward for good behavior, a gift from God.
- *Native American:* Health is living in harmony with nature.

- *African–American:* The mind, body, and spirit are inseparable. Health is maintained by living in harmony with nature, a gift from God.

Cultural groups may view illness as resulting from a pathologic process within the body or from external sources such as the "evil eye." Illness definitions from various cultures include the following:

- *Chinese:* Illness represents an upset in the balance of yin and yang. Yang is the male or positive energy, producing light, warmth, and fullness. Yin is female or negative energy, producing darkness, cold, and emptiness. To heal disharmony, yin and yang must be brought into harmony. Yin treatments are for yang illnesses, and vice versa. Yin treatments include acupuncture, herbal teas, and vegetables. Yang treatments include spicy foods and burning incense.
- *Hispanic:* Illness represents either physiologic imbalance or punishment for wrongdoing. Imbalances may be viewed as "hot" or "cold." Hot illnesses are treated with cold substances, and vice versa. It is believed that imbalances may occur because of dislocation of body parts, resulting, for example, in abdominal cramping (empacho) or depression of the anterior fontanel in infants (caida de la mollera). Supernatural forces such as witchcraft and bad eye (mal ojo) also may cause imbalances, as may fright (susto). Finally, causing others to envy oneself (envidia) can produce an imbalance and cause bad luck.
- *Native Americans:* The sources of illness are defined in various ways, such as the result of evil spirits, disharmony between positive and negative forces, cause-and-effect relationships, displeasure of holy people, and misuse of sacred ceremonies. Illness affects the person's spiritual as well as physical nature; both must be treated.
- *African–Americans:* Illness may be viewed as a disharmony of the mind, body, and spirit with nature, or the will of God. Prayer, laying of hands, and home remedies (folk medicine) may be used for treatment.

For members of many religious groups, such as Church of the Nazarene, Church of Christ, Scientist, and Assemblies of God, divine intervention through prayer is sought during illnesses.

Although these definitions should only serve as a guide and are broad generalizations, they represent an overview of the different perspectives about health and illness. The perception and experience of health and coping with illness are based upon cultural values and beliefs and provide an expectation of health care (Meleis, Lipson, and Paul, 1992). Therefore, the client's viewpoint and expectations are important and need to be considered when health care is provided. Incorporating culturally appropriate beliefs into the treatment plan encourages the client to accept the plan and participate in its implementation.

Cultural Health Customs and Rituals. In addition to shaping views about health and illness, cultural beliefs serve as the basis of customs and rituals. Customs include sexual identity practices, such as circumcising males or wearing certain clothing or ornaments; dietary regulations, such as avoiding meat or certain combination of foods; and folk remedies, such as wearing garlic necklaces or copper bracelets to guard against certain illnesses or conditions. Folk medicine represents a system of self-care, even if not formally recognized, that relieves the health care system. For example, people will eat chicken soup, take aspirin, and increase fluid intake for a cold rather than seeking professional care. If people sought professional care for every illness or adverse condition, there would be no space in the physician's waiting room. Folk medicines are used for promoting health, and dealing with short-term conditions, chronic and incurable conditions, and psychosomatic conditions (Bushy, 1992).

Dietary practices and beliefs about folk medicines are especially important considerations when collecting assessment data and designing plans of care. Here, too, recognizing a person's preferences and beliefs can assist in planning interventions and facilitating a client's acceptance with a prescribed treatment. Dietary customs and usual mealtimes should be considered if a client is taking medications with meals.

Some families use folk or home remedies to prevent and cure health problems. Folk remedies may be made by the family or require the help of special folk practitioners such as lay midwives, herbalists, curandera and curandero, medicine men and women, and faith healers. Folk practitioners have various educational backgrounds and usually learn their skills and obtain their knowledge through apprenticeships. Chicken soup exemplifies a popular American folk remedy for the common cold and flu. Other remedies include drinking herbal teas, cleansing the system with enemas or laxatives in the spring, taking extra vitamin C in the winter, eating raw onions and garlic, rubbing goose fat on the chest, drinking hot lemonade with whiskey and honey, wearing charms or medals, praying, and sitting in sweat baths or saunas.

Because individuals from many ethnic minorities have a foreshortened life span and increased prevalence of chronic illnesses, careful assessment of cultural beliefs and practices becomes important to establish effective and efficient nursing services. In the United States, life expectancy for the overall population is 75 years and approaches 80 years for Caucasians; for African–Americans, however, life expectancy is 69.4 years, and statistics show that many Native Americans die before age 45 (DHHS, 1991). Statistics also show that Native Americans are more likely to die from diabetes, cirrhosis, and pneumonia/influenza; Hispanics are more likely to die from diabetes, HIV (AIDS), and perinatal conditions; and African–Americans are more likely to die from heart disease, cancer, and stroke (DHHS, 1991).

In addition to such genetically predisposed ethnic risk factors, poverty is an added risk factor for many minorities. Poverty often denies people access to health care. Even for those who do manage to gain access to health care services, many are reluctant to seek health care because of fear and distrust of the health care system and providers who may seem unfamiliar, impersonal, or strange to them. There may be a language barrier or lack of understanding when interventions are described. When interventions are first presented to people, many will seem polite and agreeable, but often they fail to follow through with prescribed interventions or regimens, particularly if interventions are complicated, expensive, or long term. The nurse should know that just because a person agrees to a plan of care at the outset does not always mean that the individual fully understands or is willing to follow through with prescribed care.

Spirituality

The dimensions of spirituality include a continuous interrelationship between the inner being of a person, the supreme values that guide the person, and the relationship with self, others, and the environment (Carson, 1989). Spirituality interacts with all aspects of the person and is "expressed through interpersonal relationships between persons and through a transcendent relationship with another realm; [it] involves relationships and produces behaviors and feelings which demonstrate the existence of love, faith, hope, and trust, therein providing meaning to life and a reason for being" (Labun, 1988). Supreme values are most commonly placed with God but may be placed in science, nature, or whatever the individual believes. Most people have spiritual beliefs in some form, whether these believe are part of a formal religious creed or a more amorphous component of a general philosophy of life.

Emblen (1992) defined religion as a system of organized beliefs and worship that the person practices. Organized religions provide a set of values, beliefs, norms, a frame of reference, and a perspective that can be used to organize information and govern daily activities. When numerous cultures exist within one society, religious values, beliefs, and norms will vary. In many societies, one set of religious beliefs dominate, such as Judaism in Israel and Islam in Saudi Arabia.

Religious beliefs can have a strong influence on views about health and illness. In some instances, illness may be interpreted as punishment for certain deeds. Conversely, some religious codes, such as the Latter Day Saints of Jesus Christ (Mormons), promote healthy life-styles by advocating that certain potentially harmful substances such as tobacco and alcohol be avoided. Most religions have beliefs and practices that influence health and illness, such as dietary habits, birth control, birth, and death (beliefs regarding autopsies and cessation of life support). Religion may also provide a sense of identity and equilibrium, promoting the development of a person's strengths and a positive life-style.

Individuals throughout their life-span experience spiritual and religious development. Spiritual development is a dynamic process of gaining awareness of the meaning, purpose, and values in life. Religious development is the process of accepting a specific system of beliefs, values, norms, and rituals. Spiritual and religious development may or may not parallel each other. At the heart of religious or spiritual beliefs is the faith that one's beliefs are true and valid. The concept of faith can be viewed in a broader context of intellectual, philosophical, and developmental growth. Several stages of faith development have been advanced. Fowler (1983) has identified seven developmental stages of faith (see Display 17-2). It is Fowler's belief that most people do not move into the higher stages of development.

Knowing a person's present developmental stage of faith can provide insight into his or her spiritual needs and can serve as a guide in planning appropriate interventions of care. Once spiritual and religious beliefs are developed, they usually do not change significantly. A crisis such as serious illness or the death of a loved one, however, may cause spiritual distress. At the same time, such a crisis can provide an opportunity for growth by forcing the person to rethink beliefs and values. Understanding a person's spirituality and religious beliefs can assist the nurse in providing support during such a crisis.

Display 17–2
Fowler's Stages of Faith Development

- *Primal faith* (Stage 0—infancy) Prelanguage; characterized by the formation of trust relationships with significant others.
- *Intuitive-projective faith* (Stage 1—early childhood): Beliefs based on imagination, perception and feelings; beliefs involve positive and negative powers affecting the child.
- *Mythic-liberal faith* (Stage 2—childhood and beyond). Characterized by development of logical thinking, which assists with understanding world order and meaning of life. The perspectives of others, especially family and religious figures, are usually accepted.
- *Synthetic-conventional faith* (Stage 3—adolescence and beyond). Personal, mostly unreflective, synthesis of values and beliefs evolves as the person attempts to reduce internal conflict by relying on conventional belief systems.
- *Individualistic-reflective faith* (Stage 4—young adulthood and beyond). Characterized by critical reflection on values and beliefs and understanding of self and the social system. Choices made about ideology and life-style.
- *Conjunctive faith* (Stage 5—middle life and beyond). The recognition of multiple interpretations of reality; reinterpretation of life and appreciation of symbols, metaphor, and myth for understanding truth.
- *Universalizing faith* (Stage 6—middle life and beyond). Grounded in oneness with the powers of being. Visions free the individual to devote self to overcoming division, oppression, and brutality.

THE INTERVIEW AND HEALTH HISTORY

A person's values and beliefs are revealed throughout the health assessment interview and become apparent through language, behavior, and appearance. You will be interviewing individuals from different cultures and with different levels of English fluency. Display 17-3 contains suggestions on how to enhance the effectiveness of interviewing individuals from cultures different from your own. Assessment of value and belief components includes collecting information about the following cultural and spiritual factors:

Culture

- Ethnic background
- Beliefs about health and illness
- Dimensions of orientation

Spirituality

- Philosophy of life
- Spiritual beliefs and values
- Spiritual support

If a person does not indicate any difficulties with spirituality, only a screening assessment may be necessary. However, if a person does report a problem, or is at risk be-

---

Display 17–3
Enhancing Communication with Individuals of Other Cultures

- Determine the level of English fluency—if necessary arrange for an interpreter.
- Speak to the *client,* not to the interpreter.
- Allow the client to choose his or her own seating for comfort, with private space and eye contact.
- Choose a speech rate and sentence structure that promotes understanding and demonstrates respect.
- Avoid slang, jargon, and metaphors.
- Use open-ended questions; may need to rephrase in several ways to obtain desired information; ask for explanation.
- Provide reading material in appropriate language.
- If an interpreter is used, try to use the same interpreter with every encounter.
- Avoid offensive body and verbal language.

(Adapted from Spector, R. [1991]. *Cultural diversity in health and illness.* Norwalk, CT: Appleton & Lange)

Interview Guide **Value and Beliefs**

Culture

What culture or ethnic group do you identify with? _____

If you are unaware or have limited knowledge of the group identified, then ask:

Could you describe for me some of the beliefs and values important in your culture? _____

Describe for me your beliefs regarding illness and the causes of illness _____

Describe for me your beliefs regarding health and the causes of health _____

When you make plans do you primarily look to the future, concentrate on the present, or look to the past for guidance? (For clarification, have the individual describe his or her response, such as "Could you please give me an example" or "Could you describe what you mean by . . .")

Spirituality

Do you generally get out of life what you want? (describe)

What are the most important things for you?

Is religion or a belief in God important to you? If *yes,* can you describe how? If *no,* can you describe your beliefs regarding the meaning and purpose of life?

If Appropriate

Would you describe any religious practices that are important to you _____

Are there any religious books you like to read or find comforting? _____

Do you find prayer or meditation helpful? _____

Has being sick affected your beliefs in your religion or God? _____

When you need spiritual support or help what do you do? (who do you talk with)? Would you like to talk with that person now?

---

cause of life circumstances, or is having difficulty following through with an agreed-upon plan of action, then a more thorough assessment is indicated. It is important to remember that values and beliefs are related to other health patterns, including coping and stress tolerance, roles and relationships, and health perception and health management.

The Interview Guide shown in the accompanying display may be used to direct the interview.

Culture

Ethnic Background. The impact of ethnic background upon the life-style and beliefs of an individual will vary depending on the degree to which the person follows the values and beliefs of the culture. Assuming that a person from an ethnic group will automatically share that group's views can lead to incorrect conclusions. With each succeeding generation from the original immigrants, individuals tend to be less affiliated with the original culture and more affiliated with their surrounding culture. At times, this difference between generations causes family strain. Families whose members have more than one set of cultural values, beliefs, and customs generally experience more distress than families with one cultural orientation.

Data related to ethnic background can be collected through a combination of open and closed questions. If the person does not speak a language adequately known by the nurse, an interpreter may be needed. Except in emergency cases, the client's children should not interpret for the client because their presence and involvement can inhibit the discussion of certain topics. Ideally, the interview

should be rescheduled for a time when an interpreter is available. If you are interviewing a person who by dress and/or speech seems to be a recent immigrant, you may ask the following type of questions:

> Have you lived in this area long?
> Where are you originally from?
> In (insert country) what did you do for health care?
> I don't know much about the way of life in (insert country). Could you tell me a little about that?

If clothing or mannerism provides you no clue to an ethnic background, you may wish to use the following type of questions:

> Have you lived in this area long?
> Where are your parents and grandparents from?
> How closely do you identify with the culture of your parents or grandparents?
> Do you practice any special activities that you identify as part of your cultural heritage?

Health Beliefs. Many individuals use folk remedies before seeking assistance from western health professionals. Belittling a client's reliance on folk remedies is detrimental to the nurse–client relationship. It is much more productive to explore what remedies the client uses for common health problems such as colds, fevers, and headaches, and what remedies are used for chronic illnesses such as hypertension. Preventive folk remedies, such as wearing charms, eating special foods such as ginseng, or drinking teas, should be identified. A nonjudgmental attitude is recommended because some of these practices have been identified as effective and because prohibiting such practices could cause physical and emotional anguish and distrust of the provider.

Usually wives or mothers are the providers of health care in the family. In some cultures, older women assume responsibility for dispensing health care advice to the extended family. Families may also rely upon cultural health providers. Knowledge of who assumes responsibility for the health of the individual and the providers used for specific problems can assist in a greater understanding of the individual's health practices. Cultural rituals are usually associated with major life events such as birth, puberty, marriage, and death and should be discussed whenever possible. Dietary customs that advocate or prohibit eating certain foods should also be investigated.

Open-ended questions will reveal more information regarding health practices. You may ask the following type of questions:

> Many people use home remedies when they don't feel well. Could you describe what you do when you aren't feeling well?
> Are there any special things you do when a baby is born?
> When you are not feeling well, who do you consult with first? Usually how effective is their advice?
> Could you describe remedies you use to help you stay healthy?

Time Orientation. To develop appropriate nursing interventions and health teaching, an understanding of time orientation is helpful. Assess how the client views past, present, and future; does time walk or run?

Locus of Control. Consider the client's beliefs about control, health, and illness. For example, a client who views human beings as having little control over life events may not value illness-prevention behaviors. For a more detailed discussion, see Chapter 13 and Table 13-1.

Spirituality

Philosophy of Life. How a person views life can affect physical and emotional well-being. Life philosophies are culturally influenced and are related to time orientation, beliefs about the relationship of human beings to nature, interpersonal relationships, and life purposes. Assessing this dimension includes determining whether the client is satisfied with life, has plans for the future, and sees a purpose for own life. Also important is the degree of harmony that exists between the person's philosophy and his or her culture. Such congruence, known as heritage consistency, enhances spirituality.

To gather data regarding a client's philosophy, you may ask a question such as "Would you describe for me what you believe is the meaning and purpose of life?" Use follow-up questions to clarify and verify your understanding.

Spiritual Beliefs. Spiritual beliefs and values may or may not be linked with an organized religion. Atheists and agnostics have spiritual beliefs and values to the same extent as devout Baptists and Moslems. Individual values and beliefs vary greatly. Although many spiritual assessments tools exist, most explore only a person's relationship with God or a supreme being. Spiritual values and beliefs go beyond belief in a "being" or "force" and include beliefs about death, sin, illness, health, the existence of a soul, life after death, and responsibilities to others.

Most health history forms contain a question about religious preference. Additional questions to ask during the interview concern actual religious activities and the degree to which the client ascribes to religious beliefs or values. Such questions reveal whether the religion cited on the form is actively practiced and if it is an integral part of the person's life and philosophy.

Religious values and beliefs affect health and health decisions. Jehovah's Witnesses, for example, forbid receiving transfusions of blood or blood products. Christian Scientists avoid using medications. Birth control strategies are restricted in some religious groups, such as Catholics and Islamics. The Amish and Christian Scientists avoid immunizations. Information should be sought about whether the client avoids certain foods or drink or engages in spiritual rituals such as praying a certain number of times per day or wearing special garments.

Established health care practices can interfere with or complicate religious practices. For example, gelatin capsules cannot be ingested by Jews and Seventh Day Adventists, who practice Old Testament dietary laws. Pork insulin is prohibited for Jews and Islamics. Diabetic diets that require eating three meals a day may interfere with religious fasts. Taking daily medication for a chronic condition may conflict with a devout Christian Scientist's belief in "Divine Mind" and spiritual truth.

Interview questions that would elicit data about spirituality beliefs would include the following:

> Are there any foods you eat or avoid because of your religious beliefs?
> Is there anything that is forbidden by your beliefs I should be aware of?
> Would you describe how important your religious beliefs are to you?
> Has anything recently changed your belief in your religion or God?

Spiritual Support. People who lack sufficient spiritual support or a sense of spirituality are at greater risk for spiritual distress during a crisis. Exploring other philosophical areas can help identify means of providing psychological support. Inquire about family values, stage of faith development, spiritual support from others, and spiritual self-support. Many individuals receive spiritual support from prayer, reading a religious book such as the Bible, wearing or having near special symbols such as rosary beads, and wearing special garments.

The following open-ended questions are useful to collect data regarding spiritual support:

> Who else in your family shares your religious beliefs?
> What religious books or religious articles are helpful to you?
> When you need spiritual help, who assists you?
> Do you find prayer or meditation helpful? (describe)

DIAGNOSTIC STUDIES

There are no specific diagnostic studies for spiritual distress. Several assessment tools are available that are similar to the interview guide display—for example, "Guidelines for Spiritual Assessment" (Stoll, 1979); "Spiritual Well-Being" (Ellis, 1983); and "Spiritual Assessment Guide" (O'Brian, 1982). Sector (1991) has developed a comprehensive Heritage Assessment Tool, which may be used if more information is desired; however, there are similar components in the interview guide.

NURSING OBSERVATIONS RELATED TO VALUES AND BELIEFS

Observation Focus

While conducting the interview and performing a physical examination, a number of observations may be meaningful for values, beliefs, and spirituality. Because of the quality of these dimensions, however, the nurse must verify objective data with subjective information. Without client verification, the nurse can only assume problems with spiritual distress and conflict of beliefs and values.

General Appearance

The nurse can gather much information from general appearance; however, one must be careful not to jump to conclusions before validating observations.

Dress. The way an individual dresses may indicate cultural or religious background. For example, orthodox Jewish men wear a yarmulke (skullcap), adult Mormons wear sacred undergarments, Mennonite women wear long-sleeved dresses and a cap, Indian women may wear native dress, and Islamic Arab women cover their hair.

Facial Expressions. Facial expressions can provide information during the interview and physical examination. For example, a questioning expression, frown, or grimace may lead you to wonder if the individual really understands what is being asked. Lack of eye contact may represent normal behavior in some Native American people.

Touch. A person's avoidance of a handshake or other touching may indicate cultural customs. For example, the only women Orthodox Jewish men touch are their wives, children, and mothers, and Islamic Arabs do not touch anyone considered unclean (Carson, 1989).

Speech. An individual's speech can provide much information, such as the presence of an accent, fluency in verbal English, English reading level (the types of words spoken should provide a clue regarding what could be read), and the use of other languages.

Associated Body System Alterations

Physical indicators that may assist you to diagnose responses to spiritual distress include signs and symptoms of stress or anxiety. Some related body system alterations may be observable in the cardiovascular, respiratory, and gastrointestinal systems (see Chap. 16). One obvious physiologic cultural difference is the male penis, for which some religions practice circumcision (Jewish, Islamic), whereas others do not (Hindu). Circumcision is a common practice in the United States but not in other countries, such as Mexico and most Third-World countries.

Nursing Observations   *Values and Beliefs*

General Principles	Conclusions about values and beliefs are primarily based upon interview data. Observations are used to verify some interview data; however, observations need corresponding interview data to be accepted as factual.
Preparation for Assessment	Interview the client in a quiet, comfortable, private area. Make eye contact as appropriate and provide enough private space for the person to feel comfortable. You should be at the same level as the client—that is, if the client is sitting or lying, you should be sitting.
Examination and Documentation Focus	• Cultural and ethnic background • Use of folk remedies • Verbalization regarding spiritual beliefs • Participation in religious activities

Examination Guidelines   *Values and Beliefs*

Procedure	Clinical Significance
1. OBSERVE FOR CULTURAL AND ETHNIC BACKGROUND.	
a. Note cues in dress, speech, and body language.	Men are more likely to adopt Western dress than women; therefore, be alert to subtle cues.

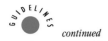 *continued*

Values and Beliefs

Procedure

b. Note how knowledgeable client is about customs and rituals when explaining them.

c. Actively listen for cues of past and potential conflict between client, nurse, health regimen options, and health care system.

2. OBSERVE FOR OBVIOUS SIGNS OF FOLK REMEDY USE.
   a. Observe for physical signs.
   b. Actively listen for remarks about folk remedies

3. EVALUATE SPIRITUAL BELIEFS.
   a. Actively listen for remarks regarding spiritual beliefs.

4. PARTICIPATION IN RELIGIOUS ACTIVITIES:
   a. Observe for evidence of religious activity.

   b. Observe for abrupt change in religious practices

Clinical Significance

If a client can tell of ethnic rituals and customs but cannot describe or explain those practices, the client may not actually engage in those activities.

Statements that may indicate past or potential conflicts:

"I've tried that and it doesn't work."

Smiling while saying "yes, yes, yes."

"I'll have to ask my (husband, mother)."

No response or an apparently inappropriate response to a question.

Physical signs of folk remedies used include copper bracelets, a coin on the navel wrapped with a belly binder in a Mexican-heritage infant, strong garlic breath smell, a small pouch tied to a cord around the neck or attached to a belt, and a bracelet made of hair.

Types of statements indicating spiritual distress (Carson, 1989):

Expressions of anger, hurt, disappointment in God, religious representatives, church/temple/synagogue

Verbalization of inability to sleep, stay asleep, or nightmares

Questions regarding reason for illness, suffering ("Why is God letting this happen to me?")

Questions about belief system or meaning/purpose of life.

Verbalizing inability to exercise usual religious practices

Asking for spiritual guidance/assistance

Expressions of unworthiness

Evidence of belief and participation in organized religion includes the presence of such items as a holy book; the wearing of a crucifix, star of David, or other religious symbol; praying; rosary beads; presence of religious statues and paintings; speaking in "tongues;" taviz (a black string with words of the Koran attached worn by Islamics); wearing sacred undergarments (Mormons)

Indications of abrupt change in religious practice: A person who has traditionally read the Bible or watches specific religious programs suddenly stops. Conversely, a person who claims to have no religion suddenly begins to read holy books or watch religious programs.

Documenting Assessment Findings

Assessment data and clinical judgments are documented from the client interview and nurse observations. Assessment pertaining to values and beliefs may be documented as a part of a comprehensive assessment, entered in progress notes, or incorporated into problem-oriented records. Examples of narrative and problem-oriented types of documentation follow.

Example 1

Mrs. H, age 24 years, delivered a 32-week-gestation female 18 hours ago. Surgery is indicated for the infant. The surgeon leaves the room as the nurse enters, and the nurse discusses the situation further with Mrs. H. The documentation, which pertains to values and beliefs, is as follows:

Crying, "I don't want my baby to die. The doctor said she has to have surgery and will need blood. Receiving blood is against my religion. He said that he will get a court order if I don't agree. Can he do that? What will happen to my baby?" Starts sobbing. Jehovah

Witness belief. Hospital social services contacted to assist. Encouraged to call the family.

These findings may be recorded in a problem-oriented format as follows:

S: I don't want my baby to die. The doctor said she needs surgery and blood. Receiving blood against religion. Doctor will get court order if I don't agree. Can he do that? What will happen to my baby? Jehovah Witness belief.

O: Spiritual distress related to crying, sobbing

A: Conflict between religious belief and medical care needs of newborn

P: Conference with physician, notify hospital social worker, encourage contact of family members for support, reevaluate within 1 hour

Example 2

Mr. A, aged 64 years, was admitted to the hospital to control diabetes mellitus and learn insulin administration. The nurse takes the vial of insulin and other supplies into the room to begin implementing the teaching plan. The following was recorded:

After observing insulin vial, states "Get that dirty bottle out of here. I can't take anything made from a pig. Is all insulin made from pigs?" Physician notified. Order for human insulin obtained.

These findings may be recorded in a problem-oriented format as follows:

S: Get that dirty bottle out of here, I can't take anything made from a pig. Is all insulin made from pigs?

O: Comments made after seeing pork-base insulin vial, pork prohibited in Islamic religious belief.

A: Spiritual distress related to conflict between religious belief and insulin order

P: Notify physician for insulin order acceptable to client. Human insulin order is received.

Example 3

Mr. J, aged 73 years, is newly admitted to the intensive care unit with myocardial infarction. On the admission note, the nurse documents the following:

Concerned regarding religious undergarment, devout Latter Day Saint; all clothes removed in ER; wearing hospital gown only. "My chances of making it are better with my garments on," wringing hands, restless.

These findings may be recorded in a problem-oriented format as follows:

S: Where are my garments? My chances are better with my garments on. States garments were removed in ER; devout Latter Day Saint.

O: Spiritual distress related to wearing hospital gown only, wringing hands, restless

A: Hospital custom of wearing hospital gown only interferes with practice of wearing religious garments, which provide emotional support.

P: Find garments. Discuss with client possibility of putting garments on but leaving chest exposed for possible emergency access in the ICU.

Example 4

The J family is interviewed as a result of a hospice referral. Mr. J, aged 39 years, is dying. The family was seen in the hospital. The nurse made a home visit to Mrs. J to evaluate the home environment and equipment needed. The nurse documents the following:

"Why does he have to die? To suffer? Why is God doing this to us? Pete never hurt anyone. Why would God punish my family? It just tears my heart to see him." Crying. Bible on dining room table open to Psalms.

These findings may be recorded in a problem-oriented format as follows:

S: Why does he have to die? To suffer? Why is God doing this to us? Pete never hurt anyone. Why would God punish my family? It tears my heart to see him.

O: Crying; Bible on dining room table open to Psalms.

A: Spiritual crisis related to spouse's illness and anticipated death

P: Collect further data next visit about religious beliefs and values. Listen and communicate willingness to discuss spiritual beliefs. If appropriate, encourage spiritual support from spiritual leader, extended family, or friends.

Example 5

Nancy, aged 22 years, was interviewed about values and beliefs as a part of her initial visit to a health maintenance clinic. Documentation was as follows:

Reports a belief in a supreme being who is benevolent, attends church irregularly, satisfied with life as it is. Of German heritage. Identifies with middle class America.

These findings may be recorded in a problem-oriented format as follows:

S: Believes in benevolent supreme being, attends church irregularly, satisfied with life as it is, German heritage, identifies with middle class Americans

O: Midwest US accent, dress appropriate for age and lifestyle

A: Functional value and belief system

P: Follow-up with routine screening in 1 year

NDx

Nursing Diagnoses Related to Values and Beliefs

The only nursing diagnosis for values and beliefs is Spiritual distress.

Spiritual Distress

Spiritual distress occurs when there is a disruption in the life principle that pervades a person's entire being and integrates and transcends one's biologic and psychosocial nature (NANDA, 1990).

History

The individual would express a disturbance in his or her belief system. This may be expressed by questioning credibility or fairness of beliefs, inability to perform previous religious activities, sense of emotional vacuum, anger at life events, and requests for spiritual assistance.

Physical Findings

Physical findings may be totally absent. Signs and symptoms of anxiety or stress, such as palpations, sleeplessness, and gastric upset, may be present. You might observe a sudden increase or decrease in the amount of spiritual interest or activity.

Clinical Problems Related to Values and Beliefs

Assessment of values and beliefs is useful for making nursing diagnoses and to determine appropriate interventions for clinical problems. Clinical problems such as miscarriage, death, and diagnosis of a potentially fatal disease can be factors in the nursing diagnosis of spiritual distress.

Understanding values and beliefs will allow the nurse to determine areas of potential conflict between the client's values and beliefs and the health care options. Selecting and modifying appropriate options that reinforce or at least do not conflict with the client's values and beliefs enhance adherence to a health regimen. Charting out the client's beliefs and the possible health regimen options may be useful in determining the most appropriate intervention

> *Display 17–4*
> ## Comparing Values and Beliefs with Health Options
>
> | Values and Beliefs | Option #1 | Option #2 | Option #3 |
> |---|---|---|---|
> | Value #1 | +++ | + | – – |
> | Value #2 | + | + | + |
> | Value #3 | +++ | + | 0 |
> | Belief A | – | + | – – – |
> | Belief B | +++ | +++ | + |
> | Belief C | + | + | – |
> | Belief D | + | + | + |
>
> Key: agreement with client +, disagreement, –, neutral 0
> (Adapted from Tripp-Reimer, T., Brink, P., & Saunders, J. [1984]. Cultural assessment: Content and process. *Nursing Outlook, 32* (2), 78-82)

(see Display 17-4). In the example, option 3 has less of a chance for adherence even if scientifically that is the best option. The nurse may desire to use the same chart to insert his or her own values and beliefs and/or that of the health agency to determine where conflicts may occur between the client and nurse, client and agency, and nurse and agency.

ASSESSMENT PROFILE 1

* *

Mr. and Mrs. Hong are recent immigrants to the United States from a refugee camp in Thailand. They currently live in a city composed mostly of Christians. The Hong family practices Buddhism. While in Thailand, Mrs. Hong was found to have tuberculosis and placed on INH. She recently stopped taking her medication, stating that the pills were upsetting the yin and yang balance.

Profile Analysis

The Hong family are at risk for spiritual distress related to the following factors: religious beliefs (Buddhist) uncommon in community, health providers potentially unaware of cultural and spiritual beliefs, potential conflict between client belief system and medical regimen, and probable inadequate community spiritual support to family.

When reviewing Mrs. Hong's record before the interview, the nurse identified the focus of data collection and made inferences about probable nursing diagnoses. Previous failure to consider values and beliefs may have accounted for

Mrs. Hong's reluctance to comply with the medication regimen. In preparing for the appointment, the nurse reviewed the health beliefs of Buddhism and Southeast Asians, especially beliefs about yin and yang. With this limited knowledge base, the nurse was able to initiate a more meaningful assessment about the conflict between the client's belief system and the health care she needed.

Based on data in the chart and knowledge about the values and beliefs of the client, the nurse made a tentative diagnosis of Spiritual distress. Further data collected during the interview revealed difficulties such as inability to purchase desired incense for the altar at home, unfamiliar foods, and lack of spiritual support from family members remaining in Thailand. These problems had lead Mrs. Hong to believe the upset in her yin and yang was adding to the family's problems. During the interview, the nurse learned more about the Hong's beliefs so that future conflicts could be reduced. A final diagnosis was made of Spiritual distress related to conflict of the health regimen with beliefs and related to difficulty in practicing religious rituals.

ASSESSMENT PROFILE 2

• •

Tim, aged 16, was diagnosed 1 year ago during a pre-sports physical with insulin-dependent diabetes mellitus. During the last 6 months, he has frequently forgotten to check his blood glucose levels, take his insulin, and stay on his diet. His mother called the clinic expressing concern that, in addition to problems with his health, he argues with his siblings more, refuses to attend church with the family, and has stated that "I don't believe in God. If there was a God then I wouldn't have diabetes." Tim has an appointment the next day at the clinic.

Profile Analysis

Before Tim's appointment the nurse reviewed his health record and focused on the possible problems, as well as additional data that might be needed to support or rule out a tentative diagnosis. A possible diagnosis of Spiritual distress evidenced by expressed religious doubts related to life style requirement needed to control diabetes was made by the nurse. In selecting this possible diagnosis, the nurse also considered Tim's stage of spiritual and faith development.

Additional data would be needed to support such a diagnosis. Primarily, the nurse needs to know whether Tim's perception is the same, similar to, or different from his mother's. After data collection and analysis, a final diagnosis can be made.

ASSESSMENT PROFILE 3

• •

Sarah, aged 75 years, was admitted to the hospital after a fall at home. She has had hip surgery and has been progressing as expected. One morning, Sarah refused her morning meal of toast, coffee, eggs, and bacon. The nurse observed that Sarah was unusually quiet and had numerous small complaints.

Profile Analysis

Upon reviewing Sarah's chart, the nurse discovered that Sarah was Jewish. No one had asked Sarah about her religious beliefs and rituals; however, she had previously eaten all her meals without problems. The nurse thought of several possible diagnoses, including Spiritual distress related to inability to practice spiritual rituals. During a focused assessment, the nurse discovered that today was the first day of Passover and Sarah always ate only kosher and unleavened (without yeast or other leavenings) foods during Passover. Kosher dietary laws forbid the eating of pork, milk, and meat together and the use of utensils and plates that have had nonkosher foods on them. In talking with Sarah, the nurse learned about Jewish dietary customs and the significance of Passover. The nurse confirmed her diagnosis of Spiritual distress. With collaboration from the dietary department and pastoral care, the nurse developed a plan of care to lessen the spiritual distress experienced by Sarah.

Chapter 17 SUMMARY

The assessment of values and beliefs focuses on the following:

• Person's values, beliefs, and spiritual dimensions, especially in relation to health and illness
• Relationship of values, beliefs, and spirituality to health care regimens
• Identification of spiritual problems that require nursing interventions or referrals
• Assessment of own values, beliefs, and spirituality.

When assessing values and beliefs, you should consider the following:

• All people have some type of spiritual dimension.
• Your own spirituality, culture, and values may influence the care provided to others.
• Assessment of spirituality is important regardless of age, mental status, cognitive ability, and health status.

• Some spiritual problems are best treated by others, such as spiritual leaders, prayer groups, or another nurse. You should make appropriate referrals.
• Your understanding of the accepted norms for various cultures, ethnic groups, or religious groups enhances the ability to identify cultural or spiritual conflicts.
• You should avoid generalizing and stereotyping, and respect the values and beliefs of all clients.

Data pertaining to values and beliefs are obtained by the following means:

Interview

• Spiritual beliefs, and rituals and related dietary habits, if any

RESEARCH *Hi*GHLIGHT

How does spiritual well-being affect the hardiness of an individual?

Hardiness, a personality characteristic, is an inner resource used to resist the undesirable effects of stress, thereby reducing the occurrence and severity of stress-related illnesses. The more hardy an individual is, the better he or she is able to cope with stress and survive under adverse conditions (Carson and Green, 1992).

In a recent research study, Verna Carson and Harry Green explored the relationship between spiritual well-being and hardiness. They studied 100 individuals (mostly males) with the diagnoses of HIV-positive and AIDS. The mean age was 37.18 years. Most viewed their physical health as fair to good, and 47 did not have any religious affiliation. Spiritual well-being was measured by totalling scores from 20 items of a religious well-being subscale and an existential well-being subscale. Findings included a statistically significant correlation between the total spiritual well-being score and the existential well-being subscale score with hardiness. The relationship between religious well-being and hardiness was not reported.

What significance does the study have for health assessment?

Spirituality is one of the most frequently omitted assessment components of health examinations. If spiritual well-being increases one's chances of survival during adversity by increasing hardiness, then its importance to health assessment is relevant. The premise of this study—that spiritual health is linked to psychological health—was supported. On the basis of this finding, then, one could conclude that health assessment is incomplete without spiritual assessment.

Can the study's findings be applied to practice?

Although the sample of this study comprised only those individuals with an incurable condition/illness (HIV-positive and AIDS), many other clients that the nurse encounters also have incurable health problems. Additionally, if spiritual well-being is related to hardiness in adversity, it may also be related during times of apparent wellness. Although this study was an exploratory study with a select population and must be used cautiously, it does support the premise that nurses cannot practice holistic health care if spiritual well-being is omitted.

- Identification of cultural heritage, including beliefs about health and acceptable treatment for illness
- Possible perceived conflict between prescribed health-illness regimens and beliefs
- Expressed disturbance of belief system

Nursing Observations

- Assessment of dress, accent, language use, and presence of religious or spiritual articles
- Observation of consistency between stated cultural membership and behavior
- Observation of spiritual practices

Assessment of value and beliefs based on these principles and methods assists you in identifying the following defining characteristics (cues) for the nursing diagnosis Spiritual distress (distress of the human spirit).

The following related nursing diagnoses may be identified during the assessment:

Anxiety
Ineffective individual coping
Altered family processes
Anticipatory grieving
Hopelessness
Knowledge deficit
Altered self-concept

✳ CRITICAL THINKING

A 65-year-old Native American man is admitted to the hospital for treatment of pneumonia and active tuberculosis. He has a large extended family who desire to spend a great deal of time at his bedside. He and his family request that the tribal medicine man be actively involved in his care.

Learning Exercises

1. You are not familiar with the Native American culture. Propose how you would proceed to assess cultural perspectives pertaining to the patient and his family.

2. Explain how you would know if a cultural conflict existed between this patient and his health care providers.

3. Explain how you would guard against cultural stereotyping as you care.

4. Identify and describe observations you would make about interactions between this patient and his visitors that would be relevant to culture.

BIBLIOGRAPHY

Baldi, S. & Puglisi, S. (1985). Spirituality. In L. Hill & N. Smith (Eds.). *Self-care nursing* (pp. 186–216). Norwalk, CT: Appleton-Century-Crofts.

Bauwens, E. & Anderson, S. (1984). Social and cultural influences on health care. In M. Stanhope & J. Lancaster (Eds.). *Community health nursing: Process and practice for promoting health* (pp. 89–108). St. Louis: C.V. Mosby.

Betz, C. (1981). Faith development in children. *Pediatric Nursing, 7,* 22–25.

Burnard, P. (1987). Spiritual distress and the nursing response: Theoretical considerations and counseling skills. *Journal of Advanced Nursing, 12* (3), 377–382.

Bushy, A. (1992). Cultural considerations for primary health care: Where do self-care and folk medicine fit? *Holistic Nursing Practice, 6* (3), 10–18.

Carson, V. (1989). *Spiritual dimension in nursing process.* Philadelphia: W.B. Saunders.

Charnes, L., & Moore, P. (1992). Meeting patients' spiritual needs: The Jewish perspective. *Holistic Nursing Practice, 6* (3), 64–72.

Charonko, C. (1992). Cultural influences in "noncompliant behavior and decision making." *Holistic Nursing Practice, 6* (3), 73–77.

Clark, A. (1978). *Culture, childbearing, health professionals.* Philadelphia: F.A. Davis.

Clark, M. (1984). *Community nursing: Health care for today and tomorrow.* Reston, VA: Reston Publishing.

Dawes, T. (1986). Multicultural nursing. *International Nursing Review, 33* (5), 148–150.

Ellis, C. (1983). Spiritual well-being: Conceptualization and measurement. *Journal of Psychology and Theology, 11* (5), 330–340.

Embers, J. (1992). Religion and spirituality defined according to current use in nursing literature. *Journal of Professional Nursing, 8* (1), 41–47.

Fleming, J. (1981). An evaluation of the use of the Denver Developmental Screening Test. *Nursing Research, 30* (5), 290–293.

Fowler, J. (1983). Stages of faith. *Psychology Today, 17* (11), 56–62.

Frankenburg, W.K. & Dodds, J.B. (1967). The Denver Developmental Screening Test. *Journal of Pediatrics, 71*:180–191.

Gordon, M. (1987). *Nursing diagnosis: Process and application* (2nd ed.). New York: McGraw-Hill.

Haase, J., Britt, T., Coward, D., Leidy, N., & Penn, P. (1992). Simultaneous concept analysis of spiritual perspective, hope, acceptance, and self-transcendence. *Image, 24* (2), 141–152.

Harmon, Y. (1985). The relationship between religiosity and health. *Health Values, 9* (3), 23–25.

Henderson, G., & Primeaux, M. (Eds.) (1981). *Transcultural health care.* Menlo Park: Addison-Wesley.

Hill, L. & Smith, N. (Eds.) (1985). *Self-care nursing.* Norwalk, CT: Appleton-Century-Crofts.

Hoff, L. (1984). *People in crisis* (2nd ed.). Menlo Park: Addison-Wesley.

Kluckholn, F. (1961). *Variations in value orientation.* New York: Row Peterson.

Kluckholn, F. (1976). Dominant and variant value orientations. In P. Brink (Ed.). *Transcultural nursing* (pp. 63–91). Engelwood Cliffs: Prentice-Hall.

Leininger, M. (Ed.). (1978). *Transcultural nursing: Concepts, theories, and practice.* New York: John Wiley & Sons.

McLane, A. (Ed.) (1987). *Classification of nursing diagnoses: Proceedings of the seventh national conference.* St. Louis: C.V. Mosby.

Meeks, L. (1977). Roles of spiritual health in achieving high level wellness. *Health Values, 1* (5), 222–224.

Meleis, A., Lipson, J., & Paul, S. (1992). Ethnicity and health among five Middle Eastern immigrant groups. *Nursing Research, 41* (2), 98–103.

Murray, R. & Zentner, J. (Eds.) (1993). *Nursing concepts for health promotion* (5th ed.). Englewood Cliffs, Prentice-Hall.

North American Nursing Diagnosis Association. (1990). *Taxonomy I revised 1990 with official nursing diagnoses.* St Louis: North American Nursing Diagnosis Association.

O'Brian, M. (1982). The need for spiritual integrity. In H. Yura & M. Walsh (Eds.). *Human needs and the nursing process* (pp. 85–116). Norwalk, CT: Appleton-Century-Crofts.

Olade, R. (1984). Evaluation of the Denver Developmental Screening Test as applied to African children. *Nursing Research, 32* (4), 204–207.

O'Pray, M. (1980). Developmental screening tools: Using them effectively. *Maternal-Child Nursing, 5,* 126–130.

Pender, N. (1987). *Health promotion in nursing practice* (2nd ed.). Norwalk, CT: Appleton-Lange.

Peterson, E. (1985). The physical . . . the spiritual . . . can you meet all of your patient's needs? *Journal of Gerontological Nursing, 11* (10), 23–27.

Pitch, J.J. (1988). Wellness spirituality. *Health Values, 12* (3), 28–31.

Spector, R. (1991). *Cultural diversity in health and illness* (3rd ed.). Norwalk, CT: Appleton & Lange.

Stanhope, M., & Lancaster, J. (Eds.) (1992). *Community health nursing: Process and practice for promoting health* (3rd ed.). St. Louis: C.V. Mosby.

Steele, S.M. & Harmon, V.M. (1979). *Value clarification in nursing.* New York: Appleton-Century-Crofts.

Steiger, N. & Lipson, J. (1985). *Self-care nursing: Theory and practice.* Bowie, MD: Brady Communications.

Stoll, R. (1979). Guideline for spiritual assessment. *American Journal of Nursing, 79* (11), 1574–1577.

Tripp-Reimer, T. (1984). Cultural assessment. In J. Bellack & P. Bamford (Eds.). *Nursing assessment: A multidimensional approach* (pp. 226–246). Belmont, CA: Wadsworth Publishing.

Tripp-Reimer, T., Brink, P., & Saunders, J. (1984). Cultural assessment: Content and process. *Nursing Outlook, 32* (2), 78–82.

Wilson, R. (1978). Religiosity and health: Implications for health promotion. *Health Values, 2* (3), 144–146.

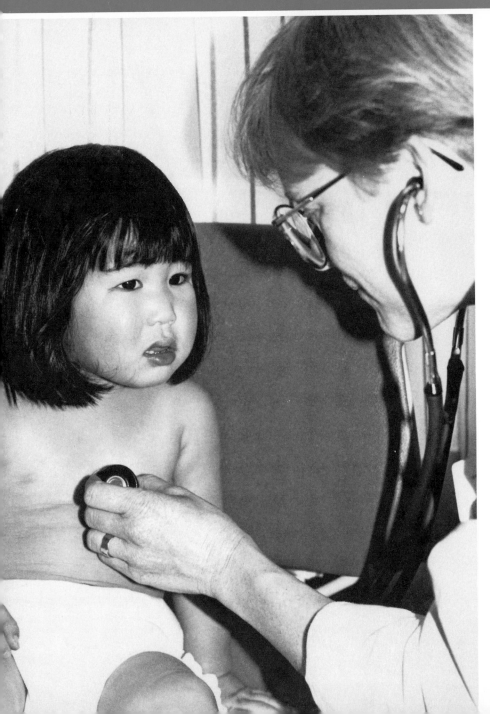

Unit III

Health Assessment Across the Life Span

Chapter 18

Growth and Development Concepts for Health Assessment

Assessment Terms

Ages And Stages Theories
Life Event Theories
Variability Theories
Developmental Screening

Anticipatory Guidance
Ageism
Object Permanence
Egocentricism

INTRODUCTORY OVERVIEW

A person's growth and development level should be evaluated to promote health and identify dysfunctional areas that require intervention. Growth and development are evaluated relative to the person's stage in the life cycle. Several theories explain development patterns across the life cycle.

Growth refers to quantitative physical and physiologic changes that occur over time. Development refers to changes that are more qualitative in nature, such as the development of functional, psychosocial, and cognitive behaviors over the life span. Growth and development are integrated processes. For example, physical growth may be necessary before a child can develop certain skills and abilities. Growth and development also influence interaction, self-concept, and coping patterns. Therefore, developmental assessment provides an indication of how people are adapting to personal changes and changes in the environment.

Certain physical characteristics and psychosocial and cognitive behaviors are expected at different levels of growth and development, and provide the criteria for developmental assessment. Developmental assessment is a means of determining a person's actual levels of growth and development and comparing them to norms and expected behaviors. An individualized assessment is imperative because chronologic age is not a reliable predictor of a person's growth and development. Assessment of an individual's growth and development level enables the nurse to make additional judgments about the appropriateness of the person's behaviors, predict expected behaviors, and plan nursing care in a manner that supports the person in meeting developmental tasks.

Jill Fuller and Jennifer Schaller-Ayers:
HEALTH ASSESSMENT: A NURSING APPROACH, Second Edition.
© 1990, 1994 by J. B. Lippincott Company.

PURPOSES OF DEVELOPMENTAL ASSESSMENT

Evaluating human growth and development is a complex process, but one that can be facilitated by considering the purpose of the assessment. The purpose, in turn, helps to determine the approach that is appropriate for assessing a particular client.

Providing Anticipatory Guidance

Understanding human development can help the nurse to provide anticipatory guidance, such as teaching parents of infants and children to anticipate and identify normal developmental changes and advising elders that peripheral vision decreases with age so that when driving an automobile they need to turn their heads to check for on-coming vehicles. It is also important to realize that some developmental patterns and problems are in fact more likely to occur in certain age groups. For example, fear of strangers begins around 6 to 9 months and presbyopia begins around age 40 years. Appropriate screening tests may be included in the health assessment process such as the Denver Developmental Screening Test II (DDST2) (see Appendix D).

A developmental assessment for purposes of anticipatory guidance might result in recommendations being made regarding accident prevention, nutrition, dental care, and discipline (Fig. 18-1). The examiner can help the parents of infants and children recognize particular developmental milestones, tasks, and crises, and discuss the parents' plans for dealing with each stage. Similarly, anticipatory guidance also applies to other age groups.

Assessment of Physical Changes

Physical growth and the development of body systems are readily evaluated during the physical examination. Certain normal physical changes occur during infancy, childhood, adulthood, and late adulthood. The nurse should be aware of what constitutes normal physical features for persons at different ages to evaluate normal growth, development, and maturation signs. Body system variations for infants, children, and older adults are discussed in Chapters 19 and 20.

Developmental Screening

Developmental assessment may focus on evaluating a person's mastery of motor and social skills, as well as language, speech, and intellectual development. Because these skills develop rapidly in young children, developmental screening is especially important for clients in these age groups. Early identification of delays is essential so that interventions can be started to correct or minimize problems. Adults continue to develop their intellectual and social skills, so a screening evaluation of these skills should

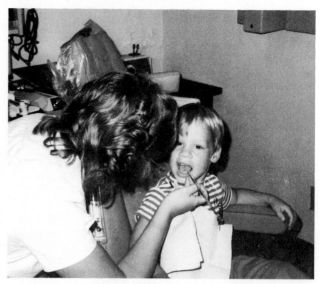

Figure 18–1. Recommending that a child begin dental visits between 3 and 3 1/2 years of age is a way of providing anticipatory guidance to a parent.

be performed. A knowledge of current screening recommendations, which change on occasion, is essential when evaluating both children and adults.

Developmental screening procedures differ from diagnostic procedures. Developmental screening is a means of quickly and reliably identifying persons whose developmental level is below normal for their age, indicating the need for further investigation. Diagnostic procedures are designed to identify the nature, extent, and severity of a developmental delay or disability. The nurse's role includes conducting the initial screening and consulting with other health care professionals for more specific diagnostic testing.

GROWTH AND DEVELOPMENT THEORIES

Several theories have been developed to explain or predict human growth and development. Major differences in theoretical perspectives focus on whether to consider human growth and development as related to one of the following:

- A series of sequential ages and stages
- Life events, crises, or transitions
- Individual timing and variability of roles within age groups

You may use any of the growth and development theories as a guide to collecting and interpreting data about a person's behavior. No one theory is broad enough to cover all aspects of human growth and development. Moreover, some theories, by stressing one aspect of growth over another, lack the holistic perspective valued by nursing. The "ages and stages" theories of human development have been most widely applied in clinical assessment situations.

Ages and Stages Theories

Theories based on ages and stages focus on biologic changes that occur with age or the completion of a series of psychological, social, or moral developmental tasks (stages). These theoretical perspectives assume that people experience similar physical and psychological developmental changes at the same ages. For example, a child's growth can be assessed by comparing height and weight to age-specific norms presented in standardized growth charts or tables. Similarly, norms for head and chest circumference for infants have been developed that accurately indicate normal growth patterns for the first 2 years. Standardized weight for height and bone structure charts are also available for adults.

Ages and stages perspectives may be especially helpful when evaluating the growth and development of infants and children. The chronologic categories associated with development from infancy through adolescence (*e.g.,* neonate, infant, toddler, preschooler, school-age, preadolescent, and adolescent) are easily distinguished because physical and psychological growth occurs in a predictable and highly visible manner in each age group.

Among adults, however, the differences are not so exact. Although physical, psychosocial, and cognitive changes occur in each phase of adult life, the changes are not consistent or predictable enough to be used to distinguish between adult age groups.

Theories describing age-related changes in adult age groups have been further challenged as experts debate the nature of normal physical changes that occur with the aging process. Some critics believe that norms for older people are based on changes observed in elderly people receiving extended health care and therefore do not truly represent normal healthy aging of the general population (McElmurry and LiBrizzi, 1986). With increased focus and research on diverse groups of healthy elderly people, more accurate information concerning normal physical aging should emerge.

Theories that explain the human life cycle in relation to stages of development with associated developmental tasks have also been criticized for incorporating sexual, cultural, and age-related biases. For example, Levinson's model is based on life events of adult men and identifies a male-oriented work role as an index for normal development (Levinson, 1980). This model indicates that work roles develop in the early 20s; however, for women who delay working outside the home until their children are grown, or who simultaneously fulfill work and family roles, Levinson's model may be inappropriate. In other words, if you apply this model to a woman who has just taken her first job at age 40, you might erroneously conclude that the woman's developmental growth has been delayed.

Developmental stage theories may be culturally biased. The conclusions made about normal development are often based on a longitudinal (across time) study of a particular group of subjects. Often, the group is not only predominantly male, but also, as in the case of Erikson's research, predominantly white and middle class. To avoid negative stereotyping, you should be cautious about applying the developmental norms associated with this group to clients with different cultural backgrounds when, in fact, other developmental norms may be applicable.

Stage theories, which emphasize "normal" age-related behaviors, may promote age stereotypes and "ageism" (a negative attitude toward a particular age group). For example, a stage theory may advocate a particular age range for marriage, such as by the third decade of a person's life. Applying a stage theory could lead you to conclude that a person who first marries at age 50 is developmentally delayed.

Ages and stages perspectives are evident in the growth and development theories of Erikson, Levinson, Piaget, and Kohlberg. Each theorist associates a set of developmental tasks with different ages.

ERIKSON'S THEORY

Erik Erikson is one of the leading theorists who represent human development as a passage through sequential stages characterized by developmental crises and tasks. Erikson's Developmental Stages (1963) are eight sequential stages of human development. Each stage is characterized by a core problem or crisis that must be resolved to some extent before a person can progress to the next stage. A person who successfully passes through each developmental stage will eventually attain ego integrity. This state is associated with high self-esteem and a positive outlook on life. Conversely, inadequate resolution of developmental crises may lead to despair rather than ego integrity. In this case, the person suffers low self-esteem, feelings of inadequacy or anger, and impaired coping patterns. Erikson's theory may be especially useful when evaluating a person's self-concept.

Developmental assessment based on Erikson's theory involves observing behaviors and responses associated with developmental tasks. Successful completion of each developmental task is associated with resolving the following conflicts.

Trust Versus Mistrust (Infancy or Birth to Age 1 Year). Trust develops as the infant develops a sense of confidence and reliance on self, others, and the environment. These attributes develop as a result of interaction with others and the environment. Specifically, the infant develops a sense of trust if his or her needs are met promptly, consistently, and predictably.

Autonomy Versus Shame and Doubt (Toddlerhood or Age 1 to 3 Years). Autonomy includes exercising self-control over motor abilities and toileting, handling decisions, and adequately coping with problems. Pride, patience, and self-reliance begin to develop. Parental encouragement and approval rather than strict control help children accomplish this task. Autonomous children begin to assert their independence and demonstrate a will. The words *me, mine,* and *no* are often verbal expressions of autonomy. Children in this age group often refuse to cooperate on the DDST.

Initiative Versus Guilt (Preschool Period or Age 3 to 6 Years). Initiative is reflected in energetic and enterprising behaviors such as assertiveness, learning, imagination, increasing dependability, and the ability to plan. Initiative fosters exploration of the environment outside the home. Observable behaviors associated with initiative include mastering tasks and learning new skills.

Industry Versus Inferiority (School-age Period or Age 6 to 12 Years). Industry includes identifying and solving problems, and forming responsible work habits and attitudes. A sense of industry is demonstrated by confidence, self-control, mastering tasks (such as the multiplication table) and perseverance, as well as an interest in activities beyond the moment and the self.

Identity Versus Role Diffusion (Adolescence or Age 12 to 18+ Years). The process of forming an identity involves developing a sense of self that resists extreme change during periods of stress or challenge. Developing an identity enables a person to develop self-confidence and self-esteem. Identity or self-concept is influenced by many factors, including interactions with peers, parents, and others; gender identity; sociocultural beliefs and practices; and adult role models.

Intimacy Versus Isolation (Young Adulthood or Age 18 to 30 Years). Intimacy refers to establishing an intense, lasting relationship with another person or persons. Individuals attempt to adjust behavior and needs for mutual satisfaction within the relationship. Such relationships contribute to a sense of belonging and further contribute to a person's self-esteem and self-identity.

Generativity Versus Stagnation (Middle Adulthood or Age 30 to 65 Years). Generativity involves making contributions to family, society, and succeeding generations through activities such as parenting and pursuing careers. The generative adult demonstrates consideration, productivity, charity, and perseverance.

Ego Integrity Versus Despair (Age 65 till Death). Ego integrity is characterized by acceptance of self and the roles one has fulfilled. A person with ego integrity usually has a positive self-concept that enables him or her to maintain meaningful interactions with others. Of all of Erikson's stages, this can be the longest; for example the person who lives to be 100 (not unusual today) remains in this stage for 35 years.

LEVINSON'S THEORY

Levinson's (1980) developmental theory emphasizes sequential stages of adult development. Each adult developmental stage is associated with a particular age group and specific developmental tasks. Levinson developed his theory by studying life patterns of adult men, including hourly workers, corporate executives, academic biologists, and writers. The stages of development and associated developmental tasks he identified are as follows.

Early Adult Transition (Ages 17 to 22). Early adulthood tasks include establishing independence, making choices regarding career and life-style, and modifying existing family and social relationships.

Entrance into the Adult World (Ages 22 to 28). As a person becomes an adult, the primary tasks include establishing an independent living situation and exploring, preparing for, and making a commitment to adult roles.

Age 30 Transition (Ages 28 to 33). Members of this age group are faced with the task of evaluating current lifestyle, values, family situation, and career choices.

Settling Down (Ages 33 to 40). Settling down is characterized by affirming personal integrity, becoming a full-fledged adult, and striving for goal achievement.

Midlife Transition (Ages 40 to 45). At this stage, the adult engages in a critical examination of life-style. The developmental task is to recognize time limitations for goal achievement and to integrate polarities such as young–old, destruction–creation, and masculine–feminine.

Entering Middle Adulthood (Ages 45 to 50). Middle adulthood is a period of restabilization after the midlife transition period.

Age 50 Transition (Ages 50 to 53). This stage involves a set of developmental tasks similar to those of the midlife transition. The person reassesses life-style and major goals.

Middle Adulthood Culmination (Ages 53 to 60). Developmental tasks include continued work toward achievement of life goals and making contributions to society.

PIAGET'S THEORY

Jean Piaget's theory describes age-related development of cognitive abilities in infants, children, and adolescents. Cognitive abilities are mental capacities that allow a person to learn new skills and behaviors, communicate with others, think abstractly and conceptually, exercise judgment, and use knowledge. An understanding of a person's cognitive abilities is important when planning individualized nursing care. Piaget's framework may also enable you to screen for developmental delays.

Piaget stresses the following four sequential stages of intellectual development.

Sensorimotor Stage (Ages 0 to 2). The infant is in the sensorimotor stage of cognitive development. The infant perceives the world through the senses of sight, hearing, taste, smell, and touch, and responds to such perceptions by simple motor activities. Cognitive development progresses as the infant learns from repeated sensimotor experiences and is further influenced by innate intellectual capacity, maturation, nutrition, exposure to language, and social interaction.

A major cognitive developmental task associated with this stage is learning about object permanence. Between ages 7 and 8 months, the infant begins to retain a mental image of an object that has been removed from view. Consequently, he or she will search for rather than forget objects that have disappeared. Understanding object permanence enables the child to develop a broader view of the world, because he or she learns that the environment is separate and distinct from self. Additional developmental tasks include beginning to conceptualize time and the relationship of cause and effect.

Preoperational Stage (Ages 2 to 7). By age 2, the toddler enters the preoperational stage of cognitive development. A toddler views the world in terms of self (egocentricism); no other viewpoints make sense. The child judges his or her actions in terms of the consequences they have for self rather than others.

Children at this stage usually learn by imitating others. The child is curious and seeks information by asking many questions and exploring the surroundings. Thought processes become more complex, but the child still interprets the world in terms of parts rather than wholes; in concrete rather than past or future. A major developmental task is basic language skills.

Concrete Operations Stage (Ages 7 to 12). A child who reaches the stage of concrete operations is less egocentric and appreciates others' views. Talking becomes a means of communicating thoughts and understanding others' viewpoints. The child begins to classify objects, solve concrete problems, read, understand clock time, and understand the concept of cause and effect. Alternative means to achieve the same outcome are considered. During this stage, cognitive development progresses rapidly because the child is usually motivated to learn and is intellectually active through school experiences. The primary developmental task is to further strengthen language and writing skills.

Formal Operations Stage (Ages 12 to 16). The preadolescent moves from concrete, matter-of-fact thinking to the cognitive development stage called formal operations. During this period, the ability to think abstractly develops; thinking becomes more imaginative; and young persons learn to view situations in relation to the past, present, and future. He or she begins to develop a philosophy of life.

Adolescents begin to develop adult thinking patterns, including the ability to consider hypothetical situations and abstractions, verbal problem-solving abilities, and searching for possible solutions to problems.

KOHLBERG'S THEORY

Lawrence Kohlberg, utilizing the theory of Piaget, developed a theory of the development of moral reasoning and judgment. He described moral development as occurring in three stages: preconventional, conventional, and postconventional morality (Kohlberg, 1976, 1981). Each moral stage is based or dependent upon the level of cognitive ability. Moral reasoning focuses upon the process of decision making when values conflict and necessitate a choice and justification of action.

Preconventional. (Age 1 to 7). Culturally established rules determine what is labeled good, bad, right, and wrong. This stage is divided into two phases: punishment and obedient orientation, and individual instrumental orientation. *Punishment and obedient orientation* generally occurs from ages 1 to 7. Children make moral decisions to avoid punishment. The parent figure defines what is good and bad. It is the perceived consequences of the parental reaction to a particular behavior that guides the child.

In some situations, the preschool child (3 to 6 years) will begin to replace the fear of punishment with a desire for pleasure or satisfaction in moral reasoning; this is referred to as *individual instrumental orientation*. The child makes a decision based upon getting something desired in return for action or behavior. This phase generally lasts through school age (12 years).

Conventional. (Age 6 Through Adulthood). The expectation of family, peers, and society guide moral reasoning.

The individual desires to conform to ideals of good behavior; conformity, loyalty, and social order are valued. This stage is divided into the phases of mutual interpersonal expectations and respect for authority (law and order orientation). Moral reasoning in the *mutual interpersonal expectations phase* (also called approval seeking) is based upon meeting expectations of others. There is a desire to receive approval from others. This type of moral reasoning occurs from age 6 through adulthood. Kohlberg (1981) believes that most women in the United States never progress beyond this phase. Carol Gilligan (1982) and others dispute this conclusion.

Moral reasoning in the *respect for authority* phase is based upon the individual's desire to conform to laws, meet responsibilities, and respect the underlying principles of the laws and obligations. Wearing a car restraint belt because it's the law and not because of the benefit it confers is an example of this level of reasoning. Kohlberg believes that most individuals in the United States never progress beyond this phase of moral reasoning and judgment (1981).

Postconventional. (Middle Age or Older). The individual in the postconventional stage of moral development makes autonomous decisions according to universally accepted principles that the individual believes are appropriate. This stage is divided into two phases: the social contract and universal ethical principles. In the *social contract phase,* the individual has an awareness that people have a variety of values and beliefs that are related to one's culture. There is a belief that not all laws and obligations are just. In moral reasoning, the individual utilizes freedom of choice and selects appropriate principles to use as a guide and seeks change within the social system.

The highest stage of moral development is *universal ethical principles*. The individual utilizes abstract ethical principles and not social norms in moral reasoning. The individual is willing to violate a rule believed to be wrong even without the support of others and without regard for his or her own well-being. Decisions are based on conscience and internal rules.

OTHER AGES AND STAGES THEORIES

Havinghurst (1972) developed a set of developmental tasks for different age groups with the development of psychological and motor skills. In addition to a person's chronologic age, however, culture and concurrent social events are significant influences on development and the completion of developmental tasks. Fowler (1983; see Chap. 17) proposes that faith also develops in conjunction with the development of cognitive abilities, according to identifiable stages.

Life Event Theories

Proponents of life event or transitional developmental theories contend that human development occurs because of specific events, such as career changes, retirement, or new roles, including parenthood and marriage. This view places less emphasis on the relationship between chronologic age and development, because certain tasks are associated with specific events regardless of the person's age. For example, becoming a new parent is associated with certain developmental tasks whatever the parent's age. Therefore, the developmental assessment should focus on how the person develops as a parent rather than at what age and in what sequence this development occurred. Furthermore, other life events and transitions may occur simultaneously with parenthood and should be considered during developmental assessment. For example, knowing that a new parent is recently divorced, unemployed, and the mother of two school-aged children is more relevant than knowing her age.

Evaluating life events and transitions is especially appropriate for disciplines such as nursing. By assessing how the person is coping with various life events, you can determine whether intervention is indicated. Lazarus (1984) emphasizes that how a person copes with life events and transitions has more impact on growth and development than when such events occur.

Lazarus's developmental theory is an example of a life events perspective (Lazarus, 1984). This theory stresses that coping with life events is necessary for healthy development. The theory classifies various types of life stresses and coping responses that influence development (see Chap. 16).

Variability Theories

Variability theories of human development are applied more frequently to adults than to adolescents and children. According to variability theories, development is related to individual timing or influences, such as gender, economic status, education, and occupation. Variability theories have been developed from Neugarten's research, which indicates that as people age, their behaviors are determined by personality factors and past behavior patterns (Neugarten, 1964). This theory also proposes that as people age, they become more dissimilar from one another. Thus, generalizing that one set of behaviors represents normal development is difficult. Such dissimilarity or "fanning out" explains why one could easily see similar behaviors in a group of 10-year-olds but could not readily generalize about behavior in a group of 60-year-olds. Variability theories do not tie developmental tasks to a specific time in life, such as marriage at age 25 or financial security at age 50, but rather, emphasize that personalities determine life-long behaviors.

Vaillant (1977), another variability theorist, concludes from his research that previously successful completion of developmental tasks does not influence adult development as much as sustained relationships with others. Early traumatic events in a person's life are not considered reliable predictors of behavior later in life.

Variability theories have been criticized for fostering attitudes that people cannot change because their basic personalities determine behaviors. As a result, people may be negatively stereotyped as belonging to a particular personality type. Such assumptions could affect nursing interventions.

Chapter 18 SUMMARY

A person's developmental level is evaluated as part of a complete health assessment in order to determine adaptation during the life span to personal changes and changes in interaction with the environment. Growth refers to quantitative physical changes, whereas development refers to qualitative changes. Growth and development are closely interrelated processes.

The purposes of developmental assessment include the following:

- Provision of anticipatory guidance
- Assessment of physical changes
- Developmental screening

Several growth and development theories are available to help you interpret developmental assessment findings. Major growth and development theoretical perspectives include the following:

- Age and stage theories
- Life event, crisis, and transition theories
- Variability theories

Because no one theory is considered broad enough, you may apply several theories to interpret developmental assessment data.

✳ CRITICAL THINKING

You are admitting a 79-year-old woman to a long-term care facility. She is recently widowed following her husband's sudden and unexpected death from a myocardial infarction. She is alert and oriented but has sig-

Learning Exercises

1. Determine and discuss which one of the developmental theories would be most useful to you as you plan an admission assessment of this woman.

nificant mobility restrictions secondary to osteoarthritis. She is upset about living in the nursing home but can no longer manage at home without the help of her husband.

2. Develop several interview questions to evaluate this woman based on this theoretical perspective.

3. Explain how developmental data could be used to develop a plan of care for this woman.

BIBLIOGRAPHY

Erikson, E.H. (1963). *Childhood and society* (2nd ed.). New York: W.W. Norton.

Fowler, J. (1983). Stages of faith. *Psychology Today, 17* (11), 56–62.

Gilligan, C. (1982). *In a different voice*. Cambridge, MA: Harvard University Press.

Havinghurst, R.J. (1972). *Developmental tasks and education* (3rd ed.). New York: David McKay.

Kohlberg, L. (1981). *The philosophy of moral development: Moral stages and the idea of justice*. New York: Harper and Row.

Kohlberg, L. (1976). Moral stages and moralization: The cognitive developmental approach. In T. Lickkona (Ed.). *Moral development and behavior*. New York: Holt, Rinehart & Winston.

Lazarus, R.S. (1984). *Stress, appraisal, and coping*. New York: Springer Publishing.

Levinson, D.J. (1980). Toward a conception of the adult life course. In N.J. Smelser & E.H. Erikson (Eds.). *Themes of work and love in adulthood*. Cambridge, MA: Harvard University Press.

Lowenthal, M.E., & Chiriboga, D. (1973). Social stress and adaptation: Toward a life course perspective. In C. Eisdorfer & M. P. Lawton (Eds.). *The psychology of adult development and aging*. Washington, DC: American Psychological Association.

Murray, R.B., & Zenter, J.P. (1993). *Nursing assessment and health promotion through the life span* (5th ed.). Englewood Cliffs, NJ: Prentice-Hall.

McElmurry, B.J., & LiBrizzi, S.J. (1986). The health of older women. *Nursing Clinics of North America, 21* (1), 161–171.

Neugarten, L. (1964). *Personality in middle and late life*. New York: Atherton Press.

Piaget, J. (1969). *The theory of stages in cognitive development*. New York: McGraw-Hill.

Piaget, J., & Inhelder, B. (1969). *The psychology of the child*. New York: Basic Books.

Schlossberg, N.K. (Ed.) (1984). *Counseling adults in transition: Linking practice with theory*. New York: Springer Publishing.

Stevenson, J. (1977). *Issues and crises during middlescence*. New York: Appleton-Century-Crofts.

Vaillant, G. (1977). *Adaptation to life*. Boston: Little, Brown.

Health Assessment of Infants, Children, and Adolescents

Examination Guidelines

Newborns

Infants

Younger Children

Older Children and Adolescents

Assessment Terms

Tailor Position	Cognitive Functions
Bonding	Moral Development
Engrossment	Gag Reflex
Apgar Score	Fencing Response
Anthropometric Evaluation	Blink Reflex
Barlow's Test	Doll's Eye Response
Puberty	Moro Reflex
Secondary Sexual Characteristics	Stepping Reflex
Adolescence	Palmar Reflex
Menstruation	Grasp Reflex
Identification	Plantar Grasp Reflex
Self-Concept	Babinski Reflex
Colic	Rooting Reflex

INTRODUCTORY OVERVIEW

Health assessment of infants, children, and, to a lesser extent, adolescents differs from assessment of adults in approach, techniques, and interpretation of findings. Infants and children grow physically and develop cognitively and emotionally at a rapid pace. You are challenged to evaluate growth and development in the pediatric population in relation to developmental norms that may be quite different for children only a few months apart in chronologic age.

Healthy children should be assessed at frequent time intervals that change as the child ages. For example, during the first year of life, the child, who is rapidly growing and changing, is usually assessed five to six times, whereas the school-aged child is assessed yearly. Developmental and anthropometric changes are evaluated in relationship to previous assessments of the child, in comparison to standards of growth and development, and are conducted to detect deviations from normal ranges as soon as possible. In extreme cases, screening can mean the difference between mental retardation and normalcy. For instance, a child with a hepatic enzyme deficiency (phenylalanine

Jill Fuller and Jennifer Schaller-Ayers:
HEALTH ASSESSMENT: A NURSING APPROACH, Second Edition.
© 1990, 1994 by J. B. Lippincott Company.

hydroxylase) has abnormal amino acid blood and tissue levels, which can lead to brain damage and mental retardation. If the child is placed on a special diet during brain development, however, mental retardation can be avoided.

Health assessment of the child also involves evaluating other family members. Because most children are accompanied by one or more family members, you have the opportunity to assess many aspects of family functions that affect the child, including family relationships, values and beliefs, and health management practices. Parents or other caretakers may need nursing intervention regarding their concerns for, and their ability to meet, the needs of the child. The needs of caretakers will change as the child grows and develops.

Assessment Focus

This chapter focuses on well-child assessment, not deviations related to congenital, acquired, or genetic anomalies, or the preterm newborn. In such cases, a comprehensive assessment should be performed by a pediatrician specialist, and the child then may be followed by a pediatric nurse practitioner.

Your ability to interpret observations of children is facilitated by an understanding of normal growth and development processes. For example, findings such as lordosis, Snellen screening of 20/40, and umbilical hernia are considered normal at one age but abnormal at another age. Being aware of normal ranges for various ages will help you determine if intervention or referral is necessary.

The wide variation among individual children in growth and development makes interpretation of assessment findings especially difficult. For example, although most children learn to walk between ages 11 and 15 months, some children walk as early as 9 months and others not until 22 months. The range of 9 to 22 months is considered normal for learning to walk. Furthermore, children vary greatly in height, weight, and rates of developing motor, language, and social skills. Also, individual variations and ranges of normal become greater as people age.

Age Classifications

From a growth and development perspective, children are evaluated with respect to norms for a particular age range. The following categories are widely used:

- Newborn: birth to 1 month
- Infancy: 1 month through 11 months
- Toddler: 12 months through 35 months
- Preschool: 3 years through 5 years
- School age: 6 years through 12 years
- Adolescence: 13 years through 17 to 20 years

Nursing Diagnoses

Although all nursing diagnoses are appropriate for children, not all nursing diagnoses are used for each age group. For example, Self-care deficit and Incontinence would be the maturational norm for infants and toddlers. In place of the nurse emphasizing what the child cannot naturally accomplish, the nurse would be assessing parenting skills. Some nursing diagnoses applicable to children that are often overlooked include Rape-trauma syndrome, Potential for violence, Alteration in parenting (especially the adolescent mother), and Grieving.

Some nursing diagnoses focus on the family, thereby implying an effect on children. These diagnoses include Altered parenting, Alteration in family process, and Ineffective family coping. Additionally, children at specific ages are at higher risk for some nursing diagnoses than at other ages. For example, infants and toddlers are at higher risk for poisoning and suffocation than school-aged children or adults. Adolescents are at higher risk for disturbance in personal identity, self-esteem, and body image than the preschool and school-aged child.

The nursing diagnosis altered growth and development is used almost exclusively with children under 22 years. If an adult has not accomplished a developmental task, the focus is then on what has been altered because of this delay (Carpenito, 1991). For example, the individual with altered motor development may have the diagnoses of Impaired physical mobility and/or Self-care deficits.

For the diagnosis Altered growth and development, the child must exhibit an inability to perform or difficulty performing a task or behavior typical of his or her age group, and/or the child's weight must be two standard deviations below what it should be for height, and/or the child has experienced an undesired drop in weight–height ratio. Reasons for altered growth and development can be related to health problems of the child or environmental conditions. Health problems might include congenital heart defects, neurologic impairments (cerebral palsy, mental retardation), muscular dystrophy, nutritional deficits (inadequate intake or disease processes such as cystic fibrosis), and prolonged casting of an extremity. Environmental factors may include lack of stimulating environment; parental lack of nurturing knowledge; abuse or neglect; loss or separation of family member, friend, or pet; hospitalization; and stress.

KNOWLEDGE BASE FOR ASSESSMENT

Judgments are made about the health status of newborns, infants, children, and adolescents on the basis of observations made during the interview and physical assessment. In babies and young children, functional abilities are rapidly evolving. Health assessment is focused on determining the acquisition and mastery of necessary skills such as motor and social skills, including language, speech, and intellectual development. Developmental screening tools such as the Denver Developmental Screening Test 2 (DDST2) and the Denver Articulation Screening Examination (DASE) may provide a reliable means of determining the development of motor, cognitive, social, and speech abilities (see Appendix D).

Health Perception and Health Management

For *babies* and *young children,* the responsibility for health promotion and health maintenance activities lies with parents or other caregivers. Health-promotion activities for infants begin with the mother's health habits and exposure to harmful substances before and during the prenatal period. *Adolescents* usually have developed a perception of their own health status and generally assume more responsibility for their health maintenance.

The assessment of health perceptions and health-promoting activities requires an evaluation of the following:

* Common health concern or problems
* Immunization status
* Screening for diseases and disease risk factors
* Safety practices

Common Health Concerns or Problems. Healthy infants may experience few problems except for common colds and ear infections. First-time parents may have more questions and concerns about their children because of lack of previous experience and not knowing what is normal and what is not. As children interact with other children in environments such as day care, school, and play grounds, the incidence of communicable diseases increases. More frequent colds, ear and throat infections, skin infections, and parasite infestation (pediculosis or lice) may occur. School-aged girls may develop urinary tract infections related to improper hygiene following bowel elimination. In addition, young children often develop vision and hearing problems. The most common adolescent health problems are accidents, nutritional disorders (including obesity, anorexia nervosa, and bulimia), acne, substance abuse, pregnancy, sexually transmitted diseases, and stress-coping problems.

Immunizations. Childhood immunizations are commonly initiated shortly after birth for protection against communicable diseases such as hepatitis, diphtheria, pertussis, tetanus, poliomyelitis, measles, mumps, and rubella. Table 19-1 presents a recommended immunization schedule for infants and children. The recommended immunization schedule has had several revisions in the last 2 years. You are encouraged to use this as a guide only, because other revisions may follow. Parents should be encouraged to keep written immunization histories or charts to remind them of the schedule and for proof of immunization status for entry into school and college.

Screening for Disease or Disease Risk Factors. Children from families with positive histories for genetic-related diseases such as cardiovascular disease and diabetes mellitus should receive appropriate screenings such as blood pressure and education regarding the effects of lifestyle. Cholesterol screening of young children is considered controversial in part because normal range of cholesterol is not known for children. Adolescents should begin to practice self-examination techniques such as breast self-examination or testicular self-examination. Sexually active

Table 19-1. Recommended Immunization Schedule: Infancy Through Adulthood

Recommended Age	Vaccine(s)	Comments
Shortly after birth	Hepatitis B*	Usually given prior to discharge.
1 month	Hepatitis B	
2 months	DPT[†], TVOPV[‡] and HbOC or PRP-OMP[¶]	DPT and TVOPV can be initiated earlier in areas of high endemicity.
4 months	DPT, TVOPV, and HbOC or PRP-OMP	2-month interval desired for TVOPV.
6 months	DPT, HbOC and Hepatitis B (TVOPV)	TVOPV optional; usually given in areas where polio might be imported (e.g., some areas of southwest U.S.)
12 months	PRP-OMP	Only if PRP-OMP series has been used.
15 months	MMR[||], HbOC, and tuberculin test	May give DPT and TVOP at same time.
18 months	DPT and TVOPV	May be given at 15 months with MMR and HbOC. DPT and TVOP considered as part of original series.
4–6 yr	DPT, TVOPV, and MMR	DPT is not given after 7 years. MMR can be given any time between 4 and 12 years.
14–16 yr	Td[#], hepatitis	Repeat Td every 10 years for lifetime.

*Hepatitis B vaccine. After the initial series of three, a booster may be given every 5 to 7 years depending upon titer level and associated risk (high-risk hemodialysis clients, international travelers, resident of long-term facility such as institutions for mentally retarded, health care providers, and household contacts of hepatitis B carriers).

[†]Diphtheria and tetanus toxoids with pertussis vaccine.

[‡]Oral attenuated poliovirus vaccine contains poliovirus types 1, 2 & 3.

[¶]HbOC and PRP-OMP Haemophilus influenza b conjugate. A child should receive either HbOC or PRP-OMP, not both. The vaccinated child should complete the series started and not switch.

[||]Live measles (rubeola), mumps, and rubella viruses in a combined vaccine.

[#]Adult tetanus toxoid (full dose) and diphtheria toxoid (reduced dose) in combination.

For all products used, consult manufacturer's brochure for instructions for storage, handling, and administration. Biologics prepared by different manufacturers may vary, and those of the same manufacturer may change from time to time. The package insert should be followed for specific products.

female adolescents should have a pelvic examination and Papanicolaou's (Pap) smear.

Safety Practices. Accidents are the leading cause of morbidity and mortality of babies, children, and adolescents. Home safety should be carefully evaluated for infants and young children. Measures should be taken to prevent falls, burns, and ingestion of poisons. Learn whether the preschool-aged child knows how to avoid traffic. Check whether the child can recite his or her name, address, and telephone number. How does the child perceive police and firefighters; are they feared or seen as helpful adult figures? You may directly interview older children about safety measures. Ask the child questions such as, "What would you do if a fire started in the kitchen? What would you do if a stranger wanted you to go with him or her?"

Automobile safety is a concern for all age groups. Is the child restrained in an automobile and is the restraining device appropriate for the child's age and size? Infants and toddlers should be restrained in infant seats with a five-point harness. The infant seat should face the back of the car seat until the infant is several months old or above a particular weight. Children more than 4 years of age or weighing more than 40 pounds may use a standard lap belt. The shoulder harness should not be used until the child is taller than 55 inches because the strap may cause neck injuries.

For children and adolescents who participate in sports activities, are appropriate measures taken to prevent sports-related injuries? Do adolescents drive under the influence of drugs or alcohol? Driving while intoxicated is a common risk for trauma or death.

Nutrition and Metabolism

Evaluation of nutritional status in the infant, child, or adolescent can be accomplished by the following methods:

- Interview parents or older child to obtain diet history and insight into any nutritional problems
- Use anthropometric evaluation, including height, weight, and head and chest circumferences in infants. Midarm muscle circumference and skinfold thickness may be measured in older children.
- Perform physical assessment to detect problems interfering with nutritional process and to detect signs of malnutrition.

Development of Eating Functions. At birth, babies can only suck and swallow liquids that are introduced into the back of the throat, as occurs with nipple feeding. By age 2 months, the infant is usually able to swallow semisolid foods because the tongue can be brought against the palate. Between age 4 and 6 months, the gag reflex decreases, which facilitates swallowing solid foods. Teeth eruption usually occurs before the infant can ingest solid foods. The first teeth to erupt, between ages 5 and 6 months, are the lower central incisors. By 1 year, the infant usually has 6 to 8 teeth. Problems related to the development of eating functions include problems with weak sucking, bottle/breast weaning, appetite control, and food allergies.

Eating Behaviors. According to Erikson's developmental theory, the conflict facing children from ages 1 to 3 years involves autonomy versus shame and doubt. The young child usually resolves this conflict by asserting independence from parental control. Eating behaviors exemplify this need for autonomy beginning with weaning, when the child no longer takes breast or bottle feedings and begins to use a cup and eat at the table. These changes usually occur by the end of the first year. Early self-feeding is frequently associated with messiness, with almost as much food on the child as in the child. By the end of the second year, the rate of physical growth decreases, and children can tolerate longer periods between meals. The young child may also demonstrate autonomy by refusing certain foods or insisting on self-feeding.

Older children may find mealtime distracting because they are preoccupied with other activities. As children become older, their eating habits and food preferences are increasingly influenced by advertising and social/peer pressure. Children on special diets, such as diabetic diets, may experience difficulty in adhering to the diet while attempting to eat foods their friends eat, especially at special events such as birthday parties.

Adolescents are particularly likely to engage in fad diets or unusual eating habits. Self-esteem is often tied to self-image; female adolescents often seek the ideal model-thin appearance, male adolescents often aspire to a muscular athletic appearance. These perceptions and other pressures place adolescents at risk for eating disorders of anorexia (not eating), bulimia (gorging followed by forced vomiting), and steroid abuse to build muscles with increased weight.

Caloric Needs. Caloric needs and nutrient requirements change throughout the life span. Caloric and nutrient needs for different age groups are in Appendix A. Caloric needs are further evaluated in relation to the child's rate of physical growth, stage of sexual maturity, and usual levels of physical activities.

Anthropometric Measurements. Anthropometric measurements of infants include measurement of height, weight, and head and chest circumference. In older children, height and weight are evaluated, and skinfold thicknesses may be evaluated. Measurements should be graphed. On a graph, children establish a normal curve for growth that should be consistent. Regardless of height and weight measurements, height should be proportional to weight. Because of age-related variations in the amount and distribution of subcutaneous fat, anthropometric norms vary across age groups and gender. Tables are available with norms for different age groups (see Appendix E).

Elimination

Patterns of bowel and bladder elimination should be evaluated in relation to age-related norms and expectations. You should determine the following:

- The child's pattern of bowel and bladder elimination
- Characteristics of feces and urine
- Development of control of bowel and bladder elimination and related behaviors
- Problems with bowel and bladder elimination

Elimination Patterns. The character of feces is evaluated in infants to determine if the gastrointestinal tract is functioning normally and if bowel elimination problems such as diarrhea or constipation are present. Meconium, a tarry, odorless stool, is usually the first bowel movement after birth. Passage of meconium prior to birth is usually indicative of fetal distress and places the baby at risk for pneumonia. During the first week of life, the baby usually has transitional stools, which may be loose, green or yellow in color, and infiltrated with mucus. Two to four bowel movements a day is considered normal.

Differences in the infant's stool may be attributed to diet. Babies receiving formula will usually have feces that are more yellow and harder than the feces of breast-fed babies. Formula-fed infants average one to two bowel movements a day, whereas breast-fed babies may have as many as four per day. As other foods are added, the infant's feces becomes more adult-like. Initial voiding usually occurs within the first hour after birth; frequency depends on the total fluid intake and hydration status.

Control of Elimination. Children usually indicate a readiness for bowel and bladder training between ages 2 and 3 years. Bowel training usually occurs before bladder training, and daytime bladder control is usually achieved before nighttime dryness. Periodic loss of daytime bowel and bladder control is considered normal in young children and may occur during stressful periods or intense play. Complete control of elimination is usually achieved by age 4 to 5 years, although bedwetting may occur through the preschool and school-age years.

Once bowel and bladder control are developed, children generally have few problems related to elimination. Young girls may develop occasional urinary tract infections because of poor hygienic practices.

Activity and Exercise

The developmental aspects of activity and exercise functions one should consider when evaluating children include the following:

- Nature of play, exercise, and leisure activities
- Developmental and maturation of self-care abilities in relation to eating, dressing, and attending to personal hygiene
- Actual or potential problems that may be associated with activity

Motor Development. Motor functions develop rapidly and eventually mature during adolescence and young adulthood. Motor functions are easily evaluated during the physical assessment of the child and by the administration of screening tools such as the DDST2 (see Appendix D). With the development of motor abilities, increasing independence occurs in the performance or self-care activities such as feeding, dressing, and attending to personal hygiene.

School-age children and adolescents are usually completely independent in their performance of self-care activities.

Play. Play is the major activity of early childhood, providing opportunities for social interaction, learning, and developing gross and fine motor function. Playing house, for example, encourages role playing with socialization, and computer games increase hand-eye coordination. Toy safety and age-appropriate toys and leisure activities should be discussed with parents. Inappropriate toys can be harmful or fatal, especially for young children.

By the end of the second year, children begin to exhibit parallel play, which involves playing near other children but not always interacting with them. Preschoolers (ages 3 to 5 years), move to cooperative play patterns and begin to participate in group activities that require mutual cooperation with other children.

Cognition and Perception

Evaluation of cognitive and perceptual functions can be accomplished by the following:

- Administration of appropriate screening tools such as the DDST2 and DASE
- Interaction with the child
- Interview of parents about any cognitive and perceptual problems
- Physical assessment of sensory and hearing systems, and special senses

Cognitive Functions. Piaget's theory of cognitive development (1969) describes four sequential stages of cognitive development in infants, children, and adolescents (see Chap. 18 for a discussion of Piaget's theory). Application of this theory assists in understanding how children of different ages think and learn, which has implications for anticipatory guidance as well as nursing interventions of a teaching–learning nature.

According to Piaget, infants are in the sensorimotor stage of cognitive development. Learning occurs by repeated exposure to stimuli that are perceived through the senses of sight, hearing, smell, and touch. As the infant grows, other factors influence the learning process, especially the child's innate intellectual capacity, exposure to language, social interactions, and physical health.

The development of the infant's cognitive functions is evaluated by determining the age when certain learned responses first occurred. For example, by age 3 months the infant should recognize and respond to the primary caregiver; at age 4 months the bottle-fed infant can associate the appearance of a bottle with feeding; at age 6 months, the infant can recognize people as familiar or strange. Also at 6 months the infant begins to imitate behaviors demonstrated by others. Some of these behaviors, such as waving bye-bye, are not well developed until the infant has developed greater coordination. The infant learns object permanence by 7 months and will demonstrate this understanding by looking briefly for a hidden object. The search for hidden objects will continue for a longer period at 9 months and makes "peek-a-boo" a fun game.

Children aged 2 to 7 years are viewed by Piaget as being in the preoperational stage of cognitive development. The child is inquisitive and learns by imitating others. Thought processes are concrete, and the child's attention span is short. Children in this age group should be screened for problems with vision and hearing that may interfere with cognitive development. Physical problems, mental deficits, and shorter-than-usual attention span may also influence the rate of cognitive development.

Older children and adolescents enter the stages of concrete and formal operations, respectively. Cognitive development usually proceeds without major problems as long as appropriate adaptions have been made to any sensory deficits, the child is motivated to learn, and the child is exposed to stimulating, learning environments. Consideration should be given to school performance as well as the effects that watching television and preoccupation with computer/video games may have on learning.

Language Development. The ability to comprehend and speak the dominant language develops with cognitive abilities. Language comprehension precedes the ability to speak or write the language.

Several screening tools, Early Language Milestone Scale (ELM Scale) and Denver Articulation Screening Exam (DASE), are available to assess speech abilities. The ELM Scale is used for children from birth to 36 months, and the DASE is used for children from 2.5 to 6 years. The DDST2 also has a language development component. Generally, the DDST2 is sufficient unless a more extensive screening is desired (*e.g.,* correct articulation of specific word sounds). The DASE is presented in Appendix D.

It is helpful to evaluate the age that the child acquired various verbal skills. For example, almost all children should coo by 2 to 3 months and babble beginning at 4 months. Infants begin verbalizing "ma" or "da" sounds around 7 months. After 12 months, children begin to verbalize rather than cry some of their needs, although this communication may be in the form of jargon that may only be understood by family members.

Understandable speech begins between 15 and 24 months in the form of two- to three-word phrases and plurals. By age 2 years, the receptive vocabulary consists of about 900 to 1200 words and expressive vocabulary consist of approximately 250 words. The child knows some 2000 words by 6 years (this doubles by sixth grade); some of these words may include profanities learned by imitating others. Verbal communication skills and the ability to write continue to develop during the school-age years and adolescents.

The development of language skills is influenced by factors other than innate cognitive abilities. It is especially important to determine the possible influences of other factors when speech development appears delayed. Factors that optimize language development include a consistent and satisfying relationship with a parent or other caregiver, a sense of security, verbal stimulation (*e.g.,* storytelling, descriptive conversation), and positive response to attempts to verbalize. Speech delays may be secondary to hearing problems and lack of verbal communication within family.

Sleep and Rest

Evaluation of sleep and rest in babies, children, and adolescents should focus on the following:

- Amount of time the child sleeps each day, including naps and nighttime sleep
- Child's or parent's perceptions of sleep pattern disturbances

- Identification of factors that contribute to sleep and rest problems

Sleep Patterns. Sleep patterns vary greatly from the newborn period through adolescence (for a description of the normal sleep cycle, see Chap. 12). Newborns generally spend more time asleep than awake, requiring as much as 18 hours of sleep per day. Such long sleep periods are believed to support the infant's rapid growth rate.

Infants gradually develop individual nocturnal sleep patterns. Some infants may sleep through the night as early as 6 weeks of age, and most sleep all night by age 3 months. Premature infants may develop nocturnal sleep patterns more slowly than full-term infants. Morning and afternoon naps are common through the first year. The infant may sleep 12 to 14 hours during the night and 1 to 4 hours during the day.

Toddlers and preschool-aged children generally sleep 12 to 14 hours a day, including one or two daytime naps. By age 5, children may need only one daytime nap or rest period. Nighttime awakenings are normal. Presleep routines such as bath, snack, or bedtime story may help ease the transition from activities to sleep and rest. Sleep pattern disturbances related to nightmares, bedtime fears, sleepwalking, and bedwetting may develop in preschool-aged children and may persist through early school-aged years.

School-aged children may require only 9 hours of sleep per day, although great variability exists among children. School-aged children commonly resist bedtime at a specific hour because they want to continue favorite activities such as watching television and playing games.

The adolescent's sleep–rest needs usually increase because the rate of physical growth accelerates. Daytime naps and late awakening on weekends are not unusual because this age group is subject to fatigue.

Sexuality and Reproduction

Sexuality and reproduction are evaluated in children and adolescents primarily to determine the following:

- Parental and child teaching needs in relation to sexual development and sexual myths
- Development and maturation of secondary sex characteristics
- Sexuality self-esteem

Sexual Development. The development of a person's sexuality begins during infancy and continues throughout the life span. Infants derive bodily pleasure from sucking and being touched. The manner in which the infant is fed, washed, stroked, kissed, and hugged provides messages related to sexuality. Infants explore their own bodies, including genitalia.

Toddlers explore their own bodies and begin to differentiate between males and females at about age 2. They develop an interest in viewing the genitals of adults and other children of either gender. Normally, gender identity is firmly established by age 3 as the child explores bodily functions, especially elimination. Between the ages of 3 and 4, children may begin to masturbate; this may represent one way the young child deals with stress.

Preschool children develop a curiosity about reproduction and the differences between men and women, boys and men, and girls and women. Children continue to ask questions through early school-age years about such topics as where babies come from, breast-feeding, and why women have breasts and men have penises. During this developmental phase, children require simple and factual explanations.

School age is generally a quiet time for sexual development. Children generally have same-sex friends. They continue to learn more about the anatomy of their bodies and experiment with different sexual roles.

Puberty. Anticipatory guidance for school-age children may focus on preparing the child for the physical changes associated with puberty. You may ask parents questions about how they plan to prepare their children for changes such as menstruation. Generally, girls begin puberty between ages 10 and 12, and boys between ages 12 and 14. For girls, sign of puberty include changes related to breast development, pubic and axillary hair growth, menarche and menstruation, and height increases (Table 19-2). For boys, puberty changes include genital development; ejaculation from masturbation or nocturnal emissions (wet dreams); pubic, axillary, chest and facial hair growth, voice changes; and height increases (Table 19-3).

Adolescent Sexuality. The development of sexuality involves more than experiencing and responding to the physical changes of puberty. During adolescence, the further developments of one's personal identity and sexuality are closely associated. Adolescents are concerned with attitudes, behaviors, and feelings toward themselves and the opposite sex; relationships, affection, and caring between

people; and recognition and acceptance of themselves and others as sexual beings. They also must deal with incorporating the physical changes of sexual development into their self-image and sexual identity. Adolescents may question their sexual identities and sexual orientations.

Adolescents usually have educational needs in relation to sexuality and reproduction. Parents may or may not be able to meet these needs. You should determine if parents and children discuss sexual matters, including sexual values, sexual roles, and related behaviors. Additional evaluation may include determining the adolescent's knowledge about risks of sexual intercourse, including pregnancy and sexually transmitted diseases.

Coping and Stress Tolerance

During assessment of children in relation to stress and coping, you should focus on the following:

- Common stressors associated with childhood stages of growth and development
- The child's perception of stressors
- Behavioral manifestations of coping or responding to stress
- Support systems during times of stress or crisis

Stress Response. The infant's response to stress is commonly manifested by crying. By age 2, children can respond to simple stresses by expressing impatience and imitating some adult displays of emotions. When overwhelmed, the response to stress can be excessive and manifested in a "temper tantrum." Preschool children begin to

Table 19–2. Physical Changes with Puberty and Adolescence in Girls

Age	Physical Changes
8–13 yr (average 11 yr)	Breast development
	Sequence:
	Stage 1: Preadolescent—no glandular tissue
	Stage 2: Breast bud stage
	Stage 3: Further breast tissue growth with nipple protrusion
	Stage 4: Nipple and areola form a mound distinct from breast tissue
	Stage 5: Mature breast (average age 14 to 16 yr)
8–13 yr (average: 1 yr after breast bud stage)	Pubic hair growth
	Sequence:
	Stage 1: Preadolescent—no pubic hair
	Stage 2: Sparse, long, silky, pigmented hair mainly along the labia
	Stage 3: Coarser, darker, curlier hair spreading sparsely over pubic symphysis
	Stage 4: More hair growth and distribution than stage 3, but hair does not yet extend to medial surface of thighs
	Stage 5: Adult pattern with hair growth to medial aspect of thighs
9–14 yr (average: 1 yr after stage 2 pubic hair)	Axillary hair growth
10–15 yr (average: during stage 3 or 4 breast development)	Menarche: initial cycles may be anovulatory; ovulatory cycles begin within 2 yr of menarche
	Height increase: average American adolescent grows 24 cm (9 in), with peak growth spurt at age 12 yr
Puberty through adolescence	Increased apocrine gland secretion, sometimes resulting in acne

Table 19–3. Physical Changes with Puberty and Adolescence in Boys

Age	Physical Changes
10–13 yr (average: 11 yr)	Genital development *Sequence:* 　Stage 1: Preadolescent—no enlargement of testes or penis 　Stage 2: Enlargement of testes; scrotal skin becomes more pigmented; no significant enlargement of penis 　Stage 3: Penis enlarges in length; continued enlargement of testes 　Stage 4: Penis grows in length and width with glans development; enlargement of testes 　Stage 5: Mature genitals (average age 15–16 yr)
10–13 yr (average onset with stage 2 genital development)	Pubic hair growth
14–15 yr	Facial hair growth
	Voice changes
	Height increase: Average American adolescent grows 34 cm (13.5 in), with peak growth spurt at age 14 yr
Approximately 3 yr after onset of stage 2 genital development	Ejaculation (masturbation or nocturnal emissions); mature sperm produced between ages 14–16 yr
Puberty through adolescence	Increased apocrine gland secretion, sometimes resulting in acne

use adaptive mechanisms such as denial, reaction formation, regression, projection, suppression, and sublimation, which help the child develop stress tolerance as well as a sense of independence. Because physical activity is a method of handling stress, children with high levels of stress may be hyperactive.

Young children usually learn to imitate the feelings, emotions, and responses to stress from family members. This process, called *identification,* helps children learn how persons of like gender experience and cope with stress. Imagination, as well as play and participation in sports activities, may be used to alleviate stress.

School-age children can identify stressors, and they begin to reason with others regarding how to cope, using past experiences and advice from others. They may also engage in ritualistic behavior to reduce anxiety. Fantasy can compensate for feelings of inadequacy or inferiority. Projection, rationalization, regression, sublimation, and malingering may help protect the ego when children are unable to perform at expected levels. Using such defense mechanisms in moderation can help children handle anxiety and grow emotionally.

Adolescence is a transition period from childhood to adulthood and is generally considered a stressful period for both adolescents and their families. Coping styles are fairly established by mid-adolescence, although they can learn new ways to cope from peers and adult role models. Alcohol and other chemicals may be used by adolescents in attempts to cope with stressors.

Roles and Relationships

During the health assessment of infants, children, and adolescents, determine the following pertaining to roles and relationships:

- Nature of the child's important relationships and who fulfills the child's needs for nurturing, protecting, and helping
- Dynamics among family members
- Roles enacted by the child

Important Relationships. The infant's most important relationships are usually with the parents or primary caregiver. A major developmental task for a new family involves attachment. *Bonding,* the most significant relationship between mother and infant, refers to the attachment that is usually initiated following the infant's birth. *Engrossment* refers to the father's initial parental response to the baby. Instruments are available to assess the quality of mother–infant bonding (*The Neonatal Behavioral Assessment Scale* and *Neonatal Perception Inventory;* see Bishop, 1976; Clark, 1976; Brazelton, 1973).

Behavioral indicators of a positive relationship between the infant and primary caregiver include the following:

- Response to caregiver's voice by making sounds (by age 2 months)
- Visual recognition of caregivers (by age 3 months)
- Preference for being with other during waking hours, and initiation of social interaction by smiling (by age 4 months)
- Separation anxiety, or fear of being with strangers (by age 6 months) or fear of being separated from primary caregiver (between 7 and 10 months)

The most important relationship for the toddler usually continues to be with parents. During this developmental phase, separation anxiety resurfaces and is most stressful, especially between 18 and 24 months. A major developmental task for the toddler is learning that parental separation does not mean abandonment and can be tolerated for short periods. By age 3, most toddlers can tolerate short separations but may still cry when first left in the care of another. Toddlers begin to establish play relationships with other children, although some parallel play continues.

Preschool children begin to participate more fully as family members but may prefer to spend play time with same-age children. Cooperative play is the primary interaction with other children. Preschool children frequently play games such as house that imitate future roles. By ages 4 or 5, children usually identify strongly with the parent of the same gender and focus of love may be with parent of the opposite gender. Other significant adults include relatives, parental friends, and adult caregivers or babysitters.

School-age children begin to demonstrate decreased dependency on family and increased interaction with peers, especially neighborhood children and other adults such as teachers. Even so, family relationships are important and continue to influence emotional and social development. Interactions and frustrations with peers and adults outside the home help the child in this growth phase to learn more complex social responses.

The preadolescent usually spends more time in the community. At this age children begin to develop pride in family, school, and community. Older children may earn a small income for services such as yard care or newspaper delivery. They learn to appreciate that parents are individuals with different ideas as well as specific attributes. Gender or sex roles usually develop or are identifiable by school age. The best friend becomes very important, and friends are usually of the same gender.

Adolescent relationship patterns include interacting with peer groups and forming relationships with members of the opposite gender. Dating behaviors vary considerably across cultures and among families. The adolescent becomes very concerned about appearance and looking like others in the peer group. Achieving independence from parents and other adults while maintaining affection is an important concern. Adolescents may have many conflicts with parents, especially between ages 13 and 15. Such conflicts may develop because of crisis or the child's need to express his or her own identity. Conflicts may decrease later as adolescents begin to view parents as acceptable role models.

Adolescents may form strong relationships with other adults such as teachers, clergy, sport coaches, and parental friends. Adolescents may further identify with adult roles through part-time work or career plans.

Self-Concept

Self-concept can be evaluated by doing the following:

- Observing the child's overall appearance and body language
- Interpreting self-disclosing statements about self and self-esteem
- Observing quality of social interactions
- Identifying potential threats to self-esteem and the child's response patterns

The development of a child's self-concept (beliefs and feelings about self) is influenced by cognitive and intellec-

tual abilities, the actions and reactions of others (especially the family), moral development, and emotions.

According to Erikson, a positive self-concept in the child is achieved through successful resolution of developmental crisis experienced as the child passes through sequential stages of human development (see Chap. 18 for a discussion of Erikson's theory). Evaluation of self-concept is difficult when the child is too young to verbalize feelings about self. Young infants do not differentiate self from others. Infants establish the basis of a positive self-concept by learning to trust others through the communication of love and acceptance by caregivers. Infants who demonstrate weight loss, excessive colic, and difficulty sleeping may be apprehensive and have difficulty establishing trusting bonds with others.

Toddlers know themselves as separate beings, although the boundaries of self may be vague. Toddlers who are frustrated in their attempts to establish autonomy may have feelings of self-doubt and anger toward themselves and others. Between 18 and 36 months children conceptualize themselves as being either "good" or "bad." The self-concept of the preschool-age child may be threatened by feelings of guilt that occur when the child senses doing something wrong. Guilt feelings may be indicated by the child's behaviors, including lack of coordination, verbalization of fears, stammering speech, eating and elimination problems, fear of strangers, or a disinterest in playing with other children. The preschool child may start comparing his or her own accomplishments with those of older siblings or feel threatened by new siblings.

The greatest threats to self-esteem of school-age children include a sense of inferiority, inadequacy, difficulty learning or performing tasks, or an inability to concentrate. If the child is not doing well in school, he or she may perceive self as stupid. When evaluating self-concept in school-age children, it may be helpful to ask children to draw a picture of themselves. You and the child can then discuss the child's interpretation of the drawing.

Adolescents encounter many potential threats to self-esteem as they go through the process of forming a unique identity and adjusting to a new body image. Failure to become independent and responsible and have friends during adolescence may threaten self-confidence and self-esteem.

Values and Beliefs

Evaluation of values and beliefs can be accomplished by doing the following:

- Identifying signs of interpersonal conflict and confusion
- Identifying level of faith and moral development
- Identifying anticipatory learning needs of parents

Theories that suggest developmental norms in relation to children's values and belief systems include Fowler's (1983) theory of stages of faith development and Kohlberg's (1981) theory of level of moral development (see Chap. 7 and 18 for discussion of these theories).

Stages of Faith. Fowler classifies the infant as being in the primal stage of faith. The infant does not have values or beliefs but does understand bodily comfort and the relief of tension. "Good" and "bad" are defined in terms of physical consequences to the self.

Preschoolers and young children go through the intuitive stage of faith. The child develops an awareness of parental values, beliefs, and any associated religious practices, conforming to such patterns to gain acceptance and love. Preschoolers may misinterpret parental value and belief patterns because of limited experience or concrete thinking patterns.

School-age children enter the mythical–literal stage. The child's value and belief system can be influenced by storytelling. Symbolic meanings are still difficult to interpret for this age group. Adolescents enter the synthetic-conventional stage and may never advance further in faith development.

Moral Development. The conscience begins forming about age 4 years and is analytical as well as judgmental in relation to moral development. Kohlberg classifies sequential levels of moral development. The first level (pre-conventional stage) is characterized by a punishment and obedience orientation. The orientation is characteristic of young children who engage in right or wrong behavior depending on the consequences of the behavior. Children at this stage generally view rules as unchanging and imposed by adults. Children begin to value fairness, agreement, and equal exchange, although self-interests are still the most important.

The second level (conventional stage) is characterized by conformity to the expectations and behaviors of others. The child's conduct is influenced more by social expectations than by the threat of punishment. School-age children display these types of behaviors. As the child enters adolescence, a law-and-order orientation to right and wrong may develop. Rules may be accepted without question, because the person believes that the particular rule is best for all concerned.

THE HEALTH HISTORY
General Principles

Interviewing is an important means of obtaining health assessment data pertaining to infants, children, and adolescents. The degree to which the child can participate during the interview process will depend on the child's age, and verbal communication and social skills. For the most part, infants and toddlers will be inactive in the interview process, whereas school-age children and adolescents can be very involved. Children as young as 2.5 to 3 years of age comprehend a great deal of what is being said around them. When interviewing the child's parent or caretaker, you should be alert to the interaction between the child, adult, and other individuals present. The length of the interview and history taking will often be shorter for the young child than the adolescent.

Establishing Rapport. Regardless of the child's age, you should always make an effort to address the child directly as well as people accompanying the child during the interview. Through such direct verbal interaction, you can convey interest in the child as well as communicate comfort and safety. When the child is a newborn or infant, you will usually greet and introduce yourself to the parents first. For school-age children and adolescents, who may participate actively in the interview process, you should address the child first.

Introductions should be sufficient to establish your name, title, and role; the child's name and preferred nickname; and the identity and relationships of people accompanying the child. If parents are not accompanying the child, it is important to determine the reason.

Both verbal and nonverbal communication influence the establishment of rapport. Take care that verbal and nonverbal behaviors communicate to the child that the surroundings are safe. Many children feel threatened by white uniforms or lab coats, strange equipment, or harsh lighting. In addition, a hurried, abrupt, or uncaring attitude may be threatening to the child. Praising the child during the health assessment is one way to make the child feel more comfortable (*e.g.,* "You're helping by holding so still" or "Thank you for opening your mouth so big").

You should make a special effort to establish an atmosphere that is nonjudgmental and noncritical. This effort is especially important when establishing rapport with those accompanying the child. If parents are made to feel guilty or inferior, they are less likely to share their perceptions with you. Parents, who can detect subtle changes that may go unrecognized by others, need to believe that their observations are valid and warrant discussion.

Evaluating Verbal Abilities. An understanding of the development of a child's verbal abilities will help you during the interview process. Both comprehension and the ability to communicate verbally are related to age and emotional status. In general, the younger the child, the more concrete is his or her thinking. Also, the more anxious the child is about the health assessment visit and the real or imagined threat of a "shot," the less likely it is that the child will converse with you.

Important Interview Topics

For interviewing and performing physical examinations, there is little difference in approach for the toddler and preschool child. The preschool child has a longer attention span and may be more cooperative than the toddler; however, the approach to the interview and examination is similar. The same is true for the school-age and adolescent child. However, the adolescent does become more independent from parents and relies less on parents in answering health questions. Therefore, for interview topics and examination guidelines, the following four age groups are used: newborn, infant, young children, and older children and adolescents.

Newborns. The health history of the newborn primarily addresses prenatal care; labor and delivery; Apgar scores at birth, 1, and 5 minutes; and anthropometric measurements. The maternal history should include the following data: general health, number of pregnancies (gravida and para), prenatal diseases or conditions (such as hypertension, eclampsia, vaginal bleeding, and infectious diseases), use of medication, exposure to radiation, attitude toward pregnancy and children, and perceptions of fetal movement. Labor and delivery data should include duration of pregnancy and labor, place of delivery, nature of labor (analgesia or anesthesia use, and any spontaneous or induced complications), nature of delivery (presentation, unassisted or assisted, and any complications), and any concerns of the parents.

The child's history should include Apgar scores, height, weight, head circumference, complications or anomalies noted, feeding characteristics, type of feeding (breast or formula—specify type), duration of hospitalization, use of medications, usual daily schedule, and any illnesses or problems such as jaundice or convulsions.

Infants and Toddlers. If the interview is initiated to assess the health status of an infant, you should obtain the same data as for the newborn, as well as developmental milestones. You may ask parents open-ended questions such as "Tell me what your child is doing now". Such an approach will elicit information without alarming parents if the child is not able to perform a particular skill. After determining the child's present developmental status as perceived by the parent, you should obtain data regarding appropriate milestones such as when the child smiled, rolled over, sat unsupported, stood unsupported, used words, and cut deciduous teeth.

During the interview, you should also try to become familiar with the infant and assess parent–child interactions. Toddlers, who have a short attention span and are busy exploring their environment, may find it difficult to be held during the interview and prefer to explore. Ensure that the environment during the interview is safe for the child.

Preschool Children. The preschool child will probably be able to participate in the interview, although very young or shy children may have limited interaction. Ask questions directed toward the child that are appropriate for the child's age. In addition to the usual data, record data on the age when the child first walked, language development, and toilet training. If the child has no history of congenital problems or developmental delays, you may decide to collect little or no information about pregnancy, labor and delivery, and Apgar scores. If abnormal findings are noted during the assessment, however, you may then decide to record such information.

School-Aged Children. Usually, a great deal of interaction occurs between the examiner and the school-aged child during the interview. Although this child is capable of relaying a current history, the parent should validate data and provide remote history. When interviewing a child, you should ask questions simply and directly. Stories and dolls may be helpful if the child is experiencing difficulty with providing information (this technique is especially useful if sexual, emotional, or physical abuse is suspected and the parent is not present). If the child is not experiencing congenital problems or developmental delays, you may choose to eliminate the birth data. Early developmental milestones can be determined during the assessment. At the end of the interview, you should ask both child and parent to contribute any further information that may be

helpful. You should also discuss any concerns or problems. Spend some time alone with an older child to determine if he or she has any concerns that require privacy.

Adolescents. Usually the adolescent can participate fully in the interview process without parental assistance. You should ask the adolescent whether discussion may include parents. If parents are present, direct interview questions to the adolescent and not the parent. Often adolescents have questions or concerns they would like to discuss with you privately about sexual activities or concerns, alcohol, tobacco, or drugs. In such cases, advise the adolescent what information must be shared with other health professionals or parents.

At some point in the interview, parents should be included and afforded the opportunity to discuss concerns either with or without the adolescent present. The joint interview period may be the only time you will be able to assess the parent–child relationship. In some instances, however, an adolescent may seek health care without a parent's presence or knowledge.

Display 19-1 is a sample form for recording pediatric interview and examination data using functional health patterns in acute care settings.

DIAGNOSTIC STUDIES FOR NEWBORNS

Some diagnostic studies are mandated by state law. Generally, these are measurements phenylketonuria (PKU) and thyroxine (T_4) levels. Other studies, such as bilirubin, blood type, sickle cell, HIV testing, hearing, Apgar score, and gestational age, are often performed.

Phenylketonuria. This test is performed 1 to 4 days after the newborn has ingested breast milk or formula. This is a blood test that measures the amount of phenylalanine amino acids in the blood. Excessive phenylalanine in the body causes tissue and brain damage resulting in mental retardation.

Thyroxine. This test is performed at the same time as the PKU. Thyroxine is a thyroid hormone necessary for normal growth, development, and metabolism. Newborns with low values (hypothyroid) risk permanent brain defects.

Bilirubin. Bilirubin is a result of red blood cell breakdown. The liver cannot metabolize all of the bilirubin produced; therefore, plasma bilirubin increases. The high plasma bilirubin results in jaundice (a yellowing of the skin). Most infants experience normal physiologic hyperbilirubinemia beginning about the third day. If bilirubin level rises above 12 mg/dL, it is considered excessive, and central nervous system damage may occur.

Blood Type. A newborn's blood type may be tested, especially if the mother is Rh-negative and the father is Rh-positive. Blood type may also be tested if ABO incompatibility is suspected.

Sickle Cell. Sickle cell disease is a genetic blood disease that primarily affects individuals of African heritage. Sickle cell testing detects the presence of hemoglobin S. If hemo-

(Text continues on pg. 569)

Display 19–1
Guidelines for Recording the Pediatric Data Base Using Functional Health Patterns

This form was developed for use in acute care settings but could be adapted to other health care settings.

Functional Health Status

Nursing History/Examination—Children

Date: _____ Time: _____ Name: _____ Source of Information: _____
Admitting Diagnosis: _____ Age: _____
Reason for Admission: _____

I. Health Perception and Health Management = Subjective Data	Objective Data
A. What is the problem? Why did you seek help today? Describe the problem. How has the problem been managed at home?	General appearance Child/parents
B. Current health Preventive and safety practices Health today as related to past months, years Family/parent health	

    C. Past health
       1. Birth history
          Prenatal: Planned pregnancy

Emotional response	Wt. gain
Complications	Alcohol use; medication

          Natal: Length of labor   Spontaneous/induced

Vaginal/cesarean	Anesthesia
Complications	
Bonding	Support person

          Neonatal: Wt.: _____ Length: _____ Head circ.: _____
            Apgar
            Nursery course:
       2. Immunizations: DPT   Polio   Measles   Mumps
                    Rubella   TB test   Flu   Hib
       3. Growth and development:
          Motor: Rolling over _____
                    Sitting _____
                    Crawling _____
                    Standing _____
                    Walking _____
                    Sports _____
          Social-cognitive:
                    Smiling _____
                    First word _____
                    Sentences _____
                    Playing _____
                    School _____
          Early behavior patterns as viewed by parents
       4. Frequency of health assessments and checkups—date of last visit
       5. Hospitalizations: Date, reason, length, diagnosis
       6. Accidents or injuries: Time, place, reactions, physical response
       7. Allergies/reactions: Drugs, foods, contactants, inhalants
    D. Family history: Familial, inherited, genetic disorders (use back of sheet to illustrate)

Parents	Heart
Siblings	Hypertension
Aunts, uncles (maternal, paternal)	Arteriosclerosis

(continued)

Display 19–1
Guidelines for Recording the Pediatric Data Base Using Functional Health Patterns (continued)

D. Family history (*continued*)

Cousins   Coronary artery disease
Maternal grandparents   Blood disorders
Paternal grandparents   Renal disease
       Cancer
       Diabetes
       Obesity
       Arthritis
       Gout
       Mental illness
       Epilepsy
       Allergies
       Migraines

Race-culture
Environmental history:
  Type of housing
  Seasonal changes
  Pollution effects
Economic
  Employment of parents
  Adequate means for family needs
Community resources used: Associations, organizations, foundations, HHC, CHNC, PHN

II. Nutrition

Recall of intake past 24 hours: Food, fluids, vitamins   Wt.: _____

Ht.: _____

Meal patterns   Head: _____
(attach growth chart)
Temp: _____ AX-R-O
B.P.: _____

Eating behavior   Skin
First tooth   How many now?   Teeth
Likes   Dislikes   Rash; odors
Food allergies/behavioral changes toward certain food   Nodes

III. Elimination Patterns

Bowel and bladder pattern: Daytime; nighttime control   Bowel sounds
Usual time of BM   Appearance of feces, urine
Words used for BM;   Urination
Recent changes in elimination   Hernia
Excess perspirations? Odor?

IV. Activity-Exercise Patterns

Describe usual day   Reflexes, ROM, gait, strength
Level of self-care/routine
  Feeding   Pulses
  Dressing   Capillary refill
  Toileting   Breath sounds
  Bathing   Respiratory sounds
       Heart sounds
  Mobility   Coordination
Use of free time   Motor skills

VI. Sleep-Rest Patterns

Usual pattern   Naps   Appear rested?
  Child/parent

(continued)

Display 19–1
Guidelines for Recording the Pediatric Data Base Using Functional Health Patterns (continued)

VI. Sleep-Rest Patterns (*continued*)	
Sleeping arrangements	Attentive
Bedtime items Blanket/stuffed toy	
Easy to awaken?	
VI. Cognitive-Perceptual Patterns	
Variations in vision, hearing, taste, smell, touch, pain	PERRLA
Response to noise, touch, talking, music	Cover test
Educational experience (includes infant stimulation)	Acuity Glasses
Speech pattern	Hearing Ears
Ability to cooperate, communicate	Speech DASE
	Pain
Behavior as viewed by parents	Sensory functions
	Oriented
VII. Self-Perception-Self-Concept Patterns	
Outstanding personality trait	Body posture/movement
Overall behavior	Eye contact
Interests	Behavior changes
What causes fears, strong emotions How handled?	Self-confidence
Sense of humor	
VIII. Role Relationship	
Usual care-giver/parent-child interaction	Observed interaction with
Siblings:	significant others
Sibling-child relationship	
Grandparents	
Peer interactions	
Favorite person	
Security objects	
Additional members of household	
Response to separation	
Dependency	
School adjustment	
IX. Sexuality–Reproductive Patterns	
Knows if she/he is a girl/boy (feelings of maleness, femaleness)	Testicles examination
Basic language for body parts and functions	Breast examination
Direct teaching regarding sexuality	Genitalia
Response to questions	
Best friend	
Menarche	
X. Coping–Stress Tolerance Patterns	
Response to stress changes	Problem solving/coping
New environment/people	observed
Illness	
Hospitalization	
Frequent illness(es)	
Experience of separation from parents	
Occurrence of dependent behavior	
Method of discipline	
Reaction	
Response to criticism, correction	
Family stressors	
Community resources used by the family	
XI. Value–Belief Patterns	
Goals for future	Varied health practices

(continued)

Display 19–1
Guidelines for Recording the Pediatric Data Base Using Functional Health Patterns (continued)

XI. Value–Belief Patterns (*continued*)
   What qualities are important in life
      Parents/child
   Is religious belief important/supportive to family?
      Religion   Sunday school

Other Diagnostic Screening Tests   *Other Laboratory Tests*
DDST2
Preschool Readiness: Experimental Screening Scale
Draw-a-Person
Neonatal Perception Inventory
Anticipatory Guidance Need
Others

Summary Statement: (Cluster cues—Nursing diagnosis)

(Developed by Marita Hoffart, Assistant Professor of Nursing, Minot State University, Minot, North Dakota)

---

globin S is present, then hemoglobin electrophoresis should be performed to determine if the newborn has the trait or the disease.

HIV Testing. Newborns of mothers with HIV or at risk for HIV are usually tested for presence of HIV. The *polymerase chain reaction test* differentiates between newborns who do not have HIV from those who do. Maternal HIV may remain in the newborn's blood for up to 15 months (not all of these newborns will develop HIV disease).

Hearing. Special audiometric testing of newborns is available, and some hospitals routinely test hearing of all newborns.

Apgar Score. This screening is done at 1, 5, and sometimes 10 minutes after birth. The neonate receives a score from zero to 2 for each of the 5 assessment areas. A score below 6 is considered abnormal. The five assessment areas are heart, respirations, muscle tone, reflex response, and color. Zero scores would be absent heart rate, absent respirations, limp muscle tone, no response to catheter in nostril or to foot slap, and blue or pale color. A score of 1 would be heart below 100, weak cry, some flexion of extremities, grimace to catheter in nostril and foot slap, body pink, and blue extremities. A score of 2 would be heart over 100, good cry, well-flexed muscles, cough or sneeze to nasal catheter, cry and withdrawal of foot to slap, and completely pink. Each assessment area receives a score; the score range is 0 to 12.

Gestational Age. Normal gestation is between 38 and 42 weeks. A newborn of less than 38 weeks' gestation is considered to be premature. Some newborns are large for gestational age (occurs commonly when mother has diabetes mellitus), and some are small for gestational age. Determining gestational age is an important consideration. Several gestational screening tools are available, such as Clinical Estimation of Gestational Age (Brazie and Lubchenco, 1977) and Gestational Age of Newborn (Dubowitz and Dubowitz, 1977). These or similar screening tools are available in newborn care units.

DIAGNOSTIC STUDIES FOR INFANTS

Routine diagnostic and screening studies performed on infants include developmental screening, urine screening, and hemoglobin.

Developmental Testing. Because infants grow and develop, regular developmental testing should occur. The DDST2 is an example of such a tool. If delays are noted, the child should be referred for diagnostic testing by a specialist. Possible diagnostic tests are numerous and relate to the specific delay.

Urine Screening. A complete urine analysis can be performed to determine the presence of any anomalies such as glucose, protein, and red or white blood cells. Generally, a urine dipstick screening test is sufficient. If any of the above is positive, then a routine urinalysis should be performed. This is usually performed when the infant is 6 months.

Hemoglobin or Hematocrit. Hemoglobin tests measure the amount of hemoglobin in the blood. Hemoglobin is a protein found in red blood cells that carries oxygen. A hemoglobin level below 10 g/dL is considered to be low, and the infant would be anemic. Hematocrit measures the percent of red blood cells in a blood sample. Low hematocrit levels are frequently associated with anemia. For infants, a reading below 29% is considered low.

DIAGNOSTIC STUDIES FOR YOUNG CHILDREN

Diagnostic and screening studies routinely performed during young childhood include developmental testing, urine screening, and hemoglobin/hematocrit measurement as discussed in the section for infants. Developmental testing generally occurs at each visit, whereas the others are generally performed annually. At age 4, vision and hearing screening occur (see discussion of these tests in Chap. 11). A dental examination is usually recommended between ages 2 and 3 years and then every 6 months. A tuberculin skin test is a diagnostic screening to determine the presence of tuberculosis antibodies. This is usually recommended at 24 months and whenever the child is exposed to tuberculosis. A false-positive result is possible if the skin test is given up to 3 months after a measles, mumps, and/or rubella immunization. The two can be given simultaneously.

DIAGNOSTIC STUDIES FOR OLDER CHILDREN AND ADOLESCENTS

The only routine diagnostic or screening studies performed on older children are tuberculin skin testing, hemoglobin, and urine screening (these have been discussed previously in this chapter). Other diagnostic tests may be appropriate because of risk factors such as sexual activity. Most diagnostic tests appropriate for adults are also appropriate for adolescents if indicated.

NEWBORNS
Anatomy and Physiology Overview

Birth to the first 29 to 30 days of life is considered the newborn or neonate period. Birth requires rapid adjustment to a new environment. The lungs must inflate, and the heart must change from fetal to systemic circulation (the foramen ovale closes, the ductus arteriosus closes, and the umbilical vein closes). Heart and respiratory rates may be irregular for the first month. Because of their large surface area and immature thermoregulation, risk for hypothermia is high.

The normal newborn weight is between 2500 and 4000 gm (5 lb 8 oz to 8 lb 13 oz), and length is between 45 and 55 cm (18 to 22 in). Asymmetry of the head is common due to molding of the head during the birth process (the bone plates shift to accommodate the maternal pelvic outlet and birth canal). At birth, the newborn is assessed for heart rate, respiratory rate, muscle tone, reflex responses, and color (these form the basis of the Apgar score). Although all organs are present at birth, some are immature, such as the intestines and liver.

Physical Examination | *Newborns*

General Principles	A complete head-to-toe assessment of the newborn is usually conducted within the first 24 hours of birth and again at age 4 weeks. The newborn is at risk for developing hypothermia because of a large surface area and immature thermoregulation mechanisms. Therefore, you should assure a warm environment and only expose body parts as necessary during the physical assessment (Fig. 19-1). Examination of the circulatory and respiratory systems should be performed while the newborn is quiet. All manipulative or intrusive procedures should be performed last. Whenever possible, the assessment of the newborn should occur with the parents present so that you can inform the parents about normal growth and development and appearance, and also answer any questions (Fig. 19-2).
Preparation	Before performing the physical examination, you should fully explain to the parent or parents what you will be doing. The examination should be performed in a location where both parents and nurse are comfortable. This can be accomplished at the mother's bedside or in an examination room. Adequate lighting is essential, as is privacy for parents to ask questions. Have available an extra diaper in case a change is needed during or after the examination.
Equipment	• Scale • Tape measure to measure length • Head circumference tape measure • Stethoscope • Otoscope or pen light
Examination and Documentation Focus	• Identify physical findings within normal parameters. • Identify deviations from normal. • Identify possible risks. • Assess physiologic changes associated with birth.

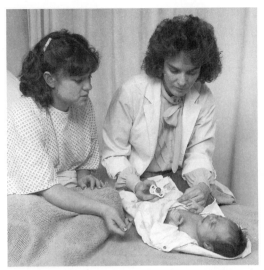

Figure 19–1. The newborn baby is kept warm during the examination by exposing body parts only as necessary.

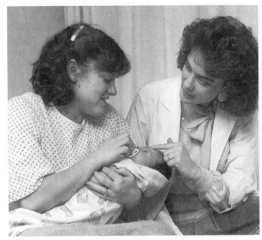

Figure 19–2. The parent may discuss concerns with the nurse during the newborn examination.

Examination Guidelines   *Newborns*

Procedure

1. ANTHROPOMETRIC MEASUREMENTS.

    a. With newborn on examining table or in mother's arms, measure head and chest circumference by applying a tape measure around the widest part of the head (just above the eye brows) or chest (at nipple line) as shown in the figure. Maintain records of serial measurements on standardized graph tables and compare to normal ranges. Tables for head and chest are shown in Appendix E.

Clinical Significance

Normal Findings
The full-term newborn's head circumference should be about 33 to 35 cm, the chest circumference 30 to 33 cm.

Deviations from Normal
Head circumference should not be more than 3 cm larger or smaller than the chest circumference. If larger, may be hydrocephalus; if smaller, may be microcephaly.

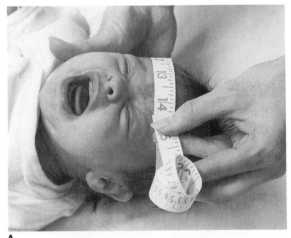

A

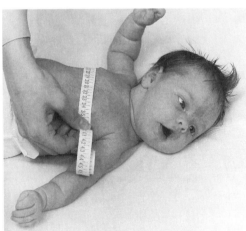

B

Measuring head circumference (A) and chest circumference (B)

    b. Measure length of newborn from head to heels; extend legs as much as possible without forcing.

    c. Weigh newborn without any clothing, including diaper. Record weight on growth chart. Record height to weight on growth chart. (See Appendix E for examples.)

Normal Findings
Length usually between 45 and 55 cm (18–22 inches)

Normal Findings
Weight is generally between 2500 and 4000 grams (5 lbs 8 oz and 8 lbs 13 oz). Weight to height should be proportional.

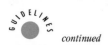

continued

Newborns

Procedure	Clinical Significance

Clinical Significance

Deviations from Normal

Less than 2500 grams may represent prematurity; more than 4000 grams is frequent when mother is diabetic and newborn may be large for gestational age.

2. ASSESS HEAD.

  a. Assess hair.

Normal Findings

Hair may vary in amount and color; more copious amounts of hair are seen on preterm infants. Lanugo (fine hair) may appear on the body, especially the shoulders and back.

  b. Face and skull:

  (1) Observe for symmetry and position of head.

  (2) Try to transilluminate skull if newborn has high-pitched cry. This is evaluated by holding a flashlight with a protective foam collar against the baby's head from several different angles.

Normal Findings

Asymmetry of the face or skull may be associated with molding caused by accommodation of the skull to the birth canal. This problem usually resolves within 1 week. The newborn is unable to hold the head erect. The head will lag when the baby is pulled to a sitting position. The skull should not transilluminate.

Deviations from Normal

Caput succedaneum, swelling of soft scalp tissue from birth trauma, may be noted. *Cephalhematoma,* unilateral edema over parietal bones, may occur after birth and resolves in 6 weeks. *Complete transillumination* of the skull is abnormal. Localized bright spots or glowing of the entire skull may indicate severe pathology.

  (3) Palpate fontanelles (soft, flat depressions); use fingers to palpate skull, noting anterior and posterior fontanelles.

Normal Findings

The fontalles may pulsate at same rate as heart. The anterior fontanelle is 2.5 to 4.0 cm across; the posterior fontanelle is not greater than 2 cm across and may even be closed. The posterior fontanelle usually closes at about 2 months, and the anterior closes between 12 and 18 months.

Deviations from Normal

A depressed fontanelle may indicate dehydration, and bulging may indicate hydrocephalus or increased pressure within the brain. Closed anterior fontanelle is not normal.

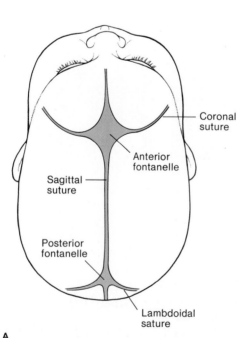

A

Palpating the fontanelles

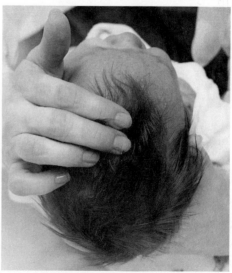

B

continued

Newborns

Procedure

c. Examine the oral cavity. Examination of the newborn's oral cavity is important to determine if congenital anomalies exist. Inspecting the newborn's oropharynx may be difficult because of the strong reflex protrusion of the tongue when depressed with a tongue blade. Although the uvula may be retracted upward and backward during crying, observations of the oral cavity may still be possible.

  (1) Inspect and palpate the palate with your finger; inspect, when possible, using a tongue blade and light.

Clinical Significance

Normal Findings

The palate is slightly higher and narrower than in the adult. The palate and oral cavity is moist; generally no salivation is present.

Deviations from Normal

A high palate or narrow arch or holes in the palate are considered abnormal, and referral is indicated. *Epstein's pearls* (Bohn nodules) may be observed along both sides of the hard palate midline. These small, whitish nodules cause no problems and usually disappear by age 2 or 3 months.

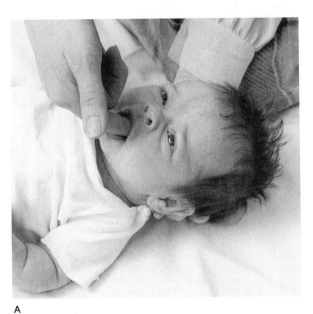
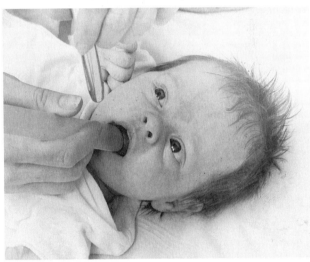

A   B

Examining the oral cavity. (A) Palpating the palate with the finger. (B) Inspecting the palate using a tongue blade and light.

  (2) Inspect the tongue.

Normal Findings

The tongue should fit in the mouth and be pink in color and not coated. Sucking reflex should be strong and coordinated.

Deviations from Normal

A large, protruding tongue may be a sign of congenital defects and should be referred. A white, cottage cheese–like coating on the tongue and cheeks may be thrush, caused by *Candida albicans.*

  (3) Inspect and palpate the gums.

Normal Findings

The gums of dark-skinned babies may have accumulations of patchy brown pigment; this is usually insignificant.

Deviations from Normal

Epstein's pearls may be noted on the gums. Occasionally an infant will be born with a tooth or one erupts shortly after birth, but this is not significant.

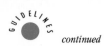
continued

Newborns

Procedure

(4) Look for the tonsils. The tonsils generally cannot be seen.

d. Inspect the nose. Observe the nares for patency and flaring. The newborn's sinuses are poorly developed and generally are not assessed.

e. Inspect the eyes.

(1) The external eye may be assessed by holding the infant supine with the head gently lowered, which causes the eyes to open. Bright light will interfere with an effective eye assessment.

(2) Inspect eyelids. Upper and lower lid eversion is usually not performed during newborn assessment.

(3) Inspect the lacrimal apparatus.

(4) Inspect the bulbar conjunctiva and sclera.

(5) Elicit light reflexes. The corneal light reflex, red reflex, and pupillary constriction to light should be observed. A funduscopic examination is not usually performed on newborns unless some type of anomaly is present, in which case an ophthalmologist should conduct the examination.

(6) Check for visual acuity.

Clinical Significance

Normal Findings
Generally the tonsils cannot be seen.

Normal Findings
The nose may be flattened. There should be no flaring of the nares. The newborn is an obligatory nose breather. Sneezing may be frequent and is a normal attempt to clear nasal passages.

Deviations from Normal
Bruising of the nose may occur during delivery. Any flaring of the nares may indicate respiratory distress; evaluate immediately.

Normal Findings
Newborns generally keep their eyes closed most of the time. As with adults, eye color varies. Light-skinned babies usually have gray to blue eyes, and dark-skinned babies usually have brown eyes. Eyes should move in all directions.

Normal Findings
Eyelids may be edematous for the first 2 days; frequent blinking is normal. Epicanthal folds are normal in Asian infants.

Deviations from Normal
If epicanthal folds are large in Asian babies or are noted on children of other ethnic backgrounds, Down's syndrome may be suspected.

Normal Findings
No tearing is evident for the first month.

Normal Findings
Bulbar conjunctiva and sclera may be blue tinged; small vessels may be visible in the sclera.

Deviations from Normal
Yellow discoloration occurs with jaundice. Subconjunctival hemorrhage may be present, caused by rupture of vessels during birth.

Normal Findings
The baby should blink at bright light. Red reflex and bilateral symmetric corneal light reflex can be noted.

Deviations from Normal
The absence of a red reflex may indicate congenital cataracts.

Normal Findings
Nystagmus may be present. The older neonate may be able to follow an object to midline; however, you may be unable to assess acuity. Visual acuity is about 20/500.

Deviations from Normal
Lack of blinking or sensitivity to bright light may indicate blindness.

continued **Newborns**

Procedure

f. Inspect the ears and assess hearing.

(1) Determine the position of the external ears. An imaginary line is drawn from the inner and outer canthus of the eye to the vertex. The pinna of the ears should be at the level of this line.

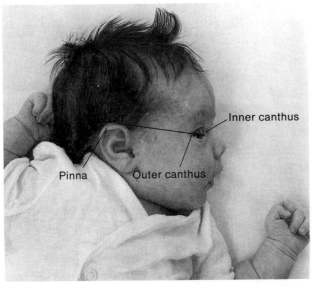

Checking ear position

(2) To assess the newborn with the otoscope, the baby should be held immobile, with special effort taken to maintain head immobility during the assessment. The following positions may be helpful: (1) prone with arms restrained at side and head secured by another or (2) supine with arms over head and head secured. The otoscope should be held with the handle directed toward the top of the head. Children less than age 3 years have an upward curvature of the canal. Therefore, to visualize the structures, you should pull the lower auricle or pinna down and back.

(3) Hearing screening. Check hearing by ringing a bell or making a similar noise near the newborn.

3. EXAMINE THE CHEST AND BACK.

a. Inspect and palpate the shoulders and neck, including the clavicular area.

b. Inspect the back.

Clinical Significance

Normal Findings

The pinna of the ears should be at the level of the eye-to-ear line.

Deviations from Normal

Low-set ears are associated with congenital kidney defects and other problems.

Normal Findings

Tympanic membrane visualization is usually not performed on newborns because the canal is usually filled with vernix caseosa and amniotic fluid. When the canal is clear, the tympanic membrane and other structures should be visualized.

Normal Findings

The newborn should display the startle reflex in response to a bell or other loud noise.

Deviations from Normal

If no startle reflex occurs, refer the baby for further hearing evaluation.

Normal Findings

The neck is short, and it is difficult to determine landmarks or the thyroid gland; the neck should be able to turn 80 degrees to the left and right.

Deviations from Normal

A broken clavicle is a common complication of birth; signs include local swelling, visible dislocation, crepitus, and tenderness.

Normal Findings

Spinal curvature is convex; there are no cervical or lumbar curves. The newborn has a C-shape appearance when held from the abdomen.

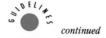

continued

Newborns

Procedure

    c. Examine the sacral area for dimpling, bulging, masses, or tufts of hair.

4. ASSESS THE LUNGS.

    a. Observe rate with chest exposed and auscultate for lung sounds, using appropriate-size diaphragm and bell attachments.

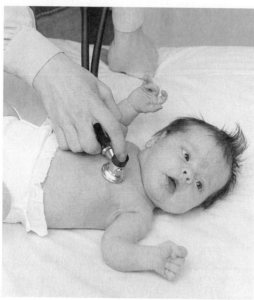

Auscultation of the anterior chest. Note the small bell and diaphragm attachments on the stethoscope.

    b. Palpate the back with two fingers while the newborn is crying.

    c. Percuss the chest lightly with one finger.

5. ASSESS HEART.

    a. Observe apical impulse.

Clinical Significance

Normal Findings

There should be no blemishes.

Deviations from Normal

Any dimpling, bulging, masses, or tufts of hair may indicate a neurotube defect.

Normal Findings

The newborn has abdominal respirations at a rate of 30–60 breaths/minute. Brief periods of apnea may be present for the first 4 weeks. Clear bronchovesicular breath sounds are normal.

Deviations from Normal

Apnea for longer than 20 seconds accompanied by lower heart rates is associated with sudden infant death syndrome. A pattern of seesaw breathing (abdominal thorax breathing), flaring of the nostrils, and noisy respirations indicated respiratory distress.

Normal Findings

Fremitus findings are similar to those in the adult.

Normal Findings

Hyperresonant sounds are normal.

Normal Findings

Should be seen at fourth intercostal space to the immediate left of the mid-clavicular line.

continued

Newborns

Procedure

b. Auscultate the heart while the baby is quiet and before proceeding to more intrusive methods. Use an appropriate-size diaphragm and bell to auscultate the newborn. Auscultate the five precordial landmarks: (1) aortic, second right intercostal space by the sternum; (2) pulmonary, second left intercostal space near the sternum; (3) third left intercostal space right and left of the sternum; (4) tricuspid area, fifth interspace, right of the sternum; and (5) apex, lateral to mid clavicular line at fourth–fifth interspace.

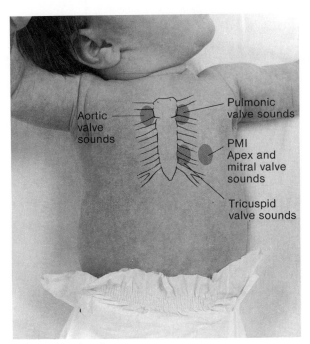

Precordial landmarks

c. Assess blood pressure and peripheral pulses—carotid, brachial, femoral, and pedal—using only one finger to avoid obliterating the pulse. Vasoconstriction from chilling will make pulses less intense. Blood pressure should be taken with Doppler or 1-inch blood pressure cuff.

Clinical Significance

Normal Findings

A normal heart rate is 120 to 170 beats/minute. The rhythm may be slightly irregular, with an increased heart rate on inspiration and a decreased heart rate on expiration. Heart sounds of newborns are louder than adults because the thinner chest wall and the larger-size heart in proportion to the chest. Heart sounds are also shorter in duration and higher in pitch. An S3 may be heard as a normal finding and occurs in 30% of all newborns.

Deviations from Normal

An S4 is never considered a normal finding. Murmurs are frequently heard in newborns until age 48 hours. Most murmurs resolve with the transition from fetal to systemic pulmonary circulation. Murmurs can also represent congenital heart malformations, especially if persisting more than 2 days and accompanied by other signs such as cyanosis. All murmurs persisting more than 2 days require further evaluation.

Normal Findings

Pulses should be of same intensity in corresponding limb; amplitude should be same in limbs.

Deviations from Normal

A difference in the amplitude of pulses between the lower and upper extermities is considered abnormal and may represent coarctation of the aorta.

Normal Findings

A newborn's blood pressure ranges between 40 and 50 mm Hg systolic but will vary depending on cuff size and if a Doppler is used. By age 4 weeks the baby's blood pressure averages 80 systolic and 40 diastolic.

Deviations from Normal

If the systolic blood pressure is 96 or greater for the first 7 days or 104 or greater between 8 and 30 days, referral is warranted for significant hypertension. Before referral you should get three elevated readings while the child is quiet and not crying.

GUIDELINES *continued*

Newborns

Procedure	Clinical Significance

Procedure

6. ASSESS THE ABDOMEN.

Assessing the abdomen will be easier if the newborn's abdomen is relaxed. Allowing the crying or restless baby to suck a pacifier and flex the knees relaxes the abdomen.

a. Inspect the abdomen.

b. Auscultate the abdomen using appropriate-size stethoscope attachments.

c. Percuss the abdomen.

d. Palpate the abdomen. Perform light and deep palpation, gently, with finger tips. It may be difficult to differentiate pain and tenderness, especially if the baby is already crying. If fluid is suspected in the abdomen, use a flashlight to transilluminate the abdomen.

7. EXAMINE THE HIPS AND LOWER EXTREMITIES.

a. Inspect the foot.

Clinical Significance

Normal Findings

The contour of the abdomen is rounded and dome shaped. The umbilical cord should be dry in 5 days and drop off by 2 weeks. The end of a fresh cord should have three vessels visible. A fine venous network may be observed.

Deviations from Normal

Protrusion of the abdomen above the chest may be the result of feces, masses, or organ enlargement. Further evaluation is required. Visible peristalsis may indicate pyloric stenosis. Prominent venous networks along with taut skin appearance is abnormal, and in such cases the abdomen should be transilluminated. Small (1–2 cm) umibilical hernias may be noted and are usually considered normal in children before age 2 years and normal in black children until age 7 years. If the skin is open around the hernia, immediate attention is required from a pediatrician. Herniation throught the diastasis rectus muscle may result in a midline bulging between the xiphoid and umbilicus, especially when the baby is crying. This hernia usually disappears during the early school years. Inguinal and femoral hernias are not normal.

Normal Findings

Bowel sounds are heard every 10 to 30 seconds.

Deviations from Normal

Absent or hypoactive bowel sounds.

Normal Findings

Tympany is heard and may be increased secondary to air swallowing. The upper edge of the liver should be located by percussion within 1 cm of the fifth intercostal space. The spleen may be located by percussion 1 or 2 cm below the costal margin.

Deviations from Normal

Hepatomegaly is associated with congestive heart failure secondary to congenital heart defect.

Normal Findings

The abdomen should feel soft during inspiration. There should be no transillumination.

Deviations from Normal

The light will glow through the skin if fluid or air is present but will not glow if solid masses or blood is present.

Normal Findings

The foot appears flat and the soles have creases. Shortly after birth the feet may remain in the same position they were in utero, appearing deformed. Full range of motion and manipulation can bring the foot back to normal position if a true deformity is not present.

Deviations from Normal

Lateral deviation of the forefoot (metatarsus varus) and inversion of the foot with the forefoot adducted (Talipes varus), polydactyly, or syndactyly.

continued **Newborns**

Procedure

b. Inspect legs with the newborn supine on the examining surface; place the knees together and note how far apart the legs are at the ankles.

c. Test range of motion. Perform range-of-motion testing of the lower extremities while palpating over involved joints.

d. Examine hips. There are two tests for the hips: Ortalani's test and Barlow's test. Both are used to detect congenital hip dislocation because it is often missed at first examination; repeat these tests through infancy. *Ortolani's test:* With the baby supine on the examining surface and the knees and hips flexed, place your first two fingers over the greater trochanter and your thumb over the lesser trochanter. With both hands placed in this manner, abduct both hips by pulling the knees toward the examining surface.

Clinical Significance

Normal Findings
Some bowing of the legs is considered normal. The legs should be equal in length. Creases of legs and gluteal folds should be symmetric and even.

Deviations from Normal
Severe bowing is not normal; uneven creases may indicate congenital hip dislocation.

Normal Findings
The hip abducts to 170 degrees and can be put through full range of motion. The knees and ankles should perform full range of motion.

Deviations from Normal
Clicking sounds or crepitus are considered abnormal, as is the inability to abduct the hip past 160 degrees.

Normal Findings
You should not feel over the greater trochanter a click or slip of the femoral head.

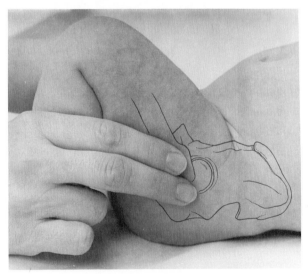

A

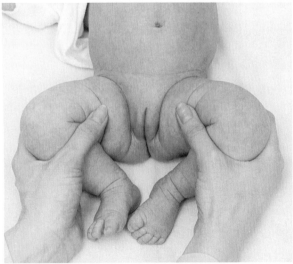

B

Ortolani's test for congenital hip dislocation. (A) Placement of examiner's hands. (B) Abduction of infant's hips.

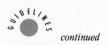

continued

Newborns

Procedure

Barlow's test: Place the baby supine on the examining surface. Use one hand to steady the pelvis by placing the fingers over the greater trochanter of the hip being tested and gently pressing your hand over the symphysis pubis. Grasp the outer thigh with your other hand, placing your thumb over the lesser trochanter. Test by applying backward and outward pressure in a motion that moves the femur away from the joint socket.

Clinical Significance

Deviations from Normal

If you feel slipping movements, the hip may be unstable or dislocated.

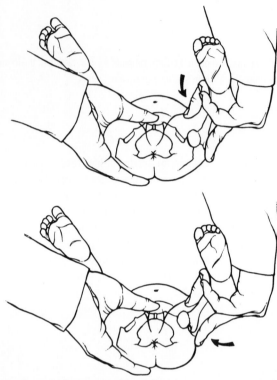

Barlow's test for congenital hip dislocation

8. EXAMINE THE GENITALIA.

  a. Males:

    (1) Inspect the penis.

Normal Findings

The shaft of the penis should be straight. Erections are common, with the usual nonerect length of the penis being 2 or 3 cm. The urethral opening should appear as a midline slit. The foreskin is loose and may cover the urethral opening in the uncircumcised baby.

Deviations from Normal

A dorsal or ventral urethral opening on the shaft of the penis is abnormal.

    (2) Inspect and palpate the scrotum. If testes are not felt, place a finger over the inguinal ring and push gently toward the scrotum. The testes may descend into the scrotal sac with this maneuver.

Normal Findings

Each scrotal sac should be 1 or 2 cm across and contain a testicle. Normally, the spermatic cord is smooth on palpation.

Deviations from Normal

If the testes are palpable in the inguinal canal but will not descend, consider then undescended and refer. Scrotal rugae may be absent in preterm infants. Edema and bruising of the scrotum are commonly observed with breech delivery. A deep cleft in the scrotum may be related to genitourinary anomalies or ambiguous genitals. Transillumination of the scrotum may be conducted to differentiate fluid from mass lesions. Lumps or roughness in the scrotum may indicate a hernia.

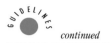

Newborns

Procedure	Clinical Significance

Procedure

b. Females:

(1) Inspect the external genitalia. Assess the genitals by placing the baby supine with the hips abducted (frog position).

c. Assessment of pelvic structures

9. EXAMINE THE ANUS AND RECTUM.

For newborns, this part of the assessment is restricted to inspection. The rectum is not usually digitally assessed.

10. EXAMINE THE UPPER EXTREMITIES.

a. Inspect arms and hands.

11. EXAMINE THE SKIN.

a. Inspect the skin as each body part is assessed. During the assessment of specific body parts, all creases and skin folds should be carefully examined.

Clinical Significance

Normal Findings

The labia majora and minora may be edematous but should separate. The size of the labia is influenced by maternal hormones, and decreases in size may be noted within 2 or 3 weeks. If the baby was born breech, more edema and possibly bruising of the labia may be observed. The color of the labia will be light pink in light-skinned newborns and darker than the skin of the abdomen in dark-skinned newborns. The clitoris appears large (0.3–0.5 cm) in proportion to the rest of the genitalia. A vaginal opening is present in newborns and may drain a mucoid, white discharge for 4 weeks. Vaginal secretions may be blood tinged the first week after birth. Skene and Bartholin glands are not visible or palpable in newborns and should not have discharge. The urethral meatus is usually midline, anterior to the vagina, and emits an uninterrupted stream when the baby is voiding.

Deviations from Normal

If the clitoris is larger than 0.5 cm, the appearance ambiguous, or the vaginal orifice unusual, the baby should be evaluated further. The absence of a vagina is abnormal.

Pelvic structures are not usually evaluated in newborns and young children.

Normal Findings

The passage of meconium stool is associated with patency of the gastrointestinal tract. Feces from breast-fed babies are mustard colored and watery to soft in consistency, whereas formula-fed babies have yellowish-green feces that are more formed.

Deviations from Normal

A child who has not passed a meconium stool or seems to pass meconium through the urinary meatus or vagina, or who does not have an anal opening (imperfect anus) should be referred immediately.

Normal Findings

The nails are soft and pliable, usually longer than wide. Nails may be long enough to scratch the skin. Vernix caseosa may be observed under the nails.

Deviations from Normal

These include polydactyly (extra fingers) and syndactyly (fused or webbed fingers). Transverse palmar creases (simian lines) with a curving and shortened fifth finger are associated with Down's syndrome.

Normal Findings

The skin color may change rapidly in response to activity and temperature changes. Normal variations in skin color and pigmentation include the following:

- An *erythematous flush* may be noted, especially during the first 8 to 24 hours.

- Children of *dark-skinned* parents may appear lighter in the newborn period because melanin concentrations have not developed except on nail beds and the scrotum.

- *Cyanosis* or *acrocyanosis* (cyanosis of hands and feet) may appear, especially if the baby is chilled.

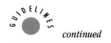

continued

Newborns

Procedure	Clinical Significance
	• *Physiologic jaundice* occurs in about half of all newborns and is noted as slight yellowing of the skin occurring 3 or 4 days after birth. It usually disappears within 1 week. Physiologic jaundice is more common in breast-fed newborns.

Clinical Significance

- *Physiologic jaundice* occurs in about half of all newborns and is noted as slight yellowing of the skin occurring 3 or 4 days after birth. It usually disappears within 1 week. Physiologic jaundice is more common in breast-fed newborns.
- *Transient mottling* (*cutis marmorata*) is noticed on the trunk and extremities in response to cold.
- *Mongolian spots* are areas of dark blue or black pigmentation that are observed more frequently in dark-skinned infants, especially in the sacral and gluteal regions.
- *Vernix caseosa* is a white, cheeselike substance that covers the skin of the fetus. It is present in varying degrees and is almost always seen in skin folds and creases.
- *Lanugo* is a fine, silky covering of hair present in varying degrees after birth, more commonly in preterm newborns.
- *Telangiectatic nevi* (commonly called "stork bites" or "angel kisses") are macular red or deep pink lesions at the back of the neck, eyelids, or forehead. These lesions may blanch to touch and usually fade with age but may be noted when excessive skin flushing occurs, even in adults.

Deviations from Normal

A beefy red color lasting more than 24 hours may be related to hypoglycemia. Persistent cyanosis may represent a congenital heart problem. If jaundice occurs earlier than 3 days or is a darker yellow, it may represent hemolytic disorders. Transient mottling may be pronounced in preterm bodies or Down's syndrome infants. Common benign lesions that may be noted on the newborn's skin include the following:

- *Milia* appear as small white papules on the face, especially on the nose, cheeks, and chin. Milia represent sebaceous cysts and usually disappear within 2 months.
- *Cavernous hemangiomas* are cystic lesions with a reddish-blue hue. The lesion may grow at variable rates and may require medical treatment.
- *Strawberry hemangiomas* are red or purple, raised areas on the skin caused by dilated capillaries. Although the lesion may increase in size, it is usually no greater than 2 or 3 cm wide. The lesion may appear at birth or shortly thereafter and disappear by age 5 years.
- *Port wine stains* are purplish, sharply demarcated macular lesions that can occur on any skin surface or mucous membrane. The lesion is related to excessive proliferation of the capillary bed of the skin; the lesion may invade the nervous system, and additional evaluation may be necessary.
- *Café au lait spots* are small, light-brown (coffee with cream color) macules. If fewer than six are noted over the entire body, the lesion has little clinical significance. If six or more are present, a high correlation exists with neurofibromas; further evaluation is warranted.
- *Erythema toxicum* (flea bite rash) is a diffuse rash characterized by small, red papules, 2 to 4 mm in size, with small, white, pinpoint centers. Commonly appears within 24 hours after birth on the trunk and diaper area and disappears spontaneously in 7 to 10 days.

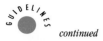
continued

Newborns

Procedure

b. Assess moisture and turgor. Skin turgor of the newborn should be evaluated using the skin of the lower abdomen. Skin turgor is a good indicator of the degree of hydration.

12. PERFORM A NEUROLOGIC EXAMINATION.

a. Assess muscle strength and function. Hold the newborn upright at the axilla with feet on a flat surface.

b. Assess sensory functions.

c. Assess reflex movements. It is not always necessary to test all the newborn reflexes. The most important reflexes to elicit include the Moro, stepping, palmar grasp, plantar grasp, Babinski, and rooting reflexes. The methods of testing these reflexes and the expected responses are shown in the display, "Newborn and Infant Reflex Evaluation."

d. Assess cranial nerves. The cranial nerves are difficult to evaluate in newborns and infants because cooperation is usually required. Observation of certain behaviors may help you make judgments about cranial nerve function.

Clinical Significance

Normal Findings

The skin of the newborn should appear soft and smooth. Dry, flaky skin may indicate prolonged gestation. It is not uncommon to observe a transient puffiness or edema of the hands, feet, legs, eyelids, pubis, or scrotum. This condition usually disappears within 2 or 3 days.

Deviations from Normal

Any alteration in neurologic findings, such as weakness, absence of normal reflexes, or asymmetry, may reflect neurologic problems.

Normal Findings

If the baby can maintain this position, muscle strength is considered adequate.

Deviations from Normal

Muscle weakness is apparent if the baby slips through the nurse's hands. Some muscle paralysis may occur as a result of pressure during vaginal delivery. Paralysis may disappear spontaneously or may disappear within 3 months with therapy, or may be limited to no recovery. Paralysis of any area needs to be assessed by a physician.

Normal Findings

The sensory assessment of newborns is nonspecific; vision and hearing screening is discussed earlier. The response to painful stimuli may be the only sensory function tested during the newborn assessment. Limbs should withdraw in response to painful stimuli.

Normal Findings

Several reflex movements are noted in newborns that are not present in other age groups. These primitive reflexes normally disappear by a specific age range. Failure to elicit one of these reflexes or persistence of the reflex beyond the usual time may be related to neurologic problems.

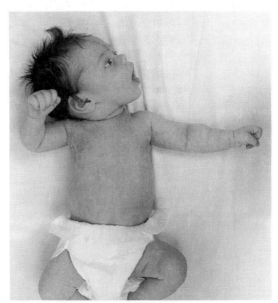

The fencing response, or tonic neck reflex, elicited by turning the infant's head to the side when the infant is supine. Note the skin mottling secondary to cold exposure.

Newborn and Infant Reflex Evaluation*

Reflex	Method of Testing	Expected Response	Appearance	Disappearance
Moro	Hold the infant, supporting the head and neck with one hand and the buttocks and lower legs with the other; lower head by several cm, suddenly, being careful not to hyperextend	1. Sudden, symmetrical abduction of arms and shoulders 2. Elbows extend 3. Hands open with semiflexion of index finger and thumb to form a C 4. Arms return over body with clasping motion	Birth	Diminishment in 3 or 4 mo, disappearance by 6 mo
Startle	Expose to loud noise, sudden position change (see Moro testing); jar crib	Similar to Moro but hands are clenched	Birth	4 mo
Tonic neck	Hold the infant supine and turn the head to one side so the jaw is over the shoulder	1. Extension of arm and leg on the side to which head is turned 2. Flexion of opposite arm and leg	Birth	3–4 mo
Stepping (dancing or walking)	Hold infant under axillae, allowing feet to contact firm surface	Legs move up and down as though infant were walking	Birth	4 mo
Placing	Hold infant under axillae and move one foot to touch the edge of a table	Flexion of knee and hip, and placement of stimulated foot on table surface	Best after 4 days	Variable
Palmar grasping	Place finger or small object in infant's palm	Fingers curl tightly around finger or object	Birth	4 mo
Plantar grasping	Place thumb firmly against ball of infant's foot	Plantar flexion (curling) of all toes	Birth	12 mo
Babinski	Stroke lateral aspect of foot from heel toward little toe with tongue blade or other edged object	Big toe rises (dorsiflexion) and other toes fan out (positive Babinski sign)	Birth	24 mo
Rooting	Touch edge of infant's mouth or lightly stroke cheek	Mouth opens, and head turns toward stimulus	Birth	Usually 4 mo, but variable
Sucking	Touch infant's lips	Sucking movements	Birth	3–4 mo
Blinking	Expose to sudden, bright light	Eyelids close	Birth	12 mo
Acoustic blinking	Expose to sudden, loud noise	Bilateral eyelid closing	Birth	Variable
Parachuting	Thrust body downward, suddenly in head-first position	Arms and fingers extend in a protective motion	4–6 mo	Indefinite
Neck righting	Turn head to one side and observe body movement	Body will turn toward same direction as neck	3 mo	
Body righting	Turn hips or shoulders to one side and observe body movement	Other body parts turn in same direction as hip or shoulder	6 mo	24–36 mo
Landau	Hold infant suspended prone, in horizontal position; raise head	Extension of legs and spine	6–8 mo	12–24 mo

*Failure to elicit a reflex may be abnormal. Try again to elicit the reflex before deciding it is absent. Persistence of reflexes beyond usual time of disappearance may indicate neurologic dysfunction. Refer infants if abnormal findings exist.

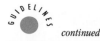 *continued*

Newborns

Procedure

(1) Assess cranial nerves III, IV, and VI by observing a blink reflex and eliciting a doll's eye response (rotation test). To check this response, hold the baby up under the axillae at arms' length facing you. Turn the body in one direction and then the other; the head is restrained by your thumbs.

(2) Assess cranial nerve V by observing the newborn's rooting and sucking reflexes.

(3) Assess cranial nerve VII.

(4) Assess cranial nerves IX and X.

Clinical Significance

Normal Findings

The eyes should turn in the same direction as the body.

Movements of the facial muscles should appear smooth, symmetric, and without tremors or spasticity.

Normal function of cranial nerve VII is indicated by wrinkling of the forehead when the baby is crying and by symmetric mouth movements.

The ability to swallow and a gag reflex indicate normal functioning of cranial nerves IX and X. Function of cranial nerve XII is required for the coordination of sucking and swallowing.

Documenting Newborn Examination Findings

Example 1: Normal Findings

S: Mother reports no difficulty with pregnancy (gravida i, para i), labor (12 hours), or delivery. Family history negative for genetic disorders. Intends to breast-feed.

O: 3 hours old, Apgar 8 at 1 minute and 10 at 5 minutes. Heart rate 142, no murmurs, respirations 40, weight 3500 g, length 50 cm, head circumference 34 cm, chest circumference 31 cm, anterior and posterior fontanel soft, good sucking reflex, mouth without defects, ears at same angle as eyes, spine intact—no hair tufts, extremities, symmetric, urinary meatus at center of glans, testes descended, meconium stool present, urinated.

A: Normal newborn

P: Provide discharge teaching to mother
  a. Care of circumcision (to be performed later)
  b. Breast-feeding
  c. Newborn care
  To be reassessed by regular health care provider in 4 weeks

Example 2: Deviation from Normal

For a complete newborn assessment a check sheet is beneficial. Normals are checked, and abnormalities are described. This is an example of this type of documentation.

S: Mother denies any difficulty with pregnancy, labor (8 h), or delivery. Two living children with no congenital defects. No history of genetic disorders.

O: See Newborn Assessment Form for normals. Heart rate 152 while sleeping; S3 heart sound loudest at third left intercostal space; lips, hands, and feet blue. Respirations 50 at rest.

A: Heart murmur needs follow-up.

P: Advise pediatrician of findings.

Clinical Problems Related to Newborn Examination

Common clinical problems related to newborns include normal physiologic jaundice (see discussion under diagnostic tests), heart murmurs, respiratory distress syndrome, prematurity (see discussion under gestational screening), and diseases transmitted from the mother. Newborns experience numerous congenital disorders; refer to any nursing pediatric textbook for a complete description of these problems.

Heart Murmurs

Heart murmurs are usually transitory (see Chap. 10 for discussion of murmurs). They are frequently heard in newborns until age 48 hours. The murmurs resolve with the transition from fetal to systemic pulmonary circulation. S3 sounds are normal and occur in 30% of all newborns; however, S4 sounds are never normal in newborns. Murmurs lasting more than 48 hours or associated with cyanosis can represent congenital heart malformations.

Respiratory Distress Syndrome

Respiratory distress syndrome occurs in newborns when the lungs are not mature. Signs of respiratory distress syndrome include difficulty with inspiration, see-saw pattern of breathing (thorax then abdominal), flaring of the nostrils, and noisy respirations. Respiratory distress syndrome can be life-threatening.

Diseases Transmitted from Mother

In utero or during delivery, neonates can be exposed to numerous diseases. Of the sexually transmitted diseases, gonorrhea can cause blindness, herpes simplex can be life-threatening, and syphilis infection can occur. The HIV virus can be transmitted (most cases of AIDS in children are a result of in utero transmission).

INFANTS

Anatomy and Physiology Overview

Infancy begins at 30 days of life and continues until age 1 year. During this time, the infant will triple birth weight and grow about 9 inches. The infant will go from a completely dependent being to an interactive being that can sit alone, crawl, possibly walk, feed self, and express wants and dis- pleasures. Infancy is marked by rapid and predictable growth and development. Maturation of organs occurs so that the infant can digest foods other than milk, the im- mune system can provide some protection, and heart and respiratory rates are no longer irregular. Muscles and re- flexes develop so the infant can pinch, scribble, swallow solid foods, and protect self when falling. This is the great- est growth and development age for the individual; there- fore, frequent assessment of growth and development is necessary to detect possible problems early.

Physical Examination　　*Infants*

General Principles

The approach used in assessing infants depends on the age of the baby. Before age 6 months, the infant may be assessed on an examining table in much the same manner as a newborn. Babies at this age are not generally afraid of strangers and will quickly forget the more intrusive parts of the assessment. After age 6 months, the infant is more fearful of strangers and may be anxious about separation from the parent. As the infant develops better body control, he or she may become uncooperative. Therefore, the assessment may be less threatening if the infant is held on the parent's lap as much as possible. Clothing need only be removed to assess specific body parts. Your conversation will be directed mostly toward the parents if the baby is less than 6 months old, and will include both parents and child after age 6 months. For older in- fants, try to create a game-like atmosphere to encourage cooperation. Performing the DDST2 before the physical examination often provides the infant a chance to get used to surroundings, and many examination findings can be observed.

The cardiovascular and respiratory systems should be evaluated when the infant is quiet; this may occur at any time during the assessment. Intrusive procedures, such as assessment of the ears and throat, and laboratory testing should probably be per- formed at the end of the assessment.

The American Academy of Pediatrics (1988) recommends the following components for health assessment of infants: interval history, height and weight, head circumfer- ence, vision and hearing by history, development screening, a complete physical as- sessment, hemoglobin (9 months), immunizations, urinalysis (6 months), and anticipa- tory guidance. Health assessment of infants should occur at ages 2, 4, 6, 9, and 12 months.

Preparation

The infant should be examined when the parent is present and comfortable. Adequate lighting and sufficient chairs are essential. Parents should be advised of what you will be doing. Privacy is important so that parents can feel free to ask questions. The room should be sufficiently warm so that the infant will not chill.

Equipment

- Measuring tape for length and head circumference
- Scale
- Stethoscope
- Otoscope and ophthalmoscope
- Tongue blade
- Equipment to measure blood pressure
- DDST2 Kit
- Materials necessary for hemoglobin and urinalysis testing

Examination and Documentation Focus

- Assess growth and development
- Identify deviation from normal
- Identify risk factors
- Monitor any deviations for improvement or worsening or no change

Examination Guidelines *Infants*

There are many similarities between newborn and infant assessment. Some findings are the same; others change as a result of growth and development. For some procedures you will be referred to Examination Guidelines for the newborn or to other sections.

Procedure

1. ANTHROPOMETRIC MEASUREMENTS.

   1. Measure the head and chest circumference, using the same procedure as for newborns. Older infants may be afraid of the tape measure; have the parent assist you in restraining arm if necessary, and perform as quickly and as accurately as possible.

   2. Measure height and weight to evaluate physical growth. Chart all measurements on an appropriate growth chart; this will allow you to evaluate growth according to standardized ranges and determine the child's own growth curve.

2. EXAMINE THE HEAD.

   a. Inspect the cranial scalp, hair, face, and ear pinnae. Note the symmetry of facial structures as the baby cries or smiles.

   b. Palpate the fontanelles.

   c. Assess the eyes.

   (1) Evaluate visual acuity. Much of visual acuity can be tested while performing the DDST2. The funduscopic assessment may be difficult or impossible to perform if the infant is uncooperative. To focus on the retina, the initial lens settings on the ophthalmoscope should be between 0 and 5 diopters. If you are unable to perform a funduscopic assessment, test for the red reflex, corneal light reflex, and pupillary constriction and blinking.

   (2) Assess lacrimal apparatus.

   (3) Assess eye color.

Clinical Significance

Normal Findings
The head circumference normally increases by 1.5 cm each month for the first 6 months and by 0.5 cm per month between 6 and 12 months. Chest circumference is almost equal to head circumference by age 12 months.

Normal Findings
Birth weight should double by 5–6 months and triple by 9–12 months. Height should increase by 50% by 12 months.

Normal Findings
The face, skull, and hair distribution should be fairly symmetric. The amount of scalp hair varies.

Normal Findings
The posterior fontanelles should be closed by age 2 months. The anterior fontanelle is usually closed by age 18 months.

Deviations from Normal
A sunken fontanelle may indicate dehydration, whereas a bulging fontanelle may indicate increased intracranial pressure. Premature closing of the anterior fontanelle is not normal.

Normal Findings
The infant's eyes should be able to rotate 180 degrees to follow an object in the field of vision by age 3 months. By age 5 months the infant will focus on objects that are 3 feet away or further. Normally, infants have full binocular vision, depth perception, and visual acuity of 20/100.

Deviations from Normal
Inability to follow or fix the eyes on objects may be abnormal. Strabismus may be noted at age 3 months but should resolve by age 6 months. Persistence of strabismus after 6 months is abnormal and should be evaluated. Internal eye structures appear smaller than they would in the adult, and the macula is poorly developed and not discernible until age 1 year. Blinking is frequent and bilateral.

Deviations from Normal
Unilateral blinking is considered abnormal; other abnormal findings same as newborn.

Normal Findings
The lacrimal apparatus continues to develop, and true tearing begins between 1 and 2 months.

Deviations from Normal
If no tearing occurs after 2 months the lacrimal apparatus may be plugged, and additional intervention is necessary to unplug it.

Normal Findings
The infant's permanent eye color is developed by age 12 months. Bulbar conjunctiva and sclera that were blue tinged in the newborn period gradually lose this coloration. A slight yellow cast may be noted over the sclera and conjunctiva of dark-skinned infants.

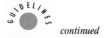
continued

Infants

Procedure

d. Inspect the ears. Assess the inner ear with the otoscope (perform this procedure near the end of the assessment because of its intrusive nature). Place the infant supine on the examining table. The parent may help restrain the baby by holding the arms over the head and holding the head between the hands. Children younger than 3 years have an upward curvature of the ear canal; therefore, pull the auricle down and back to visualize the tympanic membrane.

Using a small speculum, closely assess the tympanic membrane for abnormalities. Pneumotoscopy is performed by gently forcing air into the ear canal by squeezing a bulb that is attached to the otoscope via a small rubber tube.

Clinical Significance

Deviations from Normal

Continuation of blue coloration may indicate osteogenesis imperfecta.

Normal Findings

Findings should be the same as with adults. With pneumotoscopy the normal tympanic membrane will move in and out as positive and negative pressure is applied.

Deviations from Normal

Tympanic membrane redness, bulging, and loss of the light reflex or other landmarks are abnormal. When inflammation or fluid is behind the tympanic membrane, it will move little or not at all with penumotoscopy.

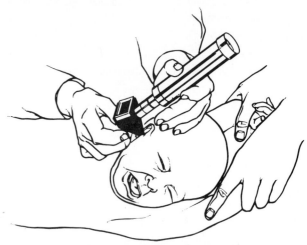

Restraining the infant during the physical examination

e. Assess oral cavity and throat. With the infant supine on an examining table or parent's lap, have the parent restrain the baby by holding arms overhead. If the infant will not open the mouth, you may hold the nose closed, which causes the mouth to open. Gently insert a tongue blade between the upper and lower teeth/gum line, moving toward the midline of the tongue. The gag reflex will be stimulated when the blade is back far enough. The infant should quickly open the mouth, and oral structures may be inspected. Use of a penlight facilitates inspection. Observe the palate, teeth, tonsils, and oral mucosa, and note any lesions.

3. EXAMINE THE CHEST AND BACK.

Assessment of the chest is similar to that in the newborn.

Normal Findings

Tooth eruption begins with the lower central by age 6 months. The pattern of tooth eruption is summarized in the accompanying display. Tonsils may seem large but should be the same color as surrounding tissue.

Deviations from Normal

Tooth eruption delayed beyond 12 months should be evaluated. Deviations for infants are the same as for newborns and adults.

Normal Findings

The cervical curve of the spine develops at age 3–4 months; lumbar curve develops and lordosis becomes evident as the baby begins to walk (12–18 months).

Deviations from Normal

Same as with newborn.

4. EXAMINE THE HEART AND LUNGS.

a. Observe the ventilatory rate and pattern.

Normal Findings

The infant has abdominal respirations at a rate of 20–40 breaths/minute. Apnea is less common in infants than in newborns.

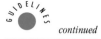

continued

Infants

Pattern of Tooth Eruption in Infants and Children

Time of eruption of deciduous teeth

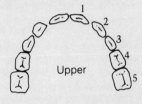

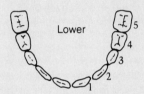

		(Upper)	(Lower)
1	Central incisor	8–12 mos.	5–9 mos.
2	Lateral incisor	8–12 mos.	12–18 mos.
3	Cuspid		18–24 mos.
4	First molar		12–18 mos.
5	Second molar		24–30 mos.

Time of eruption of permanent teeth

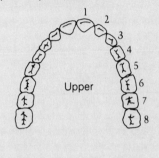

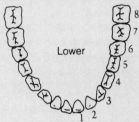

		(Upper)	(Lower)
1	Central incisor	6–7 yr.	7–8 yr.
2	Lateral incisor	7–8 yr.	8–9 yr.
3	Cuspid	9–10 yr.	11–12 yr.
4	First bicuspid	10–11 yr.	10–11 yr.
5	Second bicuspid	11–12 yr.	10–12 yr.
6	First molar	6–7 yr.	6–7 yr.
7	Second molar	11–13 yr.	12–13 yr.
8	Third molar	17 yr.	17–18 yr.

Procedure

b. Auscultate the heart and lungs while the baby is quiet, before proceeding to more intrusive procedures. The infant may remain on the parent's lap or be held in the parent's arms in a chest-to-chest position for posterior auscultation.

Auscultate heart sounds with a small-sized bell and diaphragm attachments. The infant's heart is generally in the same position as the newborn's heart; therefore, the locations of the apical impulse and auscultatory landmarks are similar (see physical assessment of newborn).

Clinical Significance

Normal Findings

The infant's heart rate ranges from 80–160 beats/minute. The heart rhythm is frequently irregular (sinus dysrhythmia), especially during sleep.

Heart sounds: A physiologic or normal third sound may be auscultated. This is most frequently heard at the second left intercostal space.

Deviations from Normal

An infant who is a poor sucker and who is gaining weight slowly may have a cardiovascular problem. Murmurs may be detected. Innocent murmurs, a soft blowing sound that is not heard in other areas, may be insignificant; however, it is difficult to determine seriousness by auscultation alone. Murmurs heard for the first time should receive further evaluation.

Normal Findings

Clear bronchovesicular breath sounds are normal.

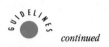

continued

Infants

Procedure

c. Measure blood pressure. With infants and some small children, it is difficult or impossible to auscultate Korotkoff's sounds without a Doppler. If a Doppler is not available, the flush method of blood pressure measurement may be used. The value obtained represents the approximate mean blood pressure. To perform the flush method, a proper-size cuff is applied to the infant's arm or leg just above the wrist or ankle. While holding the limb above the level of the heart, the hand or foot is squeezed or wrapped snugly with an elastic bandage to empty the underlying capillaries and veins. The skin below the level of the cuff will appear blanched. Inflate the cuff, then unwrap the hand or foot and allow the extremity to return to the infant's side. Slowly deflate the cuff and read the manometer when the color of the extremity changes from blanched to flushed.

5. EXAMINE THE ABDOMEN.

a. Inspect the abdominal contour and look for hernias in the supine position and as the infant is held in a standing position. Also inspect for abdominal hernias when the baby is crying. Avoid vigorous deep palpation if the baby has just finished feeding.

b. Auscultate the abdomen using appropriate bell and diaphragm.

c. Percuss the abdomen to identify abdominal organs.

6. EXAMINE EXTERNAL GENITALIA.

Place the infant supine and hold the hips abducted (frog position). Carefully inspect the genitals and perineum for skin lesions and rashes. Many findings are similar to the newborn (see Examination Guidelines for newborns).

a. Females:

   (1) Inspect labia

   (2) Inspect vaginal and urethral orifices. Part the labia with the thumb and forefinger.

   (3) Internal structures are not assessed unless molestation is suspected, and then a qualified physician should perform the assessment.

Clinical Significance

Normal Findings
Normal systolic pressure is 70–80 mm Hg.

Normal Findings
The infant's abdomen is dome shaped and moves with respiration. The diastasis recti muscle remains split as in the newborn period. A fine venous network may be observed over the abdomen. The umbilicus should appear dry and inverted.

Deviations from Normal
Visible peristaltic waves moving across the upper abdomen are abnormal and may be secondary to pyloric stenosis. Prominent venous networks along with a taut skin appearance are abnormal. In such cases, the abdomen should be transilluminated (see newborn). Umbilical eversions over 2 cm wide represent hernias and may require further evaluation. Smaller umbilical hernias, however, are common in this age group.

Normal Findings
Bowel sounds are normally heard every 10 to 30 seconds. Percussion may reveal increased tympany, which is secondary to air swallowing during feeding.

Normal Findings
After age 6 months, the liver span is 2.4–2.8 cm at the midclavicular line; by age 12 months, the span is 2.8–3.1 cm at the midclavicular line.

Normal Findings
The labia minora are more prominent than the labia majora.

Deviations from Normal
Redness and swelling of the labia may indicate sexual molestation or infection.

Normal Findings
No redness or discharge should be noted.

continued

Infants

Procedure	**Clinical Significance**

Procedure

b. Males:

   (1) Inspect penis.

   (2) Inspect and palpate scrotum. If testes are not descended, try to descend them by placing fingers over the inguinal ring and gently pushing the testes toward the scrotum.

7. EXAMINE THE ANUS AND RECTUM.

   Generally these is not assessed except externally.

8. EXAMINE THE SKIN.

   Inspect the skin as each body part is being assessed. Examine skin creases and folds carefully.

Clinical Significance

Normal Findings

Erections are common during infancy. The foreskin may not be fully retractable until age 1 year in the uncircumcised male.

Deviations from Normal

Severe inflammations of the skin of the penis may occur with diaper rash.

Normal Findings

Testes may move back and forth between the inguinal canal and scrotum until age 4 years. If the undescended testes easily descend into the scrotum, this finding may be normal.

Deviations from Normal

Hernias and hydroceles are common problems in this age group. The scrotum may appear enlarged or asymmetric. The scrotum may be transilluminated. Transillumination occurs across a hydrocele (fluid) but not across hernias (mass). Failure to palpate or descend the testes is abnormal and should be evaluated.

Normal Findings

Infant should be having bowel movements without difficulty; there should be no anal fissures or tears.

Normal Findings

The skin should be moist, have good turgor, and be without blemishes.

Deviations from Normal

Any scars, bruises, or abrasions in various stages of healing, particularly above the knees and below the elbows and in the diaper area, may indicate child abuse. Skin pallor and cyanosis are abnormal in the infant. Pallor may be a sign of anemia. Cyanosis is often associated with congenital malformations of the heart or great vessels. The most common skin deviations in infants include the following:

- *Diaper dermatitis* (diaper rash) is noted early as erythema in the diaper area. If severe, papules and skin excoriation may be noted. The skin folds in the inguinal and gluteal areas are especially sensitive to the irritating effects of urine. Secondary infections with Candida (yeast) may occur. Candida lesions appear as bright red, circumscribed, scaling patches. Satellite lesions may be present.

- *Seborrheic dermatitis* (cradle cap) appears on the scalp or diaper area as flat, adherent, greasy scales. This condition is fairly common, and exact causes are unknown; however, a relationship to infrequent shampooing of the hair may exist. Secondary bacterial infection may occur, especially if pruritus causes scratching of the lesions.

- *Atopic dermatitis* (eczema) is noted in infants with skin hypersensitivity and allergic tendencies. Exposure to various allergens, irritants, moisture, temperature changes, excessive dryness, and even fear and stress can cause the skin to itch intensely. Itching causes scratching, and eventually the skin develops eczematous lesions and lichenification. Eczematous lesions appear as erythematous papules and vesicles that may have a discharge and become crusted. In infants, eczema usually appears on the face and in skin folds.

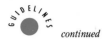

continued

Infants

Procedure

9. ASSESS MUSCULOSKELETAL STRUCTURES AND FUNCTIONS.
   The musculoskeletal system is best evaluated with the infant supine and unclothed except for a diaper.

   a. Examine the upper extremities. Assess the upper extremities and the manner in which the infant uses the hands and fingers. Many of the hand and finger functions can be evaluated during the administration of the DDST2 (see Appendix D).

   b. Examine the lower extremities. The infant's hips should be assessed for dislocation and deformities at every health assessment until age 1 year. The diaper should be removed for this assessment. Perform Ortolani's and Barlow's tests (see Examination Guidelines for newborns).

   c. Assess other musculoskeletal functions. Move the infant through several position changes to evaluate other musculoskeletal functions.

   (1) First, gently pull the infant from the supine to the sitting position. If necessary, prop the infant into a sitting position.

   d. Test appropriate reflexes for the infant's age (see previous display, "Newborn and Infant Reflex Evaluation").

Clinical Significance

Normal Findings
The hands will be held in tight fists until after age 1 month, when they are held loosely fisted. The infant's grasp should be strong and equal. After age 3 months, the infant can hold objects placed in the hands, and by age 4 months, objects in the hands will be taken directly toward the mouth. At age 5 months, the infant will voluntarily grasp objects and clasp the hands together. Objects will be transferred from one hand to the other by 7 months. The ability to pick up objects between the thumb and forefinger (pincer grasp) begins to develop at age 8 months. The ability to hold a crayon is developed by age 11 months.

Deviations from Normal
Bone dislocations may be the result of pulling, lifting, or twirling the infant up by the arms.

Deviations from Normal
Other indicators of hip problems include asymmetry of hip abduction, unequal leg lengths, and unequal skin creases and folds of the legs. The legs have a bow-legged appearance throughout infancy.

Normal Findings
By age 4 months the infant can maintain balance when propped. Observe the infant's ability to maintain the position, hold the head upright, and control back position. Most infants can sit unsupported by 6–7 months. Crawling movements begin by age 6 months. By age 7 months, greater mobility is possible by crawling. By 9 months most infants begin to pull themselves to a standing position and stand easily by holding onto something. Walking by holding onto furniture may be observed at age 11 months. Momentary standing without support occurs by age 1 year, and most infants walk unsupported by 14 months.

Normal Findings
Infants will lose various reflexes during this time period, such as tonic neck and Moro. However, they will gain new reflexes such as neck righting, Landau, and parachuting. Persistence of reflexes beyond normal time of disappearance or failure to elicit new reflexes at the appropriate age may indicate neurologic defects.

Documenting Infant Examination Findings

Example 1: 9-Month-Old Male

S: Mother states happy baby, standing unsupported, eats three meals/day, breast-feeds four times a day for 20 minutes, plans to wean to cup in next 2 to 3 months. No specific problems.

O: Normal DDST2—see form. Weight for height at 50th percentile, weight and height in 75th percentile—see chart. Urine negative for glucose, protein, and red blood cells and white blood cell counts. No abnormal physical findings—see exam check sheet.

A: Normal growth and development

P: Return in 3 months for follow-up. Anticipatory teaching: safety precautions for 9 to 12 months and weaning to cup.

Example 2: Deviations from Normal

S: Has been fussy all night, unusual, pulling at right ear, has had a cold for 2 days. Here for regular 6-month check up and immunizations.

O: Temperature 100. Right ear: tympanic membrane bulging and red, fluid present. Left ear: tympanic membrane red around edges, no fluid or bulging, landmarks and light reflex present. Green nasal discharge, nasal membranes bright red. Normal lung sounds—no crackles or wheezes.

A: Suspect otitis media

P: Refer to nurse practitioner in clinic this AM. Defer developmental testing and immunizations until well. Mother will reschedule appointment in 2 weeks.

Clinical Problems Related to Infant Examination

The most common clinical problems of infants are otitis media, upper respiratory infections, diaper rash, allergies, and colic.

Otitis Media

A discussion of otitis media is in Chapter 10. Infants are at high risk for otitis media because their eustachian tubes have a horizontal connection between the inner ear and the pharynx. As the child ages, this tube becomes more vertical.

Upper Respiratory Infections

Upper respiratory infections with accompanying otitis media occur frequently in infants. Most upper respiratory infections are viral and are either nasopharyngitis (involve nose and pharynx) or pharyngitis (throat and tonsils). Elevated temperature, cough, and runny nose (rhinitis) are common. Parents should avoid the use of aspirin because of the risk of Reyes syndrome (acute encephalopathy with degeneration and a high mortality rate). Types of lower respiratory infections include *bronchitis* (an inflammation of

the bronchi almost always occurs with upper respiratory problems) and *pneumonia* (an inflammation of the lungs can be viral or bacterial).

Diaper Rash

Diaper rash or diaper dermatitis results from urine and feces excoriating the skin. If urine and feces are allowed to remain on the skin, denudement and bacterial infection may occur. Plastic pants and plastic covers on disposable diapers increase warmth and decreases air circulation, enhancing conditions that promote dermatitis. Prompt changing of the diaper and adequate cleansing will inhibit diaper dermatitis.

Allergies

The most common allergy of infants is to foods. The major foods causing allergies are eggs, wheat, vegetables, and fruit. When infants start eating more foods, they are exposed to numerous new antigens and the immature intestinal tract absorbs many of these antigens, producing allergic reactions. As the intestinal tract matures, the infant may outgrow some food allergies. Symptoms of food allergies include rash, irritability, diarrhea, abdominal bloating, flatus, and respiratory coughing or wheezing. Food allergies can be controlled by avoiding foods that cause allergic reactions.

Colic

Colic is a paroxysmal abdominal pain or cramping. Infants with colic have loud crying, are irritable, and draw legs up to the abdomen; they are not easily comforted. Colic is more common in infants under age 3 months. The exact cause of colic is unknown. Parents become very frustrated with the daily routine of colic, have guilt feelings about not being able to relieve infant, and become irritable from lack of sleep and prolonged crying of infant.

YOUNG CHILDREN

Anatomy and Physiology of Young Children

This section includes the toddler (12 mo to 3 y) and the preschool child (3 to 6 y). This is the age of upright locomotion, self-expression, autonomy, and gaining independence in self-care. Physical growth is slower than that which occurs in the infant. The average weight gain for this period is about 20 pounds (about 4 to 6 pounds/year) and height gain is about 15 inches (about 3 inches/year). The head is smaller in proportion to body size, and about age 5, children can place their arm over their heads and touch their ears. Most organs are fairly mature by this age. The liver and intestines are functioning. Reproductive organs, however, are still immature.

Although physical growth has slowed, cognitive development is rapidly progressing. The ability to speak and comprehend language increases dramatically. Children learn to count, distinguish and name colors, and define simple concepts such as what is a ball or lake. Young children like to explore and discover their world. Play is a major component of these children's lives; during play, they learn roles and develop fine and gross motor movement.

Physical Examination | *Young Children*

General Principles

Children between the ages of 1 and 5 years may be the most challenging to assess because of their fear of strangers, fear of bodily injury, and the need to be in control of the situation. Some of the child's anxiety may be alleviated by talking to the child and parents throughout the assessment. You should inform the child of what you are about to do (*e.g.,* "Now I'm going to look at your tummy"). Engaging the child in a story or game may also be helpful. Older children in this age group may be anxious because they anticipate an injection. If the child asks about this possibility, honest discussion should be encouraged.

It may be helpful to demonstrate the use of equipment on the parent, a doll, or yourself to ease the child's fears. For example, place the blood-pressure cuff on the parent before using it on the child. Allow the child to handle equipment as much as possible. Using the equipment in a playful manner is also helpful. For example, allow the child to "blow out" the light on the otoscope. Let the child listen through the stethoscope to body sounds.

Younger children may feel more comfortable sitting on the parent's lap during most of the assessment. Older children may cooperate on the examining table with the parent at their side. Although it is optimal to assess children completely unclothed except for underwear, for more modest children, clothing may be removed only as necessary. You should ask the parent's permission to remove the child's underclothes. You can use this opportunity to teach both child and parent about the child's rights and protection from molestation.

The use of screening tests such as the DDST2 may be the most effective way to evaluate neurologic functions as well as fine and gross motor skills in this age group. The DDST2 may be performed at the beginning of the assessment to establish rapport and a game-like atmosphere.

As is the case when assessing babies, the more intrusive parts of the assessment should be performed last. You may wish to listen to heart and lung sounds at the beginning of the assessment when the child is quiet.

You should prepare the child for uncomfortable or painful procedures such as finger pricks. Talking to the child during uncomfortable procedures is helpful. Often the child can be distracted from discomfort with talking, singing, adhesive bandages, and stickers.

Restraint

Occasionally, it becomes necessary to restrain a young child while performing more intrusive procedures such as assessing the ears and oral cavity. You may use one of the following positions: (1) lying prone with arms restrained at side and head secured by another, (2) lying supine with arms over head and head secured, or (3) sitting on the parent's lap with the arm restrained and head held against the parent's chest and the legs restrained by the parent's legs. To avoid trauma to the ear canal, immobilize the child's head during otoscopic assessment if the child is unable to cooperate.

The American Academy of Pediatrics (1988) recommends the following components for the health assessment of young children: interval history, height and weight, blood pressure beginning at age 3, vision and hearing by observation and history until age 4 and then by a standard testing method, development and behavior assessment, physical assessment, immunizations, tuberculin test at 24 months, urine analysis at 24 months, anticipation guidance, and initial dental referral at 3 years. The scheduling of assessment should be at ages 15, 18, and 24 months and then yearly.

Preparation

Having an enclosed room available that is well lit, has chairs and appropriate size for child, and is safe for the wandering toddler and preschool child is preferred. All equipment should be out of the reach of the child. A DDST is best performed in an area where tables and chairs appropriate for the child are available, or in an area where the child can sit on the parent's lap.

Equipment	• Scale
	• Chart to measure height
	• Vision screening equipment (age 4 and above)
	• Hearing screening equipment (age 4 and above)
	• Stethoscope
	• Otoscope and ophthalmoscope
	• Pediatric blood-pressure cuff
	• Tongue blade
	• DDST2 kit
Examination and Documentation Focus	• Assess growth and development.
	• Identify deviation from normal.
	• Identify risk factors.
	• Monitor any deviations for improvement or worsening or no change.

Examination Guidelines   *Young Children*

Perform developmental screening tests before physical examination. Only those physical findings that differ from those for adults are discussed in this section.

Procedure	**Clinical Significance**
1. ANTHROPOMETRIC MEASUREMENTS.	
a. Measure height and weight. If the child is walking, standing height measurement is preferred over lying length. When the child's height as opposed to length is measured, a new graphic form for height and weight should be utilized.	***Normal Findings*** Weight should be proportional for height.
b. Head and chest circumference may continue to be evaluated until the child is 3 years old.	***Normal Findings*** Chest circumference exceeds head circumference at 24 months.
2. EXAMINE THE HEAD. Most assessments of shape and hair distribution are the same as for adults.	
a. Examine the eyes.	
(1) Inspect the external eye. Perform the cornea light reflex test by shining a light approximately 13 inches level with the eye brows; observe where the light falls.	***Normal Findings*** The external eye should have a similar appearance in adults and children. ***Deviations from Normal*** Strabismus may be noted in this age group. In a child without strabismus, the light should be observed in the center of each pupil. It is important to test for strabismus to prevent blindness in one eye secondary to amblyopia.
(2) Ophthalmoscopic assessment is difficult to perform on children in this age group. Determine if the red reflex is present. If child cooperates, the macula and retinal vessels may be visualized.	***Normal Findings*** The retina and macula should appear similar to the fundus of the adult. A red reflex should occur.
(3) Assess visual acuity. Refractive visual errors do occur in young children, so evaluation of visual acuity is an important part of the assessment. The traditional Snellen chart needs to be modified for this age group, although the procedure for Snellen testing is similar to that used with adults. The child may not be able to cooperate until age 3–4 years. The 3-year-old child should be screened for visual problems with an "HOTV" chart. At age 4 some children can use the illiterate "E" version.	***Normal Findings*** Visual acuity at age 3–4 years is 20/40; by age 5 it is 20/30.

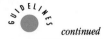

continued

Young Children

Procedure

b. Examine the ears. The child may need to be restrained while assessing the ears. Children under 3 years have an upward curvature of the ear canal; therefore, you should pull the lower auricle down and back to visualize ear structures. For older children use the same techniques as for the adult to visualize the ear structures. The speculum is inserted only ½ to ¼ inch in young children because their ear canal is short. Use the largest speculum the ear will accommodate.

Clinical Significance

Normal Findings

The appearance of the ear and related structures is similar in all age groups.

Deviations from Normal

If fluid in the inner ear is suspected or if the child is not hearing well by history or standardized testing, determine if the tympanic membrane is mobile (see pneumotoscopy in the Examination Guidelines for infants for technique).

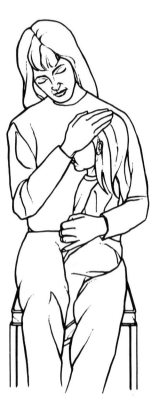

Restraining the young child during the physical examination

c. Assess the oral cavity and nose. Children in this age group may perceive this part of the assessment as threatening and refuse to cooperate. In some cases, it may be necessary to restrain the child. If the child will not open the mouth, hold the nares shut. When the mouth opens, insert the tongue blade to elicit a gag reflex. Quickly visualize the mouth and throat as the mouth opens.

d. Examine the throat and neck.

(1) Palpate the cervical lymphatic structures.

(2) Inspect the tonsils.

Normal Findings

Assessment findings are similar in infants and young children (see Examination Guidelines for infants).

Deviations from Normal

Children in this age group frequently have upper respiratory infections associated with otitis media and enlarged tonsils.

Deviations from Normal

Tender lymph nodes may be an indication of infection.

Normal Findings

Tonsils may seem enlarged but should be the same color as surrounding tissue.

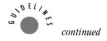

continued

Young Children

Procedure	Clinical Significance

Procedure

3. EXAMINE THE HEART AND LUNGS.

   a. Ausultate the chest. Auscultation will be easiest when the child is cooperative and quiet. Use smaller stethoscope attachments for children.

   b. Percuss the chest.

   c. Measure and evaluate blood pressure and peripheral pulses. At age 3 all children should have blood pressure measured at regular intervals. In some small children it is difficult or impossible to auscultate Korotkoff's sounds. If this is the case, the flush method of blood pressure measurement may be used (see blood pressure measurement in Examination Guidelines for infants).

4. ASSESS THE ABDOMEN.

   a. Inspect the abdomen. The general appearance of the abdomen should be observed while the child is standing, sitting, or playing in the room. Assessment of the 4- or 5-year-old may be easier with the child on the examination table rather than on the parent's lap.

   b. Percuss and palpate the liver.

Clinical Significance

Normal Findings

The average heart rate in 2-year-olds is 80 to 130 beats/minute; from 3 to 5 years it is 80 to 120 beats/minute. An irregular heart rhythm characterized by a higher rate during inspiration than expiration (sinus dysrhythmia) is normal in young children. At the second left intercostal space, a splitting of the second heart sound is common in young children. *Breathing pattern:* Young children continue to have an abdominal breathing rate of 20 to 40 breaths/minute.

Normal Findings

The lung percussion note is slightly more resonant than that noted in the adult.

Normal Findings

The blood pressure reading should be less than 116/76 for children up to 5 years. Peripheral pulses should be palpable with as 3+ quality when graded on a 4-point scale. Pulses should be equal bilaterally.

Deviations from Normal

If a child has two consecutive readings above 116/76 after a 5-minute rest period, additional evaluation is necessary. In children, hypertension is most commonly related to kidney disorders.

Normal Findings

Young children have a rounded abdomen (potbelly appearance) in standing and supine positions that appears exaggerated secondary to lordosis. Any splitting of the diastasis rectus muscle begins to resolve at this age.

Deviations from Normal

Umbilical hernias that were present during infancy begin to resolve in light-skinned children by age 2 years and in black children by age 6 or 7 years.

Normal Findings

The liver span at the mid axillary line is 3.5–3.6 cm at age 2 years and 4.3–4.4 cm at 4 years. The liver may normally be palpable 1 or 2 cm below the costal margin in this age group. Use only one hand to palpate the liver.

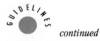

continued

Young Children

Procedure

5. EXAMINE THE GENITALS.

   a. Inspect the external genitals. A pelvic assessment is rarely performed on young girls and requires special instruments as well as expertise. The child less than 3 years of age may assume the frog-leg position. Older children may be seated on the examination table. The head is raised 30 degrees so the child may comfortably lean against the table while assuming a frog-leg position. The child may be modest and feel more comfortable with a drape. Boys older than 3 years may sit on a chair or table in the tailor position, with the knees bent and feet flat or knees bent and ankles crossed.

6. EXAMINE MUSCULOSKELETAL FUNCTIONS.

   a. Musculoskeletal functions can be evaluated during the DDST2 and by watching the child playing or moving around the room. Asking the child to demonstrate activities such as hopping on one foot, throwing a ball, and getting onto a chair will help you evaluate muscle development and skeletal functions.

   b. Note muscle strength, hands, and nails as you would for an adult.

   c. Examine the hips and lower extremities. Evaluation of the hips for deformities or dislocation continue as routine screening until age 4.

7. PERFORM A NEUROLOGIC EXAMINATION.
   The young child will not be able to cooperate with neurologic testing; however, the 3- to 4-year-old will cooperate with testing if in a game.

Clinical Significance

Normal Findings
The appearance of external genitals is similar to that noted during infancy (see Examination Guidelines for infants).

Deviations from Normal
By 4 years any male whose testicles are not continuously descended into the scrotum should be evaluated by a physician for possible treatment.

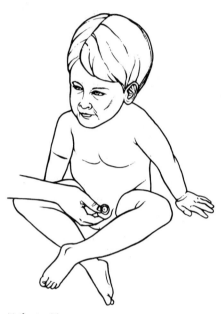

Tailor position

Normal Findings
The young child has spinal lordosis, but becomes less noticeable as the child grows. The child should be able to get up from a supine to a standing position without having to place the hands on the thighs for extra leverage.

Deviations from Normal
The inability to get into a standing from a supine position could indicate certain types of muscular dystrophy.

Deviations from Normal
Children with cardiovascular problems may have clubbing of the fingers.

Normal Findings
The bow-legged appearance of infancy disappears by age 2 to 3 years. A knock-kneed appearance is normal between the ages of 2 and 4. Feet pronation is common until age 30 months. The arch of the foot develops by age 3 years. When checking the feet, also observe the child's shoes for patterns of wear and proper fit.

Normal Findings
Neurologic findings should be similar to those for adults.

Documenting Young Child Examination Findings

Example 1: Normal Findings

S: No problems; in for regular 3-year-old visit, eats three meals per day but is now a picky eater, plays house with other children.

O: Normal DDST2—see sheet. No deviations from normal noted—see exam check list. Has remained at 60% for height and weight—see chart. Urine negative for protein glucose, red blood cells and white blood cell count. Immunizations up to date.

A: Normal growth and development

P: Return in 1 year for health assessment. Return to clinic as needed for illness or problems. Anticipatory teaching—safety ages 3 to 4.

Example 2: Deviation from Normal

S: Child 4 years old. Was 3 weeks premature, Apgar 6 and 8. Discharged from hospital at 5 days. Mother doesn't remember anything "really" being wrong with Mike. Quiet child, rarely talks, and often ignores mother.

O: Only deviations reported—see exam check list and DDST2 for normals. Unable to test vision or hearing. Caution in language, unable to relate what to do if cold or tired, does not give last name. Delay—unable to follow directions of on, in front, behind, and under. DASE only correctly pronounced 14 sounds for a score in the fifth percentile.

A: Altered growth and development, language etiology unknown.

P: Refer to Speech Hearing Clinic for hearing and speech assessment.
Mother to call after speech and hearing evaluation and nurse to follow up at that time.

Clinical Problems Related to Examination of Young Children

In addition to the clinical problems that occur in infancy except for colic, young children have health problems that include poisoning (usually the 2- to 3-year-old) and infectious diseases such as chicken pox and strep throat. Immunizations can prevent the infectious diseases of measles, rubella, mumps, poliomyelitis, pertussis (whooping cough), tetanus, diphtheria, *Hemophilus influenza* B, and hepatitis B.

Poisoning occurs in the young child when toxic substances such as medication, plants, household cleaning agents, and insecticides are within reach. The sense of taste is not well developed in the toddler, and one means to explore the world is to taste it. Poisoning is preventable, and parents should receive anticipatory guidance regarding how to childproof their homes.

Chicken pox is the only childhood disease for which there is no immunization. It is caused by the *Varicella zoster* virus, which causes shingles in adults. It has a 14- to 21-day incubation period. Communicability usually begins 1 day prior to eruption of lesions to when vesicles have developed crusts. There is a slightly elevated temperature, fatigue, and anorexia for the first 24 hours followed by highly pruritic (itchy) rash. The rash begins as a macule, and progresses to a papule and then to a vesicle.

Strep throat is caused by the group A beta-hemolytic *Streptococcus*. If untreated, it can progress to scarlet fever and cause complications or rheumatic fever with corresponding heart and glomerulus damage. Incubation is approximately 10 days. It begins with a sore throat usually covered with white patches. A throat culture should be performed with all suspicious sore throats. Treatment is usually a full course of penicillin or erythromycin.

OLDER CHILDREN AND ADOLESCENTS

Anatomy and Physiology Overview

The school years generally refer to the period between 6 and 12 years, and adolescence between the ages of 13 and 18 to 19 years. The school-age period is a stable period and tends to be a healthy period for children. They are at lower risk for otitis media and have fewer colds. Cognitive and emotional development are the hallmarks for this group. Growth again slows, so children usually gain 3 to 6 pounds per year and add 1 to 2 inches in height per year. Males and females tend to be about the same size. Head size to body proportion continues to decrease. Muscle strength increases, and muscles continue to develop until they reach maturity in adolescence. All deciduous teeth are lost during school age. During school age and adolescence, heart and respiratory rates decrease and blood pressure increases. Life-style habits are formed in school age, and obesity with sedentary life-style in the school-age child is not uncommon.

In adolescence, one sees a re-emergence of rapid physical growth and organ development. Final growth is generally attained in adolescents. During a growth spurt, young men can grow 4 to 12 inches and add 15 to 65 pounds, whereas young women increase in height 2 to 8 inches and add 15 to 55 pounds. Stature growth generally ceases in young men at age 20 and in young women at age 17. By the end of the adolescence, all organs are physiologically mature. The reproductive system becomes fully operational. Adolescent response to physical and physiologic changes can cause stress and moodiness.

Physical Examination

Older Children and Adolescents

General Principles

Older children and adolescents usually cooperate during the physical assessment; therefore, the assessment may be performed in a manner similar to adults. Thorough assessment of the neurologic and musculoskeletal systems may be performed in the same manner in this age group as in adults. Less concern exists about performing intrusive procedures such as the ear and throat assessment, at the end of the examination. Assessment of the genitals and pelvic assessment of the adolescent may represent the most distressing parts of the assessment.

School-Aged Children

The school-aged child may be cooperative during the assessment if the child knows what to expect. Although he or she may still fear receiving an injection, you can use the child's curiosity regarding his or her body and explain the function of instruments to elicit cooperation. Allowing the child to listen to body sounds is also a good teaching opportunity. The child should be dressed in underclothes and a gown for modesty, if desired. Parents may or may not be present, depending upon the wishes of the child and parent. You should assess the genitalia and teach about child molestation and primary sexual development at the end of the assessment. Laboratory tests and immunizations can also be performed at this time.

Adolescents

The adolescent may or may not wish to have parents present during the physical assessment. Such a decision may be influenced by the gender of the nurse and the parent. For example, a girl may not want her father to be present or she may want her mother present if the nurse is a man. During the assessment, teaching about health status and bodily changes that have or will occur may be beneficial. Body changes often cause the adolescent to be critical of his or her self-concept and body image. Moreover, adolescents often have unrealistic expectations about normal ranges of body development or are unaware of such changes. Assess the genitalia last, and thoroughly explain the procedure first.

The American Academy of Pediatrics (1988) recommends the following components for health assessment: interval history, height and weight, blood pressure, vision screening every 2 years, hearing screening by standardized testing at 5, 12, and 18 years and other times by history, development assessment, physical assessment, immunizations, tuberculin test at 18 years, hemoglobin and urinalysis at 8 and 18 years, and anticipatory guidance. For this age group, health assessment should occur every 2 years.

Equipment

- Scale
- Chart to measure height
- Vision screening equipment
- Hearing screening equipment
- Stethoscope
- Otoscope and ophthalmoscope
- Pediatric and/or adult blood pressure cuff
- Tongue blade
- Pen light
- If pelvic examination: vaginal speculum, gloves, water-soluble lubricant, hand-held mirror, goose neck lamp, glass slides, sterile cotton-tip applicators, wooden spatulae, and fixative

Examination and Documentation Focus

- Assess growth and development.
- Identify deviation from normal.
- Identify risk factors.
- Monitor any deviations for improvement or worsening or no change.
- Assess secondary sexual changes and sexual maturity.

Examination Guidelines *Older Children and Adolescents*

The school-age and older child is able to cooperate with the nurse during the physical examination. Findings become more like those for the adult. Only those findings and assessment techniques that vary from adults are discussed in this section.

Procedure	Clinical Significance

1. ANTHROPOMETRIC MEASUREMENTS.
 	
  a. Measure weight and height.
  b. Muscle circumference and skinfold thickness may be evaluated.
	Deviations from Normal
	Be alert for rapid weight changes. Excessive weight loss or inadequate weight gain may be signs of anorexia nervosa or bulimia.

2. EXAMINE THE HEAD. The assessment of the head is the same as in adults. a. Examine the eyes. Assess the eyes and evaluate visual acuity. This assessment is essential to ensure optimal visual acuity during cognitive development and learning. The assessment is conducted in a manner similar to that of adults. Older children will usually cooperate, follow instructions during evaluation of eye movements and visual acuity, and focus their eyes as instructed by the nurse. Children who wear corrective lenses should be tested with lenses on. Inquire as to when the last refractive change occurred. Be sure to ask about contact lenses before performing eye assessment.	***Normal Findings*** Ophthalmoscopic findings are the same as for adults. Visual acuity is 20/30 until age 8 to 10 and becomes 20/20 by age 9 or 10.
b. Examine the ears. Assess the ears in the same manner as you would for the adult. The ear pinnacle is pulled upward and outward during the otoscopic assessment. Hearing acuity is also tested, either by standard testing or the whisper test.	***Normal Findings*** Should be similar to those in the adult.
c. Examine the oral cavity. Children in this age group usually will cooperate with assessment of the oral cavity. If the child is extremely anxious, demonstrate the procedure on the parent. Inquire about teeth brushing, flossing, and regular dental assessments.	***Normal Findings*** Assessment findings are similar to those noted in adults.
d. Examine the neck. Carefully palpate the cervical lymph nodes.	***Normal Findings*** Nodes should not be enlarged.
3. EXAMINE THE HEART AND LUNGS. a. Perform auscultation, percussion, and inspection as for the adult.	***Normal Findings*** The heart rate at 6 years is 75 to 115 beats/minute, with the average being 95. From age 7 years to adolescence the heart rate is 70 to 110 beats/minute, with the average being 85. Older adolescents have heart rates similar to those of adults at 60 to 100 beats/minute, with the average being 82. The respiratory range for this age group should be 16 to 20 beats/minute. Abdominal breathing is observed until age 6 or 7 years. After this age, girls begin to develop a thoracic pattern, whereas boys continue to have an abdominal pattern.
b. Measure blood pressure.	***Normal Findings*** For children ages 6 to 9 years, blood pressure should be less than 122/78; ages 10 to 13, less than 130/80; girls age 14, less than 133/82; girls age 15, less than 137/85; girls 16 to 20, less than 140/85; boys 14 to 19, less than 128/84.
4. EXAMINE BREASTS. Examine female breasts as in the adult woman.	***Normal Findings*** The female breast develops to maturity during adolescence. See Table 19-2 for breast development.

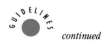

Older Children and Adolescents

Procedure

5. EXAMINE SKIN.

   Inspect the skin during the general survey and while assessing each body part.

6. EXAMINE THE ABDOMEN.

   a. Conduct the assessment of the abdomen in a manner similar to that used with adults. Ticklishness may interfere with the assessment. Placing the child's hand under yours during palpation may help reduce ticklishness. Depending upon size and abdominal musculature, you may use one or both hands for palpation.

   b. Percuss and palpate the liver.

7. EXAMINE THE GENITALS.

   Children in this age group should be assessed on an examining table and may feel more comfortable if draped. Older children and adolescents may or may not desire the parent's presence and should be given a choice after an explanation of the assessment. A frog-leg position is used for school-age children. Girls should not be placed in a lithotomy position, which may be frightening and uncomfortable. This position may be used for girls older than age 15 years. Boys may be seated and placed in the tailor position (see Examination Guidelines for younger children). Girls usually experience their first pelvic assessment during adolescence. You should explain the procedure, including any uncomfortable sensation that may be experienced (see Chap. 14). Boys should be assessed for hernias in the same manner as an adult. Prostate assessment is rarely performed on children and adolescents. Refer to Tables 19-2 and 19-3 regarding physical changes with puberty.

   a. Females:

   (1) Inspect pubic hair.

   (2) Inspect the external genitalia.

Clinical Significance

Deviations from Normal

Infectious skin disorders are noted in this age group, including impetigo, rashes, and fungal infections. Seborrhea and acne are common skin problems of adolescents.

Normal Findings

The potbelly contour may be observed in younger children in this group when the child is standing. The abdomen may have a scaphoid contour when the child is supine. All umbilical hernias should be resolved by age 7.

Normal Findings

The liver span at the midaxillary line at age 6 is 4.8 to 5.1 cm; at age 8, 5.1 to 5.5 cm; and at age 12, 9 cm. The liver may be palpated 0 to 2 cm below the costal margin in school-age children. The findings for adolescents are the same as for adults.

Normal Findings

Soft, downy hair may be first noted along the labia majora at age 9 to 12 years. Darker hair appears on the mons pubis at age 10 to 12. Abundant, coarse hair appears by age 12 to 13.

Normal Findings

The labia minora recede to their adult configuration before puberty. The clitoris is about 1 cm wide in school-age children and 2 cm wide in adolescents. The hymen membrane may develop a 1-cm opening by age 10 to 12 years. Bulging behind the hymen may indicate the presence of blood. A watery vaginal discharge may be noted 2 or 3 years before the onset of puberty. Skene's and Bartholin's glands should not be visible and should not have any associated discharge.

Deviations from Normal

With the presence of sexually transmitted diseases in older children and young adolescents or enlarged vaginal orifices, sexual abuse should be considered.

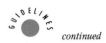
continued

Older Children and Adolescents

Procedure	Clinical Significance
b. Males: (1) Inspect pubic hair.	***Normal Findings*** Fine, downy pubic hair first appears at the base of the penis between ages 10 and 12. By age 13 darker, coarser hair is noted at the base of the penis. The distribution of pubic hair is similar to that noted in adult males between the ages of 14 and 16, with a spread to the inner thigh by age 16.
(2) Inspect the penis.	***Normal Findings*** Penil growth begins at approximately 11 years. The penis reaches adult size and shape by age 17.
(3) Inspect and palpate the scrotum.	***Normal Findings*** The scrotum enlarges starting at age 10, with the left side usually appearing longer. The scrotum reaches adult size by approximately age 17. The adolescent should be taught how to do a testicular self-examination.
9. ASSESS MUSCULOSKELETAL FUNCTION. a. Inspect and palpate the spine. It is important to evaluate the spinal configuration carefully in this age group, with an emphasis on scoliosis screening. Evaluate the child by inspecting the exposed spine with the child in standing and bending forward positions. Stand behind the child and note structural symmetry when standing. Then ask the child to bend at the waist, allowing the arms to hang forward. b. Assessment of the musculoskeletal function is similar to that in the adult, and findings are similar.	***Normal Findings*** The shoulder heights should be equal, and bony prominences such as the scapulae should be at the same horizontal level. ***Deviations from Normal*** Scoliosis is a lateral curvature of the spine. Scoliosis is most commonly noted during and after growth spurts in the adolescent.

Documenting Examination Findings

Example 1: 10-Year-Old Male

S: No problems, enjoys school, favorite subjects math and art. Occasionally has difficulty seeing blackboard. Grades are "OK." Plays soccer after school on a community team. Has one best friend of same age and gender and several other friends at school. Rarely reads but watches TV 2 to 4 hours per night. Mother states no problems, pleasant child, no colds or ear infections this year, had chicken pox last year, believes immunizations up to date.

O: Physical examination findings: no deviations except for vision—see exam check sheet. Vision on Snellen screening 20/40 right eye and 20/30 left eye. Able to follow directions, cooperative. Weight-to-height proportion has increased from 50th percentile to 60th.

A: Visual impairment possible. Weight gain greater than desired over last year.

P: Refer to eye specialist for further evaluation.
To return in 2 years for follow-up
Teaching: need to decrease empty calorie foods and increase activity, encouraged reduction in high cholesterol foods and increase in fruits and vegetables.

Example 2: 17-Year-Old Female

S: Wants to play volleyball, here for sports physical, LMP 2 weeks ago, regular cycle of 28 days, flows 5 days. Not sexually intimate with anyone. No health problems. Denies recent weight loss. Came by self.

O: Genital and pelvic examination deferred. Physical findings normal—see exam check sheet. Weight-to-height proportion 40th percentile.

A: Healthy, however possible nutritional deficiency as evidenced by low weight to height.

P: Return as needed. At next visit assess weight and height proportion and dietary intake.

Clinical Problems Related to Examination of Older Children and Adolescents

School-age children can develop the same infectious diseases as younger children. Colds, upper respiratory infections, and otitis media are less common than at younger ages. Common eye problems such as near- and far-sightedness occur (see Chap. 11).

Adolescents can experience numerous health problems. Sexually active adolescents are at risk for all sexually transmitted diseases and women are at risk for pregnancy (see Chap. 15). Other problems may include anorexia and bulimia, and drug abuse.

Anorexia nervosa is characterized by severe weight loss in the absence of a physical cause. Anorexia is more common in women, occurring most frequently around 12 to 13 years and again at 19 to 20 years. With severe weight loss, amenorrhea, bradycardia, decreased blood pressure, and cold intolerance may occur. Bulimia is a similar disorder, although severe weight loss may or may not occur. The individual may gorge herself or himself on food and then force vomiting. This disorder is more common in women; however, it has recently been recognized in men who participate in wrestling.

Drug abuse is a major concern with adolescents. Types of drugs abused include alcohol, prescription drugs, and street drugs such as crack. The use of intravenous drugs also places them at risk for HIV disease, as does prostitution to purchase drugs. Signs of drug abuse may include depression, withdrawal behavior, skipping or cutting school, change in usual behavior, friends who use drugs, and increased moodiness.

Chapter 19 SUMMARY

The health assessment of newborns, infants, children, and adolescents requires a different approach than that used for adults, and may require a different interpretation of the findings. Developmental screening in these age groups is important to determine if physical growth as well as cognitive and social abilities are proceeding as expected. Developmental screening tests such as the DDST2 are routinely administered to children less than 6 years old to detect developmental delays.

You should consider the child's fears, ability to follow directions, and physical abilities when conducting the physical assessment. Flexibility is required to accommodate each child's specific needs.

This chapter presented assessment information regarding newborns, infants, young children, and older children and adolescents. An overall knowledge base for the assessment of children was presented by functional patterns. For each age group, the following was discussed:

- Overview of anatomy and physiology
- Principles of physical examination
- Guideline for physical assessment with emphasis on difference in procedure and clinical significance for child
- Specific diagnostic studies identified
- Discussion of common clinical problems

The nursing diagnosis that applies only to children is alterated growth and development. Other nursing diagnoses that affect children are family diagnoses such as the following:

Altered parenting
Alterations in family process
Ineffective family coping

Most other nursing diagnoses can be utilized for children; however, some may not be appropriate because of the normal maturational status of young children (e.g., Incontinence and Self-care deficit).

✳ CRITICAL THINKING

Assessment of infants, children, and adolescents requires special attention to developmental stages and associated behaviors. The nurse is often required to try creative approaches to optimize the process of data collection.

Learning Exercises

1. Identify and discuss the primary similarities in assessing children and adults.

2. Explain how you would assess sexual and reproductive functions in a sexually active 13-year-old female. Create a script of the first few sentences you might say in this situation.

3. You are conducting a well-baby examination of a 16-month-old. He is crying and clings to his mother when you approach him. Describe how you would respond.

4. Explain how you would include a 5-year-old as an active participant in the health assessment process.

BIBLIOGRAPHY

Baker, C., & Wong, D. (1987). Q.U.E.S.T.: A process of pain assessment in children. *Orthopedic Nursing, 6* (1), 11–21.

Bishop, B.A. (1976). A guide to assessing parenting capabilities. *American Journal of Nursing, 76* (11), 1784–1787.

Block, G., & Nolan, J. (1986). *Health assessment for professional nursing: A developmental approach* (2nd ed.). Norwalk, CT: Appleton-Century-Crofts.

Bowlby, J. (1969). *Attachment and loss, vol. I.* New York: Basic Books.

Brazelton, P.T. (1973). *The neonatal behavioral assessment scale.* Philadelphia: J.B. Lippincott.

Carpenito, L. (1993). *Nursing diagnosis: Application to clinical practice* (5th ed.). Philadelphia: J.B. Lippincott.

Chinn, P.L. (1979). *Child health maintenance* (2nd ed.). St Louis. C.V. Mosby.

Chinn, P.L., & Leitch, C.J. (1979). *Child health maintenance: A guide to clinical assessment* (2nd ed.). St Louis: C.V. Mosby.

Clark, A.L. (1976). Recognizing discord between mother and child and changing it to harmony. *American Journal of Maternal–Child Nursing, 1* (2), 94–99.

Erikson, E.H. (1963). *Childhood and Society* (2nd ed.). New York: W.W. Norton.

Ferholt, J. (1980). *Clinical assessment of children: A comprehensive approach to primary pediatrics.* Philadelphia: J.B. Lippincott.

Fowler, J.W. (1974). Toward a developmental perspective on faith. *Religious Education, 69,* 207–219.

Frappier, P., Marino, B., & Sheshmanian, E. (1987). Nursing assessment of infant feeding problems. *Journal of Pediatric Nursing, 2* (1), 37–44.

Freiberg, K. (1992). *Human development: A life span approach* (4th ed.). Boston: Jones and Bartlett.

Hester, N.O. (1987). Health perceptions of school-age children. *Issues in Comprehensive Pediatric Nursing, 10* (3), 137–147.

Hinson, F. (1985). *Handbook of pediatric nursing.* Sydney, Australia: Williams & Wilkins.

Holmes, T.H., & Rahe, R.H. (1967). The social readjustment rating scale. *Journal of Psychosomatic Research, 11* (2), 213–218.

Hurd, J.M.L. (1975). Assessing maternal attachment: First step toward the prevention of child abuse. *Journal of Obstetric, Gynecologic, and Neonatal Nursing, 4* (4), 25–30.

Jackson, D., & Saunders, R. (1993). *Child health nursing: A comprehensive approach to the care of children and their families.* Philadelphia: J.B. Lippincott.

Kohlberg, L. (1981). *The philosophy of moral development: Moral stages and the idea of justice.* New York: Harper & Row.

McCown, D.E. (1984). Moral development in children. *Pediatric Nursing, 10,* 42.

McPherson, A., et al. (1988). What teenagers think about their health. *School Nurse, 61* (7), 224–225.

Moss, J. (1981). Helping young children cope with the physical examination. *Pediatric Nursing 7* (2), 17–20.

Mott, S., Fasekas, N., & James, S. (1990). *Nursing care of children and families: A holistic approach* (2nd ed.). Menlo Park, CA: Addison-Wesley.

Muscari, M. (1987). Obtaining the adolescent sexual history. *Pediatric Nursing, 13* (5), 307–310.

Piaget, J. (1969). *The theory of stages in cognitive development.* New York: McGraw-Hill.

Piaget, J., & Inhelder, B. (1969). *The psychology of the child.* New York: Basic Books.

Pillitteri, A. (1987). *Child health nursing: Care of the growing family* (3rd ed.). Philadelphia: J.B. Lippincott.

Pontious, S.L. (1982). Practical Piaget: Helping children understand. *American Journal of Nursing, 82* (1), 114–117.

Smith, M., et al. (1991). *Child and family: Concepts of nursing practice.* New York: McGraw-Hill.

Tauer, K.M. (1983). Promoting effective decision-making in sexually active adolescents. *Nursing Clinics of North America, 18* (2), 275–292.

Waechter, E., Phillips, J., & Holaday, B. (1985). *Nursing care of children.* Philadelphia: J.B. Lippincott.

Wieczorek, R.R., & Natapoff, J.N. (1981). *A conceptual approach to the nursing of children: Health care from birth to adolescence.* Philadelphia: J.B. Lippincott.

Zelle, R., & Coyner, A. (1983). *Developmentally disabled infants and toddlers: Assessment and intervention.* Philadelphia: F.A. Davis.

Health Assessment of Elderly Persons

Examination Guidelines

Elders

Assessment Terms

Activities of Daily Living (ADLs)
Instrumental Activities of Daily Living
   (IADLs)
Cohort Effect (Generational Effect)

Presbycusis
Osteoporosis
Kyphosis

INTRODUCTORY OVERVIEW

In many respects, the approach to assessing older persons is similar to that for observing and interviewing younger adults. Information obtained from the health history and physical examination is analyzed to evaluate functional status and to identify and monitor physical problems regardless of the person's age.

Some procedures and techniques may need to be modified when the client is older, however, especially if the person is less mobile or has some limited sensory or cognitive capacities. In addition, the assessment data should be interpreted in light of functional abilities and physical changes relative to the normal aging process.

Assessment Focus

Judgments about health status and the ability to perform activities of daily living are based upon a comprehensive assessment of an elderly individual. The individual's perceptions about and misconceptions about aging and health greatly influence the functional capability and seeking of health care when needed.

Evaluations regarding health status are based upon interview data, observations, and physical examination of the individual. In the very old or in those elders with compromising health conditions such as obstructive lung disease, the emphasis on health assessment may turn toward the physical ability to perform activities of daily living (ADLs, such as dressing, bathing, feeding, and toileting) and instrumental activities of daily living (IADLs, such as shopping, house cleaning, yard maintenance, meal preparation).

Jill Fuller and Jennifer Schaller-Ayers:
HEALTH ASSESSMENT: A NURSING APPROACH, Second Edition.
© 1990, 1994 by J. B. Lippincott Company.

The goals for assessing elders include the following:

- Obtain perception about health status.
- Assess health status.
- Identify normal changes of aging.
- Distinguish between normal aging and health problems.
- Assess ability to perform ADLs and IADLs.
- Assess medication-taking habits.

Nursing Diagnoses

No specific nursing diagnoses relate only to elders. Some nursing diagnoses do not relate to elders because of the normal aging process; these include Altered growth and development and Effective and Ineffective breast-feeding. Although we often think of elders as not having parenting responsibilities, more elders are continuing to provide care to adult children, dependent adult children (such as those with developmental disabilities and post–brain-trauma victims), and grandchildren (either as secondary or primary caregivers). Elders who obtain guardianship of grandchildren may experience intergenerational altered family process.

Elders, especially the very old (85 years and over), are at high risk for nursing diagnoses that relate to physical mobility impairment, self-care deficits, altered home management, altered health maintenance, incontinence, social isolation, and grief. Elders are also at risk for poisoning related to side effects of the numerous drugs they ingest. After very young children, elders are the next highest risk group for fire trauma and death. An elder with an acute illness is at great risk for complications such as pneumonia, which can be life-threatening.

With the very old it is not difficult to identify possible nursing diagnoses. The difficulty is in applying critical decision-making processes to select those nursing diagnoses that are primary and those that are secondary.

KNOWLEDGE BASE FOR ASSESSMENT

Difference Between Normal Aging and Pathology

Although the rate of decline may vary, irreversible, physiologic decline is an inevitable consequence of aging. Most gerontologists agree that humans begin to experience universal and progressive decline in physiologic capacities from the third decade until death. For example, longitudinal studies of aging populations provide evidence for the following age-related changes in the pulmonary system: increased residual lung volumes, decreased alveolar surface available for gas exchange, and decreased diffusion capacity across the alveolar capillary membrane. Although these physiologic changes are considered normal in the aging person, they may also be associated with disease states. For example, long-term exposure to environmental pollutants or tobacco smoke may cause similar lung changes, in which case the lung tissue should be considered diseased rather than aged. To assess the older client effectively, you must be able to distinguish such pathologic outcomes, in terms of tissue destruction or alteration that may be identical.

Tissue injury or alteration may be caused by organisms or by immunologic, chemical, or physical factors. For example, lung tissue may be irreversibly altered by the chemical and physical effects of tobacco smoke. Conversely, tissue alteration may have a genetic basis in that a key substance has been affected or omitted, such as occurs in panlobular emphysema in which a hereditary deficiency of the protein alpha-1-antitrypsin occurs. Finally, tissue alteration may be caused by intrinsic degenerative processes occurring as spontaneous biological and chemical reactions that are thermodynamically controlled. If a degenerative change occurs in all members of a population, despite diet, life-style, or genetic makeup, the change should be regarded as an aging process. Such distinctions provide the key for distinguishing pathology from normal aging.

Occasionally, an age-related physiologic change cannot be distinguished from pathologic or life-style factors because one process may be superimposed on another. For example, cardiovascular function declines with age, yet age-related changes may be difficult to distinguish from cardiovascular deconditioning associated with a sedentary life-style. Often the difficulty may be that some findings are associated with disease in younger age groups but attributed to normal aging in the elderly. For example, a 30 mm Hg increase in systolic blood pressure may signal hypertension in a 30-year-old but may be considered normal or even adaptive in an 80-year-old person.

Although aging processes should not be confused with disease processes, some physiologic aging processes, although not in themselves significant, may increase the older person's vulnerability during illness. For example, age-related declines in the pulmonary system are not causative factors for pneumonia, but pneumonia can be a more threatening illness for an older person because of age-related alterations.

Difference Between Normal Aging and a Medication Side Effect

Occasionally, you may overlook a medication effect when assessing an elderly person because adverse drug effects often mimic changes erroneously associated with aging, such as hearing loss, visual blurring, altered thought processes, muscle rigidity, and tremors. Whenever behavior or cognition changes, you should obtain a detailed drug history that includes prescribed, borrowed, or over-the-counter drugs, administration schedule, and reasons for altering recommended schedules. Furthermore, it is important to realize that some common drug side effects, such as altered thought processes, are not normal agerelated changes and require further evaluation.

Drugs commonly used by elders tend to have a narrow therapeutic range. Normal changes of aging in the kidneys, liver, gastrointestinal tract, and body fluid composition can result in toxic drug effects even if the prescribed dose is in the correct dose range. The effect of each drug separately may have been studied and is known; however, many elders experience polypharmacy (taking numerous drugs). Many elders take four prescription drugs a day (sometimes several doses of the drug are taken per day, such as twice daily). The possibility that drug interaction may produce undesirable effects is a major concern with elderly clients.

Variability of Physical Aging

Even in the absence of pathology or medication effects, physical changes associated with aging may be difficult to describe. Generally, more physical variability occurs in older persons than among younger ones. The aging process occurs at different rates and, in some cases, is modified. For example, skin wrinkling, an inevitable consequence of aging, can be affected by genetic tendencies, sun exposure, or cosmetic surgery. Chronology alone cannot be used to predict all age-related changes.

Variability exists between different age groups as well as among the same age groups. For example, many growth and development theorists classify all persons older than age 60 years as elderly or older adults, yet a 60-year-old person may differ greatly in physical appearance and abilities from a 90-year-old one. However, there may also be no differences in the health and functional status of a 60-year-old person and a 90-year-old person.

Illness in Elderly Persons: Altered Presentations

Physical signs and symptoms of illness may differ between younger and older age groups. Because the older person's signs and symptoms tend to deviate from the usual, diagnosis of some conditions may be more difficult. For example, ischemic-quality chest pain is one of the hallmarks of myocardial infarction. Elderly persons do not always experience this type of chest pain during myocardial infarction, however, or the location of the pain is atypical, and they may report pain as abdominal instead of precordial. For some elderly persons experiencing acute myocardial infarction, dyspnea may be the only symptom.

Conversely, the older person may have symptoms typically associated with a pathologic process yet without associated pathology. For example, the older person may experience voiding frequency, nocturia, urgency, and dysuria, which are classic symptoms of urinary tract infection. The person may be free of infection, however, and such symptoms may represent structural alterations of the genitourinary system. Confusion and incontinence may be the only indications of urinary tract infection in elderly persons. Table 20-1 shows additional variations in pathologic presentations in older persons.

Health Perception and Health Management

Because people are living longer, the health concerns of older adults and possible health promotion activities for

Table 20–1. Altered Presentations in the Elderly

Problem	Classic Presentation in Young Patient	Presentation in Elders
Urinary tract infection	Dysuria, frequency, urgency, nocturia	Dysuria often absent; frequency, urgency, nocturia sometimes present. Incontinence, confusion, anorexia are other signs
Myocardial infarction	Severe substernal chest pain, diaphoresis, nausea, shortness of breath	Sometimes no chest pain, or atypical pain location such as in jaw, neck, shoulder. Shortness of breath may be present. Other signs are tachypnea, arrhythmia, hypotension, restlessness, syncope
Pneumonia (bacterial)	Cough productive of purulent sputum, chills and fever, pleuritic chest pain, elevated white blood count	Cough may be productive, dry, or absent; chills and fever, and elevated white count also may be absent. Tachypnea, slight cyanosis, confusion, anorexia, nausea and vomiting, tachycardia may be present.
Congestive heart failure	Increased dyspnea (orthopnea, paroxysmal nocturnal dyspnea), fatigue, weight gain, pedal edema, night cough and nocturia, bibasilar rates	All of the manifestations of young adult or anorexia, restlessness, confusion, cyanosis, falls
Hyperthyroidism	Heat intolerance, fast pace, exophthalmos, increased pulse, hyperreflexia, tremor	Slowing down (apathetic hyperthyroidism), lethargy, weakness, depression, atrial fibrillation, and congestive heart failure
Depression	Sad mood and thoughts, withdrawal, crying, weight loss, constipation, insomnia	Any classic signs, plus memory and concentration problems, weight gain, increased sleep

(Henderson, M.L. [1985]. Assessing the elderly (part II): Altered presentations. American Journal of Nursing, 85[10], 1103–1106)

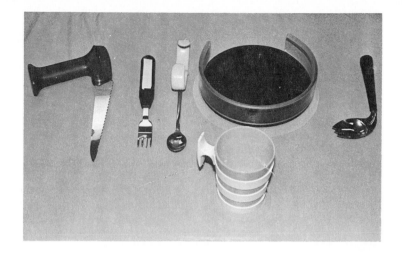

Figure 20-1. Adaptive eating utensils can help the older adult with a functional limitation to eat independently and maintain a healthy diet.

them are being studied more extensively and understood. Disease and poor health are no longer believed to be inevitable consequences of aging, even though declining physical function may be inevitable. For elderly persons, major health promotion efforts are directed toward safety, nutrition, dental hygiene, providing immunizations, and screening for chronic or debilitating diseases. Health restoration may also be an important aspect of health care for elderly persons, who suffer a higher incidence of disability and chronic illness than the rest of the population.

Common Health Concerns and Problems. Review with the person his or her perceptions of current health status, including any functional limitations or problems with performing activities of daily living. The person's knowledge and understanding of any health problems should be evaluated to determine how these problems are managed. A comprehensive recall of all past health problems, such as every childhood disease, minor injury, or hospitalization, may not be necessary if such events do not influence current health status. Determine all the medications taken by the person as well as the reasons for taking them and how the medications are obtained.

Participation in Age-Appropriate Health Promotion and Health Maintenance Activities. Determine whether or not the person engages in certain activities to stay healthy and minimize the effects of aging. Physical activity and proper nutrition are important for health promotion in any age group.

Safety Practices. The older person may require special safety practices to prevent injury, especially if age-related sensory deficits have occurred or slower response and reaction times exist. Many questions related to safety will be initiated on the basis of the person's health history or the examiner's observations. For example, if a sensory deficit such as poor depth perception is apparent, the examiner should ask about lighting levels in the home, safety of stairways, and cues the person relies on to signal a change of level when walking.

Screening Practices. The person's participation in disease screening activities should be determined and evaluated in relation to screening recommendations for older age groups. Special attention should be given to screening

activities aimed at early detection of hypertension, heart disease, and cancer, especially of the breast, colon, cervix, and prostate gland (see Chap. 6).

Nutrition and Metabolism

Several factors may predispose the older person to nutritional problems, including physiologic changes, socioeconomic status, and functional limitations (Fig. 20-1). Specific factors that may influence nutrition include the following: changes in the structure and function of the oral cavity and/or the gastrointestinal system, changes in coloric needs, inadequate income, physical limitations, and anthropometric skinfold measurements.

Changes in Structure and Function of Oral Cavity. Chewing abilities may be limited as teeth are lost or altered (a preventable condition). Decreased saliva production and decreased salivary ptyalin may be associated with less efficient breakdown of foods. Ill-fitting dentures or teeth that are in otherwise poor condition may contribute to pain with eating. Taste and smell sensations also diminish with advancing age and may predispose the person to excessive use of salt and sugar.

Changes in Gastrointestinal Structures and Functions. Esophageal disorders may be more prevalent in older persons, especially relaxation of the lower esophageal sphincter, which is associated with reflux and "heartburn," and spasm or hiatal hernia, which may interfere with the passage of food to the stomach. A decline in the efficiency of digestive enzymes and hydrochloric acid may be related to less effective absorption of nutrients from the intestine.

Changes in Caloric Needs. In general, caloric requirements decrease with advancing age because metabolism is slowed and activity levels are lower. Failure to reduce the caloric intake and maintain a quality diet on fewer calories may contribute to obesity or other forms of malnutrition. Nutritional requirements for older age groups are presented in Appendix B.

Inadequate Income. The income of many older persons may be limited, thus influencing the affordability of food. The diet of people in poverty is generally high in carbohydrates and lacking in high-protein foods and fresh fruits and vegetables.

Physical Limitations. If the older person has physical limitations, the ability to shop for and prepare food may be affected. Some persons adapt to such changes by the use of services such as those that provide home-delivered meals.

Anthropometric Skinfold Measurements. The measurement of skinfold thickness is a standard component of anthropometric assessment. Because subcutaneous fat loss occurs with aging, normal skinfold thickness is less in the older adult. You should refer to tables with norms for different age groups for the best results.

Elimination

Several conditions may contribute to problems with bladder elimination in the older person. Atrophy and weakening of the muscles involved in bladder elimination may result in either reduced bladder capacity or urinary retention. Fecal impaction or prostatic hypertrophy may also contribute to urinary retention. The incidence of urinary tract infections is higher in older age groups and may produce symptoms such as urgency, frequency, and dysuria. Tumors involving genitourinary structures are more common in older persons. Physical limitations or cognitive deficits may make toileting difficult.

Commonly, the older person will report some degree of voiding more frequently and urgently because of age-related changes in musculature. Incontinence is not considered a normal manifestation of aging. Assessment should be directed toward determining what factors are contributing to the problem.

The most common bowel elimination problem in older age groups is constipation. Constipation should not be considered an inevitable consequence of aging, however. Although colon muscle tone diminishes with advancing age, many of the risk factors for constipation are the same across age groups. These risk factors include inadequate intake of dietary fiber, minimal intake of liquids, immobility, use of constipating drugs, and ignoring the urge to defecate.

Activity and Exercise

Capacities for activity and exercises are influenced by motivation and life-style as well as by age-related alterations in body systems, especially the cardiovascular, pulmonary, and musculoskeletal systems. Age-related changes in these systems may not always be apparent by physical examination but nevertheless may influence functional abilities.

Age-related cardiovascular changes may influence functional abilities by contributing to fatigue and a diminished capacity for exercise tolerance. Except in disease processes, the older person may compensate or adapt to cardiac changes, and the electrocardiogram, heart rate, and heart sounds may reveal few changes. Declines in cardiovascular

function that may influence activity and exercise functions include the following:

- Progressive decline in cardiac output (1% per year between the third and eighth decades) secondary to cardiac muscle changes, including endocardial fibrosis and sclerosis, left ventricular wall thickening, and increased infiltration of cardiac muscle with fat
- Slowing of the heart rate and prolongation of systole secondary to fibrosis of the cardiac conduction system
- Altered cardiac response to exercise (the heart rate increases more slowly with activity and takes longer to return to baseline levels)

Degenerative lung changes in the older person may also be a factor contributing to fatigue, dyspnea, and diminished exercise tolerance. Age-related changes in lung tissue that may influence functional abilities include the following:

- Loss of lung elastic recoil
- Loss of surface area for gas exchange
- Decreased respiratory muscle strength

Finally, age-related changes in the musculoskeletal system may contribute to altered mobility and strength. The muscles may become weaker secondary to decreased skeletal muscle contraction time, decreased muscle fiber tone, and decreased effectiveness of muscle glycolytic enzymes. In addition, some of the joints become less mobile as joints and ligaments undergo ankylosis.

Despite inevitable degenerative changes in the body systems, regular exercise is believed to preserve or at least optimize cardiac, pulmonary, and musculoskeletal functions.

Cognition and Perception

No decline in IQ is noted with normal aging unless the speed of reaction time is a factor in IQ measurement. Because aging is associated with a decreased velocity of motor neuron impulse formation (a 15% decline by age 80 years), the older person will react more slowly to certain stimuli and take longer to perform certain tasks. Other age-related changes in cognitive functions include a decreased capacity for short-term memory recall, whereas long-term memory remains intact.

Usually some loss of the sensory functions occurs with aging. Sensory deficits such as impaired hearing, poor eyesight, and inability to differentiate extremes in temperature distort the environment and predispose the person to injury, social isolation, and other functional limitations.

Sleep and Rest

Changes in sleep patterns are common with aging. Elderly persons spend less of their total sleep time in stage 4 or deep sleep and frequently report sleeping less soundly. Even so, older persons generally require only 5 to 7 hours of sleep per day. Reports of insomnia are common in older age groups and are usually attributed to interruptions of sleep from nocturia, nocturnal dyspnea, attempts to sleep in an unfamiliar environment, muscle cramps or tremors, or medications.

Older people commonly awaken early in the morning with the inability to resume sleep. Although sleep requirements may be met, the person may report that he or she is sleeping poorly or not at all.

Although one nap per day may help older persons meet sleep and rest requirements, frequent daytime napping can further disrupt nighttime sleeping. Some people may not realize how often they nap if napping occurs during regular activities, such as watching television or reading.

Sexuality and Reproduction

Although an age-related decline in fertility and reproductive processes exists in both men and women, sexual functioning continues into old age. The research of Masters and Johnson (1970) suggests that older women may become disinterested in sex not because of decreased sexual desire, but because partners are unavailable or unstimulating. Generally, an active sexual life during early and middle adulthood ensures continued sexual interest and activity in later life.

Notwithstanding continued sexual desire, an illness or physical change in later adulthood may affect sexual function. Physical causes of sexual dysfunction identified by Masters and Johnson included a wide range of cardiorespiratory, genitourinary, neurologic, endocrine, and vascular problems as well as infectious diseases and obesity. Feelings of fatigue and dyspnea, which may be associated with many chronic illnesses, may interfere with sexual function. Normal age-related changes in the function of organs required for arousal and orgasm primarily result in additional time being required for sexual arousal. Each phase of the sexual response cycle—excitement, plateau, orgasm, and resolution—may be prolonged, and responses may be less intense (although not necessarily less pleasurable).

Coping and Stress Tolerance

Stressors confront people of all age groups, but the elderly person may lose some ability to adapt to stress. Repeated exposure to stressors may occur as the person is faced with the many changes and losses associated with aging. The person's perception of these stressors will greatly influence the stress response and coping patterns. Coping with stress is enhanced by a positive self-concept, having sufficient energy to deal with stress, and support systems. Without some of these resources, the person may be overwhelmed by stress, a phase of exhaustion may ensue, and the person may become vulnerable to other health threats.

Roles and Relationships

Several theories of aging address the roles associated with advancing age. The disengagement theory of Cummings and Henry (1961) proposes that old age is a time to withdraw from society and others and give up roles. This theory has been criticized for its negative perceptions of aging. Nevertheless, the loss of significant and meaningful roles is a reality for some older persons.

Havighurst's activity theory (1968) views aging more in terms of role transitions. The actively engaged older person may relinquish certain roles but usually substitutes new roles for old ones. For example, social roles associated with an increase in leisure time and activities may be substituted for occupational roles (Fig. 20-2). In general, the ability to make role substitutions is associated with a more positive self-concept.

Family relationships may change with advancing age; often, those significant others who fulfill family functions, such as providing comfort and support, may not be part of a nuclear family. Elderly, unrelated roommates may fulfill family functions.

Even in more traditional family structures, family relationships undergo several changes as a person ages. The

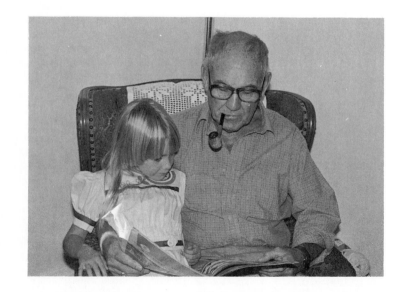

Figure 20–2. Grandparenting is a role nearly everyone enjoys.

older adult may have aging parents and a spouse to care for and may begin to lose friends and relatives through death. Dysfunctional family relationships may occur at any stage of the life-cycle. The older person in a dysfunctional family may be at greater risk for abuse, especially if the person is dependent, disabled, and living with family members.

Self-Concept

Self-concept, the person's beliefs and feelings about self, is influenced by factors such as physical status, cognitive and intellectual abilities, social and familial roles, moral and ethical inclinations, and emotions. Many factors may threaten self-esteem in the older person: the physical process of aging alters body image, roles are given up or lost, and societal or even family attitudes toward the older person may be negative, especially if the person becomes more dependent.

A positive self-concept in older persons is associated with improving physical limitations and comfort levels when possible, maintaining familiar components of one's life-style, maintaining interactions with others, coping effectively with the changes of aging, and maintaining a role as an active decision maker. According to Erikson, a positive self-concept in the older person is achieved through successful resolution of the developmental task of ego integrity versus despair. Ego integrity is characterized by acceptance of new roles in life and satisfaction with one's past life accomplishments. Despair is characterized by disappointment in one's past life and feelings of anger and bitterness.

Values and Beliefs

Value and belief patterns evolve throughout life, often becoming more complex with advancing age. Values and beliefs serve as the framework for ideas and opinions about what is appropriate, acceptable, and meaningful. Beliefs involve personal truths based on faith or conviction, whereas values focus on the worth associated with goals, actions, and other people.

A person's values may be determined by a direct approach. Ask the person to complete the statement "I value . . . " Values are also identified by observing behaviors and listening to the person's informal conversation.

Fowler (1983) discusses stages of faith development during the life span. According to Fowler, older adults may be at the same developmental stage as younger adults in relation to faith, which is called the individualtive–reflective stage of faith. This stage is characterized by critical appraisal of personal and societal belief systems. Concern with meeting family and group expectations may occur. Older adults may progress to the stage identified by Fowler as universalizing faith. At this stage, the person usually feels fulfilled by his or her faith and accepts the tenets of that faith.

Although crisis situations as well as the inevitability of death may cause the older person to analyze values and beliefs, it is not always a factor in rejecting values or beliefs.

The nurse should recognize the importance of this aspect of human function in all age groups and recognize whether or not the person is in spiritual distress and in need of additional support.

THE HEALTH HISTORY

Although obtaining the health history is the same for elders as any adult, the process may take longer. Several age-related factors may influence the communication processes used during the interview. Physical, cognitive, or social alterations may influence communication, including hearing losses (presbycusis), vision losses (presbyopia), slowed responses, short-term memory losses, the need to reminisce, slower processing of information, ageism on the part of the examiner, cohort influences, and the tendency of the older adult to be "socially appropriate" or adopt social norms. Because of such influences, you should conduct the interview with certain principles in mind.

Establish Rapport. The older person will probably be more willing to share pertinent information in an atmosphere that encourages trust and mutual respect. Open the interview courteously and give your name, title, and purpose of the interview and examination. Do not assume that the older person will be able to read such information from your name tag. Determine how the person wishes to be addressed; for example, use of first name versus being called Mr. or Mrs. Smith (many elders prefer Mr. or Mrs. Smith but may say "you can call me Dale," knowing that this is the current social custom).

Explain the purpose of eliciting information. Some older people have been conditioned to keep personal matters to themselves and may be hesitant to answer some questions. Ask the person's permission to record interview data, and explain the purpose of such records. Some people may be suspicious that written records will be used against them in insurance claims.

Ask Questions Slowly, Face the Elder, and Allow Sufficient Time for Responses. The older person may require more time to process questions and formulate thoughts and answers. You may be asking the individual for information about events that occurred 40 or 50 years ago. Give the person time to answer one question before asking the next question. Otherwise, the person may feel rushed, depersonalized, and hesitant to share important information. Allow the person to finish statements, and avoid interrupting. Family members, if present, may tend to respond for the older person. Avoid this situation by interviewing the older person and the family separately.

Face the Person and Speak Slowly and Quietly. Although some hearing loss is often present in older people, especially for higher-pitched sounds, they will be more likely to hear you if you speak slowly with a low voice tone. Speaking rapidly tends to run words together, and raising the voice only increases the pitch. Modify the environment to promote communication by providing adequate lighting for lip reading and eliminating extraneous noise, such as telephones, televisions, radios, and background conversation.

Allow the Person to Reminisce. The interview process and your questions may stimulate past memories, which can be therapeutic for the client and instructive for the examiner. For example, the person may discuss methods of handling problems that will give you insight into a particular coping style. You will need to establish a balance between the person's need to reminisce and your need to collect health assessment data in a timely manner, however.

Listen for Cohort Influences. A cohort or generational effect may often explain or influence a person's behavior. A cohort effect implies that some life event affecting an age group influences current behavior or attitudes. For example, the Great Depression influenced many lives; an elderly person may report, "In my day, everyone worked and we worked hard for a living—not like these people on welfare." Cohort effects may also influence health-related behaviors in that a person may discontinue certain medications because "they are too expensive, and no charity is going to pay for them."

Ascertain the Person's Health Perception. The person may have a different perception of health than you do. For example, the person may not hold health as an absolute value, which is legitimate. The person may not perceive the seriousness of certain health problems as long as activities of daily living are not disrupted. Many common health problems of aging, such as arthritis and memory loss, are often believed to be the effects of normal aging. Because these are considered normal, the individual may not seek health care. It is important to distinguish false and irrational perceptions of health from valid perceptions.

Look for Inconsistencies in Data. If the person responds to a question inappropriately, perhaps he or she did not hear or understand you. Conversely, the person may not understand a question but may answer anyway. Occasionally, the person may answer inappropriately because the question was threatening. In some instances, the person may be confused, and a family member may help clarify questions and responses.

Inferences are made about the person's functional status by analyzing cues detected by observation, interview, and physical examination. The parameters of a functional health assessment are essentially similar for all age groups. The person's age and developmental state as well as your knowledge of the aging process, however, all influence how you interpret health assessment findings.

ASSESSMENT OF ELDERS
Anatomy and Physiology Overview

The anatomy and physiology of aging have been discussed in the sections regarding knowledge base for assessment. Many of the changes of aging are the result of or adaptation to physiologic changes. With age, the individual may become shorter, kidney function is reduced, the cardiovascular and respiratory systems lose elasticity and efficiency, there is an increase in the proportion of fat to muscle mass, albumin levels are lower, the liver decreases in mass, there is a loss in blood volume after 80 years, and calcium is lost from the bones.

Physical Examination   *Elders*

General Principles

Certain principles and guidelines may be helpful throughout the physical examination of an older person.

- Keep the person warm. The older person may feel cold more readily because of a diminished blood flow or decreased amounts of subcutaneous fat.
- Vary positions if mobility is impaired.
- Guard against fatiguing the person. If performing a complete assessment, you may wish to perform segments at different appointments or times. Allowing the individual to provide health history over 1 to 2 days and completing the physical examination at two or more different times reduces fatigue and allows the individual to remember past events. It is especially easy to fatigue the older person during comprehensive neurologic assessment because information processing and reaction times are slowed. Do not rush the person because this approach may contribute to feelings of fatigue and frustration and could alter normal findings. Consider the appropriateness of screening examinations when possible.
- Thoroughly inspect areas at high risk for skin breakdown. This inspection includes removing dentures to examine the oral cavity and removing hearing aids to inspect the ear, if applicable.
- Vary the intensity of stimuli used for sensory testing. Because some of the tactile senses diminish with age, it may be necessary to use stronger stimuli to elicit sensory perception, especially when testing pain and temperature sensation. Be careful, however, not to induce injury.

Preparation	Select an environment that is without extraneous noise, that is well lit and without glare, and that ensures privacy. Provide a chair that is comfortable. If an examination table is to be used, a step stool may be needed. Special geriatric examination tables are available that can be lowered closer to the floor and then raised as needed. When the person is on the examination table, ensure that the individual has adequate support. You may wish to raise the table into a Fowler or semi-Fowler position.
Equipment	Equipment generally needed for a physical examination includes the following:

- Stethoscope
- Blood pressure cuff
- Otoscope and ophthalmoscope
- Tongue blade
- Unsterile gloves
- Cotton balls
- Water-soluble lubrication jelly
- For a pelvic examination, you need to assemble additional equipment (see Chap. 15).

Examination and Documentation Focus	
	• Identify normal changes associated with aging.
	• Distinguish differences between normal aging and actual or potential health problems.
	• Determine functional status.
	• These are accomplished through observation, inspection, palpation, percussion, and auscultation.

Examination Guidelines *Elders*

Procedure	Clinical Significance
1. ANTHROPOMETRIC MEASUREMENTS.	
a. Measure weight and height.	***Normal Findings*** Normal lifetime average height loss of 2.9 cm for men and 4.9 cm for women. Loss begins in the 50s. There is a decline in muscle mass and fat mass. There is an overall weight loss by age 80 to 90 years, which is highly variable.
2. EXAMINE THE HEAD.	
a. Inspect hair and distribution.	***Normal Findings*** Hypopigmentation of the hair occurs (gray), hair shaft becomes thinner, hair growth may be scant, scalp hair loss is common in both genders.
b. Examine the eyes.	
(1) Inspect external eyes and measure acuity.	***Normal Findings*** Loss of fat tissue causes eyes to appear sunken. Lids may droop, resulting in inversion (entropion) or eversion (ectropion). Pupil diameter decreases and reaction slows. Owing to decreased tearing, eyes may be dry. There may be a lipid accumulation (*Arcus senilis*) that causes a white-gray circle around cornea. Cornea may cloud with advanced age. *Visual acuity:* Visual acuity for far vision increases, and for near vision decreases. Ability to distinguish pastel colors, adapt to a dark or bright room, and accommodate to near objects (presbyopia), decreases as does peripheral vision.
(2) Inspect the inner eye with ophthalmoscope; set diopter on 10–12.	***Normal Findings*** Very little change is associated with normal aging; blood vessels may be minimally narrowed. The fundus may appear more yellow. ***Deviations from Normal*** Presence of cataracts, macular degeneration (lack of central vision), elevated eye pressure or cupping of optic disk (glaucoma), nicking of blood vessels.

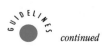
continued

Elders

Procedure

c. Examine the ear.

(1) Inspect the outer ear and inner ear with otoscope.

(2) Evaluate hearing by interviewing, observing, and administering tuning fork tests, watch tick tests, or whispering tests. Observe the elder and listen for verbalizations of the following:

- Gradual and progressive hearing loss for 2 to 10 years.
- Anxiety in response to loud sounds or noisy environments.
- Tinnitus, especially in quiet surroundings.
- Difficulty in understanding conversation (poor speech discrimination), especially in noisy environments.
- Hearing but not understanding.
- Hearing aids that fail to correct hearing losses.

d. Examine the nose and nares.

e. Examine the oral cavity.

(1) Inspect oral cavity with use of tongue blade, pen light, and unsterile gloved hand.

Clinical Significance

Normal Findings

The pinna increases in width and length; hair growth may be present near the helix, anthelix, and tagus. The skin may become dry and less elastic. Cerumen becomes dryer.

Deviations from Normal

Cerumen impaction

Normal Findings

Tympanic membrane is translucent and rigid; landmarks should be identifiable.

Normal Findings

Sensorineural hearing loss is called presbycusis. This hearing loss is gradual and progressive for high-frequency tones, particularly high-pitched consonants such as /f/, /s/, /th/, /ch/, /sh/ or in situations producing higher pitches, such as telephone conversations. Presbycusis may be secondary to atrophy of the hair cells of the organ of Corti (sensory presbycusis) or thickening of the tympanic membrane and sclerosis of the inner ear (mechanical presbycusis).

Deviations from Normal

No evidence exists that age-related physiologic changes contribute to conductive hearing losses. If a conductive hearing loss is detected, consider possible causes including cerumen impaction, Paget's disease of the bone, or otosclerosis.

Normal Findings

The nose elongates with age. Mucous membranes may seem dry. Nares should show no other aging changes.

Normal Findings

Elastin degeneration in the dermis and loss of the vermilion border of the lips may occur, which may result in a pursed-lip appearance. The gums and oral mucosa may appear paler as a result of diminished capillary blood flow. Saliva production decreases with age, which may contribute to dryness of the oral mucosa. The oral mucous membranes appear thinner and shinier secondary to decreased capillary blood flow. The gums recede slightly, because increasing bone resorption around the teeth (osteoporosis) occurs. Usually the older person has fewer than 32 adult teeth because of loss over time from decay, removal to adjust alignment, or trauma. Tooth loss is not an inevitable consequence of aging. Prosthetic tooth replacements are common. Tooth color may be yellower and darker than normal because the tooth enamel has less translucency and becomes thinner, allowing the yellow dentin to be more visible. Taste sensation may decrease as taste buds degenerate and less saliva is produced.

Deviations from Normal

Pursed-lip appearance from edentulism or jaw malalignment; pale mucous membranes secondary to anemia; decreased salivation secondary to medications, including phenothiazides and anticholinergics, moniliasis, stress, or dehydration; tooth loss secondary to periodontal disease. Tooth loss.

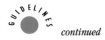

continued

Elders

Procedure

3. EXAMINE THE NECK.

4. EXAMINE THE CHEST.

   a. Inspect and palpate the breasts, using same guidelines as in Chapter 15.

   b. Inspect, auscultate, and percuss chest for respiratory findings. Procedure is the same as with younger adults.

   c. Inspect and auscultate for the precordium, including neck veins.

5. EXAMINE THE ABDOMEN.

   Follow the same procedure as for younger adults. The abdomen will be easier to palpate because of decreased abdominal muscle tone.

Clinical Significance

Normal Findings

The examination findings of the neck and related structures are similar to those in younger adults.

Normal Findings

Breasts become more elongated and flat with age. Granular tissue decreases.

Deviations from Normal

Any new lump is more likely to be cancer than any other etiology. Other deviations are the same as for younger woman. *Gynecomastia* may occur in men, related to hormone alterations or medication side-effect.

Normal Findings

Percussion of the lungs reveals more hyperresonance, which is secondary to increased residual lung volumes. Other findings should be similar to those in younger adults.

Deviations from Normal

Although the following are common, they may not be the result of normal aging. Anteroposterior chest diameter increases because of kyphosis, atrophy of respiratory muscles, and increased residual lung volumes. The transverse–thoracic diameter is decreased secondary to costal cartilage calcification. Chest expansion decreases with aging secondary to costal cartilage calcification, kyphosis, and atrophy of respiratory muscles. Breath sounds are diminished in intensity secondary to decreased ventilatory air flow.

Normal Findings

Visible pulsation may be present above right clavicle, especially in women; the aorta elongates with age, and pulsation reflects blood movement in innominate artery, which moves up into the chest. The heart sounds S1 and S2 may be less intense; S4 may be heard as ventricle becomes less compliant. Heart rate returns to resting state more slowly. Pulses may be more readily felt.

Deviations from Normal

Point of maximal impulse may be lateral to the midclavicular line; this is secondary to shoulder narrowing, kyphosis, and downward displacement of the heart. Amplitude may decrease as chest becomes more rigid. Systolic murmurs may be associated with calcification, fibrosis, and lipid accumulation on aortic or mitral valves, resulting in valve rigidity and incomplete closure. Diastolic murmurs are always abnormal in elders. Bruit over carotid arteries.

Normal Findings

Abdominal sounds may not be as frequent. The abdomen becomes more rounded or protuberant with maturity as subcutaneous fat accumulates in the abdominal region and organs are displaced because of musculoskeletal changes such as kyphosis. The lower liver border may extend past the costal margin. In the older person, this represents displacement secondary to increased lung distention and diaphragmatic flattening rather than increased liver size. Greater difficulty palpating a distended bladder will occur because the overall bladder capacity decreases with age.

Elders

Procedure	Clinical Significance

Procedure

6. EXAMINE THE GENITALIA.
   a. Female: The older woman may not be able to comfortably assume the lithotomy position and use the stirrups because of musculoskeletal changes. Modify the lithotomy position by allowing less knee flexion and foregoing the use of stirrups, or use a left lateral Sims position. Vaginal size may decrease with advancing age, especially in nonparous women, so consider using a smaller vaginal speculum. Because of a decrease in size, the vagina may accommodate only one finger instead of two during bimanual palpation.

   b. Males: If the man cannot tolerate the usual position (bending 90 degrees at the waist), examine from the left lateral Sims position.

7. INSPECT THE SKIN.
   To check turgor for dehydration, use forehead.

8. EXAMINE THE MUSCULOSKELETAL SYSTEM.
   Follow the same procedure as for young adults.

9. EXAMINE THE NEUROLOGIC SYSTEM.
   Use the same procedure as with younger adults.

Clinical Significance

Normal Findings
Age-related changes in the external genitals occur secondary to estrogen depletion and include thinning and graying of the pubic hair, flattening and increased wrinkling of the labia majora, and decrease in size of the clitoris. The vagina becomes narrower because of fibrosis. The vaginal mucosa appears drier and paler, and rugae are less prominent. These changes are related to decreased secretory activity. The cervix decreases in size, and the os may appear smaller or stenotic. The uterus and ovaries decrease in size. A 50% decline in ovary size occurs by age 60 years, so the ovaries may not be palpable.

Normal Findings
Age-related changes in the appearance of the external genitals are related to depletion of sex hormones. The pubic hairs become thinner and grayer, the size of the penis and testes decreases, the consistency of the testes is less firm, and the scrotal sac becomes pendulous with fewer rugae. The evaluation of hernias is similar in older and younger age groups.

Deviations from Normal
Prostate enlargement is not a normal age-related change, although increasing age is a major risk factor for benign prostatic hypertrophy.

Normal Findings
The skin may appear thin and translucent, related to loss of adipose tissue and degeneration of collagen. There is loss of skin turgor and body hair (which also becomes thinner). The skin may be dry and wrinkled.

Deviations from Normal
Telangiectases are the result of dilated vessels that appear on the skin as a thin, bright-red tangle of lines; also known as spider nevi. Seborrheic keratoses are benign, hyperplastic, warty lesions that begin to appear at about age 40; may be yellowish to tan in color, never dark brown or black. Actinic keratosis lesion on sun-exposed areas; pink to mildly red considered premalignant. Cherry angiomas and dilation of superficial capillaries occur most commonly after 40. Elders are susceptible to the same deviations as younger adults.

Normal Findings
Muscle strength may decrease but should be bilaterally equal. Lumbar spine tends to flatten, causing the upper spine and head to tilt forward.

Deviations from Normal
Range of motion in some joints may be restricted owing to arthritis and similar disorders. Kyphosis occurs as a result of degenerative changes to disks. Gait may become smaller and speed slower.

Normal Findings
See hearing and vision. All other neurologic findings should be similar to those in younger adults. Responses may be slower.

DIAGNOSTIC STUDIES FOR ELDERS

No special diagnostic studies are limited to elders; however, some diagnostic studies are performed more commonly in elders or more frequently. Many of the diagnostic studies performed on elders are disease-related, such as blood tests for prostate-specific antigen for prostate cancer and blood glucose studies for diabetes mellitus rather than to measure health status, such as hemoglobin levels.

Laboratory values for some diagnostic studies change with age (*e.g.,* erythrocyte sedimentation rate increases with age). However, most laboratory values differ significantly more because of gender rather than age when adulthood is achieved.

Common diagnostic tests for elders include complete blood chemistry, including a complete blood count; mammogram for women; hearing and vision testing; electrocardiograms; blood pressure; and other studies that are indicated because of individual risk, such as diabetes mellitus.

Documenting Elder Examination

90-Year-Old Woman Living Alone

S: No specific complaints, in excellent health, takes no medications, continues to mow lawn and plant vegetable garden. Friends provide transportation for shopping. Able to do own housework but not as good as few years ago. Eats only two meals a day and coffee in the morning.

O: Only deviations from normal noted; see flow sheet for normals. Weight loss of 30 pounds in last year, 10 teeth upper and 10 lower, about half in poor repair. Oral mucosa dry. Hemoglobin 12.0 g.

A: Altered nutrition: less than body requirements as evidenced by weight loss. Possible etiology—inadequate intake possibly complicated by tooth loss.

P: Return in 1 month to monitor weight. Refer to nutritionist. Make home visit in 2 weeks to evaluate environment and meal preparation in home.

Clinical Problems Related to Elder Examination

Elders experience numerous clinical problems. Some of the more life threatening are cerebrovascular accidents, cancers, myocardial infarctions, and pneumonia and influenza. Neurologic problems that frequently occur in elders include Parkinson's disease, Alzheimer's disease, and cerebrovascular accidents.

The most common health problems experienced by elders are hypertension, arthritis (see Chap. 10), diabetes mellitus, incontinence (see Chap. 9), hearing and visual loss (see Chap. 11). Hypertension is defined as a diastolic pressure greater than 90 mm Hg and/or a systolic pressure greater than 140 mm Hg. The etiology of hypertension is unknown in most individuals.

Chapter 20 SUMMARY

The physical examination of the older person is similar to the examination of younger people, especially regarding examination techniques. Even so, some skill modification may be required for optimal examination of the older person. Additionally, you should modify the manner in which physical examination findings are interpreted, focusing on functional ability and normal physical aging. Age-related changes are noted in all major body systems.

Difficulty in distinguishing normal findings and deviations from normal in the older client may be attributed to the following:
- *Physical aging processes may be difficult to distinguish from pathologic processes.*
- *Normal aging consequences may be confused with medication side effects or toxicities.*
- *The aging process is highly variable.*

Additional data are collected by interviewing the older client. You should be especially attentive to the following factors when interviewing the older client:
- *Establishing rapport*
- *Allowing sufficient time for responses*
- *Facing the client and speaking slowly and quietly*
- *Allowing time for reminiscence*
- *Listening for cohort influences*
- *Noting social influences*
- *Ascertaining the client's health perception*
- *Noting inconsistencies in the data*

Not only do older persons differ physically from younger persons in health states, but different signs and symptoms may be noted during illness. You should be aware of such differences to avoid misdiagnosis or failure to diagnose health problems in older persons.

✳ CRITICAL THINKING

Assessing the elderly requires modification of examination techniques on an individual basis and skillful interpretation of findings. The nurse needs a strong foundation in the concepts of normal aging in order to make clinical judgments about any deviations from normal or suspected pathology.

Learning Exercises

1. Identify and describe the primary differences between assessing a young adult and an elderly person.

2. Explain how you would assess sexuality and reproductive functions in an 80-year-old woman who is widowed. Create a script of the first few sentences you might say in this situation.

3. Identify some indicators of positive self-esteem in an elderly person.

4. Explain why you would interpret cardiovascular examination findings differently in an elderly person than a young person.

BIBLIOGRAPHY

Andresen, G.P. (1989). A fresh look at assessing the elderly. *RN, 52* (6), 28–40.

Bailey, P.A. (1981). Physical assessment of the elderly. *Topics in Clinical Nursing, 3* (3), 15–19.

Bowles, L.T., Portnoi, V., & Kenney, R. (1981). Wear and tear: Common biologic changes of aging. *Geriatrics, 36* (4), 82–86.

Burggraf, V., & Donlon, B. (1985). Assessing the elderly (Part I): System by system. *American Journal of Nursing, 85* (9), 974–984.

Campbell, E.J., & Lefrak, S.S. (1978). How aging affects the structures and function of the respiratory system. *Geriatrics, 33* (6), 68–74.

Carnevali, D.L., & Patrick, M. (1993). *Nursing management for the elderly* (3rd ed.). Philadelphia: J.B. Lippincott.

Carotenuto, R., & Bullock, J. (1981). *Physical assessment of the gerontologic client.* Philadelphia: F.A. Davis.

Cohen, S., & Bunke, E. (1981). Sensory changes in the elderly. *American Journal of Nursing, 80* (1), 1851–1880.

Cumming, E., & Henry, W.E. (1961). *Growing old: The process of disengagement.* New York: Basic Books.

Dreyfus, J. (1988). Depression assessment and interventions in mentally ill frail elderly. *Journal of Gerontological Nursing, 14* (9), 27–39.

Elipoulos, C. (Ed.) (1990). *Health assessment of the older adult* (2nd ed.). Menlo Park, CA: Addison-Wesley.

Fowler, J. (1983). Stages of faith. *Psychology Today,* 56–62.

Havighurst, R.J. (1968). Personality and patterns of aging. *Gerontologist, 8,* 20–23.

Henderson, M.L. (1985). Assessing the elderly (Part II): Altered presentations. *American Journal of Nursing, 85* (10), 1103–1106.

Hitzhuser, J., & Alpert, J. (1984). The elderly heart: Special signs and symptoms to watch for. *Geriatrics, 39,* 38–51.

Hoch, C., Reynolds, C., & Houck, P. (1988). Sleep patterns in Alzheimer, depressed and healthy elderly. *Western Journal of Nursing Research, 10* (3), 239–251.

Kane, R.A., & Kane, R.L. (1981). *Assessing the elderly: A practical guide to measurement.* Lexington, MA: Lexington Books.

Keeney, A., & Keeney, V. (1980). A guide to examining the aging eye. *Geriatrics, 35* (2), 81.

Milde, F. (1988). Impaired physical mobility. *Journal of Gerontological Nursing, 14* (3), 20–24, 38–40.

Santo-Novak, D. (1988). Seven keys to assessing the elderly. *Nursing, 18* (8), 60–63.

Speake, D.L., et al. (1989). Health perceptions and lifestyles of the elderly. *Research in Nursing and Health, 12* (2), 93–100.

Steinke, E. (1988). Older adults knowledge and attitudes about sexuality and aging. *Image. Journal of Nursing Scholarship, 20* (2), 93–95.

Stokes, S., & Gordon, S. (1988). Development of an instrument to measure stress in the older adult. *Nursing Research, 37* (1), 16–19.

Tichy, A.M., & Malasanos, L. (1979). Physiological parameters of aging—Part I. *Journal of Gerontological Nursing, 5* (1), 42–46.

Tichy, A.M., & Malasanos, L. (1979). Physiological parameters of aging—Part II. *Journal of Gerontological Nursing, 5* (2), 38–41.

Turner, M.L. (1984). Skin changes after forty. *American Family Physician, 29* (6), 173–181.

Williams, M., Ward, S., & Campbell, E. (1988). Confusion: Testing vs. observation. *Journal of Gerontological Nursing, 14* (1), 25–30, 40–42.

Assessing in Special Situations

Examination Guidelines

Bedside Head-to-Toe Examination

Chest Tubes

Nasogastric Tubes

Silicone Feeding Tubes

Intravascular Pressure Monitoring

Oxygen Therapy

Urinary Catheters and Bladder Irrigation

Intravenous Therapy

Cardiac Monitoring

Pulse Oximetry

Trauma

Substance Abuse

Bladder Retraining

Assessment Terms

Acute Care Setting

Trauma

Chemical Dependency Setting

Bladder Retraining

Flowsheet

Charting by Exception

Primary Survey

Secondary Survey

Trauma Score

INTRODUCTORY OVERVIEW

Different approaches to health assessment may be used depending on the setting, the condition of the patient, and the clinical situation in which the nurse practices. For example, approaches may differ with respect to the thoroughness of the physical examination. Previous chapters in this book have described detailed and comprehensive approaches to health assessment. Such approaches are important when establishing a broad clinical data base. For example, the discussion of the eye examination in Chapter 11 addresses all aspects of the examination, including visual acuity testing, inspection and palpation, and the ophthalmoscopic examination. Similarly, the cardiovascular examination in Chapter 10 presents a detailed approach for evaluating heart sounds and pulses. In some situations, however, such comprehensive approaches are neither warranted nor practical, and a more focused data base is sufficient for monitoring the person and for planning appropriate care. For example, a hospitalized patient who had an acute myocardial infarction will require ongoing, thorough evaluations of the cardiovascular and respiratory systems but may not have a need for a comprehensive eye examination. Data from the eye examination may contribute little or nothing to the plan of care for this patient. Furthermore, the nurse may not have sufficient time to conduct an all-inclusive, head-to-toe physical examination. Therefore, priorities need to be established in order to determine the most crucial components of history taking and examination given the circumstances.

The purpose of this chapter is to present examination guidelines for special situations in which a comprehensive head-to-toe examination may not be practical or when specialized approaches may be indicated. The special situations discussed in this chapter include assess-

Jill Fuller and Jennifer Schaller-Ayers:
HEALTH ASSESSMENT: A NURSING APPROACH, Second Edition.
© 1990, 1994 by J. B. Lippincott Company.

ment of patients in acute care settings such as hospitals, assessment of victims of trauma, assessment of clients in chemical dependency care settings, and assessment of people in bladder-retraining programs. Obviously, there are many more situations in which the nurse would choose to modify or specialize the approach to health assessment. In these, as well as the specific situations discussed in this chapter, the nurse should tailor history taking and examination to fit the individual and the situation. In order to plan an individualized approach to assessment in any special situation, the nurse should ask three questions:

What do I need to monitor most carefully for this person?
Why do I need to monitor these things?
How often should I evaluate this person?

Special Situations and Different Assessment Approaches

Four special situations and related assessment implications are presented in this chapter: acute care, trauma, chemical dependency, and bladder retraining. These situations were selected in order to illustrate important principles related to modifying the health assessment process. The acute care situation is a very common practice setting in which assessment must focus on detecting complications related to illness, treatment, or immobility in an efficient manner. The discussion of trauma assessment illustrates a standardized approach that is used in a potentially life-threatening situation when minutes or even seconds really count. In a chemical dependency setting, special skills are required to assess a person who is typically denying their illness, may have altered cognitive functions and may have multisystem physical disorders. Finally, the discussion of bladder retraining is included to illustrate the importance of assessment when planning a program of intervention for a specific health problem such as urinary incontinence.

Acute Care. The acute care setting usually refers to the hospital environment. Patients in acute care settings have health care needs because of acute illness, injury, surgical procedures, or special diagnostic procedures such as cardiac catheterization. Some outpatient settings, such as an outpatient surgical center or outpatient cardiac catheterization center, may also be considered acute care settings. Nonacute settings include places like nursing homes, private homes, and clinics.

In the acute care setting, as in other health care delivery settings, the nurse is required to balance quality care with efficiency. In order to do so, it is helpful to use systematic and consolidated approaches to assessment. One such approach is to modify the physical examination to focus on signs and symptoms indicating typical problems or compli-

cations associated with the person's acute illness, injury, or surgical or diagnostic procedure. Often in the acute care setting, the focus is on early detection of actual or potential problems so that any ill effects can be minimized. For example, following surgery the nurse might examine the patient for signs and symptoms of shock, pain, and bleeding from the surgical site. Bedside assessment in the acute care setting requires a special approach (see Examination Guidelines: Bedside Head-to-Toe Examination).

Another important consideration in the acute care setting is equipment that is part of the patient's treatment milieu. The nurse is responsible for assessing equipment or treatment devices for safe function as well as the patient's responses. Assessment of equipment requires special skill (see the Examination Guidelines for selected types of equipment).

Trauma. Trauma consists of physical injuries or wounds caused by external force or violence. A person who experiences severe multisystem or major unisystem injury, the extent of which may result in mortality or major disability, is classified as having major trauma. The assessment of the victim of major trauma focuses on rapid detection and simultaneous treatment of life-threatening injuries. The approach to physical examination is therefore highly specialized, and the process is standardized to assure efficient attention to life-threatening problems (see Examination Guidelines: Trauma).

Chemical Dependency. The chemical dependency setting refers to the clinical environment for the treatment of addiction to drugs or alcohol. Treatment may be provided on an inpatient or an outpatient basis. Special considerations are given to history taking in the chemical dependency setting. In addition to eliciting information pertaining to overall health status, special attention is given to the history and pattern of addiction. Considerable skill is required to elicit a history because the addicted person may typically deny his or her illness. However, special techniques may be helpful to penetrate the denial. The examination in this setting also requires special attention to cognitive function because the addicted person may have cognitive alterations as well as signs and symptoms of physical disorders associated with substance abuse (see Examination Guidelines: Chemical Dependency).

Bladder Retraining. Bladder retraining involves interventions to help a person regain control of urinary elimination. The success of any bladder-retraining program is directly related to the person's motivation and the nurse's ability to devise and implement an individualized retraining program. An individualized program begins with an accurate and thorough assessment of the person's urinary elimination patterns as well as any factors known to influence elimination patterns (see Examination Guidelines: Bladder Retraining).

Nursing Observations   *Acute Care*

General Principles

Patients in acute care settings are assessed, using physical examination techniques, on a regular basis; the frequency is determined by the patient's condition. Nurses usually conduct a focused or brief head-to-toe examination and inquire regarding any problems at the beginning of a shift. This enables the nurse to identify any immediate needs or problems and provides a baseline for making comparisons. A minimal bedside assessment includes consideration of general physical status, the safety and condition of the immediate environment, equipment being used for treatment, and psychosocial factors. Reassessment is conducted as needed based on the person's condition and/or policies of the hospital.

Evaluating Supportive Equipment and Patient Responses

Many patients in acute care settings require the use of supportive equipment during illness and recovery. Evaluation of equipment function and of the patient's response to equipment and associated treatments should be incorporated into the overall assessment process. Important assessment principles to keep in mind in relation to *any* type of equipment include the following:

- *Evaluate the person:* For example, if the patient has a chest tube, in addition to checking the equipment, auscultate breath sounds and palpate the chest for evidence of subcutaneous air.
- *Be systematic:* Incorporate the assessment of equipment into the head-to-toe examination sequence. Observe the patient and move out along the connections of the device.
- *Reassess equipment function:* Evaluate equipment at least every 4 hours and as needed whenever a question occurs.
- *Evaluate safety:* Note where lines or tubes are in relation to side rails, whether connections are taped or otherwise secured appropriately, and whether intact grounds or third prongs are on electrical plugs. Some equipment is inspected routinely by biomedical departments for safety. This requirement may be indicated by attached stickers or tags.

Examination guidelines pertaining to equipment follow the bedside head-to-toe examination guidelines. The following types of equipment are discussed: chest tubes, nasogastric tubes, silicone feeding tubes, intravascular pressure monitoring systems, oxygen therapy systems, urinary catheters and bladder irrigation systems, intravenous therapy systems, cardiac monitoring systems, and pulse oximetry.

Examination Guidelines   *Bedside Head-to-Toe Examination*

Procedure	Clinical Significance
1. INQUIRE ABOUT GENERAL LEVEL OF COMFORT AND ANY IMMEDIATE NEEDS.	
a. Observe for pain, dyspnea, labored breathing, anxiety.	These symptoms usually require additional evaluation and intervention.
2. PERFORM A GENERAL SURVEY.	
a. Note the following during the general survey: level of consciousness and mental status, the condition of the skin (color, edema, moisture), oral hygiene, and status of oral mucous membranes.	Any change in level of consciousness requires indepth evaluation. Skin alterations may be noted secondary to immobility or changes in cardiovascular function.
b. Observe the safety of the immediate surroundings and environment.	Most safety risks can be eliminated by early detection.
c. Continue the general survey as you examine each body region. Survey each body region to detect obvious problems and threats to safety.	

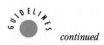

Bedside Head-to-Toe Examination

Procedure

Clinical Significance

3. MEASURE VITAL SIGNS.

   a. Evaluate blood pressure (orthostatic if indicated), pulse, respiratory rate, and body temperature.

Vital signs are general indicators of health status.

   b. Compare the most current vital signs to baseline values.

Deviations from baseline values may indicate a change in health status. For example, as elevated temperature may be an indicator of infection.

4. EXAMINE THE ANTERIOR CHEST.

   a. Note the following: the ventilatory pattern, quality of the breath sounds, and quality of the heart sounds.

Breath sounds: The presence of crackles or wheezes may indicate underlying cardiac or pulmonary disease and deserves further investigation.

5. EXAMINE THE ABDOMEN.

   a. Note the following: distention, tenderness, and quality of bowel sounds.

Hospitalized patients may have increased risk for ileus (indicated by absent bowel sounds) and constipation secondary to immobility.

6. SURVEY THE LOWER EXTREMITIES.

The lower extremities are monitored for indicators of adequate cardiovascular function and deep vein thrombosis.

   a. Inquire about calf tenderness.

Tenderness may indicate deep vein thrombosis.

   b. Note any edema of the lower extremities and palpate to evaluate degree of pitting.

Edema in lower extremities may indicate poor cardiovascular function.

   c. Dorsiflex the foot to elicit Homans' sign.

If Homans' sign is present, the person will feel calf pain with dorsiflexion. Homans' sign is an indicator of deep vein thrombosis, but the reliability of this sign is questionable since a positive Homans' sign is present in only 10% of all cases of deep vein thrombosis.

7. PALPATE LOWER EXTREMITY PULSES.

   a. Palpate the posterior tibial pulse and the pedal pulse.

Diminished pulses are associated with impaired arterial perfusion.

8. EXAMINE THE BACK.

   a. The person may be turned to the side or sit forward to expose the back. Note the skin condition, especially over bony prominences.

Patients confined to bed have an increased risk for decubitus ulcers, which most frequently develop over bony prominences.

   b. Auscultate lung sounds over the posterior thorax. Note crackles or wheezes indicative of cardiovascular or respiratory problems.

   c. Percuss the lung fields, if indicated. For example, if the person has pneumonia, you may percuss for dullness caused by consolidation of mucus; if you suspect a pneumothorax, percuss for hyperresonance caused by air in the pleural space.

9. EXAMINE ANY OTHER SYSTEMS, SYMPTOMS, OR FUNCTIONS AS INDICATED BY THE PERSON'S CONDITION.

   a. For the person at risk for or experiencing *shock,* evaluate the following:

     • Level of consciousness

Level of consciousness, cardiovascular, pulmonary, and renal functions indicate the status of vital functions.

     • Cardiovascular function—heart rate and rhythm, blood pressure, cardiac output

     • Pulmonary function—rate and quality of ventilations, arterial blood gases, breath sounds

Frequency of assessment is based on stability of the patient.

     • Renal function—urine output, electrolytes, BUN, and creatinine

   b. For the person who is *immediately postoperative,* evaluate the following:

     • Vital signs—observe for rapid pulse, rapid respiratory rate, and lowered blood pressure

These alterations may indicate shock secondary to bleeding, fluid loss, or other causes.

     • Level of consciousness

     • Pain

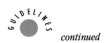
continued

Bedside Head-to-Toe Examination

Procedure

- Pulmonary status—rate and quality of ventilations, ability to maintain airway
- Wound/incision status—observe for bleeding, swelling

c. For the person reporting *distressing symptoms* (chest pain, dyspnea), conduct a complete analysis of the symptom.

  (1) Analyze *chest pain* as follows:

- Have you experienced any chest pain (ache)?
- *Description of the pain:* Burning, crushing, squeezing, heaviness, pressure, tightness, dull ache, heartburn, knife-like, stabbing, sharp, tearing, throbbing?
- *Location (ask the person to point):* Substernal, abdomen, epigastric, shoulder(s), neck, jaw, arm(s), fingers, back?
- *Onset of the pain:* When did you first notice the pain? Did it develop suddenly or gradually? How long does it last?
- *Precipitating factors:* What were you doing when the pain occurred?
- *Aggravating factors:* What made the pain worse? Deep breathing, coughing, moving, other factors?
- *Intensity:* How would you rate the pain on a scale of 1 to 10, with 10 being the most severe pain?
- *Relieving factors:* What helps alleviate the pain? Nitrates, rest, aspirin or acetaminophen, sitting upright, leaning forward, other?
- *Other symptoms associated with chest pain:* Nausea, diaphoresis, palpitations, dizziness, dyspnea, other?

  (2) Analyze *dyspnea* as follows:

- Have you experienced any difficulty breathing?
- *Onset of dyspnea:* When did you first have difficulty?
- *Aggravating factors:* What makes it worse? Activity (determine intensity of activity producing symptoms), lying flat, other?
- *Relieving factors:* What helps alleviate the dyspnea? Sitting upright (specify how long it takes for relief), rest, oxygen, other?

10. EVALUATE ANY WOUNDS, INTRAVENOUS LINES, TUBES, AND ANY OTHER EQUIPMENT IN USE (See Examination Guidelines for specific types of equipment).

Clinical Significance

Symptom analysis helps you identify the cause of the symptom and determine appropriate treatment.

Evaluation of these qualities of the pain is especially helpful when differentiating cardiac chest pain from pulmonary chest pain.

Examination Guidelines   *Chest Tubes*

What to Consider Before You Begin

- Chest tubes may be inserted into the pleural space or mediastinal space to drain air, fluid, or blood, thus restoring normal lung function after surgery, trauma, or medical conditions.
- Chest tubes frequently are attached to a closed drainage system. The most popular systems operate on a water-seal principle. A water-seal system allows drainage *from* the chest but prevents air from moving back *toward* the chest.
- Either a bottle system or commercial disposable system (*e.g.*, Pleur-Evac) may be used to establish the closed drainage system and water seal.

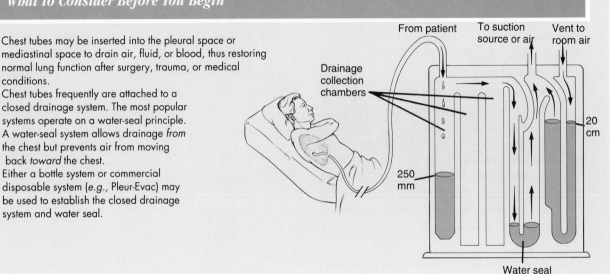

Procedure	Clinical Significance
1. INSPECT, PALPATE, PERCUSS, AND AUSCULTATE THE CHEST; NOTE ANY RESPIRATORY DISTRESS.	
a. Observe for mediastinal shift, rapid shallow breathing, and cyanosis.	These signs and symptoms may indicate a tension pneumothorax that can result from chest tube obstruction.
b. Palpate around the chest tube insertion site.	The presence of subcutaneous air, indicated by palpation of a popping or crackling sensation, could indicate an air leak from the lung.
c. Auscultate breath sounds and percuss the chest.	Improvement in the quality of breath sounds indicates reexpansion of the lung. Loss of previously heard breath sounds may be a sign of tension pneumothorax.
2. EVALUATE THE DRESSING AROUND THE CHEST TUBE INSERTION SITE.	
a. Chest tubes usually are dressed with petrolatum gauze and sterile gauze covered by occlusive cloth tape.	The dressing provides extra protection against contamination, air leakage, and accidental dislodgment of the chest tube.
b. Note whether the dressing is clean, dry, and occlusive. Note any drainage or need for reinforcement.	
c. To prevent accidental dislodgment, tape the chest tube to the chest wall where it exits the occlusive dressing.	
3. CHECK THE CONNECTION BETWEEN THE CHEST TUBE AND THE TUBING TO THE DRAINAGE SYSTEM.	The connection must be tight and taped securely to maintain a closed system and to prevent air leaks.

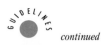

continued

Chest Tubes

Procedure

4. NOTE THE PLACEMENT OF THE DRAINAGE TUBING.

   a. Position the tubing so it will not be caught in side rails and so there are no dependent loops or kinks that allow fluid to accumulate in the tubing and interfere with drainage to the collection device.

   b. Coil and secure the tubing to the bottom sheet.

   c. Ensure that there is enough slack in the tubing secured to the bottom sheet to allow the patient to sit upright and turn.

5. NOTE ANY DRAINAGE WITHIN THE SYSTEM.

   a. Empty drainage accumulated in the tubing toward the collection system by milking the tubing.

   b. Mark the original fluid level on the outside of the drainage bottle to evaluate how fast drainage is accumulating.

   c. Observe drainage in the collection system for color and amount. Bloody drainage noted in the immediate postoperative state should decline progressively.

6. OBSERVE THE WATER-SEAL BOTTLE OR CHAMBER.

   a. Ensure that the fluid level in the water-seal bottle or chamber is maintained at 2 cm.

   b. The fluid level in the water-seal bottle should fluctuate with respirations.

   c. Note any bubbling in the water-seal chamber. Determine the source of any leaks by clamping different points of the system. Start above the first connector and briefly clamp the chest tube; if bubbling stops, the source of the air leak is the lung. If the bubbling continues, the air leak is in the system. When the bubbling stops, the leak is proximal to the clamp.

7. OBSERVE THE SUCTION BOTTLE (OR CHAMBER) AND SUCTION DEVICE.

   a. If suction has been added to the system, determine whether the suction source is turned on and connections to suction are secure.

   b. Determine whether the correct amount of suction is being delivered to the system. If a bottle is used, the amount of suction is determined by the length of the pipet (in centimeters) beneath the water surface. If a disposable chest drainage unit is used, the amount of suction is determined by the height of the column of water (in centimeters) in the suction control chamber. If evaporation has occurred, additional water may need to be added to maintain the correct amount of suction.

Clinical Significance

Proper placement of tubing is essential to drain the system and prevent accidental dislodgement of the chest tube.

The quality of the drainage is evaluated relative to the clinical status of the patient. Little or no drainage is observed with a simple pneumothorax; bloody drainage is expected if the chest tube was inserted to drain a hemothorax. Sudden, bloody drainage may indicate active bleeding.

Evaporation may lower this level so that additional water may need to be added.

This fluctuation demonstrates patency between the pleural space and drainage system. Loss of fluctuation is associated with reexpansion of the lung, obstruction of the tubing, or malfunction of the suction.

Bubbling on expiration indicates that air is escaping from the pleural space. This is expected if the chest tube was inserted to treat a pneumothorax, but such bubbling should gradually diminish. *Note:* This type of bubbling will occur with inspiration if the patient is receiving positive-pressure ventilation. Continuous bubbling indicates a leak in the system.

Bubbling in the suction chamber indicates that the suction is on. The continuous suction mode is used rather than the intermittent mode.

The typical range for water-seal suction is −20 to −30 cm of water.

Examination Guidelines *Nasogastric Tubes*

What to Consider Before You Begin

- Nasogastric tubes are used to evacuate and decompress the stomach. They may also be used to assess gastric function, administer medication, and treat other problems.
- The two most common types of nasogastric tube are the single-lumen and the double-lumen sump tubes.
- The sump lumen of the double-lumen tube is a decompression vent to prevent blockage of the suction lumen.
- Tube sizes for adults range from 14 to 18 French.

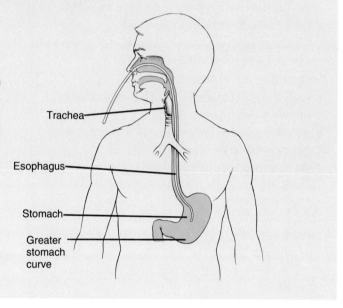

Trachea

Esophagus

Stomach

Greater stomach curve

Procedure

1. AUSCULTATE BOWEL SOUNDS AND NOTE GASTRIC DISTENTION AND DISCOMFORT.

   a. If the nasogastric tube is attached to suction, temporarily turn off the suction to avoid mistaking suction sounds for bowel sounds.

2. VERIFY POSITION OF THE TUBE IN THE GASTROINTESTINAL TRACT AFTER INSERTION, AS A ROUTINE ASSESSMENT PRACTICE, AND BEFORE INSTILLING ANY SOLUTIONS. THREE METHODS ARE RECOMMENDED FOR VERIFYING THE TUBE POSITION:

   a. Aspirate gastric contents by suction or syringe.

   b. Auscultate the gastric area while 30 mL of air is inserted into the tube. If the tube is in the stomach, a rush of air will be heard.

   c. Place the end of the tube under water to check for bubbling. Bubbling indicates that the tube is in the lung and should be removed immediately.

3. DETERMINE IF METHODS TO SECURE THE TUBE ARE ADEQUATE.

   a. Check that measures used to secure the tube to the head and gown are sufficient.

   b. Evaluate the patient's understanding and tolerance of the tube. What is the likelihood of the patient's pulling out the tube?

Clinical Significance

Nasogastric tubes may be inserted to drain gastric contents and may be removed when bowel sounds return.

Nasogastric tubes may be inserted to instill fluids and solutions. In this case, bowel sounds should be noted before using the tube. Gastric distension or discomfort may indicate blockage of the tube or dysfunction of the gastrointestinal tract.

Secure the tube to help prevent accidental removal and unnecessary pressure on the nares.

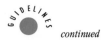 *continued* **Nasogastric Tubes**

Procedure

4. EVALUATE SKIN INTEGRITY WHERE THE TUBE OR SECURING MATERIAL (*e.g.,* TAPE) CONTACTS THE SKIN.

  a. Inspect the nares.

  b. Inspect the bridge of the nose or other surfaces where the tube is secured.

5. OBSERVE THE VENT LUMEN ON DOUBLE-LUMEN TUBES FOR SIGNS OF GASTRIC LEAKAGE.

  a. Ensure that the vent is not occluded or clamped to control leakage.

  b. To correct gastric leakage through the vent lumen, insert 20 to 30 mL of air down the vent or attach a specially designed antireflux valve.

6. EVALUATE THE SUCTION SETUP IF APPLICABLE.

  a. Verify application of appropriate mode of suction—constant or intermittent.

  b. Verify application of the proper amount of suction—low, moderate.

  c. Note the quality of gastric secretions—color, amount.

  d. Determine whether the suction canister needs to be emptied or discarded.

Clinical Significance

Tube contact with skin is a risk factor for pressure sore development.

Clamping the vent lumen contributes to a buildup of negative pressure in the system.

Examination Guidelines   *Silicone Feeding Tubes*

What to Consider Before You Begin

- Small-diameter silicone feeding tubes can be left in place comfortably and safely for several weeks to provide enteral nutrition for patients unable to eat.
- These tubes may be inserted blindly into the duodenum or introduced into the small intestine under fluoroscopy.
- Their small diameter and extreme flexibility require the use of a guide wire for placement.

Procedure

1. AUSCULTATE BOWEL SOUNDS AND NOTE GASTRIC DISTENTION AND DISCOMFORT.

2. ASPIRATE STOMACH CONTENTS TO DETERMINE AMOUNT OF RESIDUAL FEEDING SOLUTION.

  a. Temporarily discontinue tube feedings if residual amounts are high.

3. DETERMINE IF METHODS TO SECURE THE TUBE AND CONNECTIONS WITHIN THE SYSTEM ARE ADEQUATE.

Clinical Significance

Active bowel sounds indicate intestinal activity that is necessary for digestion of tube feedings. Abdominal distention may indicate intolerance or inadequate digestion of tube feedings.

High amounts of residual feeding solution are associated with increased risk for aspiration. The method of aspirating from silicone tubes to determine residual feeding solution has been questioned. It is possible that the pliable silicone tube collapses when negative pressure is applied to aspirate. In this case, residual feeding solution could not be drawn back.

Secure the tube to prevent accidental removal and optimize patient comfort.

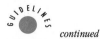

continued   ## Silicone Feeding Tubes

Procedure	Clinical Significance
4. CHECK PUMP FUNCTION AND THE ENTERAL FEEDING DELIVERY SYSTEM.	
a. Verify prescribed delivery rate on the pump.	Continuous enteral feedings usually are delivered by volumetric pump to ensure delivery of a constant volume.
b. Verify whether the prescribed solution is infusing.	
c. Note expiration date of the delivery system.	Delivery systems may be discarded and replaced every 1 or 2 days to prevent bacterial contamination, which contributes to diarrhea.

Examination Guidelines   *Intravascular Pressure Monitoring*

What to Consider Before You Begin

- Pressure monitoring systems are used to measure intravascular pressures continuously and to provide easy access for blood sampling.
- The system consists of an intravascular catheter, connecting tubing, one or two stopcocks, a continuous flush device, a transducer, and a monitor for reading pressures and waveforms.
- The most frequently monitored pressures are arterial blood pressure and pulmonary artery pressure.

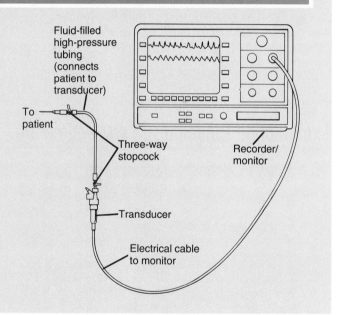

Procedure	Clinical Significance
1. EVALUATE NEUROVASCULAR STATUS DISTAL TO PERIPHERALLY PLACED INTRAVASCULAR CATHETERS. COMMON PERIPHERAL INSERTION SITES INCLUDE THE RADIAL, BRACHIAL, AND FEMORAL ARTERIES.	Neurovascular assessment is conducted in order to monitor the patient for thromboembolic complications.
a. Evaluate capillary refill time and quality of pulses distal to the catheter.	
b. Determine whether there is numbness, tingling, or loss of sensation distal to the catheter.	
c. If the pressure waveform is dampened, determine if blood flow is obstructed by catheter malposition or a tight dressing.	

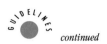

continued

Intravascular Pressure Monitoring

Procedure	Clinical Significance
2. EVALUATE THE CATHETER INSERTION SITE AND DRESSING.	
a. Arterial puncture sites have the potential to bleed, so note any evidence of bleeding.	
b. Note whether the dressing is clean, dry, and occlusive. Note any drainage or need for reinforcement.	
3. CHECK THE CONNECTING TUBING AND STOPCOCKS BETWEEN THE PATIENT AND THE FLUSH SYSTEM.	Connections should be tight to maintain a closed system and prevent air leaks. Wet dressings may indicate leaks in the system.
a. Inspect junctions joining different pieces of tubing in the same system.	
b. Check that stopcocks are turned so the system is patent between the patient and transducer.	An open system is necessary to prevent clotting and loss of pressure monitoring.
c. Inspect stopcocks and tubing for stasis of blood. If blood cannot be removed by flushing the system, consider replacing parts contaminated with blood.	Blood provides a medium for bacterial growth.
d. Examine the fluid in the pressure tubing for air bubbles.	Air bubbles should be removed because air will absorb some of the intravascular pressure before the pressure is sensed by the transducer. Air bubbles in the tubing result in underestimation of the systolic blood pressure and overestimation of the diastolic blood pressure.
4. NOTE THE SALINE FLUSH SOLUTION BAG.	
a. Ensure that there is adequate volume in the bag. There is no alarm system associated with the system to note when the solution is low or gone.	Fluid is delivered under a pressure higher than the intravascular pressure to prevent backflow of blood. Patency of the system is maintained by the delivery of fluid under 300 mm Hg of pressure, which results in delivery of a small volume (usually 3 mL/hour) continuously through the catheter.
5. BALANCE AND CALIBRATE THE SYSTEM TO ATMOSPHERIC PRESSURE IF INDICATED.	Balancing the system establishes a zero reference point that takes into account the effect of atmospheric (barometric) pressure.
6. EVALUATE THE PRESSURE WAVEFORM ON THE MONITOR.	
a. For intraarterial pressure monitoring, the arterial waveform is characterized by a rapid upstroke, a gradual downstroke, and a clear dicrotic notch (see Ch. 10, p. 253).	If these components are not present or clear, the waveform is said to be absent or dampened. Possible causes include air in the system, obstruction of the catheter or tubing, and low blood pressure.
b. For pulmonary artery monitoring, determine whether a pulmonary artery waveform is present.	Other waveforms, such as a right ventricular waveform and a pulmonary artery wedge waveform, indicate malposition of the catheter. Corrective actions should be taken according to hospital protocols.
c. Determine whether the pulmonary artery waveform is dampened; if it is, determine possible causes (see *a*).	
7. COMPARE INVASIVELY OBTAINED ARTERIAL BLOOD PRESSURE TO AUSCULTATED CUFF PRESSURE.	Direct invasive pressures are usually considered more accurate but comparable to blood pressures obtained by cuff.
	The direct invasive pressure may be equal to or slightly higher than the cuff pressure.
	If the cuff pressure is higher than the direct invasive pressure, there may be air in the system that is interfering with transmission of the blood pressure to the transducer.

Examination Guidelines   *Oxygen Therapy*

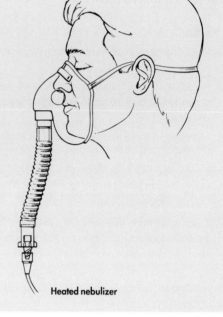

> ### What to Consider Before You Begin
>
> - Patients with acute or chronic cardiopulmonary dysfunction may require supplemental oxygen to increase oxygen loading in the lung and increase oxygen delivery to body tissues.
> - The three most common oxygen delivery systems are the nasal cannula and simple face mask, which deliver oxygen at slow rates, and the heated nebulizer, which delivers oxygen at a higher flow rate. Heated nebulizer systems include a face mask, corrugated tubing, and a heated aerosol source.

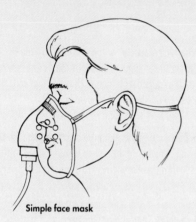

Simple face mask

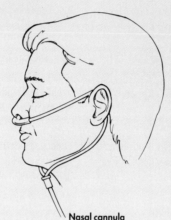

Nasal cannula

Heated nebulizer

Procedure

1. EVALUATE OXYGENATION STATUS.

    a. Observe the patient for restlessness, shortness of breath, and cyanosis.

    b. Evaluate results of arterial blood gases if available. Note whether blood gas values were measured on the current oxygen settings.

2. INSPECT SKIN SURFACES CONTACTING THE OXYGEN DELIVERY SYSTEM.

    a. *Nasal cannula:* Inspect the skin of the nares and ears for redness or impaired integrity. Examine the nasal mucosa for evidence of drying or bleeding.

    b. *Face mask:* Inspect the ears and the bridge of the nose for redness or breakdown.

Clinical Significance

These signs may indicate hypoxia. Indicators of oxygenation status on the arterial blood gases include Pao_2 and Sao_2.

Skin at tubing mask or cannula interface is at risk for pressure sore development.

continued

Oxygen Therapy

Procedure

3. VERIFY PROPER PLACEMENT OF THE NASAL CANNULA OR FACE MASK.

   a. Place a nasal cannula with the prongs in the nares. The prongs curve to fit along the floor of the nasal cavity.

   b. Ensure that the face mask fits snugly against the nose and chin with the head strap above the ears.

   c. Inspect the face mask of a heated nebulizer system during inspiration. If escaping mist disappears at the side vents of the mask, flow is inadequate. If the patient's inspiratory flow exceeds the nebulizer flow, the patient will entrain room air into the mask and decrease the oxygen percentage being inspired (FIO_2).

4. EVALUATE CONNECTING TUBING.

   a. Ensure that all connections between tubing, flow meters, and oxygen delivery device are secure.

   b. Inspect the corrugated tubing of a heated nebulizer system from the mask to the reservoir bag. Drain any accumulated water to the reservoir bag. Empty the reservoir bag as needed.

5. EVALUATE THE OXYGEN FLOW METER.

   a. A nasal cannula usually delivers 6 L/minute or less.

   b. A simple face mask usually is set at 5 L/minute or higher to deliver the desired amount of oxygen.

   c. Turn the oxygen flow meter of a heated nebulizer system all the way up and turn the special dial to the ordered FIO_2 setting (0.40, 0.60, or 1.00). Liter flow must be maximal to ensure correct oxygen delivery and flow. An inline oxygen analyzer may be required for accurate measurement of the FIO_2.

6. EVALUATE THE HUMIDIFICATION SYSTEM.

   a. Check the fluid level in the humidifier or nebulizer bottle. Does sterile water need to be added?

   b. Humidifier bottles may be omitted from low-flow nasal cannula systems.

7. DETERMINE THE TEMPERATURE OF THE DELIVERED GAS (NEBULIZER SYSTEM ONLY).

   a. Ensure that inspired gas is at body temperature.

   b. If inspired gas temperature is too high or too low, adjust the setting on the heating plate.

Clinical Significance

Proper placement assures optimal patient comfort and function of equipment.

System must be intact to assure delivery of prescribed amount of oxygen.

Water in nebulizer tubing can cause fluctuations in FIO_2 and can create an annoying gurgling sound.

The dial is set to deliver the prescribed amount of oxygen.

Lower flow rates are associated with carbon dioxide accumulation in the mask.

Water is added to some systems to humidify the patient's airway.

Proper temperature is maintained for patient comfort and to avoid tissue damage.

Examination Guidelines   *Urinary Catheters and Bladder Irrigation Systems*

What to Consider Before You Begin

- Indwelling urinary catheters are inserted for a variety of reasons but generally have one purpose—to drain urine from the bladder.
- Indwelling urinary catheters are retained by virtue of a balloon that may contain 10 to 30 mL of water inserted to inflate the balloon inside the bladder after the catheter is in place.
- Irrigation is used to give medication or keep the bladder free from clots after surgery.
- Urine output may be monitored as frequently as every hour for evaluation of the patient's physiological status or to observe the patency of a continuous irrigation system.

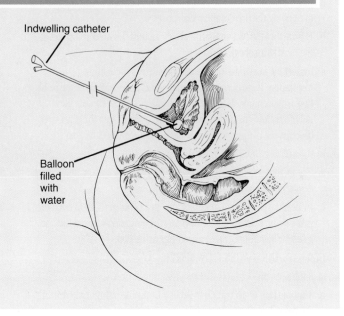

Indwelling catheter

Balloon filled with water

Procedure	Clinical Significance
1. NOTE PATENCY OF THE DRAINAGE SYSTEM AND PLACEMENT OF THE DRAINAGE TUBING AND COLLECTION BAG.	
a. Inspect, palpate, and percuss the bladder to determine whether the bladder is distended.	If the bladder is distended, the drainage system may be obstructed.
b. Observe for urine in the drainage tubing.	
c. Place the tubing so that it will not be caught in the side rails and so there are no dependent loops or kinks that allow urine to accumulate in it and interfere with drainage to the collection bag.	
d. Ensure that the catheter or tubing is taped in a manner to secure the catheter.	Securing the catheter prevents unnecessary movement.
e. Attach the collection bag to the bed frame (not the side rails), and ensure that it is off the floor.	Bags attached to side rails can be inadvertently moved by repositioning side rails.
2. EVALUATE SKIN SURFACES NEAR THE CATHETER.	
a. Inspect the urinary meatus for drainage or encrustations. Cleanse the meatal-catheter junction according to institution protocols.	
b. Inspect the meatal-catheter junction for urine leakage.	If urine leaks, a larger catheter may need to be inserted, the balloon may require more water, or the balloon may be ruptured.
3. CHECK THE CONNECTIONS BETWEEN THE CATHETER AND DRAINAGE/IRRIGATION TUBING. CHECK THAT ALL CONNECTIONS ARE TIGHT.	Connections should be tight to ensure a closed system and to help prevent infection.
4. NOTE THE CHARACTERISTICS OF URINE FLOW FROM THE BLADDER.	
a. Observe the color, odor, presence of blood or sediment, and amount of urine.	

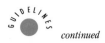
continued

Urinary Catheters and Bladder Irrigation System

Procedure

    b. If continuous irrigation is being used after surgery, observe for active bleeding (dense, dark red drainage) and clots.

    c. In continuous irrigation systems, determine the quantity of urine output. Measure the total output in the drainage system and subtract the amount of irrigation solution that was instilled.

5. FOR CONTINUOUS IRRIGATION SYSTEMS, EVALUATE THE IRRIGATION SYSTEM.

    a. Check that the irrigating solution and flow rate correspond to physician's orders.

    b. Irrigation flow rates are typically 40 to 60 mL/minute to prevent postoperative clot development.

Clinical Significance

A patient with active bleeding requires additional evaluation.

Examination Guidelines   *Intravenous Therapy*

What to Consider Before You Begin

- Intravenous (IV) therapy is initiated to provide hydration, medication, or nutrition.
- A needle or catheter is inserted either peripherally in the arms, legs, feet, or scalp, or centrally in a large vein such as the subclavian or jugular.

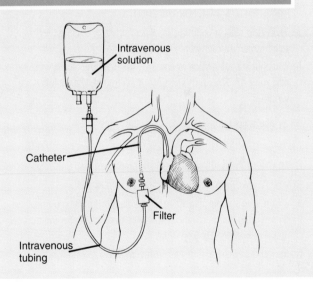

Procedure

1. EVALUATE THE PATIENT'S FLUID AND ELECTROLYTE STATUS.

    a. Examine the person for signs of overhydration or dehydration.

    b. Review input and output data.

    c. Review applicable laboratory data.

2. EVALUATE THE IV INSERTION SITE.

    a. Inspect the site for signs of inflammation or infection—redness, warmth, swelling, tenderness, discharge. Note any redness or tenderness along the cannulated vein.

Clinical Significance

Goal is to detect overall response to intravenous therapy including adverse effects.

Redness along the vein may indicate phlebitis.

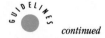 *continued*

Intravenous Therapy

Procedure	Clinical Significance

b. Ensure that the dressing is clean, dry, and occlusive. Note the date of the last dressing change. Dressing policies vary among institutions.

3. CHECK THE CONNECTIONS AND MEASURES TAKEN TO SECURE THE SYSTEM.

A closed system is required to assure optimal function and minimize bacterial contamination.

Leakage of blood or fluid indicates a faulty connection.

   a. Ensure that the connection between the IV needle or catheter and IV tubing is tight.

   b. Ensure that the IV needle or catheter and tubing is taped in a manner to prevent unnecessary movement or accidental removal.

   c. If an armboard is being used, ensure that it is stable and not compromising skin integrity or circulation.

   d. Check all other connecting sites in the system for tightness. Connecting sites may or may not be taped for additional security.

4. INSPECT THE TUBING AND IV SOLUTION.

   a. Check for air bubbles in the tubing.

Large air bubbles should be removed to minimize the risk of air embolism.

   b. Note the placement of the IV tubing.

The tubing should be placed so it will not be caught in side rails, sheets, and so forth.

   c. Inspect the drip chamber.

The drip chamber should be a half to a third full.

   d. Inspect the IV solution. Is the correct solution hanging? Is the solution clear?

   c. Note expiration dates for IV tubing and solutions.

5. VERIFY THE FLOW RATE FOR THE SOLUTION.

   a. Verify flow rates by counting drops per minute or reading the flow rate from an infusion pump.

This calculation facilitates transition to the next solution.

   b. Calculate the rate of flow by checking the IV tubing package to determine drops per milliliter (gtt/mL) delivered. Use the following formula:

$$\frac{\text{gtt/mL of tubing}}{60 \text{ min}} \times \text{total hourly volume (mL)} = \text{gtt/min}$$

   c. Estimate the time the solution will be empty based on flow rate.

6. EVALUATE INFUSION PUMP FUNCTION IF APPLICABLE.

   a. Ensure that audible alarms are turned on. Most infusion pumps have an occlusion alarm to indicate when the maximum pressure that the pump will deliver has been violated.

   b. Inspect the electrical plug and ensure an intact ground wire.

Examination Guidelines   *Cardiac Monitoring*

What to Consider Before You Begin

- Cardiac monitoring may be done by telemetry or direct attachment to a cardiac monitor.
- Telemetry systems include chest electrodes and a radio transmitter. The transmitter is compact and usually secured to the patient's gown. The electrocardiographic (ECG) signal is transmitted to a central monitoring station via the transmitter. Patients with telemetry monitoring may be mobile.
- If the patient is attached directly to a cardiac monitor by wires and electrodes, the patient is confined to an area restricted by the length of the wires and cables.

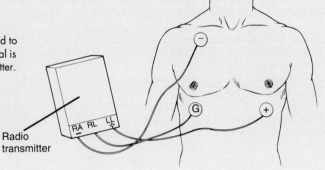

Radio transmitter

Procedure	Clinical Significance
1. VERIFY THE CARDIAC RHYTHM AND THE PATIENT'S RESPONSE.	
a. Identify the cardiac rhythm being recorded for the patient. Verify by telephone contact if remote telemetry monitoring is in effect.	
b. Note vital signs, level of consciousness, and quality of pulses.	This type of data indicates how the person is tolerating the displayed heart rhythm.
c. Auscultate the patient's apical pulse and compare that pulse rate with the pulse rate displayed by the cardiac monitor.	Indicates how well the actual heart rate correlates with the heart rate displayed by the monitor.
d. Note the quality of the transmitted signal.	Excessive artifact may indicate patient movement or poor contact of the electrode with the skin. The QRS amplitude should be at least 5 mm to ensure accurate sensing of heart rate. A poor-quality signal in a telemetry system may indicate a low battery.
2. EVALUATE THE AREAS OF SKIN IN CONTACT WITH MONITORING ELECTRODES.	
a. Inspect the skin around and under electrodes.	Conductive gel may irritate the skin and cause itching and redness after application.
b. Determine whether there is good contact between the electrode and skin.	Good contact is indicated if the electrode is secure, the gel beneath the electrode is moist, and the electrode is placed over fatty areas rather than bony or muscular areas. Electrodes may adhere poorly to moist or hairy skin surfaces.
3. EVALUATE WIRES AND CABLES IN THE SYSTEM.	
a. Observe whether there is firm attachment of wires to the electrode snaps.	This connection must be intact to transmit the ECG signal to the cardiac monitor.
b. Inspect the wires and cables for intact insulation (covering).	Insulation prevents interference from other electrical equipment in the room.
c. Note whether wires are connected firmly to the telemetry transmitter or monitor cable block.	
d. Ensure that monitor cables are placed so the patient can move freely in bed.	
e. Ensure that the monitor cable is not draped over any piece of electrical equipment that may interfere with signal transmission.	

Examination Guidelines   *Pulse Oximetry*

What to Consider Before You Begin

- Pulse oximetry monitoring is a noninvasive way to evaluate arterial oxygen saturation (SaO_2).
- The pulse oximeter includes a probe that is attached to the patient, a connecting cable, and a monitor.
- Bedside pulse oximetry monitoring enables the nurse to evaluate the patient's oxygenation status in a variety of situations such as during position changes, suctioning, physical therapy, and exercise.
- Correlate the SaO_2 value obtained via pulse oximetry with arterial blood gas results whenever available.
- The SaO_2 data is useful for seeing trends and observing changes but therapeutic changes should be based on a complete clinical assessment not on a single number.
- Many types of pulse oximeters are available, but all have similar features for assessment purposes.

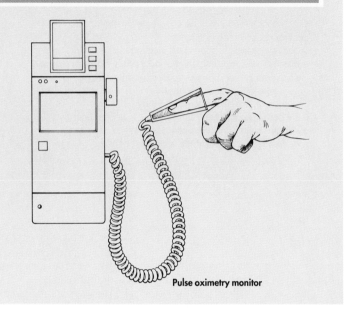

Pulse oximetry monitor

Procedure	Clinical Significance
1. EVALUATE THE OVERALL OXYGENATION STATUS OF THE PATIENT.	Increased respiratory effort, cyanosis, and dyspnea may indicate hypoxia.
a. Note the SaO_2 value on the oximeter monitor.	
b. Note respiratory effort, skin color, and reports of dyspnea.	
2. EVALUATE THE SKIN SURFACE IN CONTACT WITH THE OXIMETER PROBE.	The tissue must be perfused adequately for the oximeter to function.
a. Assess the tissue perfusion under and around the probe.	
b. Evaluate the skin for irritation.	Skin/equipment interface is at risk for impaired integrity.
3. EVALUATE THE QUALITY OF THE WAVEFORM OR READOUT ON THE MONITOR. IF THE QUALITY IS POOR:	
a. Determine whether the probe is secured adequately to the skin.	
b. Determine if the probe needs to be cleaned. Cleanse the probe with isopropyl alcohol.	Skin oils or other debris may interfere with light transmission.
c. Determine if the area in contact with the probe is perfused adequately.	
4. NOTE THE PLACEMENT OF THE CONNECTING CABLE.	Tubing should be placed so it is away from siderails and not interfering with patient movements.

Documenting the Bedside Physical Examination

It is important to maintain a record of the results of a bedside physical examination. Not only is the record a required legal document, it also serves as a means for comparing present findings with the patient's baseline or previous status. Due to the need for efficient documentation of frequent bedside assessments, as well as the status of equipment, many practitioners document in a manner that saves time. Flowsheets are widely used in clinical practice to document examination findings once an initial comprehensive admission data base has been recorded. A typical practice is to develop flowsheets that allow a "charting by exception" method (see Appendix F). Charting by exception consists of documenting only those findings defined as "abnormal." Because the definition of "normal" or "abnormal" may differ with different examiners, it is helpful to establish the criteria for "normal" findings in writing. Then when the nurse recognizes an exception to "normal," additional narrative charting is done to describe any significant findings.

Nursing Observations   *Trauma*

General Principles

The initial assessment of the victim of major trauma is divided into the *primary survey* and the *secondary survey*. The primary survey focuses on the status of the person's airway, breathing, and circulation, and the secondary survey consists of a general head-to-toe evaluation to detect additional life-threatening injuries. The secondary survey is initiated only after completion of the primary survey. Based on the results of the primary and secondary survey, a trauma score can be calculated and recorded (see Examination Guidelines: Trauma). The trauma score is used to make triage and transport decisions and to predict prognosis.

A trauma team is often used in emergency departments to evaluate and treat the victim of major trauma. The trauma team members usually have specific roles to carry out in relation to assessment that have been predetermined by hospital protocols.

During the examination of a trauma victim, exposure of all body parts is essential. Clothing should be cut away rather than pulled over the head or over legs, which may aggravate musculoskeletal injuries such as C-spine fractures, pelvic fractures, or other bone fractures. Motorcycle helmets may be kept in place until x-rays have been evaluated for evidence of C-spine integrity. Once clothing is removed, care must be taken to keep the victim warm. Use of overhead warmers or light blankets may be helpful.

Examination Guidelines   *Trauma*

Procedure

Primary Survey

1. PERFORM THE PRIMARY SURVEY IN 30 SECONDS (THINK "A-B-Cs" OR AIRWAY, BREATHING, CIRCULATION).

2. DETERMINE AIRWAY STATUS (OBSTRUCTED OR PATENT).

   a. Ask the person his or her name.

   b. Move your head close to the victim's mouth. Listen for air movement and feel the person's breath against your cheek.

   c. If you do not detect air movement, try to establish a patent airway with mechanical maneuvers such as the jaw thrust or chin lift. *Do not* hyperextend the neck.

   d. If necessary, clear debris from the airway manually or using suction.

Clinical Significance

The primary survey must proceed rapidly to detect any life-threatening conditions and initiate simultaneous treatment.

A quick way to assess airway patency is to ask the person to speak. If person speaks, the airway is patent.

Maintain neutral neck alignment until cervical spine injury has been definitively ruled out.

These actions may clear an obstructed airway.

Trauma

Procedure	Clinical Significance
3. EVALUATE BREATHING.	
a. Observe the rate, depth, rhythm, and symmetry of breathing. Expose the chest to optimize visualization.	Breathing may be significantly impaired following any of the following mechanisms of injury: striking a steering wheel, blunt or penetrating trauma to the thorax, falls or ejection from automobiles.
b. Note the use of accessory muscles (trapezius muscles, scalenes, sternocleoidomastoids).	Use of accessory muscles indicates increased work of breathing. This is noted in life-threatening conditions such as pneumothorax, hemothorax, and thoracic musculoskeletal trauma.
4. EVALUATE CIRCULATION.	
a. Conduct a rapid survey using the following techniques:	Time does not permit blood pressure measurement during the primary survey.
(1) Palpate the carotid pulse noting rate, quality, and rhythm.	If the carotid pulse is palpable, the systolic blood pressure is estimated to be at least 60 mm Hg (70 mm Hg for palpable femoral pulse; 80 mm Hg for palpable radial pulse).
(2) Measure capillary refill time. Squeeze nailbeds and count the number of seconds until blanching of the nailbed dissipates.	Capillary refill time indicates the adequacy of tissue perfusion. Normal capillary refill time is less than 3 seconds.
(3) Note the skin color.	Pallor is associated with shock.
(4) Survey for obvious bleeding.	

Secondary Survey

Procedure	Clinical Significance
1. PERFORM THE SECONDARY SURVEY IN 5 TO 10 MINUTES.	The secondary survey is a brief head-to-toe examination to determine *all* injuries, not just the obvious ones.
2. IF THE VICTIM IS CONSCIOUS, ASK ABOUT MECHANISM OF INJURY, PAIN, NUMBNESS, TINGLING, AND ABILITY TO MOVE EXTREMITIES.	This type of data provides additional information about more subtle and potentially life-threatening injuries.
a. If the victim is unresponsive, obtain this information from others such as prehospital personnel or family members.	
3. INITIATE A GENERAL SURVEY AND CONDUCT A BRIEF NEUROLOGIC EXAMINATION.	
a. Observe for guarding, stiffness, rigidity, or flaccidity. Note odors such as alcohol, gasoline, chemicals, urine, or feces.	Any of these positions may indicate injury. Odors may indicate need for special treatment or precaution. High alcohol levels could present neurologic concerns. Gasoline or chemical odors may signal need for decontamination. Urine or feces odor may indicate bladder or bowel incontinence and neurologic complications.
b. Note the following neurologic indicators: eye opening; verbal response; motor response; pupil response to light, size and equality.	Eye opening, verbal response, and motor response are assessed to determine the Glasgow Coma Scale score.

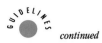

continued   ***Trauma***

Procedure

c. The Glasgow Coma Scale score may be calculated as follows:

Glasgow Coma Scale	
Finding	**Score**
Eye Opening	
Spontaneous	4
To voice	3
To pain	2
None	1
Best Verbal Response	
Oriented	5
Confused	4
Inappropriate words	3
Incomprehensible sounds	2
None	1
Best Motor Response	
Obeys commands	6
Purposeful movement (pain)	5
Withdraw (pain)	4
Flexion (pain)	3
Extension (pain)	2
None	1

4. MEASURE VITAL SIGNS–PULSE, RESPIRATORY RATE, BLOOD PRESSURE, AND BODY TEMPERATURE.

5. INSPECT AND PALPATE THE HEAD AND THE FACE.

   a. Observe for lacerations and deformities.

   b. Examine the pupils for size, shape, equality, and reaction to light.

   c. Evaluate gross visual acuity by holding up fingers and asking victim to indicate how many fingers are being shown.

   d. Palpate the head and face for tenderness and crackling of subcutaneous emphysema.

   e. Check the mouth for drainage, foreign bodies, and broken teeth. Note alignment of jaw or bite.

   f. Note any drainage from nose or ears and test for glucose.

6. INSPECT AND PALPATE THE NECK.

   a. Palpate the cervical spine and observe tenderness, spasm, or deformities.

   b. Observe for tracheal deviation.

   c. Observe for penetrating injury, ecchymosis, and edema.

   d. Observe for pulsating or distended neck veins.

Clinical Significance

Glasgow Coma Scale scores can range from 3 to 15. A score of less than 8 indicates a poor prognosis. The Glasgow Coma Scale score is incorporated into calculation of the Trauma Score (see Table 21-1). The Trauma Score is used to estimate the severity of injury.

This set of vital signs serves as the baseline as you continue to evaluate and treat the victim.

Deviations from normal may indicate neurologic injury.

These are indicators of soft tissue injury.

Any of these may compromise airway. Deformity may indicate jaw fracture.

Glucose-positive fluid represents cerebrospinal fluid.

Suspect cervical spine injury in the presence of these findings or in any victim with a head injury.

Associated with tension pneumothorax; requires immediate treatment.

Internal bleeding may compromise airway.

Distended neck veins indicate pump failure, which may be secondary to tension pneumothorax, myocardial contusion, air embolism, pericardial tamponade, or myocardial infarction.

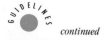

continued

Trauma

Procedure	Clinical Significance
7. INSPECT AND PALPATE THE CHEST.	
a. Observe clavicular area for tenderness, hematoma, deformity, and subcutaneous emphysema.	These finding may indicate fractures or soft tissue injury.
b. Observe sternum and rib cage for tenderness, deformity, symmetry during breathing, and breathing effort.	Paradoxic movement with breathing indicates flail chest. Asymmetric movement is associated with pneumothorax or hemothorax.
c. Auscultate briefly for breath sounds and heart sounds. Observe for absent or reduced breath sounds and adventitious sounds.	
8. INSPECT AND PALPATE THE ABDOMEN.	
a. Observe for lacerations, ecchymosis, distension, guarding, and point tenderness.	
b. Measure abdominal girth if distention is observed.	Serial measurements will detect an increase in abdominal girth, which may indicate internal bleeding.
c. Ask the victim about any tender areas. Auscultate for bowel sounds and then lightly palpate, starting in nontender areas.	Avoid aggravating injury by identifying painful areas.
d. Do not palpate splenic area if pain is reported in that area.	An injured spleen is fragile and could rupture if palpated.
9. INSPECT AND PALPATE THE PELVIS.	
a. Gently palpate over the iliac crests and the symphysis pubis.	Pain or abnormal movement may indicate pelvic fracture.
b. Examine the urinary meatus for blood.	If blood is present, *do not* insert urinary catheter.
c. Examine the rectum, noting presence of blood and sphincter control.	Loss of sphincter tone indicates neurologic injury.
10. INSPECT AND PALPATE THE EXTREMITIES.	
a. Palpate peripheral pulses—radial, femoral, pedal.	Absent pulses indicate limb injury.
b. Observe for deformities, swelling, lacerations, sensory and motor function disturbances.	
11. EXAMINE THE BACK.	
a. Reach under and palpate the spinal processes.	The victim is usually not rolled over during the secondary survey in order to protect the integrity of the cervical spine.
b. Feel along the vertebral column for differences in spacing.	Separation or compression fractures of the spine may be felt as differences in spacing.
c. Observe for deformities and lacerations.	

Documenting the Trauma Survey

The primary and secondary trauma surveys are usually documented on flowsheets in the hospital's emergency department. An example of a trauma flowsheet is shown in Appendix G. Assessment data that do not fit into flowsheet categories may be documented elsewhere on the record in narrative form.

The person assigned to record events on the trauma flowsheet during a trauma resuscitation is usually a nurse with clinical background in trauma care. The recorder must have enough knowledge of trauma care to be able to integrate and summarize data in an accurate manner.

During a trauma resuscitation, it is critical that all details of the assessment be recorded concurrently with the collection of data. Documentation based on memory is usually not as reliable. If events are happening too rapidly for the recorder to adequately use the trauma flowsheet, a separate form may be used to record events as they happen. These data are then transcribed to the trauma flowsheet when time permits.

The Trauma Score

The Trauma Score is a numerical grading system for estimating the severity of injury (Champion et al, 1981). The score is composed of the Glasgow Coma Scale (reduced to about one third total value) and measurements of cardiopulmonary function. The lowest score is 1 and the highest score is 16 (Table 21-1). Trauma victims with a trauma score less than 10 have less than a 60% survival rate. The trauma score is usually incorporated into the trauma flowsheet as shown in Appendix G.

Table 21–1. The Trauma Score

Physical Sign	Value	Points
A. Respiratory rate	10–24	4
	25–35	3
	>35	2
	<10	1
	0	0
B. Respiratory effort	Normal	1
	Shallow or retractive	0
C. Systolic blood pressure	>90	4
	70–90	3
	50–69	2
	<50	1
	0	0
D. Capillary refill	Normal	2
	Delayed	1
	None	0
E. Glasgow Coma Scale	14–15	5
	11–13	4
	8–10	3
	5–7	2
	3–4	1

Trauma score = A + B + C + D + E

Nursing Observations   *Chemical Dependency Settings*

General Principles

The assessment of the addict seeking treatment will focus on the addiction history, family and social history, review and examination of major body systems that might be affected by substance abuse, and review of laboratory tests indicating the status of involved body systems. Because the addict may be at high risk for communicable diseases, additional diagnostic testing may be obtained as part of the admission lab profile. For example, the person may be tested for tuberculosis or for human immunodeficiency virus (HIV).

Typical Laboratory Profile

Liver enzymes
Complete blood count
Platelets
Urinalysis
Blood urea nitrogen
Blood alcohol levels
Toxicology screen

Special Interviewing Techniques

Obtaining a history from the addicted person may be especially challenging because of the tendency of the addict to deny or attempt to hide his or her problems with substance abuse. One indication that the person may not be providing an accurate history is if the physical examination and laboratory profile indicate an advanced disease process but the person denies substance abuse. For example, if the liver is greatly enlarged and liver enzymes are elevated, the possibility of alcoholic cirrhosis of the liver should be considered.

It may be helpful to ask questions in a direct manner. For example, rather than asking, "Do you drink?", you may want to ask, "How many days out of seven do you drink?"

As you interview, focus on eliciting information pertaining to specific behaviors or symptoms rather than asking about general topics. For example, you might ask the person, "Do you ever wonder how you got home?" rather than asking, "Do you ever have blackouts?" On the other hand, you may ask, "Do you ever notice your hands shaking in the morning?" rather than, "Do you have withdrawal symptoms?"

Know the Language

You will communicate better with the person abusing substances if you know any special jargon the person uses to refer to their habit. For example, common street terms for solvent inhalation include "huffing" or "sniffing." Jargon may vary depending on terms used in the addict's peer group or social environment.

Examination Guidelines   *Substance Abuse*

Procedure	Clinical Significance
1. OBTAIN A HISTORY PERTAINING TO THE PATTERN OF ABUSE/ADDICTION.	
a. Determine the following:	
• Substances being abused	Assume abuse of more than one substance until you have reason to believe otherwise.
• Last time the person used	
• Frequency of use	
• Age at first use	
• Quantity used	
• Blackouts	Blackouts are considered major indicators of alcohol dependence.
• Withdrawal symptoms	Withdrawal symptoms include tremors and seizures.
• Change in tolerance	Increased tolerance: More substance is required to produce desired effect.
	Decreased tolerance: May indicate a decline in the body's ability to metabolize the substance or decreased use of a substance.
• Legal problems	History of DUI (DWI): Consider that the person may have driven drunk many times before being cited.
2. EVALUATE SUICIDE RISK. (See Chap. 16 for specific guidelines.)	Many abusive substances have depressive effects; the person may also experience despair/crisis because of related family, social, or job problems.

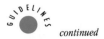
continued

Substance Abuse

Procedure	Clinical Significance
3. INQUIRE ABOUT SOCIAL AND FAMILY HISTORY.	Family and social problems are common problems in this setting.
a. Determine the following:	
• Marital status	
• History of multiple marriages	
• Employment status	
• History of job loss	
• Educational background	
• Relationship with children	
4. EVALUATE COGNITIVE FUNCTIONS. (See Chap. 11 for guidelines.)	Cognitive functions may be altered in any person who abuses drugs or alcohol.
5. REVIEW BODY SYSTEMS MOST LIKELY TO BE ADVERSELY AFFECTED BY SUBSTANCE ABUSE.	
a. Review the gastrointestinal system.	Problems associated with substance abuse: bleeding, ulcers, blood in stools, diarrhea, and loose stools.
b. Review the genitourinary system.	Problems associated with substance abuse: venereal diseases, altered urinary patterns.
c. Review the cardiovascular and respiratory systems.	Problems associated with substance abuse: hypertension, chronic obstructive pulmonary disease, chest pain.
d. Review the nervous system.	Problems associated with solvent inhalation: memory loss, loss of other cognitive functions.
6. CONDUCT A COMPLETE PHYSICAL EXAMINATION.	Physical indicators associated with substance abuse: jaundice, ascites, pedal edema, dementia, nystagmus, gait alterations, neurologic alterations, bleeding tendencies.

Documenting the Assessment in the Chemical Dependency Setting

Most of the data obtained by applying the examination guidelines in this section will be recorded as part of the admission data base for the person entering a treatment program for chemical dependency. Documentation of this information may be a one-time event rather than a series of sequential chart entries. Most facilities with chemical dependency services have standardized forms on which to record the admission data base. An excerpt from one such form is shown in Figure 21-1. Physical examination findings should be recorded using guidelines presented elsewhere in this book (see Chap. 5).

Date _____ Time _____ Referred by _____ Informant: Patient

Name _____ DOB _____ Age_____

WHY ARE YOU HERE? _____

Aspects affecting impending withdrawal:

1. Drinking history: Date & time of last use _____ Amount _____

   What _____ Length of episode _____

   Pattern of drinking for last year _____

   _____

   _____

   _____

   _____

   In the past, what reactions have you experienced when you stopped drinking?

   _____Tremors _____ Blackouts _____ Pass outs _____ Other _____

   _____ DTs _____ Seizures _____ Hear or see things _____

2. Street drug history: for each drug, list age at first use, pattern over the last year; and date, time and amount of last use:

   _____

   _____

   _____

   _____

   Have you ever used needles?_____ Shared needles? _____

Psychosocial

1. What changes, if any, have you noticed as to the amount of alcohol/chemical it takes to bring about the effect you desire?

   _____More _____Less _____Same

2. Have you ever been in legal difficulties because of drinking/using? ☐ Y ☐ N When?_____

   What? _____

3. Have you been hospitalized for alcohol/drug abuse or received treatment? ☐ Y ☐ N

   Date _____ Place _____

   Length of stay _____ Length of sobriety _____

4. Have you ever been under the care of someone for emotional behavior or depression problems?

   Date _____ Place _____

   Diagnosis _____ Meds _____

5. Have you ever attempted suicide? ☐ Y ☐ N Can you tell me about it?_____

   _____

   Do you have a plan now?_____

   _____

   What do you expect to get out of treatment? (in patient's own words)

   _____

   _____

Figure 21–1. Chemical dependency data base. An excerpt from an admission data base in a chemical dependency setting illustrating the types of data obtained pertaining to drug/alcohol addiction (courtesy of St. Joseph's Hospital, Minot, ND).

Nursing Observations   *Bladder Retraining*

General Principles

Bladder retraining involves interventions to help a person regain control of urinary elimination. Restoring urinary continence not only helps to increase the person's self-esteem and independence, it also saves countless dollars. Urinary incontinence is a leading cause of admissions to long-term care facilities and may contribute to debilitating complications such as infection, loss of skin integrity, and calculi formation. Success rates of up to 75% have been reported for bladder retraining programs, but success depends on the person's motivation and on your ability to devise and implement an individual care plan. In order to develop an appropriate program, you must first accurately and thoroughly assess the urinary elimination pattern.

Examination Guidelines   *Bladder Retraining*

Procedure

Clinical Significance

1. IDENTIFY ANY CAUSES OF INCONTINENCE THAT CAN BE TREATED MEDICALLY OR SURGICALLY OR BY DIFFERENT NURSING OR SELF-CARE INTERVENTIONS.

Conditions such as urinary tract infections must be resolved before initiating bladder retraining. Some anatomic abnormalities related to incontinence may respond to surgical treatment. For example, cystocele and urethrocele repair may eliminate Stress Incontinence. Stress and overflow incontinence (secondary to retention) may respond to interventions other than bladder retraining. For example, the person may benefit from exercises that strengthen the pelvic floor muscles or from intermittent self-catheterization.

2. DETERMINE THE PERSON'S RESPONSE TO LOSS OF CONTROL OF URINARY ELIMINATION.

   a. Determine whether the person feels helpless, frustrated, ashamed, or embarrassed.

The person may deny a bladder elimination problem. You must help the patient develop alternative coping strategies before implementing bladder retraining; otherwise, the person may refuse to participate. Cultivating self-esteem is essential for successful retraining. Encourage the person to participate in self-care activities, socialize, and wear his or her own clothes (rather than institution clothes), if appropriate.

3. OBSERVE THE VOIDING PATTERN IN RELATION TO FLUID INTAKE.

   a. Maintain records for 3 days before implementing the bladder retraining program in order to obtain baseline data about the person's incontinence pattern. Check the person frequently for continence or incontinence, and record this data along with fluid intake data (see Display 21-1 for a tool for recording data).

Although time consuming, this particular assessment technique is a crucial component of successful bladder retraining for two reasons: First, you can ascertain bladder capacity. The time noted between incontinent episodes, especially during the night when the person is at rest emotionally and physically, indicates how often the person should be taken to toilet facilities during bladder retraining. Second, fluid intake data is important because fluid is needed to stimulate the micturition reflex. A daily fluid intake of 2500 mL is recommended for successful bladder retraining. A limited fluid intake is associated with urinary tract infections, constipation and impactions, and ineffective bladder contraction. However, in some people, such as those with congestive heart failure, fluid intake should be restricted.

4. OBSERVE THE PERSON'S RESPONSE TO TRIGGER POINT STIMULATION.

   a. Stimulate trigger points, by stroking the thigh, tapping the abdomen, or pulling on pubic hair.

Trigger point stimulation may stimulate the bladder to contract and empty, especially in reflex incontinence. Because different trigger points work differently among people, ascertaining methods that help is important for bladder retraining.

5. REASSESS THE PERSON'S PROGRESS THROUGHOUT THE BLADDER RETRAINING PROGRAM.

    a. If the person does not make progress during retraining, reassess for causes such as inadequate fluid intake or new stressors.

Because setbacks are common during bladder retraining, ongoing assessment is essential to identify situations requiring intervention.

Display 21–1
Bladder Retraining Assessment Tool

	Time of Day	6 AM	8 AM	10 AM	12 AM	2 PM	4 PM	6 PM	8 PM	10 PM	12 PM	2 AM	4 AM
Day and Time	Wet												
	Dry												
Bedtime	Used urinal, commode, or bathroom												
	Amount												
Day and Time	Wet												
	Dry												
Bedtime	Used urinal, commode, or bathroom												
	Amount												
Day and Time	Wet												
	Dry												
Bedtime	Used urinal, commode, or bathroom												
	Amount												
Day and Time	Wet												
	Dry												
Bedtime	Used urinal, commode, or bathroom												
	Amount												

Documenting the Bladder-Retraining Program

The documentation focus in a bladder-retraining program is to record data that best illustrate the person's urinary elimination pattern. Regular recording, such as every 2 hours, helps the nurse accurately identify the pattern (see Display 21-1). Once the pattern is well understood, interventions, such as planned toileting, are better planned and implemented.

Chapter 21 SUMMARY

Assessment of patients in the special situations addressed in this chapter requires specific selection and application of general assessment methods. This selection is influenced by the manner in which the following questions would be answered for a particular patient:
- *What do I need to monitor most carefully for this person?*
- *Why do I need to monitor these things?*
- *How often should I evaluate this person?*

Presented in this chapter are examination guidelines for the following types of special situations:
- *The acute care setting*
- *Major trauma*
- *The chemical dependency setting*
- *Bladder retraining*

✳ CRITICAL THINKING

Students are usually taught the particulars of health assessment in great detail, with emphasis on a comprehensive health history and complete physical examination. In practice, however, there may be times when a complete examination is neither indicated nor practical; also, the clinician may encounter situations requiring specialized assessment knowledge that may not have been acquired through a general discussion of assessment principles. Good judgment must be exercised to modify a lengthy and comprehensive assessment. Specialization is required for appropriate assessment in a number of clinical situations.

Learning Exercises

1. Describe an examination sequence and associated procedures you would select to evaluate a stable, postoperative patient on the morning of discharge from the hospital. Explain the essential components of this assessment.

2. Determine and discuss the primary differences between the secondary survey of a trauma victim and a complete head-to-toe physical examination.

3. You are caring for a patient who requires a type of equipment that you and other staff members are not familiar with. Explain how you would ensure that the equipment is functioning properly.

4. Identify and discuss the pros and cons of "charting by exception."

5. A patient admitted for treatment of alcoholism tells you that he does not drink and that his wife had him committed in order to win sympathy during divorce proceedings. Explain how you would respond.

6. Explain how you would use data about urinary elimination patterns in planning a bladder retraining program.

BIBLIOGRAPHY

Cobble, J.A. (1992). Trauma assessment. *Emergency, 24* (6), 24–28.

Colwell, C.B., & Smith, J. (1985). Determining the use of physical assessment skills in the clinical setting. *Journal of Nursing Education, 24* (8), 333–337.

Lisant, P. (1991). *Substance abuse education in nursing curriculum modules. Module 1–3: Assessment of the adult client for drug and alcohol use.* Project SAEN, Volume 1, NLN Publication #15-2407, pp. 151–247.

Meusen, M. (1991). What do you think . . . bladder management. *Science of Nursing, 8* (2), 55.

Rea, R. (Ed.) (1991). *Trauma nursing core course (provider) manual* (3rd ed.). Chicago: Award Printing Corporation.

Suddarth, D.M. (1991). *Lippincott manual of nursing practice* (5th ed.). Philadelphia: J.B. Lippincott.

Appendices

Recommended Daily Calorie Intake for Adults According to Body Weight and Activity Levels as Defined by the World Health Organization

Appendix A

Recommended Daily Calorie Intake for Adults According to Body Weight and Activity Levels as Defined by the World Health Organization

Body Weight (kg)	Lightly Active* (kcal)	Moderately Active[†] (kcal)	Very Active[†] (kcal)	Exceptionally Active[§] (kcal)	Body Weight (kg)	Lightly Active* (kcal)	Moderately Active[†] (kcal)	Very Active[†] (kcal)	Exceptionally Active[§] (kcal)
Men					**Women**				
50	2100	2300	2700	3100	40	1440	1600	1880	2200
55	2310	2530	2970	3410	45	1620	1800	2120	2480
60	2520	2760	3240	3720	50	1800	2000	2350	2750
65	2700	3000	3500	4000	55	2000	2200	2600	3000
70	2940	3220	3780	4340	60	2160	2400	2820	3300
75	3150	3450	4050	4650	65	2340	2600	3055	3575
80	3360	3680	4320	4960	70	2520	2800	3290	3850

*LIGHTLY ACTIVE

Men: Most professional men (lawyers, doctors, accountants, teachers, architects, *etc.*), office workers, shop workers, unemployed men.

Women: Homemakers in houses with mechanical household appliances, office workers, teachers, most professional women.

[†]MODERATELY ACTIVE

Men: Most men in light industry, students, building workers (excluding heavy laborers), many farmworkers, soldiers not in active service, fishermen.

Women: Most women in light industry, homemakers without mechanical household applicances, students, department store workers.

[‡]VERY ACTIVE

Men: Some agricultural workers, unskilled laborers, forestry workers, army recruits and soldiers in active service, mineworkers, steelworkers.

Women: Some farmworkers (especially in peasant agriculture), dancers, athletes.

[§]EXCEPTIONALLY ACTIVE

Men: Lumberjacks, blacksmiths, rickshaw pullers.

Women: Construction workers.

(After Whitney, E.N., & Cataldo, CB [1983]. Understanding normal and clinical nutrition (3rd ed.). St. Paul: West Publishing Co)

Recommended Daily Dietary Allowances (RDAs)

RECOMMENDED DIETARY ALLOWANCES, USA

Summary Table: Estimated Safe and Adequate Daily Dietary Intakes of Selected Vitamins and Minerals*

Category	Vitamins		
	Age (yr)	Biotin (μg)	Pantothenic Acid (mg)
Infants	0–0.5	10	2
	0.5–1	15	3
Children and adolescents	1–3	20	3
	4–6	25	3–4
	7–10	30	4–5
	11+	30–100	4–7
Adults		30–100	4–7

Category	Trace Elements†					
	Age (yr)	Copper (mg)	Manganese (mg)	Fluoride (mg)	Chromium (μg)	Molybdenum (μg)
Infants	0–0.5	0.4–0.6	0.3–0.6	0.1–0.5	10–40	15–30
	0.5–1	0.6–0.7	0.6–1.0	0.2–1.0	20–60	20–40
Children and adolescents	1–3	0.7–1.0	1.0–1.5	0.5–1.5	20–80	25–50
	4–6	1.0–1.5	1.5–2.0	1.0–2.5	30–120	30–75
	7–10	1.0–2.0	2.0–3.0	1.5–2.5	50–200	50–150
	11+	1.5–2.5	2.0–5.0	1.5–2.5	50–200	75–250
Adults		1.5–3.0	2.0–5.0	1.5–4.0	50–200	75–250

*Because there is less information on which to base allowances, these figures are not given in the main table of RDA and are provided here in the form of ranges of recommended intakes.

†Since the toxic levels for many trace elements may be only several times usual intakes, the upper levels for the trace elements given in this table should not be habitually exceeded.

(Craven, R.F., & Hirnle, C.J. [1992]. Fundamentals of nursing. *Philadelphia: J.B. Lippincott*)

Food and Nutrition Board, National Academy of Sciences—National Research Council Recommended Dietary Allowances, Revised 1989*

| | | Weight | | Height[†] | | Protein | Fat-Soluble Vitamins | | | |
| | Age (yr) | | | | | | Vita-min A | Vita-min D | Vita-min E | Vita-min K |
Category	or Condition	(kg)	(lb)	(cm)	(in)	(g)	(μg RE)[‡]	(μg)[§]	(mg α-TE)[||]	(μg)
Infants	0.0–0.5	6	13	60	24	13	375	7.5	3	5
	0.5–1.0	9	20	71	28	14	375	10	4	10
Children	1–3	13	29	90	35	16	400	10	6	15
	4–6	20	44	112	44	24	500	10	7	20
	7–10	28	62	132	52	28	700	10	7	30
Male	11–14	45	99	157	62	45	1000	10	10	45
	15–18	66	145	176	69	59	1000	10	10	65
	19–24	72	160	177	70	58	1000	10	10	70
	25–50	79	174	176	70	63	1000	5	10	80
	51+	77	170	173	68	63	1000	5	10	80
Females	11–14	46	101	157	62	46	800	10	8	45
	15–18	55	120	163	64	44	800	10	8	55
	19–24	58	128	164	65	46	800	10	8	60
	25–50	63	138	163	64	50	800	5	8	65
	51+	65	143	160	63	50	800	5	8	65
Pregnant						60	800	10	10	65
Lactating	1st 6 months					65	1300	10	12	65
Lactating	2nd 6 months					62	1200	10	11	65

*The allowances, expressed as average daily intakes over time, are intended to provide for individual variations among most normal persons as they live in the United States under usual environmental stresses. Diets should be based on a variety of common foods to provide other nutrients for which human requirements have been less well defined. See test for detailed discussion of allowances and of nutrients not tabulated.

[†]Weights and heights of Reference Adults are actual medians for the U.S. population of the designated age, as reported by NHANES II. The median weights and heights of those under 19 years of age were taken from Hamill et al. (1979) (see pages 16–17). The use of these figures does not imply that the height-to-weight ratios are ideal.

[‡]Retinol equivalents. 1 retinol equivalent = 1 μg retinol or 6 μg β-carotene. See text for calculation of vitamin A activity of diets as retinol equivalents.

[§]As cholecalciferol. 10 μg cholecalciferol = 400 IU of vitamin D.

[||]α-Tocopherol equivalents. 1 mg d-α tocopherol = 1 α-TE. See text for variation in allowances and calculation of vitamin E activity of the diet as α-tocopherol equivalents.

[¶]1 NE (niacin equivalent) is equal to 1 mg of niacin or 60 mg of dietary tryptophan.

Reprinted with permission from Recommended Dietary Allowances, 10th edition, © 1989 by the National Academy of Sciences. Published by National Academy Press, Washington, DC.

			Water-Soluble Vitamins							Minerals				
Vitamin C (mg)	Thiamin (mg)	Riboflavin (mg)	Niacin (mg NE)¶	Vitamin B_6 (mg)	Folate (µg)	Vitamin B_{12} (µg)	Calcium (mg)	Phosphorus (mg)	Magnesium (mg)	Iron (mg)	Zinc (mg)	Iodine (µg)	Selenium (µg)
30	0.3	0.4	5	0.3	25	0.3	400	300	40	6	5	40	10
35	0.4	0.5	6	0.6	35	0.5	600	500	60	10	5	50	15
40	0.7	0.8	9	1.0	50	0.7	800	800	80	10	10	70	20
45	0.9	1.1	12	1.1	75	1.0	800	800	120	10	10	90	20
45	1.0	1.2	13	1.4	100	1.4	800	800	170	10	10	120	30
50	1.3	1.5	17	1.7	150	2.0	1200	1200	270	12	15	150	40
60	1.5	1.8	20	2.0	200	2.0	1200	1200	400	12	15	150	50
60	1.5	1.7	19	2.0	200	2.0	1200	1200	350	10	15	150	70
60	1.5	1.7	19	2.0	200	2.0	800	800	350	10	15	150	70
60	1.2	1.4	15	2.0	200	2.0	800	800	350	10	15	150	70
50	1.1	1.3	15	1.4	150	2.0	1200	1200	280	15	12	150	45
60	1.1	1.3	15	1.5	180	2.0	1200	1200	300	15	12	150	50
60	1.1	1.3	15	1.6	180	2.0	1200	1200	280	15	12	150	55
60	1.1	1.3	15	1.6	180	2.0	800	800	280	15	12	150	55
60	1.0	1.2	13	1.6	180	2.0	800	800	280	10	12	150	55
70	1.5	1.6	17	2.2	400	2.2	1200	1200	300	30	15	175	65
95	1.6	1.8	20	2.1	280	2.6	1200	1200	355	15	19	200	75
90	1.6	1.7	20	2.1	260	2.6	1200	1200	340	15	16	200	75

NUTRITION RECOMMENDATIONS FOR CANADIANS

Recommended Nutrient Intake Based on Age and Body Weight Expressed as Daily Rates

Age	Sex	Weight (kg)	Protein (g)	Vit. A (RE*)	Vit. D (µg)	Vit. E (mg)	Vit. C (mg)	Folate (µg)	Vit. B$_{12}$ (µg)	Calcium (mg)	Phosphorus (mg)	Magnesium (mg)	Iron (mg)	Iodine (µg)	Zinc (mg)
Months															
0–4	Both	6.0	12†	400	10	3	20	25	0.3	250‡	150	20	0.3§	30	2§
5–12	Both	9.0	12	400	10	3	20	40	0.4	400	200	32	7	40	3
Years															
1	Both	11	13	400	10	3	20	40	0.5	500	300	40	6	55	4
2–3	Both	14	16	400	5	4	20	50	0.6	550	350	50	6	65	4
4–6	Both	18	19	500	5	5	25	70	0.8	600	400	65	8	85	5
7–9	M	25	26	700	2.5	7	25	90	1.0	700	500	100	8	110	7
	F	25	26	700	2.5	6	25	90	1.0	700	500	100	8	95	7
10–12	M	34	34	800	2.5	8	25	120	1.0	900	700	130	8	125	9
	F	36	36	800	2.5	7	25	130	1.0	1100	800	135	8	110	9
13–15	M	50	49	900	2.5	9	30‖	175	1.0	1100	900	185	10	160	12
	F	48	46	800	2.5	7	30‖	170	1.0	1000	850	180	13	160	9
16–18	M	62	58	1000	2.5	10	40‖	220	1.0	900	1000	230	10	160	12
	F	53	47	800	2.5	7	30‖	190	1.0	700	850	200	12	160	9
19–24	M	71	61	1000	2.5	10	40‖	220	1.0	800	1000	240	9	160	12
	F	58	50	800	2.5	7	30‖	180	1.0	700	850	200	13	160	9
25–49	M	74	64	1000	2.5	9	40‖	230	1.0	800	1000	250	9	160	12
	F	59	51	800	2.5	6	30‖	185	1.0	700	850	200	13	160	9
50–74	M	73	63	1000	5	7	40‖	230	1.0	800	1000	250	9	160	12
	F	63	54	800	5	6	30‖	195	1.0	800	850	210	8	160	9
75+	M	69	59	1000	5	6	40‖	215	1.0	800	1000	230	9	160	12
	F	64	55	800	5	5	30‖	200	1.0	800	850	210	8	160	9
Pregnancy (additional)															
1st Trimester			5	0	2.5	2	0	200	0.2	500	200	15	0	25	6
2nd Trimester			15	0	2.5	2	10	200	0.2	500	200	45	5	25	6
3rd Trimester			24	0	2.5	2	10	200	0.2	500	200	45	10	25	6
Lactation (additional)			22	400	2.5	3	25	100	0.2	500	200	65	0	50	6

*Retinol equivalents.
†Protein is assumed to be from breast milk and must be adjusted for infant formula.
‡Infant formula with high phosphorus should contain 375 mg calcium.
§Breast milk is assumed to be the source of the mineral.
‖Smokers should increase vitamin C by 50%.
Nutrition Recommendations: The Report of the Scientific Review Committee 1990, p. 204. Published by the authority of the Minister of National Health and Welfare.

Appendix C

Height and Weight Tables for Adults

Jill Fuller and Jennifer Schaller-Ayers: HEALTH ASSESSMENT:
A NURSING APPROACH, Second Edition.
© 1990, 1994 by J. B. Lippincott Company.

Men				Women				
Height		Small Frame	Medium Frame	Large Frame	Height		Small Frame	Medium Frame	Large Frame
Feet	Inches				Feet	Inches			
5	2	128–134	131–141	138–150	4	10	102–111	109–121	118–131
5	3	130–136	133–143	140–153	4	11	103–113	111–123	120–134
5	4	132–138	135–145	142–156	5	0	104–115	113–126	122–137
5	5	134–140	137–148	144–180	5	1	106–118	115–129	125–140
5	6	136–142	139–151	146–164	5	2	108–121	118–132	128–143
5	7	138–145	142–154	149–168	5	3	111–124	121–135	131–147
5	8	140–148	145–157	152–172	5	4	114–127	124–138	134–151
5	9	142–151	148–160	155–176	5	5	117–130	127–141	137–155
5	10	144–154	151–163	158–180	5	6	120–133	130–144	140–159
5	11	146–157	154–166	161–184	5	7	123–136	133–147	143–163
6	0	149–160	157–170	164–186	5	8	126–139	136–150	146–167
6	1	152–164	160–174	168–192	5	9	129–142	139–153	149–170
6	2	155–168	164–178	172–197	5	10	132–145	142–156	152–173
6	3	158–172	167–182	176–202	5	11	135–148	145–159	155–176
6	4	162–176	171–187	181–207	6	0	138–151	148–162	158–179

(Source of basic data: 1979 Build Study, Society of Actuaries and Association of Life Insurance Medical Directors of America, 1980.Reprinted from Metropolitan Life Insurance Company, Medical Department, Health and Safety Education Division. Copyright 1900, 1900 Metropolitan Life Insurance Company)

TO APPROXIMATE YOUR FRAME SIZE

Bend arm upward at a 90-degree angle. Keep fingers straight and turn the inside of your wrist toward your body. Place thumb and index finger of other hand on the two prominent bones on either side of the elbow. Measure space between your fingers on a ruler. (A physician would use a caliper.) Compare with tables below listing elbow measurements for *medium-framed* men and women. Measurements lower than those listed indicate small frame. Higher measurements indicate large frame.

ELBOW MEASUREMENTS FOR MEDIUM FRAME

Height in 1" Heels Men	Elbow Breadth	Height in 1" Heels Women	Elbow Breadth
5'2"–5'3"	2 1/2"–2 7/8"	4'10"–4'11"	2 1/4"–2 1/2"
5'4"–5'7"	2 5/8"–2 7/8"	5'0"–5'3"	2 1/4"–2 1/2"
5'8"–5'11"	2 3/4"–3"	5'4"–5'7"	2 3/8"–2 5/8"
6'0"–6'3"	2 3/4"–3 1/8"	5'8"–5'11"	2 3/8"–2 5/8"
6'4"	2 7/8"–3 1/4"	6'0"	2 1/2"–2 3/4"

Appendix D

Denver Developmental Screening Test II (DDST2) and Denver Articulation Screening Examination

GENERAL GUIDELINES FOR DDST2

1. Find the child's chronological age on the DDST2 form. Highlight the age line across the form (a ruler is helpful). For children who were born at least 2 weeks premature and are under age 2 years, chronologically subtract the number of weeks of prematurity from the chronological age to find the appropriate testing age.
2. Discuss the test with the parents. Explain that it is not an intelligence test but rather a means of evaluating the child's current level of development and that the child is *not* expected to pass every item.
3. Provide a quiet environment without distractions for testing. It is helpful to approach the screening test as a game. Introduce only one test at a time. Keep all equipment such as blocks and ball in the kit bag until needed because these often distract the child.
4. Test the child for each item intersected by the age line. Instructions for testing each item are provided with the test. Begin with "easy" items listed to the left of the age line to promote initial success and cooperation. The items that require a response from the parent may be asked first to allow both the parent and child to become more comfortable with the surroundings and the nurse.
5. Score items by writing on the form: "P" for *pass*, "F" for *failure*, "NO" for *no opportunity* to perform this skill (can only be used for report items), "R" for *refusal*, and "C" for *caution* (a "C" is always used in combination with an "R" or "F"). Be sure to refer to the back of the form any time a number appears by the skill.
6. Score the screening test by counting the number of delays and cautions identified.

Jill Fuller and Jennifer Schaller-Ayers: HEALTH ASSESSMENT: A NURSING APPROACH, Second Edition. © 1990, 1994 by J. B. Lippincott Company.

Interpret the results as follows:

For Individual Items

Advanced: Passed an item completely to the right of the age line. The child has passed an item that most children do not pass until older.

Normal: Passed, failed, or refused an item intersected by the age line between the 25th and 75th percentile.

Caution: Failed or refused items intersected by the age line between the 75th and 90th percentile. This is used to note that the child is not performing a task that many younger children can perform.

Delay: Failed an item completely to the left of the age line; refusals to the left of the age line are delays since the refusal may be related to inability to perform the task.

For the Test with Recommendations for Follow-Up

Normal: No delays and no more than one caution for the entire test. Repeat routine screening at next well child assessment.

Abnormal: Two or more delays for the entire test. Refer for diagnostic evaluation.

Questionable: One delay and/or two or more cautions for the entire test. Rescreen in 3 months or at next well child assessment, whichever is first. Refer for diagnostic evaluation if rescreen is questionable or abnormal.

Untestable: This interpretation is based upon the number of refusals. If the number of refusals would equal an abnormal result, the child should be rescreened in 2 or 3 weeks before interpreting the results as abnormal. If the number of refusals equals questionable results, follow-up is the same as for questionable.

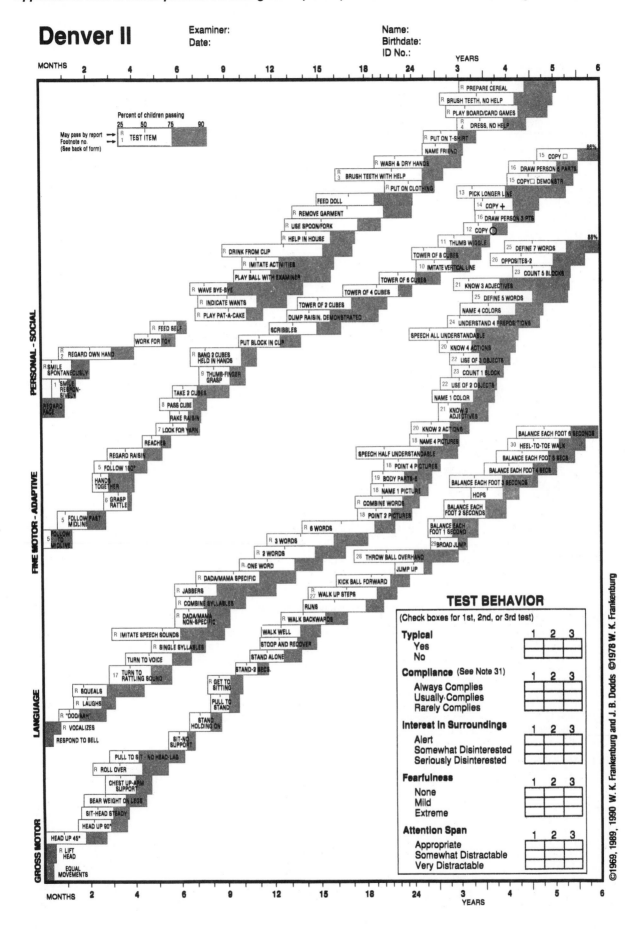

DIRECTIONS FOR ADMINISTRATION

1. Try to get child to smile by smiling, talking or waving. Do not touch him/her.
2. Child must stare at hand several seconds.
3. Parent may help guide toothbrush and put toothpaste on brush.
4. Child does not have to be able to tie shoes or button/zip in the back.
5. Move yarn slowly in an arc from one side to the other, about 8" above child's face.
6. Pass if child grasps rattle when it is touched to the backs or tips of fingers.
7. Pass if child tries to see where yarn went. Yarn should be dropped quickly from sight from tester's hand without arm movement.
8. Child must transfer cube from hand to hand without help of body, mouth, or table.
9. Pass if child picks up raisin with any part of thumb and finger.
10. Line can vary only 30 degrees or less from tester's line.
11. Make a fist with thumb pointing upward and wiggle only the thumb. Pass if child imitates and does not move any fingers other than the thumb.

  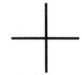 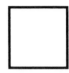

12. Pass any enclosed form. Fail continuous round motions.

13. Which line is longer? (Not bigger.) Turn paper upside down and repeat. (pass 3 of 3 or 5 of 6)

14. Pass any lines crossing near midpoint.

15. Have child copy first. If failed, demonstrate.

When giving items 12, 14, and 15, do not name the forms. Do not demonstrate 12 and 14.

16. When scoring, each pair (2 arms, 2 legs, etc.) counts as one part.
17. Place one cube in cup and shake gently near child's ear, but out of sight. Repeat for other ear.
18. Point to picture and have child name it. (No credit is given for sounds only.)
    If less than 4 pictures are named correctly, have child point to picture as each is named by tester.

 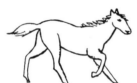 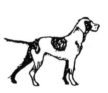 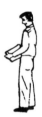

19. Using doll, tell child: Show me the nose, eyes, ears, mouth, hands, feet, tummy, hair. Pass 6 of 8.
20. Using pictures, ask child: Which one flies?... says meow?... talks?... barks?... gallops? Pass 2 of 5, 4 of 5.
21. Ask child: What do you do when you are cold?... tired?... hungry? Pass 2 of 3, 3 of 3.
22. Ask child: What do you do with a cup? What is a chair used for? What is a pencil used for? Action words must be included in answers.
23. Pass if child correctly places <u>and</u> says how many blocks are on paper. (1, 5).
24. Tell child: Put block **on** table; **under** table; **in front of** me, **behind** me. Pass 4 of 4. (Do not help child by pointing, moving head or eyes.)
25. Ask child: What is a ball?... lake?... desk?... house?... banana?... curtain?... fence?... ceiling? Pass if defined in terms of use, shape, what it is made of, or general category (such as banana is fruit, not just yellow). Pass 5 of 8, 7 of 8.
26. Ask child: If a horse is big, a mouse is __? If fire is hot, ice is __? If the sun shines during the day, the moon shines during the __? Pass 2 of 3.
27. Child may use wall or rail only, not person. May not crawl.
28. Child must throw ball overhand 3 feet to within arm's reach of tester.
29. Child must perform standing broad jump over width of test sheet (8 1/2 inches).
30. Tell child to walk forward, ⚬⚬⚬➤ heel within 1 inch of toe. Tester may demonstrate. Child must walk 4 consecutive steps.
31. In the second year, half of normal children are non-compliant.

OBSERVATIONS:

Denver Articulation Screening Examination

(For children 2.5 to 6 years of age)

Instructions: Have child repeat each word after you. Circle the underlined sounds that he or she pronounces correctly. Total number of correct sounds is the raw score. Use charts on reverse side to score results.

NAME

HOSPITAL NO.

ADDRESS

Date: _____ Child's age: _____ Examiner: _____ Raw score: _____

Percentile: _____ Intelligibility: _____ Result: _____

1. table
2. shirt
3. door
4. trunk
5. jumping

6. zipper
7. grapes
8. flag
9. thumb
10. toothbrush

11. sock
12. vacuum
13. yarn
14. mother
15. twinkle

16. wagon
17. gum
18. house
19. pencil
20. fish

21. leaf
22. carrot

Intelligibility (circle one):
1. Easy to understand
2. Understandable half of the time
3. Not understandable
4. Cannot evaluate

Comments:

Date: _____ Child's age: _____ Examiner: _____ Raw score: _____

Percentile: _____ Intelligibility: _____ Result: _____

1. table
2. shirt
3. door
4. trunk
5. jumping

6. zipper
7. grapes
8. flag
9. thumb
10. toothbrush

11. sock
12. vacuum
13. yarn
14. mother
15. twinkle

16. wagon
17. gum
18. house
19. pencil
20. fish

21. leaf
22. carrot

Intelligibility (circle one):
1. Easy to understand
2. Understandable half of the time
3. Not understandable
4. Cannot evaluate

Comments:

Date: _____ Child's age: _____ Examiner: _____ Raw score: _____

Percentile: _____ Intelligibility: _____ Result: _____

1. table
2. shirt
3. door
4. trunk
5. jumping

6. zipper
7. grapes
8. flag
9. thumb
10. toothbrush

11. sock
12. vacuum
13. yarn
14. mother
15. twinkle

16. wagon
17. gum
18. house
19. pencil
20. fish

21. leaf
22. carrot

Intelligibility (circle one):
1. Easy to understand
2. Understandable half of the time
3. Not understandable
4. Cannot evaluate

Comments:

(NK Frankenburg, University of Colorado Medical Center, Denver, 1971. Copyright © 1971. Amelia F. Drumwright)

To score DASE words: Note raw score for child's performance.   Match raw score line (extreme left of chart) with column representing child's age (to the closest *previous* age group).   Where raw score line and age column meet denotes percentile rank of child's performance when compared with other children that age.   Percentiles above heavy line are *abnormal*, below heavy line are *normal*.

PERCENTILE RANK

Raw Score	2.5 yr	3.0 yr	3.5 yr	4.0 yr	4.5 yr	5.0 yr	5.5 yr	6 yr
2	1							
3	2							
4	5							
5	9							
6	16							
7	23							
8	31	2						
9	37	4	1					
10	42	6	2					
11	48	7	4					
12	54	9	6	1	1			
13	58	12	9	2	3	1	1	
14	62	17	11	5	4	2	2	
15	68	23	15	9	5	3	2	
16	75	31	19	12	5	4	3	
17	79	38	25	15	6	6	4	
18	83	46	31	19	8	7	4	
19	86	51	38	24	10	9	5	1
20	89	58	45	30	12	11	7	3
21	92	65	52	36	15	15	9	4
22	94	72	58	43	18	19	12	5
23	96	77	63	50	22	24	15	7
24	97	82	70	58	29	29	20	15
25	99	87	78	66	36	34	26	17
26	99	91	84	75	46	43	34	24
27		94	89	82	57	54	44	34
28		96	94	88	70	68	59	47
29		98	98	94	84	84	77	68
30		100	100	100	100	100	100	100

To score intelligibility:

	NORMAL	ABNORMAL
2.5 years	Understandable half of the time or easy to understand	Not understandable
3 years and older	Easy to understand	Understandable half of the time or not understandable

Test result: 1.   Normal on DASE and intelligibility = *normal*
2.   Abnormal on DASE or intelligibility = *abnormal**

*If abnormal on initial screening, rescreen within 2 weeks. If abnormal again, child should be referred for complete speech evaluation.

Infant and Child Growth Charts

BOYS: BIRTH TO 36 MONTHS
PHYSICAL GROWTH
NCHS PERCENTILES*

NAME_____   RECORD #_____

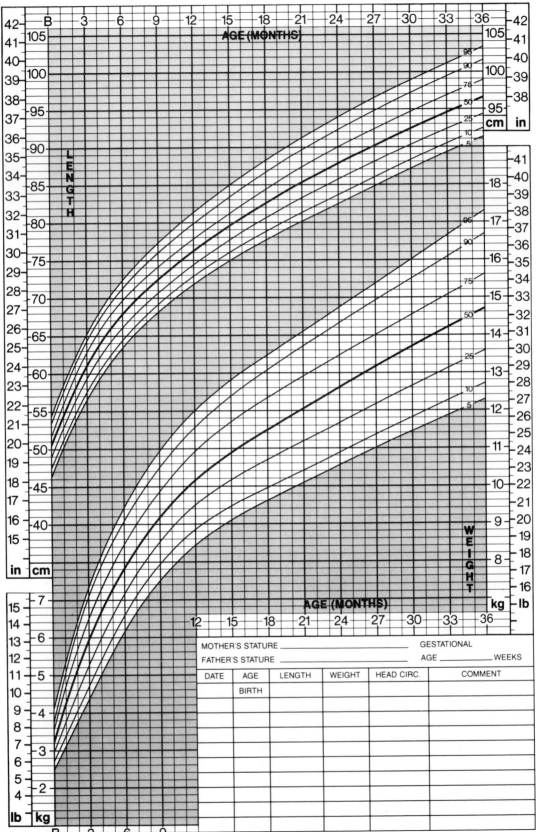

*Adapted from: Hamill PVV, Drizd TA, Johnson CL, Reed RB, Roche AF. Moore WM: Physical growth: National Center for Health Statistics percentiles. AM J CLIN NUTR 32:607-629, 1979. Data from the Fels Longitudinal Study, Wright State University School of Medicine, Yellow Springs, Ohio.

© 1982 Ross Laboratories

MOTHER'S STATURE _____   GESTATIONAL
FATHER'S STATURE _____   AGE _____ WEEKS

DATE	AGE	LENGTH	WEIGHT	HEAD CIRC.	COMMENT
	BIRTH				

BOYS: BIRTH TO 36 MONTHS
PHYSICAL GROWTH
NCHS PERCENTILES*

NAME _____   RECORD # _____

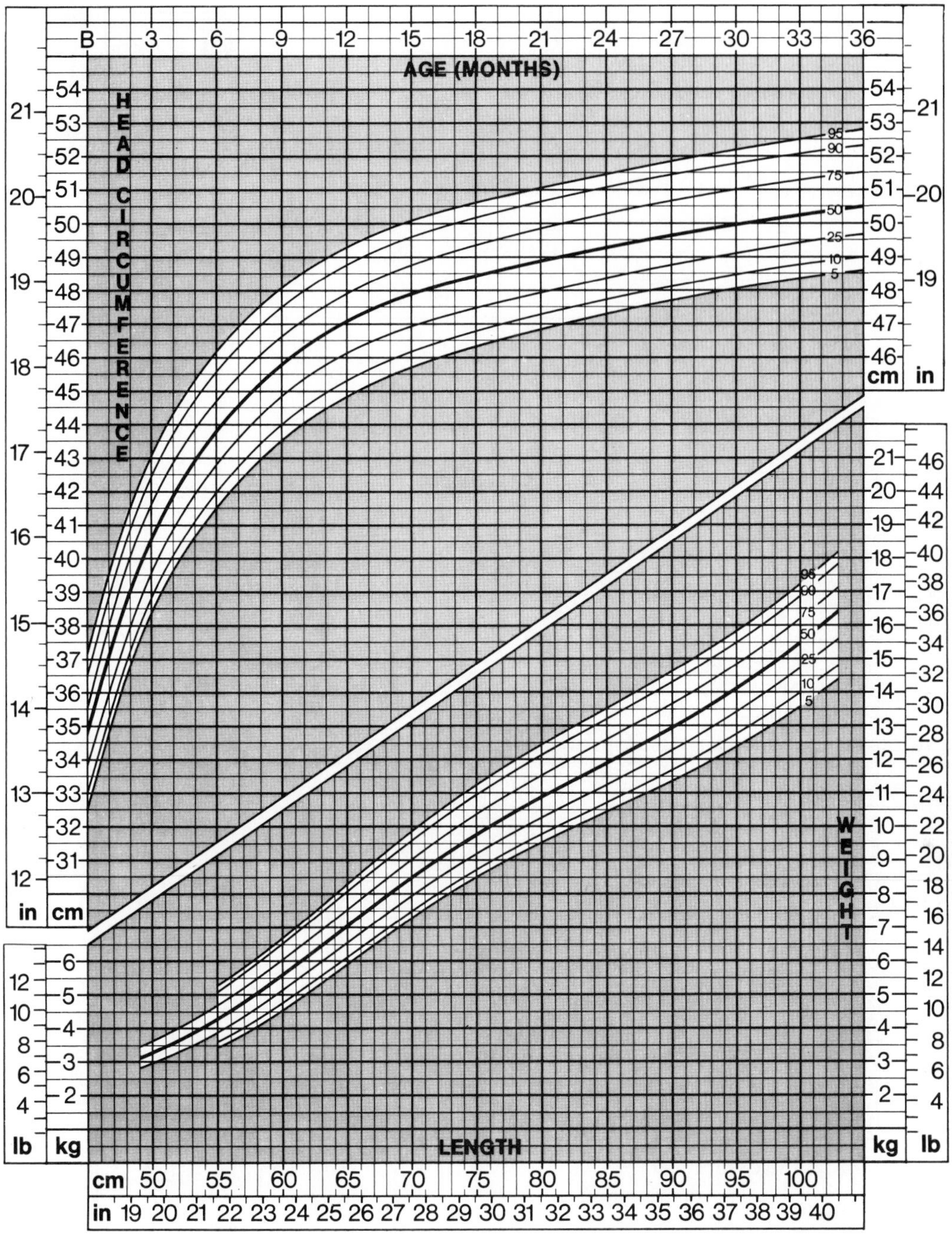

AGE (MONTHS)

HEAD CIRCUMFERENCE

WEIGHT

LENGTH

*Adapted from: Hamill PVV, Drizd TA, Johnson CL, Reed RB, Roche AF, Moore WM: Physical growth: National Center for Health Statistics percentiles. AM J CLIN NUTR 32:607-629, 1979. Data from the Fels Longitudinal Study, Wright State University School of Medicine, Yellow Springs, Ohio.

© 1982 Ross Laboratories

DATE	AGE	LENGTH	WEIGHT	HEAD CIRC.	COMMENT

BOYS: 2 TO 18 YEARS
PHYSICAL GROWTH
NCHS PERCENTILES*

NAME _____   RECORD # _____

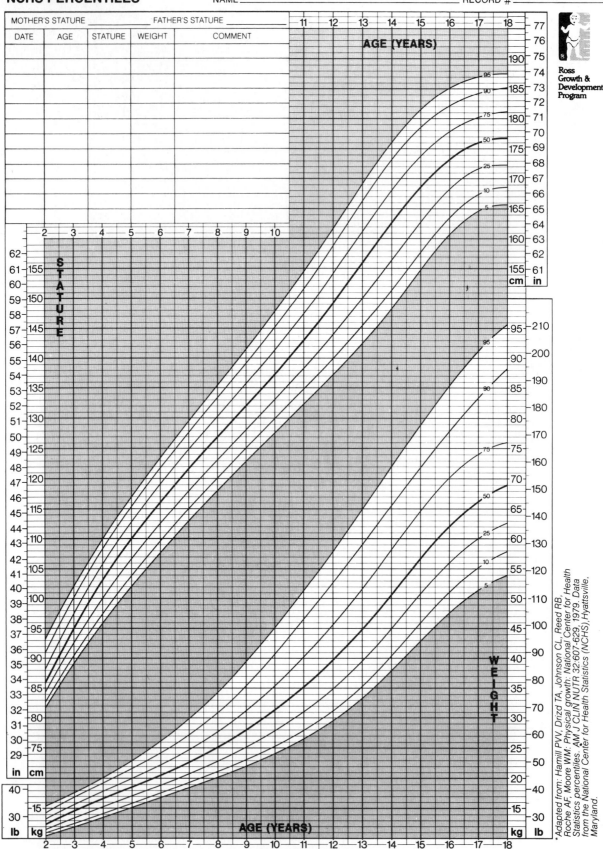

Ross
Growth &
Development
Program

*Adapted from: Hamill PVV, Drizd TA, Johnson CL, Reed RB, Roche AF, Moore WM: Physical growth: National Center for Health Statistics percentiles. AM J CLIN NUTR 32:607-629, 1979. Data from the National Center for Health Statistics (NCHS), Hyattsville, Maryland.

© 1982 Ross Laboratories

BOYS: PREPUBESCENT
PHYSICAL GROWTH
NCHS PERCENTILES*

NAME _____ RECORD # _____

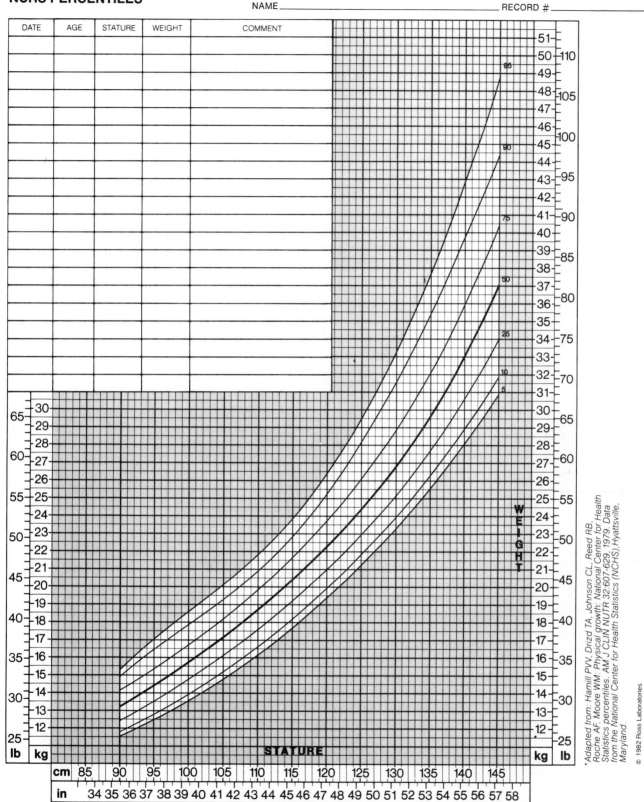

DATE	AGE	STATURE	WEIGHT	COMMENT

STATURE

cm 85 90 95 100 105 110 115 120 125 130 135 140 145

in 34 35 36 37 38 39 40 41 42 43 44 45 46 47 48 49 50 51 52 53 54 55 56 57 58

WEIGHT

lb kg

*Adapted from: Hamill PVV, Drizd TA, Johnson CL, Reed RB, Roche AF, Moore WM: Physical growth: National Center for Health Statistics percentiles. AM J CLIN NUTR 32:607-629, 1979. Data from the National Center for Health Statistics (NCHS), Hyattsville, Maryland.

© 1982 Ross Laboratories

**GIRLS: BIRTH TO 36 MONTHS
PHYSICAL GROWTH
NCHS PERCENTILES***

NAME_____ RECORD #_____

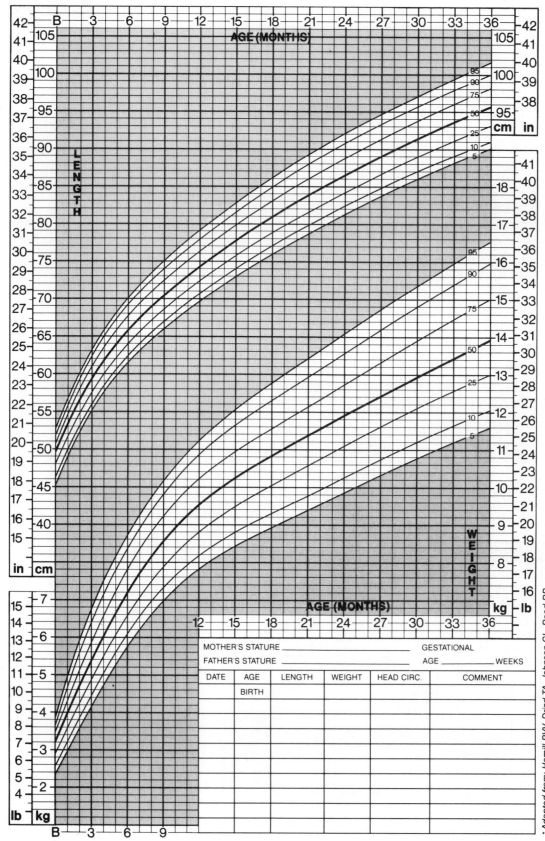

MOTHER'S STATURE _____ GESTATIONAL
FATHER'S STATURE _____ AGE _____ WEEKS

DATE	AGE	LENGTH	WEIGHT	HEAD CIRC.	COMMENT
	BIRTH				

* Adapted from: Hamill PVV, Drizd TA, Johnson CL, Reed RB, Roche AF, Moore WM: Physical growth: National Center for Health Statistics percentiles. AM J CLIN NUTR 32:607-629, 1979. Data from the Fels Longitudinal Study, Wright State University School of Medicine, Yellow Springs, Ohio.

© 1982 Ross Laboratories

GIRLS: BIRTH TO 36 MONTHS
PHYSICAL GROWTH
NCHS PERCENTILES*

NAME _____ RECORD # _____

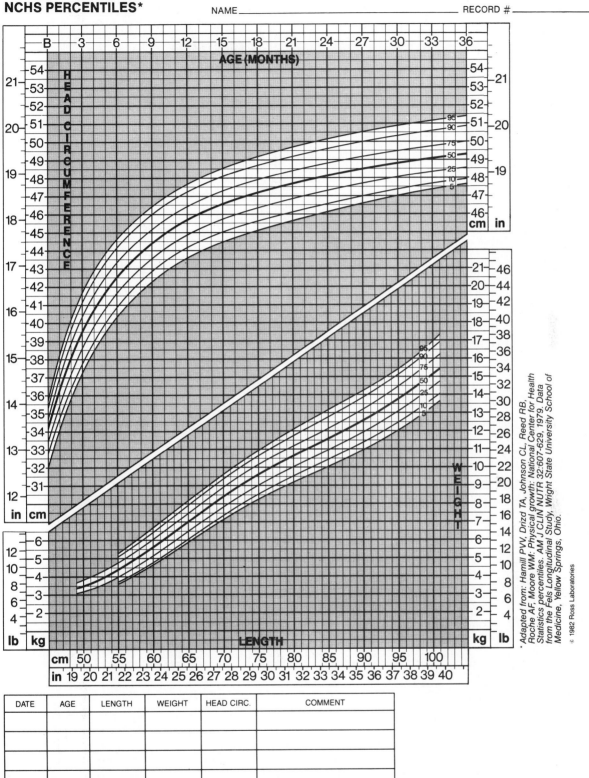

DATE	AGE	LENGTH	WEIGHT	HEAD CIRC.	COMMENT

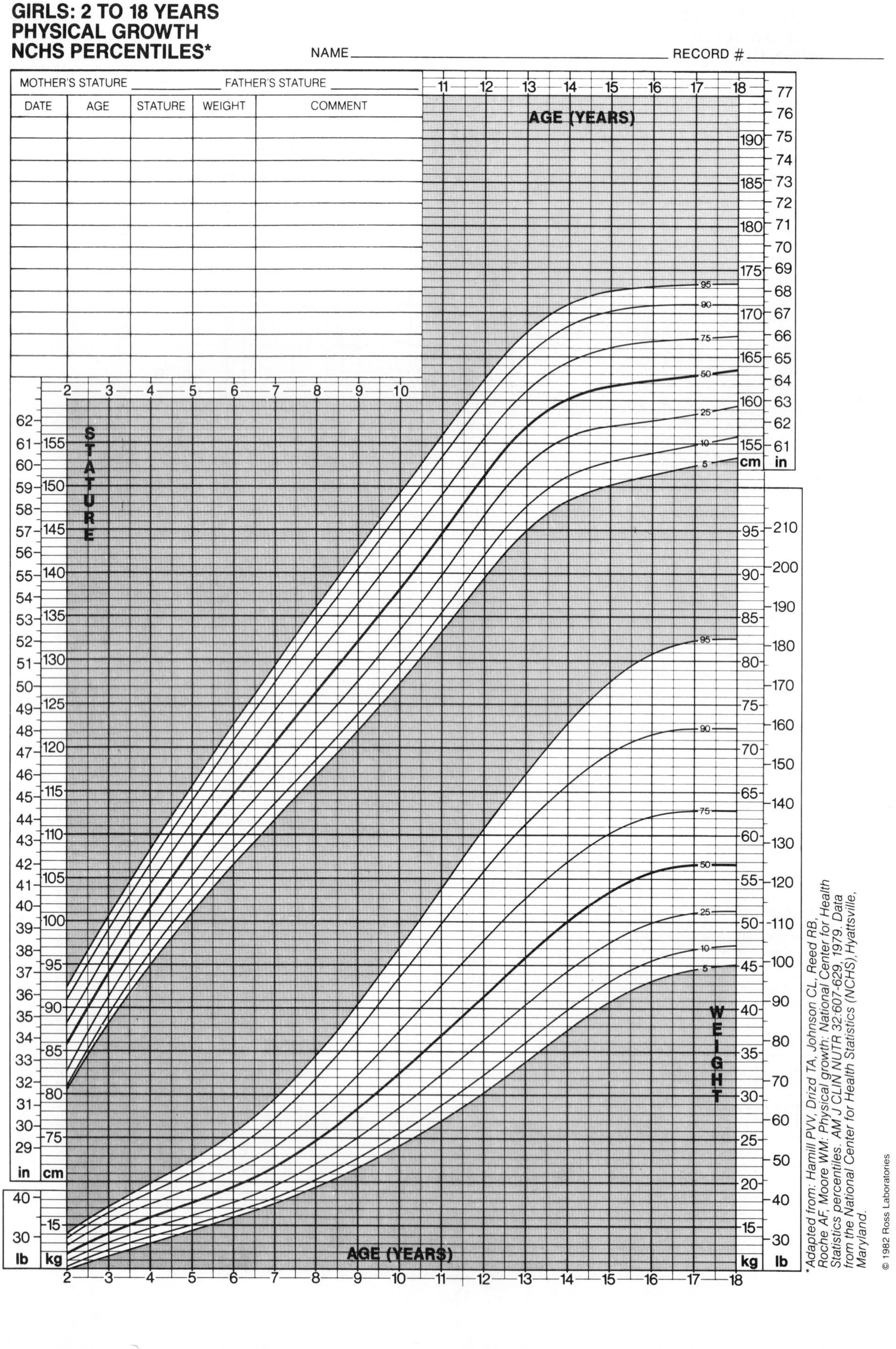

GIRLS: 2 TO 18 YEARS
PHYSICAL GROWTH
NCHS PERCENTILES*

NAME _____   RECORD # _____

DATE	AGE	STATURE	WEIGHT	COMMENT

MOTHER'S STATURE _____ FATHER'S STATURE _____

AGE (YEARS)

STATURE

WEIGHT

AGE (YEARS)

*Adapted from: Hamill PVV, Drizd TA, Johnson CL, Reed RB, Roche AF, Moore WM: Physical growth: National Center for Health Statistics percentiles. AM J CLIN NUTR 32:607-629, 1979. Data from the National Center for Health Statistics (NCHS), Hyattsville, Maryland.

© 1982 Ross Laboratories

**GIRLS: PREPUBESCENT
PHYSICAL GROWTH
NCHS PERCENTILES***

NAME _____   RECORD # _____

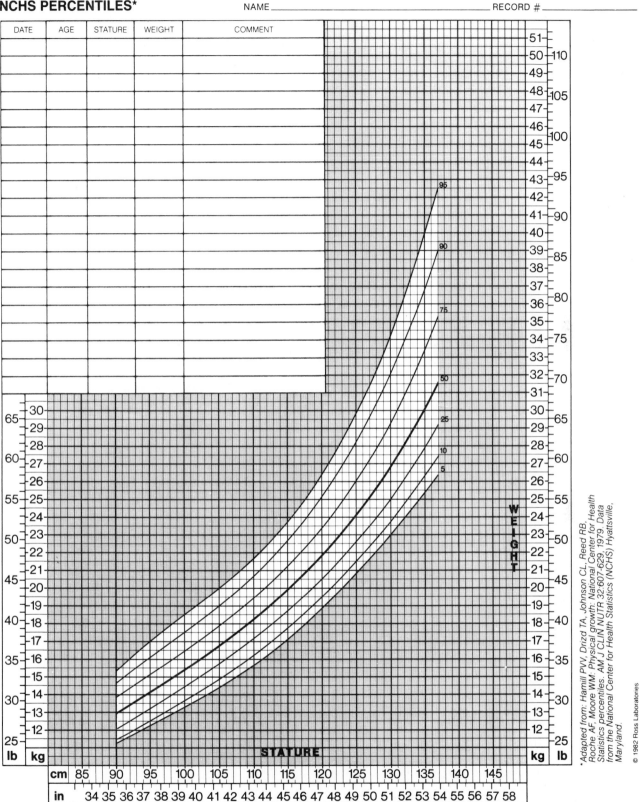

Adapted from: Hamill PVV, Drizd TA, Johnson CL, Reed RB, Roche AF, Moore WM. Physical growth: National Center for Health Statistics percentiles. AM J CLIN NUTR 32:607-629, 1979. Data from the National Center for Health Statistics (NCHS) Hyattsville, Maryland.

© 1982 Ross Laboratories

Reprinted with permission
of Ross Laboratories

Appendix F

Flowsheet for Documenting Assessment Findings in the Acute Care Setting

Jill Fuller and Jennifer Schaller-Ayers: HEALTH ASSESSMENT:
A NURSING APPROACH, Second Edition.
© 1990, 1994 by J. B. Lippincott Company.

ASSESSMENT PARAMETERS: Circle appropriate word on assessment items. All abnormal findings must be elaborated on in additional charting.

DATE:	NIGHTS	DAYS	EVENINGS
NEUROLOGICAL: Alert and oriented x 3. Equal strength to extremities and coordinated movement. Speech clear. Swallowing intact.	WNL / Abnormal Unassesed _____	WNL / Abnormal Unassesed _____	WNL / Abnormal Unassesed _____
CARDIOVASCULAR: Regular apical pulse. Denies CP. Peripheral pulses palpable. No edema noted.	WNL Abnormal Telemetry Unassessed	WNL Abnormal Telemetry Unassessed	WNL Abnormal Telemetry Unasessed
RESPIRATORY: Resp. 10-24 per min. at rest. Resp. even and unlabored. Good air exchange. Lungs clear. Nail beds pink. Oxygen: Inspirometer/Tidal Volume:	WNL Abnormal Unassessed _____ _____ _____	WNL Abnormal Unassessed _____ _____ _____	WNL Abnormal Unassessed _____ _____ _____
GASTROINTESTINAL: Abd. soft. Bowel sounds present x 4. No pain or tenderness with palpation. Diet tolerated without nausea or emesis. note NG, if applicable.	WNL / Abnormal / Unassessed _____ _____ _____	WNL / Abnormal / Unassessed _____ _____ _____	WNL / Abnormal / Unassessed _____ _____ _____
BOWEL ELIMINATION: Stool/Ostomy:	☐ Y ☐ N WNL Abnormal _____	☐ Y ☐ N WNL Abnormal _____	☐ Y ☐ N WNL Abnormal _____
GENITOURINARY: Able to empty bladder without dysuria. No bladder distension after voiding. Urine clear yellow to amber. No abnormal vaginal/penile drng. CBI's:	WNL / Abnormal Catheter Unassessed _____ _____	WNL / Abnormal Catheter Unassessed _____ _____	WNL / Abnormal Catheter Unassessed _____ _____
MUSCULOSKELETAL: Normal ROM to all joints. Absence of swelling or tenderness. No muscle weakness observed.	WNL Abnormal Unassessed	WNL Abnormal Unassessed	WNL Abnormal Unassessed
NEUROVASCULAR: Extremities pink, warm with normal mobility. No numbness or tingling reported. Peripheral pulses palpable. Neg. Homan's sign.	WNL _____ Abnormal_____ Unassessed _____ TEDS/Aces/SCD	WNL _____ Abnormal_____ Unassessed _____ TEDS/Aces/SCD	WNL _____ Abnormal_____ Unassessed _____ TEDS/Aces/SCD
INTEGUMENTARY: Skin W/D, pink. Note deviations from patients normal	WNL / Abnormal / Unassessed _____	WNL / Abnormal / Unassessed _____	WNL / Abnormal / Unassessed _____
WOUND: Dry/Intact: Changed: Wound Appearance:	_____ _____ _____	_____ _____ _____	_____ _____ _____
PHYSICAL COMFORT: Pain Medication: Time: Patient Response:	Severe/Moderate/Mild _____ _____ _____	Severe/Moderate/Mild _____ _____ _____	Severe/Moderate/Mild _____ _____ _____
Signature:			

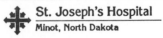

St. Joseph's Hospital
Minot, North Dakota

Medical/Surgical Flowsheet

881-2-560
1-92, 11-92

ASSESSMENT PARAMETERS: Circle appropriate word on assessment items. All abnormal findings must be elaborated on in additional charting.

DATE:	NIGHTS	DAYS	EVENINGS
NUTRITION: Placement Checked: Residual:	Tube Fdg? ☐ Y ☐ N N/A ☐ Y ☐ N Amt._____Time_____ Amt._____Time_____ Other_____	Tube Fdg? ☐ Y ☐ N N/A ☐ Y ☐ N Amt._____Time_____ Amt._____Time_____ Other_____	Tube Fdg? ☐ Y ☐ N N/A ☐ Y ☐ N Amt._____Time_____ Amt._____Time_____ Other_____
TUBES: Type: Location:	_____ _____	_____ _____	_____ _____
IV INFUSIONS: No reaction at site. No swelling or tenderness noted. Fluids infusing without difficulty Location:	WNL_____ Abnormal_____ IV/Lock/Dsg_____ _____	WNL_____ Abnormal_____ IV/Lock/Dsg_____ _____	WNL_____ Abnormal_____ IV/Lock/Dsg_____ _____
SLEEP/REST:	_____	_____	_____
ACTIVITY: Type: Assist of: Tolerance/gait:	_____ _____ _____ TCDB q2H ☐ Y ☐ N ☐ Self	_____ _____ _____ TCDB q2H ☐ Y ☐ N ☐ Self	_____ _____ _____ TCDB q2H ☐ Y ☐ N ☐ Self
SAFETY PRECAUTIONS: Side rails x2, bed low & locked, call light & table in reach, slippers & room in order	WNL	WNL	WNL
PATIENT EDUCATION/ DISCHARGE	re: _____ _____ Family present ☐ Y ☐ N	re: _____ _____ Family present ☐ Y ☐ N	re: _____ _____ Family present ☐ Y ☐ N
SPIRITUAL/ PSYCHOSOCIAL: Mood/Attitude:	_____ _____	_____ _____	_____ _____
SPECIAL EQUIPMENT:	K-pad CPM_____° Eggcrate Trapeze Other_____ _____	K-pad CPM_____° Eggcrate Trapeze Other_____ _____	K-pad CPM_____° Eggcrate Trapeze Other_____ _____
SIGNATURE:			

Nurses Notes: _____

_____

_____

_____

_____

_____

_____

_____

_____

_____

St. Joseph's Hospital
Minot, North Dakota

Medical/Surgical Flowsheet

881-2-560
1-92, 11-92

Appendix G

Trauma Flowsheet

Jill Fuller and Jennifer Schaller-Ayers: HEALTH ASSESSMENT:
A NURSING APPROACH, Second Edition.
© 1990, 1994 by J. B. Lippincott Company.

	MEMBERS	ETC PHYSICIAN	TRAUMA SURGEON	NEUROSURGEON	ANESTHESIA	CONSULT MD: TYPE:	CONSULT MD: TYPE:	ETC RN TRAUMA RN	MED RN / SURG RN	ICU RN	PASTORAL CARE
TRAUMA TEAM	Name										
	Time of arrival in ETC										

PRE-HOSPITAL DATA AND TREATMENT

DESCRIPTION OF INCIDENT

Time of Incident_____

Time of Arrival (ETA)_____

Trauma I activated ☐

FLUID RESUSCITATION PTA

TIME	FLUID TYPE	VOLUME	OUTPUT

MODE OF TRANSPORTATION
- ☐ Fire Rescue
- ☐ Police
- ☐ Ambulance
- ☐ Air Ambulance
- ☐ Self
- ☐ Other _____

TRANSPORT FROM
- ☐ Scene   ☐ Home
- ☐ Hospital _____
- ☐ Other _____

RESTRAINTS
- ☐ Seat Belt   ☐ NA
- ☐ Air Bags   ☐ Child Seat
- ☐ Air Bag & Belt   ☐ None
- ☐ Helmet   ☐ Unknown
- ☐ Padding/Protective Gear

MECHANISM OF INJURY
- ☐ Pedestrian
- ☐ Motor Vehicle Occupant
- ☐ Driver   ☐ Thrown from Vehicle
- ☐ Rollover
- ☐ Passenger - Front Seat
- ☐ Passenger - Back Seat
- ☐ Motorcycle
  - ☐ Driver   ☐ Passenger
- ☐ Pickup Truck   ☐ Semi/Bus
- ☐ Gun Shotgun
  - Calibre/Gauge_____
- ☐ Fall from Height_____feet
- ☐ Farming Accident
- ☐ Industrial Accident
- ☐ Burn
- ☐ Explosion
- ☐ Other_____
- ☐ Recreational Accident
  - ☐ Bicycle
  - ☐ All Terrain Vehicle (ATV)
  - ☐ Horse
  - ☐ Snow Ski
  - ☐ Water Ski
  - ☐ Tubing/Sledding
  - ☐ Diving
  - ☐ Other_____

VITAL SIGNS

TIME	BLOOD PRESSURE Manual Cuff	A/L or Autocuff	PULSE	RESP.	TEMP.	CARDIAC RHYTHM	OXIMETER	PUPILS R L

TIME - Pre-Hospital/Medication-Dose-Route-Site By

PRE-HOSPITAL TREATMENT

1	Airway Inserted	13ᵇ	I.V._____gauge
2	Assisted Ventilation	14	Central Line
3	Bleeding Controlled	15	Intraosseous Access
4	Burn Care	16	P.A.S.G. Inflated
5	Cervical Immobilization	17	P.A.S.G. Not Inflated
6	CPR	18	N.G. Tube
7	Defib._____	19	O.B. Care
8	External Pacemaker	20	Oxygen - Mask
9	Cricothyroidotomy	21	Oxygen - Cannula
10	Endotracheal Intub.	23	Needle Thoracentisis
11	Esophageal Obturator	24	Spinal Immobilization
12	Turn on Side	25	Splinting
13	I.V._____gauge	26	Suctioning

REVISED TRAUMA SCORE

		GLASCOW		Pre-Hospital	Arrival in ETC	Discharge from ETC
C O M A S C A L E	A Eyes Open	Spontaneous	= 4			
		To Voice	= 3			
		To Pain	= 2			
		None	= 1			
	B Best Verbal Response	Oriented	= 5			
		Confused	= 4			
		Inapprop. Words	= 3			
		Incomprehen. Sounds	= 2			
		None	= 1			
	C Best Motor Response	Obeys Commands	= 6			
		Localizes to Pain	= 5			
		Withdraws to Pain	= 4			
		Abn. Flex-decorticate	= 3			
		Abn. Ext.-decerebrate	= 2			
		Flaccid	= 1			

(A + B + C) = D   GCS TOTAL_____

E Glascow Conversion Score	13 - 15 =	4		
	9 - 12 =	3		
	6 - 8 =	2		
	4 - 5 =	1		
	> 4 =	0		
F Respiratory Rate	10 - 24/min	4		
	25 - 35/min	3		
	> 35/min	2		
	1 - 9/min	1		
	None	0		
G Systolic Blood Pressure No Pulse = no carotid pulse	90mmHG	4		
	70-89mmHg	3		
	50-88 mmHg	2		
	0 - 49 mmHg	1		
	No Pulse	0		
Trauma Score (E + F + G)				

Recorder of Pre-Hospital Data

St. Joseph's Hospital
Minot, North Dakota

Trauma Flow Sheet
Page One

678-1-018
2-93

PRIMARY ASSESSMENT

AIRWAY: ☐ Clear ☐ Obstructed ☐ Partially Obstructed
C-SPINE: ☐ Immobilized
BREATHING: ☐ Normal ☐ Labored ☐ Apneic
CIRCULATION: ☐ Pulse Present ☐ Cardiac Rate_____
 Rhythm_____
HEMORRHAGE: ☐ None ☐ Location
NEURO: ☐ Alert ☐ Responds to Verbal stimuli
 ☐ Responds to Pain ☐ Unresponsive

LAB

		TIME DRAWN				TIME DRAWN
☐	CBC		☐	BA		
☐	MD-20		☐	T & S		
☐	UA		☐	T & XM		
☐	PT/PTT		☐	# OF UNITS		
☐	CPK		☐	MISC		
☐	AMYLASE		☐	MISC		
☐	BETA CG		☐	ABG		
☐	TOX		☐	EKG		

FLUID RESUSCITATION

TIME	NO.	IV FLUID-SITE-SIZE	BY	AMT. INF

Current Medications _____
_____
_____

Allergies_____
_____
_____

PMHx_____

Menstrual Hx _____

Tetanus Status _____

Last Meal _____

Private MD_____

MEDICATION GIVEN

MEDICATION GIVEN	DOSE	ROUTE	TIME	TIME	GIVEN BY
Tetanus and Diphtheria Toxoids	0.5 CC	IM		N/A	

X-RAYS

STUDIES	PORTABLE	IN DEPT.	TIME IN	TIME OUT
☐ C-Spine	☐	☐		
☐ Chest	☐	☐		
☐ Pelvis	☐	☐		
☐ Abdomen	☐	☐		
Extremities - specify				
☐ #1_____	☐	☐		
☐ #2_____	☐	☐		
☐ IVP		☐		
☐ CT HEAD		☐		
☐ CT ABDOMEN		☐		
Oral Contrast	☐ Yes	☐ No	_____cc	
Other - specify				
☐ #1_____	☐	☐		
☐ #2_____	☐	☐		

PROCEDURE

PROCEDURE	TIME	APPEARANCE/RESPONSE
O2		
Endotracheal intub.		
Cricothyroidotomy		
C-collar		
Backboard		
C-monitor		
I.V. access		
I.V. access		
Central I.V.		
Arterial line		
NG tube Size: ____		
Foley Size: ____		
Peritoneal lavage		
Chest tube size ____	Site:	
Chest tube size ____	Site:	

VITAL SIGNS

TIME	BLOOD PRESSURE Manual Cuff	A/L or Autocuff	PULSE	RESP.	TEMP.	CARDIAC RHYTHM	OXIMETER	PUPILS R	L	E	V	M	GCS Total

_____
M.D. Ordering Tests / Procedures

_____
Recorder of Page Two

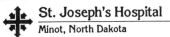

St. Joseph's Hospital
Minot, North Dakota

Trauma Flow Sheet
Page Two

678-1-018
2-93

SECONDARY ASSESSMENT

NEURO
☐ No Impairment
Pupil Size in mm   L _____   R _____

7   6   5   4   3   2   1

(+) Reacts   (—) No Reaction   (c) Closed d/t edema

Evident Deficits _____
Evident Trauma _____

HEAD
☐ No Evident Trauma
☐ Check for Contacts   Removed: ☐ Yes ☐ No ☐ N/A

Evident Trauma _____

NECK
☐ No Evident Trauma
☐ Spinal Immobilization

Evident Trauma _____

CHEST
☐ No Evident Trauma
Breath Sounds _____
Crepitus _____

Evident Trauma _____

ABDOMEN
☐ No Evident Trauma
Bowel Sounds _____

Evident Trauma _____

PELVIS
☐ No Evident Trauma
Blood at meatus: ☐ Yes ☐ No   Urine Color_____

Evident Trauma _____

EXTREMITIES
☐ No Evident Trauma
Distal Pulses/Cap Refill _____

Evident Trauma _____

BACK
Evident Trauma _____

FRONT   BACK

R   L   L   R

LEGEND

A	Abrasion	F	Fracture
Am	Amputation	Fb	Foreign Body
Av	Avulsion	GS	GSW/SGW
B	Burn	H	Hematoma
C	Ecchymosis	L	Laceration
E	Edema	S	Stab/Puncture

INTAKE AND OUTPUT

CRYSTALLOID	BLOOD	COLLOID	OTHER	OTHER	TOTAL INTAKE
URINE	NG	CHEST	EBL	OTHER	OUTPUT

DISPOSITION AND DISCHARGE PLAN

☐ DC ☐ TRANSFER ☐ ADMIT ☐ OR ☐ EXPIRED ☐ AMA
REPORT CALLED TO_____ RN___ UNIT_____ TIME_____
TRANSPORT: ☐ SELF ☐ FAMILY/SO ☐ CAB ☐ WC ☐ GURNEY
OTHER ☐ _____
TRANSFER: ACCEPTING MD _____ TIME_____
ACCEPTING HOSPITAL_____
TIME OF DISCHARGE FROM ETC _____
CONDITION ON DC: ☐ SAME ☐ IMPROVED ☐ DETERIORATED ☐ EXPIRED

TIME	NURSING NARRATIVE

Nurse's Signature

✠ **St. Joseph's Hospital**
Minot, North Dakota

Trauma Flow Sheet
Page Three

678-1-018
2-93

Index

Note: Page numbers in *italics* indicate illustrations; page numbers followed by *t* indicate tables; page numbers followed by *d* indicate display material.